Check out the additional content online at MediaCenter.Thieme.com!

Simply visit MediaCenter.Thieme.com and, when prompted during the registration process, enter the code below to get started today.

68CK-G885-2555-42KC

	WINDOWS & MAC	TABLET
Recommended Browser(s)	Recent browser versions on all major platforms and any mobile operating system that supports HTML5 video playback. *All browsers should have JavaScript enabled.*	
Flash Player Plug-in	Flash Player 9 or higher. *For Mac users, ATI Rage 128 GPU doesn't support full-screen mode with hardware scaling.*	Tablet PCs with Android OS support Flash 10.1.
Recommended for optimal usage experience	Monitor resolutions: • Normal (4:3) 1024×768 or higher • Widescreen (16:9) 1280×720 or higher • Widescreen (16:10) 1440×900 or higher A high-speed internet connection (minimum 384 Kps) is suggested.	WiFi or cellular data connection is required.

Thieme

Cutaneous Malignancies

A Surgical Perspective

Brian R. Gastman, MD
Director
Cleveland Clinic Foundation Melanoma Program
Associate Professor of Surgery
Cleveland Clinic Lerner College of Medicine
Cleveland Clinic
Cleveland, Ohio, USA

Sub-editor

Neilendu Kundu, MD
Medical Director
Plastic and Reconstructive Surgery
Mercy Health Physicians
Cincinnati, Ohio, USA

445 illustrations

Thieme
New York • Stuttgart • Delhi • Rio de Janeiro

Managing Editor: Elizabeth Palumbo
Editorial Assistant: Haley Paskalides
Director, Editorial Services: Mary Jo Casey
Production Editor: Torsten Scheihagen
International Production Director: Andreas Schabert
Editorial Director: Sue Hodgson
International Marketing Director: Fiona Henderson
International Sales Director: Louisa Turrell
Director of Institutional Sales: Adam Bernacki
Senior Vice President and Chief Operating Officer: Sarah Vanderbilt
President: Brian D. Scanlan

Library of Congress Cataloging-in-Publication Data
Names: Gastman, Brian R., editor.
Title: Cutaneous malignancies : a surgical perspective / [edited by] Brian R. Gastman.
Description: New York : Thieme, [2018] | Includes bibliographical references.
Identifiers: LCCN 2017038939 (print) | LCCN 2017039913 (ebook) | ISBN 9781626231481 (e-book) | ISBN 9781626231474 (print)
Subjects: | MESH: Skin Neoplasms–surgery | Dermatologic Surgical Procedures
Classification: LCC RD655 (ebook) | LCC RD655 (print) | NLM WR 500 | DDC 616.99/477059–dc23
LC record available at https://lccn.loc.gov/2017038939

Thieme Publishers New York
333 Seventh Avenue, New York, NY 10001 USA
+1 800 782 3488, customerservice@thieme.com

Thieme Publishers Stuttgart
Rüdigerstrasse 14, 70469 Stuttgart, Germany
+49 [0]711 8931 421, customerservice@thieme.de

Thieme Publishers Delhi
A-12, Second Floor, Sector-2, Noida-201301
Uttar Pradesh, India
+91 120 45 566 00, customerservice@thieme.in

Thieme Publishers Rio de Janeiro, Thieme Publicações Ltda.
Edifício Rodolpho de Paoli, 25º andar
Av. Nilo Peçanha, 50 – Sala 2508
Rio de Janeiro 20020-906 Brasil
+55 21 3172-2297 / +55 21 3172-1896

Cover design: Thieme Publishing Group
Cover illustration by Andrea Hines
Typesetting by DiTech Process Solutions

Printed in India by Replika Press Pvt. Ltd. 5 4 3 2 1

ISBN 978-1-62623-147-4

Also available as an e-book:
eISBN 978-1-62623-148-1

I would like to dedicate this book to my life partner and wife, Addie, whose love and support have allowed me to focus on this important endeavor. To my children, Rachelli, Dovid, Binyomen, and Esi, who I never see enough of but are growing up to be individuals any parent would be proud of. I hope this book attests that my time away is for the best of causes.

As a simple servant of a higher power, I hope this book will help the few that are here on this earth to help the many through the countless challenges of skin cancer.

Contents

Video Contents

Preface

This book is designed to meet a growing need for the modern surgeon treating skin cancer. Cutaneous malignancies are currently treated by a variety of surgical specialties. As a result, there lacks a strong unified description of how these cancers should be approached. Additionally, many recent developments in non-surgical therapies have been developed, affecting surgeons who treat these pathologies.

Surgery is one aspect in the spectrum of cutaneous malignancies treatment, beginning with prevention and detection and ending with long-term follow-up and possibly systemic therapies. Any surgeon in the position of handling any oncologic patients needs to have a robust understanding of these important aspects of skin cancer care. Often, the surgical interventions in this patient population are the least complex aspect of their treatment. In the modern era, there exist many new aspects of these cancers that may not be well known to all surgeons—for example, the increasing use of immunosuppressive therapies for transplantation and rheumatologic diseases, which predisposes patients to these tumors. There are also increasing numbers of lesser-known malignancies, such as Merkel cell carcinoma and dermatofibrosarcoma protuberans (DFSP), to name a few.

Many aspects of surgical care itself need to be considered when contemplating comprehensive care for these patients. This may include: Mohs surgery, sentinel node biopsy, appropriate margin size, method of reconstruction, and quality dermatopathology. Finally, increasing advances in targeted therapy, immunotherapy, and radiotherapy are affecting when, how, and even if a patient needs to undergo surgery.

With a multitude of new advancements in cutaneous cancers, especially for patients who progress after surgery, this is a fortuitous time to complete a comprehensive book on the management of these tumors. As national referral patterns to surgeons are ever changing, having a reference that can appeal to all types of surgeons is both timely and essential. Nonetheless this book has been written in a fashion that allows nonsurgical practitioners the ability to understand the role surgeons play in these diseases, as well as a substantial amount of information that will be beneficial for their practice. Thus, this can affect when and to whom to refer these patients, as well as what a referring physician should expect from the surgical consult. Finally, for any physician—surgeon or not—who chooses to treat these diseases, we hope this book will serve as an important reference based on the newest standards of care derived from many perspectives.

The development of a comprehensive text on the management of cutaneous cancers is overdue. This need is derived from a combination of lack of consistency amongst surgical specialties and a paucity of books devoted for the modern surgeon treating skin cancer. By employing high-volume surgeons and other skin cancer specialists who are knowledgeable in both standard of care and cutting-edge technologies, we fully expect that this book will serve as an important reference that surgeons can utilize for years to come.

Contributors

Andrea M. Abbott, MD, MS
Division of Oncologic and Endocrine Surgery
Medical University of South Carolina
Charleston, South Carolina, USA

Karri Adamson
PGY5 Resident
Plastic and Reconstructive Surgery
Medical College of Wisconsin
Milwaukee, Wisconsin, USA

Philip L. Bailin, MD
Dermatologist
Cleveland Clinic Dermatology
Cleveland, Ohio, USA

Trevor Batty, DO
Fourth Year Resident
Midwestern University
Rochester, Minnesota, USA

Elizabeth M. Billingsley, MD
Professor of Dermatology
Director
Mohs Micrographic Surgery & Dermatological Surgery
Penn State Hershey Dermatology
Hershey, Pennsylvania, USA

Jerry D. Brewer, MD
Associate Professor
Dermatology
Mayo Clinic
Rochester, Minnesota, USA

Morgan Brgoch, MD
Resident, PGY III
Division of Plastic Surgery
Penn State Health
Milton S. Hershey Medical Center
Hershey, Pennsylvania, USA

Klaus J. Busam, MD
Staff and Director, Dermatopathology
Department of Anatomic Pathology
Memorial Sloan Kettering Cancer Center
New York, New York, USA

Matthew P. Doepker, MD
Assistant Professor of Clinical Surgery/Surgical Oncology
Palmetto Health/USC Medical Group
Columbia, South Carolina, USA

William W. Dzwierzynski, MD, FACS
Professor and Program Director
Department of Plastic Surgery
Medical College of Wisconsin
Milwaukee, Wisconsin, USA

Oliver Eng, MD
PGY-4 Resident
Rutgers Robert Wood Johnson Medical School
New Brunswick, New Jersey, USA

Brian R. Gastman, MD
Director
Cleveland Clinic Foundation Melanoma Program
Associate Professor of Surgery
Cleveland Clinic Lerner College of Medicine
Cleveland Clinic
Cleveland, Ohio, USA

Nikhil Purushottam Joshi, MD
Assistant Professor of Medicine
Department of Radiation Oncology
Cleveland Clinic Taussig Cancer Institute
Cleveland, Ohio, USA

Howard L. Kaufman, MD, FACS
Professor and Chief
Division of Surgical Oncology
Chief Surgical Officer
Associate Director for Clinical Science
Surgical Oncologist
Rutgers Cancer Institute of New Jersey
New Brunswick, New Jersey, USA

Jennifer S. Ko, MD, PhD
Dermatopathology Medical Director
Cleveland Clinic Central Biorepository
Department of Anatomic Pathology
Pathology and Laboratory Medicine Institute
Cleveland Clinic
Cleveland, Ohio, USA

Vadim P. Koshenkov, MD
Professor of Surgery
Rutgers Robert Wood Johnson Medical Group
The Cancer Institute of New Jersey
New Brunswick, New Jersey, USA

Shlomo A. Koyfman, MD
Assistant Professor of Medicine
Departments of Radiation Oncology and Bioethics
Cleveland Clinic Taussig Cancer Institute
Cleveland, Ohio, USA

Neilendu Kundu, MD
Medical Director
Plastic and Reconstructive Surgery
Mercy Health Physicians
Cincinnati, Ohio, USA

Charlene Lam, MD, MPH
Assistant Professor of Dermatology
Dermatology Department
Penn State Hershey
Hershey, Pennsylvania, USA

Bindu V. Manyam, MD
PGY-1 Resident
Radiation Oncology Department
Cleveland Clinic
Cleveland, Ohio, USA

Eugen C. Minca, MD, PhD
Department of Pathology
Pathology and Laboratory Medicine Institute
Cleveland Clinic
Cleveland, Ohio, USA

Deepak Narayan, MD
Professor
Plastic and Reconstructive Surgery
Yale University School of Medicine
New Haven, Connecticut, USA

Rogerio I. Neves, MD, PhD
Professor of Surgery, Dermatology, Pharmacology, and Medicine
Melanoma and Cutaneous Malignancies Disease Team Leader
Penn State Hershey Plastic Surgery
Hershey, Pennsylvania, USA

Amrita Pandit, MD
Research Fellow
Section of Plastic Surgery
Yale University School of Medicine
New Haven, Connecticut, USA

Christine Poblete-Lopez, MD
Vice-Chairman
Dermatology Department
Cleveland Clinic
Cleveland, Ohio, USA

Sashank K. Reddy, MD, PhD
Administrative Chief Resident
Department of Plastic and Reconstructive Surgery
Johns Hopkins School of Medicine
Baltimore, Maryland, USA

Michael Schowalter, MD
Dermatologist
Cleveland Clinic Dermatology
Cleveland, Ohio, USA

Vernon K. Sondak, MD
Chief of the Division of Cutaneous Oncology
Director of Surgical Education
H. Lee Moffitt Cancer Center and Research Institute
Tampa, Florida, USA

Anthony P. Tufaro, MD, DDS
Director
Head and Neck Program for General Surgery
Vice Chief
Plastic & Reconstructive Surgery
Associate Professor
Plastic and Reconstructive Surgery
Johns Hopkins Hospital
Baltimore, Maryland, USA

Allison Vidimos, RPh, MD, FACMS
Chairman
Department of Dermatology
Vice Chairman
Dermatology and Plastic Surgery Institute
Cleveland Clinic Professor of Medicine
Cleveland Clinic Lerner College of Medicine
Case Western Reserve University
Cleveland, Ohio, USA

Sue S. Yom, MD, PhD
Associate Professor
Departments of Radiation Oncology and Otolaryngology
Head and Neck Surgery
Helen Diller Family Comprehensive Cancer Center
UCSF
San Francisco, California, USA

Calvin J. Young MD, MHS
General Surgery Resident
Department of Surgery
Yale-New Haven Hospital
New Haven, Connecticut, USA

1 Prevention of Future Skin Cancer

Trevor Batty and Jerry D. Brewer

1.1 Introduction

Nonmelanoma skin cancer (NMSC) is the most common malignancy in humans. More than 3.5 million NMSCs in more than 2 million people are diagnosed in the United States annually.[1] In fact, the incidence of skin cancer is higher than new cases of breast, prostate, lung, and colon cancer combined.[2] Melanoma incidence rates have been increasing over the past three decades. Most recent data suggest an increase of 2.7% from 2006 to 2010.[2] In 2014, melanoma is estimated to be the third and fourth most common cancer in men and women, respectively.[2] The total estimated cost of treatment for skin cancer (including melanoma, basal cell carcinoma [BCC]), and squamous cell carcinoma [SCC]) is $8.1 billion each year in the United States.[3] Aside from treatment, cost due to lost workdays and restricted-activity days is estimated at $106.2 million annually.[2] The high incidence of skin cancer—in addition to the cost and toll on society—is astounding considering that an estimated daily application of only sun protection factor (SPF) 15 in the first 18 years of life would reduce the lifetime incidence of NMSC by 78%.[4] These statistics highlight the importance and beneficial effects of skin cancer prevention.

1.2 Role of Dermatology

1.2.1 Primary Prevention

Dermatologists have an opportunity to play an active role in the prevention of skin cancer. Primary prevention, as defined by the United States Preventive Services Task Force (USPSTF), involves measures provided to individuals to prevent the onset of a targeted condition, in this case skin cancer.[5] Primary prevention methods in general have included counseling patients, involving other physicians, participating in community outreach programs, and endorsing school sun-safety programs and policy. Chemoprevention is also considered a primary preventive measure and will be discussed in greater detail later in this chapter.[5] Since NMSC and melanoma share the risk factors of exposure to ultraviolet (UV) radiation and history of severe sunburns, following primary preventive measures aimed at UV protective habits can maximize great outcomes regarding skin cancer prevention.

Skin cancer prevention can be enhanced by dermatologists asking patients if they are protecting themselves from the sun and counseling them about the importance of sun protection. The National Ambulatory Medical Care Survey found that only 1.6% of dermatologists reported mentioning sunscreen during patient visits.[6] The ability to counsel and distribute educational pamphlets gives dermatologists the opportunity to change a patient's perspective and understanding of skin cancer. During dermatologic examinations, it would be important to discuss close monitoring and personal protective clothing with patients who have exposure to known chemical risk factors for melanoma such as coal, tar, pitch, creosote, arsenic, radium, and pesticides. It is important to educate patients during visits about skin cancer warning signs and morphology for both melanoma and NMSC. Cheng et al found 59% of self-detected melanomas in situ had an established dermatologist, and many patients attributed this to education obtained during a dermatology appointment.[7]

Skin cancer prevention can be even more effective in a multidisciplinary approach. Dermatologists have the opportunity to enlist the help of fellow physicians, especially primary care providers, to emphasize the importance of the basics of skin cancer prevention including sun and tanning bed avoidance, as well as regular sunscreen use to their patients. The American Academy of Dermatology (AAD) has created a free basic dermatology curriculum that is available to the public (▶ Table 1.1).[8] This curriculum is aimed toward physicians and students. Learning modules include actinic keratosis (AK), SCC, BCC, evaluation of pigmented lesions, and melanoma. These modules are very helpful given they provide instruction and guidance on when to assure or refer the patient. The USPSTF conducted a systematic review of evidence on the effectiveness -of behavioral counseling to prevent skin cancer and found in primary care settings where counseling was given there was a decrease in intentional

Table 1.1 Helpful websites

Sponsor	URL	Information
American Academy of Dermatology	https://www.aad.org/education/basic-dermatology-curriculum	Basic dermatology curriculum for physicians and medical students
The Skin Cancer Foundation	http://www.skincancer.org/prevention	Educational links and helpful tips for skin cancer prevention
The Skin Cancer Foundation	http://www.skincancer.org/get-involved	Ideas for getting involved in fundraising, advocacy, schools, and your community
American Academy of Dermatology	https://www.aad.org/spot-skin-cancer	Links to find a dermatologist, free cancer screening, and educational information
The American Cancer Society	http://www.cancer.org/healthy/morewaysacshelpsyoustaywell/acs-skin-cancer-prevention-activities	Skin cancer awareness campaigns and education resources
The American Cancer Society	http://www.cancer.org/healthy/toolsandcalculators/quizzes/sun-safety/index	Quiz on sun safety
Centers for Disease Control and Prevention	http://www.cdc.gov/cancer/dcpc/resources/features/SkinCancer/	Facts about skin cancer, educational links, and sun-safety tips
National Council on Skin Cancer Prevention	http://www.skincancerprevention.org	News, ideas to get involved, advocacy, and educational links

Source: http://www.skincancerprevention.org.

tanning and an increase in sun-protective behaviors.[9] Another finding of this review was that appearance-focused messages were the most successful at reducing late-adolescent women's intent to pursue indoor training.[9] Following this review, in May 2012, the USPSTF recommended counseling fair-skinned children, adolescents, and young adults aged 10 to 24 years about minimizing their exposure to UV radiation to reduce their risk for skin cancer.[9] The National Ambulatory Medical Care Survey found that only 0.07% of patient visits had mention of sunscreen and only 0.9% of patients with a history of skin disease were counseled on the importance of sunscreen.[6] The results of this survey demonstrate that dermatologists and other health care providers can improve efforts to increase awareness of the importance of skin cancer prevention.

Another responsibility of dermatologists is to promote skin cancer prevention and awareness in our communities. National surveys found that only 3 out of 10 adults practice routine sun protection themselves, and approximately 60% of parents applied sunscreen and 25% used shade to protect their children.[10] The results of this survey demonstrate the need to raise community awareness of skin cancer by participating in national or local sun protection campaigns. For example, the American Cancer Society has a national skin cancer awareness campaign called "Slip! Slop! Slap! and Wrap." This slogan promotes slipping on a shirt, slopping on sunscreen, slapping on a hat, and wrapping on sunglasses to protect the eyes. The American Cancer Society has also designated the Friday before Memorial Day as "No Fry Day." Pool Cool is a sun-safety education program with eight brief sun-safety lessons taught during regular swimming lessons for children and parents.[11] Pools that use this program have been found to have better protected pool environments and better sun protection habits among swimmers and lifeguards that result in fewer sunburns.[3] A randomized controlled trial conducted in Australia showed that a population screening that included melanoma awareness campaign led to a decrease in thickness of the melanomas diagnosed during the campaign.[12,13] A study done in 1999 evaluating the previous 20 years of primary health prevention programs in Australia found a very large shift in knowledge, attitudes, beliefs, and behaviors about sunlight exposure and suntans.[14] Participation and support of national campaigns, such as these, could increase the community's awareness and application of sun-safety.

Studies of immigrants to Australia point to sun exposure during childhood and adolescence as a major risk factor for developing NMSC.[15,16] Sunburns in children are a risk factor for development of skin cancer later in life, and it has been shown that building healthier sun protection habits at an early age can lead to better sun protection as adults.[17,18] Dermatologists and other health care providers have the opportunity to promote formation of policy in local schools to educate students on healthy sun protection habits. Dermatologists and other health care providers can have a positive impact in school policy by encouraging the creation of school sun-safety strategies such as allowing students to apply sunscreen at school, having play equipment in shaded areas, scheduling recess to avoid peak sun intensity, and encouraging students to wear sun-protective clothing such as hats, long-sleeved shirts, and pants. Sun-safety curriculum has also been shown to play an important role in skin cancer prevention. Such curriculums have been shown to be effective in school-aged children as early as preschool.[19] A randomized trial found that interactive multimedia programs in conjunction with teacher instruction improved sun-safety in primary school-aged children.[20] Arizona was among the first to require skin cancer prevention as part of their health education curriculum. Since 2004, Arizona has implemented SunWise in grades K-8 in all public schools.[21] SunWise is a health and environmental education program that offers participants free materials to promote cross-curricular learning about sun-safety, UV radiation, and ozone science. The SunWise program has had success in raising awareness and increasing sun-safety behaviors.[22] This program has also been shown to prevent approximately 11,000 skin cancer cases among participants resulting in saving $4 for every $1 spent.[23] Involvement in endorsing local school policy and curriculum that affects younger individuals has great potential to further decrease the incidence of skin cancer.

Patients with previous solar damage and/or existing precancerous lesions can be treated by several means to prevent future skin cancer. The risks and benefits of the preventive treatment should be discussed and agreed upon with the patient to encourage compliance and awareness. The subsequent sections will discuss various methods of prevention and their respective efficacy. Treatments include cryotherapy, light therapy, topical medications, lasers, and chemical peels.

1.2.2 Chemoprevention

Chemoprevention is considered as primary prevention by the USPSTF.[5] The subject of chemoprevention is extensive and multiple methods deliver impressive efficacy.[24] For the purposes of this chapter, chemoprevention is the treatment of AKs. AKs account for 5.2 million office visits per year and $920 million in treatment.[25] The progression of AKs to primary invasive or in situ SCC was found to be 0.6% at 1 year and 2.57% at 4 years.[26] Dodson et al estimated a 10-year risk of AKs transforming to SCC to be around 6.1 to 10.2%.[27] Hypertrophic AKs measuring less than 1 cm in diameter located on the dorsum of the hand, wrist, or forearm in white patients were found to have a transformation rate of 50%.[28] Criscione et al found that approximately 65% of primary SCC and 36% of BCC were originally diagnosed as AKs.[26] Treatment can be directed at single or multiple AKs. If multiple less well-defined AKs are present over large areas, then field therapy can be very beneficial. Field therapy targets clinically visible and subclinical AKs. Ultimately, the choice of the method of chemoprevention should be individualized to each patient.

Cryotherapy

Cryotherapy is the treatment of choice for individual AK lesions.[29] A multicenter study found a 67.2% clearance rate 3 months after treatment when lesions were frozen for at least 2 seconds, and greater than an 80% clearance rate when AKs were frozen for at least 10 seconds.[30] Krawtchenko and colleagues reported 68% clinic clearance and 32% histological clearance 6 weeks after one or two treatments lasting 20 to 40 seconds for each lesion.[31] At a 12-month follow-up, 6% of patients who were initially cleared remained clear,[31] in contrast to a study done by Lubritz and Smolewski that reports a cure of 98.8%

treated lesions with up to 8.5-year follow-up.[32] Adverse effects include redness, blistering, crusting, oozing, and ulceration.[29] Thai et al reported hypopigmentation resulted in up to 29% of patients treated with a freeze time greater than 20 seconds.[30] In a Cochrane review, cryotherapy was found to be significantly inferior to 5-fluorouracil (5-FU) and aminolevulinic acid (ALA) photodynamic therapy (PDT).[24]

Photodynamic Therapy

PDT involves the selective accumulation of photosensitizing agents that generate reactive oxygen species when exposed to light, which causes selective apoptosis in premalignant and/or malignant cells. ALA and methyl aminolevulinic acid (MAL) are topical photosensitizing agents that are applied for a certain period prior to exposure to blue or red light. A Cochrane review found that neither the topical photosensitizing agent nor the type of light produced significantly different results.[24] The review did find that longer incubation periods of 4 hours with ALA resulted in better outcomes compared to shorter incubation times of 0.5, 1, and 2 hours.[24] In a randomized clinical trial, PDT showed a 14% better chance of complete clearance compared to cryotherapy after 3 months.[33] A single application of 5-ALA patches applied 4 hours prior to light exposure resulted in 89% clearance 12 weeks after treatment.[34] At the 12-month follow-up, this same treatment regimen was associated with 24% recurrent lesions.[34] Common adverse events include photosensitivity, pain, erythema, and pruritus.[33] PDT was found to produce a better cosmetic outcome than cryotherapy and 5-FU.[24] Other than cosmetic outcome, PDT is a good choice for patients where compliance may be an issue due to its single application.

5-Fluorouracil

5-FU decreases cell proliferation and induces cell death by interfering with deoxyribonucleic acid (DNA) and ribonucleic acid (RNA) synthesis in cells with high mitotic rates.[24] A Cochrane review found that the efficacy of 0.5 and 5% 5-FU was similar when directly compared.[24] The review also found that 5-FU efficacy was similar to PDT and superior to cryotherapy.[24] A review of studies demonstrated an average complete clearance of 52%.[35] Treatment with 5% 5-FU applied twice a day for 4 weeks showed an initial clearance of 96% and a histological clearance of 67%.[31] At 12-month follow-up, 35% of the initially clear patients remained clear.[31] The Cochrane review found that patients treated with 5-FU treatment experienced substantial skin irritation, but in general was not cause for withdrawal from treatment.[24] Possible adverse effects of 5-FU are erythema, erosions, edema, and dryness at the site of application.[36,37] The recommended treatment and duration of 5-FU varies with strength and location of application, but usually is between 1 and 4 weeks.

Diclofenac

Diclofenac is a nonsteroidal anti-inflammatory drug in a 2.5% hyaluronic acid gel vehicle. Although the precise mechanism is not understood, the current hypothesis is that the inhibition of cyclooxygenase-2 (COX-2) leads to a decrease in prostaglandin synthesis and may be responsible for inhibition of cell differentiation, induction of apoptosis, alteration of cell proliferation, and inhibition of angiogenesis.[38,39,40,41] A meta-analysis of three studies that included 364 patients found cumulative and total lesion scores of zero in 50% of patients treated for 90 days and 33% clearance of patients treated for 60 days.[42] A study of six organ transplant patients reported three out of the six completely cleared clinically and histologically after applying diclofenac 3% twice a day for 16 weeks, while the rest achieved at least 30% clearance.[43] Akarsu et al reported a complete clearance of 19.1% 24 weeks after starting diclofenac twice daily for 12 weeks, and reported no withdrawals from the study secondary to adverse effects.[44] Common adverse effects included itching, scaling, dryness, rash, and erythema, and rarely paresthesia and hyperesthesia.[44] One disadvantage of diclofenac is the lengthy treatment period of twice daily application for 60 or 90 days.

Imiquimod

Imiquimod is an immune modulator that enhances innate and acquired immune responses resulting in antiviral and antitumoral activity.[45] A meta-analysis of four studies and 393 subjects showed an average complete clearance of 70% in patients treated with 5% imiquimod cream.[35] Application of 5% imiquimod three times weekly for 4 weeks and repeating this regimen if initial lesions did not clear after a 4-week rest period produced a histological and clinical clearance of 73 and 86%, respectively, 8 weeks after final treatment.[31] Other studies report a complete clearance rate ranging from 48.3 to 57.1%.[46,47,48] At a 12-month follow-up, 86% of patients who were initially clear showed sustained clearance.[31] Patients with initial clearance were found to have a 25% recurrence rate when applying imiquimod three times per week and a 47% recurrence rate with twice a week application at 16 months.[49] Krawtchenko et al also reported that 81% of the patients treated with imiquimod had an excellent cosmetic outcome.[31] Complete clearance rates are higher with 5% imiquimod versus 3.75% imiquimod following 8 weeks of treatment.[50,51] A Cochrane review found treatment with 5% imiquimod resulted in more participant withdrawal secondary to adverse effects than treatment with 2.5 and 3.75% imiquimod.[24] Common adverse events were erythema, scabbing, and flaking (▶ Table 1.2).[47]

Chemical Peels

Chemical peels are another option for treating widespread AKs. A variety of chemical peels can be used to treat AKs and should be selected according to the histological level or severity of skin pathology in order to achieve optimal results.[61] Medium-depth chemical peels such as 70% glycolic acid with 35% trichloroacetic acid (GA-TCA) and Jessner's solution with 35% trichloroacetic acid (JS-TCA) penetrate to the papillary dermis and can be used to treat AKs.[57] The exfoliative effect of chemical peels stimulates new epidermal growth and collagen formation.[61] Chemical peels have shown to alter the epidermis restoring a more normal pattern of columnar cells with increased polarity.[61] JS-TCA and GA-TCA at day 60 post peel showed a hyperplastic epidermis and an expanded papillary dermis.[57] This study also reported 7% of JS-TCA peels and 15% of GA-TCA peels developed

Table 1.2 Common therapeutic options for skin cancer prevention in patients with actinic damage

Treatment modality	Length of treatment	Initial clinical clearance	Long-term efficacy	Common adverse effects	Comments
Photodynamic therapy	Best results seen with incubation periods of 4 h[24]	86% complete clearance[52]	24% recurrence at 12 mo[34]	Photosensitivity, pain, erythema, and pruritus[33]	Better cosmetic outcome compared to 5-FU and cryotherapy[24]
5-fluorouracil (5-FU)	1–4 wk	52%[35] compared to 96%[31] complete clearance	35% maintained clearance at 12 mo[31]	Erythema, erosions, edema, and dryness[36,37]	0.5 and 5% have similar efficacy[24]
Diclofenac	60–90 d	50% when treated for 90 d, and 33% when treated for 60 d[42]	19.1% complete clearance at 24 wk[44]	Itching, scaling, dryness, rash, and erythema[44]	
Imiquimod	2–3 times/wk for 1 mo	86% complete clearance[31]	25% recurrence 3 times/wk, 47% recurrence 2 times/wk[49]	Erythema, scabbing, and flaking[47]	81% of patients reported an excellent cosmetic outcome[31]
Cryotherapy	Greater efficacy for freezing lesion longer than 10 s[30]	80% complete clearance when frozen for 10 s compared to 67.2% when frozen for 2 s[30]	6[31] to 98.8% complete clearance[32]	Redness, blistering, crusting, oozing, and ulceration[29]	29% of patients experienced hypopigmentation after freeze times of 20 s or longer[30]
Medium-depth chemical peels	One-time application	75% reduction in AKs[53]	No recurrent AKs after 1 y[53] 40-fold decrease in developing subsequent NMSC[54]	Pigmentary changes for dark-skinned individuals, infections, allergic reactions, improper healing, hypersensitivity, and disease exacerbation.[55,56]	Effective in treating photodamage[57]
Laser ablation	One-time procedure	93% reduction in AKs[58]	80[59] to 87%[60]lesion free for 1 y	Infection, pigmentary changes, acne, milia, scar formation, and atrophic and/or easily bruising skin[59]	On average 64% of recurrences occur 32.7 mo posttreatment[59]

Abbreviations: AKS, actinic keratoses; NMSC, nonmelanoma skin cancer.

new elastic fibers. In a split face study, JS-TCA was found to produce equivalent results when compared to 5-FU.[53] Subjects in this study had a 75% reduction in AKs and experienced no recurrence of AKs for at least 1 year. In addition to treating AKs, Abdel-Daim et al suggest chemical peeling with glycolic acid, salicylic acid, and trichloroacetic acid could serve tumor prevention by removing photodamaged cells.[62] This was shown in a study done by Hantash et al which demonstrated a 40-fold lower rate of developing subsequent NMSC after treatment with 30% trichloroacetic acid peel compared to 5-FU and Carbon dioxide (CO_2) laser.[54] This study also comments on the excellent cosmetic results produced by trichloroacetic acid peels. JS-TCA and GA-TCA peels resulted in erythema, crusting, and swelling within 24 hours with crusting and swelling resolving by day 7.[57] Medium- and deep-depth peels have been associated with pigmentary changes for dark-skinned individuals, infections, allergic reactions, improper healing, hypersensitivity, and disease exacerbation.[55,56]

Lasers

Different ablative laser systems are used to treat AKs. CO_2 lasers work by collateral heat which causes collagen synthesis and the sealing of blood vessels and nerve endings leading to less pain and bleeding, whereas Erbium:yttrium aluminum garnet (Er:YAG) lasers work with high water absorption resulting in little collateral heat.[63] Re-epithelialization and resolution of erythema following Er:YAG treatment occurred in 5 to 8 days and 3 to 6 weeks, respectively.[58] In comparison, re-epithelialization and resolution of erythema following CO_2 laser treatment occurred on an average of 7 days and 6 weeks, respectively.[64] Jiang et al treated five patients with a mean of 24 lesions per patient with the Er:YAG laser, resulting in a 93% reduction in AKs.[58] In a retrospective study, Iyer et al treated 24 patients with an Er:YAG or CO_2 laser or a combination of the two lasers, resulting in a 94% reduction of AKs.[60] Also in a retrospective study of 25 patients treated in the same manner, Ostertag et al found 80% of patients remained lesion free for 1 year,[59] which is similar to the 87% clearance reported by Iyer et al.[60] On average, 64% of recurrences occurred 32.7 months after treatment.[59] This study also failed to identify a statistical difference in the apparatus used in relation to the recurrence. Histological studies 3 months after Er:YAG treatments showed reversal of epidermal actinic damage, as well as an increase in collagen formation and decreased elastosis in the superficial papillary dermis.[58] Ablative laser treatment is believed to provide prophylaxis against future keratosis and cancers.[58,59,60,65] Immunohistochemistry analysis 4 weeks after treatment with a CO_2 laser found a decrease in expression of p53 and Ki-67.[63] A study reported a decrease in the p53 mutation 6 months after CO_2 laser treatment, and the authors concluded this treatment theoretically could decrease the risk of malignant transformation.[66] Ablative laser techniques offer dramatic improvement of actinic damage of the skin.[59] A comparison study of 5-FU and Er:YAG laser resurfacing found laser resurfacing to be more effective in relation to recurrence rates.[67] The most common side effects of ablative lasers are infection, hypopigmentation, hyperpigmentation, acne, milia, scar formation, and atrophic and/or easily bruising skin.[59] Since Er:YAG lasers cause less tissue damage, they have fewer associated side effects such as scarring and pigmentary changes, along with a decreased recovery period.[58]

Cyclooxygenase-2 Inhibitors

Epidemiological studies suggest COX-2 may be involved in the pathogenesis of NMSC.[68,69,70,71,72,73,74,75] COX-2 is not constitutively expressed in most tissues,[76] but can be induced by UV radiation.[70,73,77] Celecoxib has been shown to be a selective inhibitor of COX-2.[78] Animal models have shown treatment with celecoxib inhibits the development of UV-induced premalignant skin papillomas in mice, which are believed to correspond to AKs in humans.[68,69,70,71,72,73] A randomized, double-blind, placebo-controlled trial with oral celecoxib over 11 months in 240 subjects with biopsy-proven NMSC or AK reported a decrease of 58% of NMSC in the treatment group, but failed to show a decrease in AKs.[79] Tang et al performed a trial in which patients with basal cell nevus syndrome received celecoxib or a placebo, and found that the treatment group had 26% fewer new BCCs compared to the placebo group at the end of 2 years.[80]

Antioxidants

Selenium is necessary for the functioning of glutathione peroxidase,[81] which acts to reduce DNA-damaging hydroxyl-free radicals.[82] Increased dietary selenium in mice has been shown to provide protection from UV-induced skin tumors.[83] A prospective study of 485 adults found patients with 1.3 to 2.8 µmol/L of selenium had a decreased incidence of both BCC and SCC.[84] However, no significant effect to the incidence of BCC or SCC was found in a randomized controlled trial of patients who were treated with 200 µg/d of selenium for a mean of 4.5 years and a total follow-up of 6.4 years.[85] A Cochrane review that included this study found the selenium group was 17% more likely to develop NMSC, in particular SCCs.[81] The review also reported a 35% reduction in the risk of other cancer in the treatment group.

Beta carotene has provitamin A (retinol) activity, and is an antioxidant that may reduce free radical damage of DNA after UV exposure.[81] Beta carotene supplementation is believed to work by reducing immunosuppression induced by UV radiation.[86] In a study of 1,805 patients with a recent history of NMSC, patients received 50 mg of beta carotene daily for up to 5 years without a significant effect on the incidence of new NMSC.[87] Oral vitamin A supplements, however, have been shown to significantly reduce the 5-year probability of developing a new SCC.[88]

1.2.3 Dietary Modifications

Unsaturated fatty acids are major targets for free radical attack[81]; therefore, it is possible that decreased dietary fats could reduce free radical attack and carcinogenesis.[89] A series of animal studies showed a high level of dietary fats intake markedly shortened the time between UV exposure and tumor appearance, and increased the number of tumors that developed.[90] Based on diet alone, patients on a higher fat diet were found to be at 4.7 times greater risk for developing AKs during a 2-year period than those on a lower fat diet.[89] A comparison study of normal diet and a reduced fat diet over 24 months in 115 people with a history of no more than 2 NMSC found a trend toward significant reduction in the incidence of NMSC at 2 to 5 years.[91] Jaax et al further analyzed the results of the study and found a significant difference of new NMSC in subjects on a low-fat diet compared to a normal diet.[92]

1.2.4 Chemoprevention in Organ Transplant Recipients

Rates of developing AKs and Bowen's disease in organ transplant recipients (OTR) are 50 to 100 times higher than the general population.[93] OTRs are 250 and 10 times more likely to develop SCC and BCC, respectively, than the general population.[94] SCC and BCC account for more than 90% of skin cancers in transplant recipients.[95,96,97,98] The incidence of skin cancer in renal transplant patients increases with number of years posttransplantation, starting at 7% after 1 year, and increasing to 45% after 11 years, and 70% after 20 years.[97] In addition, the incidence of skin cancer is related to age of transplantation with a mean of 8 years posttransplant for those who received transplants at approximately 40 years of age,[99] and only 3 years for patients who received transplants after the age of 60.[95] Skin cancer development is proportional to the level of immunosuppression.[97] Significantly lower CD4 counts have been associated with OTRs with cutaneous carcinomas compared to those without skin lesions.[100] SCCs appear to be more aggressive in OTRs.[101,102,103,104] This point is demonstrated in a study of cardiac transplant recipients where 27% of all deaths 4 years posttransplant were attributed to skin cancer.[105] These studies emphasize the importance of taking preventative measures in this high-risk population to significantly impact morbidity and mortality rates.

Systemic Retinoids

Retinoids are vitamin A derivatives that work by inhibiting cell growth and inducing normal differentiation in malignant cells.[106] Although indications for systemic retinoids are not conclusive, it has been suggested that retinoids are most effective in patients with a history of multiple NMSCs.[107] Acitretin is a retinoid and has been shown to be effective in the prevention of SCC in renal transplant recipients with a history of NSMC.[108] A double-blinded placebo-controlled study demonstrated 42% reduction in premalignant lesions and a 78% risk reduction in developing NMSC within the first year of treatment of acitretin.[109] In a crossover study, George et al reported an average increase of 42% of SCCs during drug-free period compared to acitretin period.[108] Studies have shown a statistically significant decrease in skin cancers with a robust effect in patients with multiple prior NMSCs.[109,110] Systemic low-dose retinoids have been shown to significantly reduce the mean number of SCCs for up to 3 years.[111] Systemic retinoids can cause cheilitis, headache, rash, photosensitivity, dry eyes, palmoplantar desquamation, epistaxis, elevate triglycerides, "stickiness," aggravation of existing musculoskeletal symptoms, nail changes, gastrointestinal side effects, and pruritus.[108] A systematic review of oral retinoids found that headaches, rash, musculoskeletal symptoms, and hyperlipidemia were the most common causes of withdrawal from treatment.[112] No significant difference in adverse effects was found when comparing 0.4 mg/kg/d acitretin for 12 months versus 0.4 mg/kg/d for 3 months, then 0.2 mg/kg/d for the remaining 9 months.[113] Retinoids are effective only during treatment.[111] A "rebound" effect on the development of SCCs when acitretin is discontinued has been reported,[107,108,109,111] and is most marked in patients taking retinoids longer than 12 months.[111] Continued use of systemic retinoids can accelerate osteoporosis, calcification of tendons and ligaments, osteophytes, and bone spurs around joints.[114,115]

Besides recommending treatments to prevent the transformation of precancerous lesions, dermatologists also perform skilled physical exams that allow for early detection of skin cancers and educate patients on mole mapping and self-skin exams (SSE).

1.2.5 Secondary Prevention

The USPSTF defines secondary prevention as preventive measures that identify and treat asymptomatic persons who have already developed risk factors or preclinical disease, but in whom the condition has not become clinically apparent.[5] Dermatologists consistently perform secondary prevention methods in their practice by performing skin examinations, mole mapping, and teaching patients how to perform skin self-examinations. Since Breslow thickness is the strongest prognostic indicator,[116] it is important to detect melanoma at the earliest stage possible.

Dermatologists have a positive impact on early detection of melanoma with an increase in incidence of melanoma and a decrease in mortality.[117] This study found that the increase in incidence was mostly due to an increase in the diagnosis of stage I cancers.[117] Authors attributed this finding to the ease of access to health care due to the high ratio of dermatologists per capita and increased public awareness.[117] In addition, patients with an established dermatologist were more likely to be given a diagnosis of melanoma in situ and to have thinner invasive melanoma.[7]

Although currently the USPSTF does not recommend SSE for the general population,[118] there is evidence that supports SSEs, especially in high-risk groups. Risk factors for melanoma include personal history of melanoma (5–8%),[119,120] family history of melanoma in two or more family members,[121] numerous nevi and presence or history of atypical/dysplastic nevi,[122,123,124] fair skin (fourfold),[125] red hair and blue eyes (twofold),[126] history of NMSC (twofold to threefold),[127,128] history of sunburns or excessive UV light exposure (twofold),[129] and indoor tanning (twofold to threefold).[130] The National Comprehensive Cancer Network (NCCN) recommends SSE in patients with a history of melanoma and NMSC.[37,131,132] It is estimated that 75% of melanomas are detected by patients themselves or by spouses, friends, or other lay persons.[133,134,135,136,137] A retrospective cross-sectional study reported patients detected 41.7% of melanomas in situ, 51% of melanomas, and 62.4% of invasive melanomas.[7] A study of 816 melanoma patients found patients who conducted SSE were associated with early diagnosis.[134] In a separate study, patients who conducted SSE were found to have significantly thinner melanomas.[138] In a large study of 1,062 melanoma patients, 19% had a recurrence that was most often self-detected.[139] This study also observed that self-detection independently predicted survival. A literature review showed a wide range of sensitivity and specificity for SSE ranging from 25 to 88% sensitivity and 57 to 97% specificity.[140] A randomized controlled trial showed an increase in accuracy and specificity of SSEs when patients received a leaflet with photos of nevi, seborrheic keratoses, and early melanomas.[141] ▶ Fig. 1.1 is taken from the AAD's website demonstrating the appropriate method to perform a SSE.[142] The SSE can create a feeling of joint responsibility with the dermatologist in early detection of melanoma.[143] It is recommended that SSEs be performed frequently at first to become familiar with their nevi and then monthly (▶ Table 1.3).[143]

Patients with multiple nevi are at increased risk for developing melanoma compared to the general population. A study found a relative risk of 1.6 for patients with 11 to 25 nevi, 4.4 for 26 to 50 nevi, 5.4 for 51 to 100 nevi, and 9.8 for patients with more than 100 nevi.[147] Patients with atypical nevi are also at high risk. The same study reported relative risks of 3.8 and 6.3 for patients with 1 to 5 atypical and more than 6 atypical nevi, respectively.[147] It is estimated that 22 to 50% of melanomas show nevus origin.[123,148,149] Mole mapping is especially helpful in these individuals. Simply drawing a mole on a mole diagram improved accuracy of reporting new lesions on SSE.[150] The ADD has provided an excellent mole map with a lesion log that is demonstrated in (▶ Fig. 1.2).[142] Other studies have demonstrated that the use of digital photography increases the diagnostic accuracy of SSEs.[150,151,152] Total nevus number usually peaks by the third decade of life and declines in the seventh or eighth.[153] With this in mind, dermatoscopic monitoring can be performed for concerning lesions in younger individuals and total body photography to monitor for new lesions in the elderly.[143]

1.3 When to Treat

1.3.1 Nonmelanoma Skin Cancer

The primary goal of treatment of BCC is the cure of the tumor along with maximal preservation of function and cosmesis. In order to achieve this goal, each case should be individualized based on treatment cure rate, preservation of function and cosmesis, and patient's preference. Tumors with low-risk characteristics and uncomplicated high-risk patients can be effectively treated by dermatologists. Indications, risks, and benefits for different treatment modalities will be discussed later in the book, so this section will focus on characteristics of low-risk tumor characteristics found in ▶ Table 1.4.

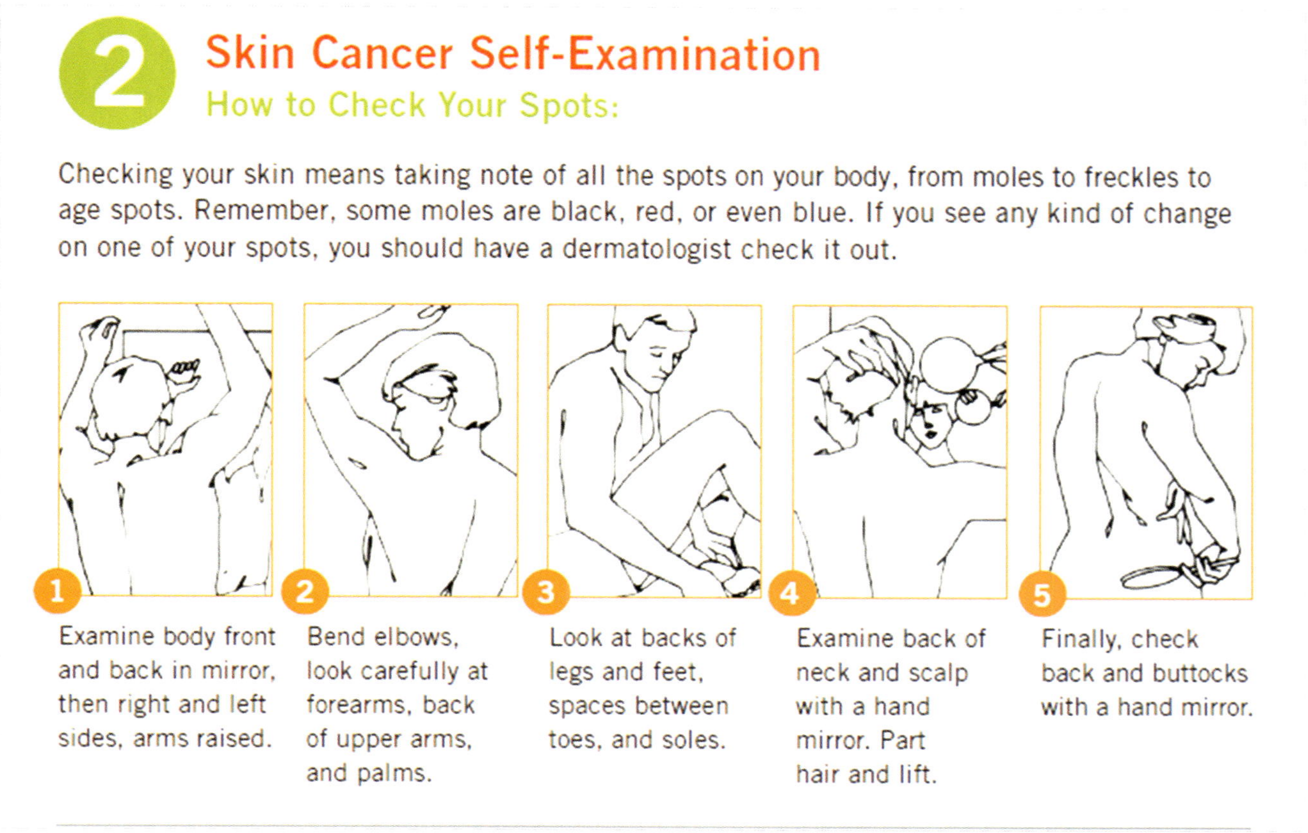

Fig. 1.1 Self-skin exam. (Reproduced with permission from the American Academy of Dermatology.[142] Copyright ©2015. All rights reserved.)

Table 1.3 Risk factors for cutaneous melanoma

Risk factor	Odds ratio	Information
Personal history of melanoma		Standardized incidence ratio 4.5–25.6
Family history of melanoma	1.8	
11–50 common moles > 2 mm	1.7–1.9	
55–100 common moles > 2 mm	3.2–3.7	
> 100 common moles > 2 mm	7.6–7.7	
1–4 atypical nevi	1.6–7.3	Atypical moles: ill-defined or irregular border; irregular pigmentation; diameter > 5 mm; erythema (blanchable in lesion or at edge); accentuated skin markings
Reported growth of a mole	2.3	
Giant congenital melanocytic		Relative risk range 239–1,224 for nevi > 20 cm in diameter extra cutaneous as well as cutaneous melanoma
Skin that does not tan easily	1.98	
Light-colored Skin	1.40–1.42	
Light-colored eyes	1.55–1.60	
Red or light-colored hair	1.4–3.5	
Presence of actinic lentigines	1.9–3.5	
History of nonmelanoma skin cancer		Twofold to threefold increased risk[127,128]
Female		Female:male standardized incidence ratio is 1.3:1

Table 1.3 continued

Risk factor	Odds ratio	Information
Age		Melanoma is rare in childhood and adolescence but risk increases with age
Affluence		Relative risk approximately of 3 for least deprived compared to most deprived on Carstairs deprivation category
Unusually high sun exposure	2.6	
Indoor tanning		A single session can increase the risk of melanoma by 20%[144]
Occupational exposure to coal tar, pitch, creosote, arsenic, or radium[145]		
Pesticide use more than two times per year[145]		

Source: Modified from Scottish Intercollegiate Guidelines Network 2004.[146]

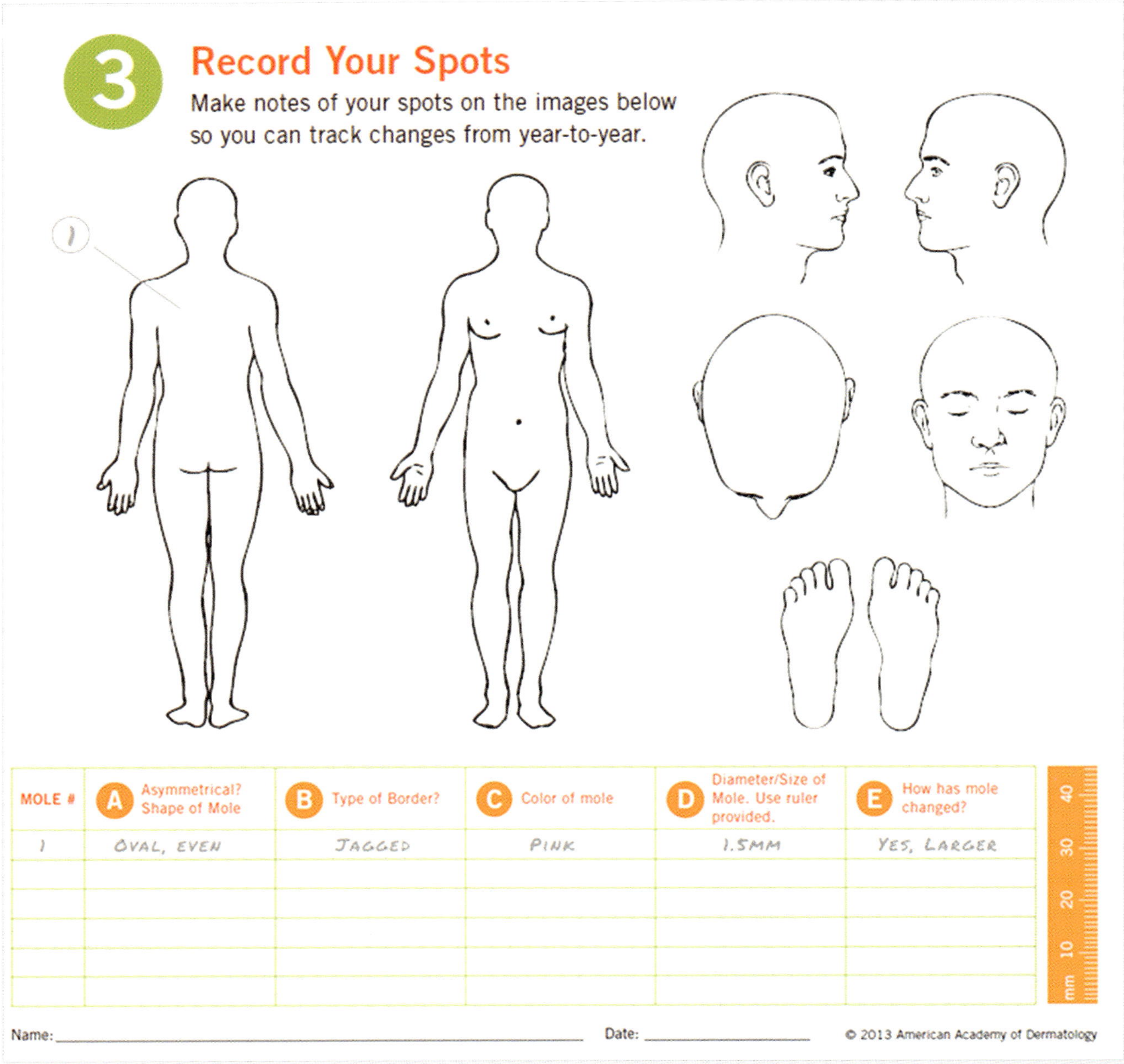

Fig. 1.2 Mole map and log example. (Reproduced with permission from the American Academy of Dermatology.[142] Copyright ©2015. All rights reserved.)

Table 1.4 Characteristics of low-risk recurrence

Basal cell cancer	Squamous cell cancer[142]
Area < 20 mm on trunk and extremities (excluding pretibia, hands, feet, nail units, and ankles)	Area < 20 mm on trunk and extremities (excluding pretibia, hands, feet, nail units, and ankles)
Area < 10 mm on cheeks, forehead, scalp, neck, and pretibia	Area < 10 mm on cheeks, forehead, scalp, neck, and pretibia
Area < 6 mm on central face, eyelids, eyebrows, periorbital, nose, lips, chin, mandible, preauricular and postauricular skin/sulci, temple, ear, genitalia, hands, and feet (location independent of size may constitute high risk in certain clinical settings).	Area < 6 mm on central face, eyelids, eyebrows, periorbital, nose, lips, chin, mandible, preauricular and postauricular skin/sulci, temple, ear, genitalia, hands, and feet (location independent of size may constitute high risk in certain clinical settings).
Primary tumor	Primary tumor
Not a site of prior radiation therapy	Not a site of prior radiation therapy or chronic inflammatory process
Immunocompetent	Immunocompetent
Well-defined borders	Well-defined borders
Nodular, superficial, keratotic, infundibulocystic, and fibroepithelioma of Pinkus	Well or moderately differentiated on pathology
Absence of perineural involvement	Absence of perineural or vascular involvement
	Slow-growing tumor
	Absence of neurologic symptoms
	Thickness < 2 mm or Clark levels I, II, III

Source: Modified from National Comprehensive Cancer Network 2014.[131]

Note: Risk factors are also increase likelihood metastasis.

1.3.2 Melanoma

Understanding when to treat or when to refer melanoma can be difficult since there are no hard and fast rules. Dermatologists can perform a wide local excision on lesions with a Breslow depth of less than 1 mm and less aggressive histological features. Ulceration and mitoses are also important to consider. A T1b melanoma can be referred to a general surgeon for sentinel lymph node biopsy and/or a medical oncologist for further work-up. Tumor, node, metastasis (TNM) staging criteria are listed in ▶ Table 1.5.[154]

1.4 When to Refer

1.4.1 Nonmelanoma Skin Cancer

The NCCN recommends that complicated high-risk tumors, regional recurrence, or the development of distant disease be managed by a multidisciplinary tumor board.[131] Characteristics of high-risk basal and squamous cell tumors can be found in ▶ Table 1.6. Metastasized SCC to regional lymph nodes has been associated with lymphovascular invasion, poor differentiation, and perineural invasion.[155] In addition, patients with regional

Table 1.5 AJCC TNM criteria for cutaneous melanoma

Tis	Thickness	Ulceration status/mitosis
T1	N/A	N/A
	≤ 1 mm	a: w/o ulceration and mitosis < 1/mm²
		b: with ulceration and mitoses ≥ 1/mm²
T2	1.01–2 mm	a: w/o ulceration
		b: with ulceration
T3	2.01–4 mm	a: w/o ulceration
		b: with ulceration
T4	> 4 mm	a: w/o ulceration b: with ulceration
N classification	Number of metastatic nodes	Nodal metastatic mass
N0	0 nodes	N/A
N1	1 node	a: Micrometastasis[a]
		b: Macrometastasis[b]
N2	2–3 nodes	a: Micrometastasis[a]
		b: Macrometastasis[b]
		c: In-transit met(s)/satellite(s) without metastatic nodes
N3	4 or more metastatic nodes, or matted nodes, or in-transit met(s)/satellite(s) with metastatic node(s)	
M classification	Site	Serum LDH
M0	0 sites	N/A
M1a	Distant skin, subcutaneous, or nodal metastases	Normal
M1b	Lung metastases	Normal
M1c	All other visceral metastases	Normal

Abbreviation: AJCC, American Joint Committee on Cancer; LDH, lactate dehydrogenase; TNM, tumor, node, metastasis.

Source: Modified from Balch et al 2010.[154]

[a]Micrometastases are diagnosed after sentinel lymph node biopsy and completion lymphadenectomy (if performed).

[b]Macrometastases are defined as clinically detectable nodal metastases confirmed by therapeutic lymphadenectomy or when nodal metastasis exhibits gross extracapsular extension.

Table 1.6 Characteristics of high-risk recurrence

Basal cell cancer	Squamous cell cancer
Area ≥ 20 mm on trunk and extremities (excluding pretibia, hands, feet, nail units, and ankles)	Area ≥ 20 mm on trunk and extremities (excluding pretibia, hands, feet, nail units, and ankles)
Area ≥ 10 mm on cheeks, forehead, scalp, neck, and pretibia	Area ≥ 10 mm on cheeks, forehead, scalp, neck, and pretibia
Area > 6 mm on central face, eyelids, eyebrows, periorbital, nose, lips, chin, mandible, preauricular and postauricular skin/ sulci, temple, ear, genitalia, hands, and feet (location independent of size may constitute high risk in certain clinical settings)	Area > 6 mm on central face, eyelids, eyebrows, periorbital, nose, lips, chin, mandible, preauricular and postauricular skin/ sulci, temple, ear, genitalia, hands, and feet (location independent of size may constitute high risk in certain clinical settings)
Recurrent tumor	Recurrent tumor
Site of prior radiation therapy	Site of prior radiation therapy or chronic inflammatory process
Immunosuppressed	Immunosuppressed
Poorly defined borders	Poorly defined borders
Pathology showing morpheaform, basosquamous (metatypical), sclerosing, mixed infiltrative, or micronodular features in any portion of the tumor	Poorly differentiated on pathology
Perineural involvement	Adenoid (acantholytic), adenosquamous (showing mucin production), or desmoplastic subtypes
	Rapidly growing tumor
	Neurologic symptoms
	Thickness or Clark level ≥ 2 mm or IV, V
	Perineural or vascular involvement

Source: Modified from National Comprehensive Cancer Network 2014.[131]

nodal involvement are at a significant increased risk for recurrence and mortality.[156] The NCCN recommends patients with palpable lymph nodes or suspicious lymph nodes on imaging receive a fine needle or core biopsy, and that negative findings be confirmed by re-biopsy and/or re-evaluation.[131] In the rare instance of metastasized cutaneous BCC, the NCCN suggests that a trial of vismodegib may be helpful even in the case of metastatic basosquamous carcinoma.[131] In the case of metastatic SCC, the NCCN recommended cisplatin monotherapy, cisplatin plus 5-FU, epidermal growth factor inhibitors, or clinical trials.[131]

1.4.2 Melanoma

In general, tumors with a Breslow depth of greater than 1 mm should be referred to a surgeon for sentinel lymph node biopsy. It is also important to discuss a general surgeon referral with patients who have T1b cancers and/or a Breslow depth between 0.75 and 1 mm with 1 or more mitoses/mm^2. A medical oncologist is an important part of patient care for those with stage II melanoma that exhibits aggressive features such as micrometastases and a deep Breslow depth, or greater than stage III cancer.

1.5 Follow-Up

1.5.1 Nonmelanoma Skin Cancer

It is estimated that 30 to 50% of patients with NMSC will develop another NMSC within 5 years.[157] In addition to a 10-fold increased risk of developing a subsequent NMSC compared to the general population,[158] they are also at increased risk for developing cutaneous melanoma.[159] Nearly 70 to 80% of all cutaneous SCC recurrences develop within 2 years of initial treatment.[160] Consequently, it is important to closely follow these patients.

NCCN recommendations for nonmelanoma skin cancer

- Complete skin exam every 6–12 months for life in patients with a history of BCC.
- Complete skin and regional lymph node exam every 3–12 months for 2 years, then every 6–12 months for 3 years, then annually for life for patients with a history of local SCC.
- Complete skin exam with regional lymph node exam every 1–3 months for 1 year, then every 2–4 months for 1 year, then every 4–6 months for 3 years, then every 6–12 months annually for life for patients with regional SCC.
- Patient education on sun protection and self-skin examination regardless of type of skin cancer.

Abbreviations: BCC, basal cell carcinoma; SCC, squamous cell carcinoma.

Source: Modified from National Comprehensive Cancer Network 2014.[131]

1.5.2 Melanoma

Approximately 30% of stage I to III melanomas that are completely resected will develop a recurrence.[161,162,163] The recurrence rate of melanoma is highest in the first 2 to 3 years after treatment.[164,165] Recurrence rates of 5.2% with stage IA, 18.4% with stage IB, 28.7% with stage IIA, 40.6% with stage IIB, and 44.3% with stage IIC have been reported.[166] An overall 5-year relapse-free survival for stage IIIA, IIIB, and IIIC patients was 63, 32, and 11%, respectively.[167] Another study found the site of first recurrence with stage I to III melanoma was local in 13% of patients, in-transit in 17%, regional lymph nodes in 46%, and distant in 24%.[168] Among 340 relapsing stage III patients, 28% had local/in-transit recurrence, 21% had regional node recurrence, and 51% had systemic recurrence.[167] The risk of recurrent disease makes appropriate follow-up essential. Unfortunately, due to the absence of clear data, there are various opinions for appropriate follow-up of patients with melanoma.[132]

NCCN recommendations for melanoma skin cancer

- At least annual skin exam for life.
- Radiologic imaging for specific signs and symptoms.
- Regional lymph node ultrasound may be considered for equivocal lymph node physical exam, patients who were offered but did not undergo sentinel lymph node biopsy, or patients with a positive sentinel lymph node biopsy who did not undergo complete lymph node dissection. However, nodal basin ultrasound is not a substitute for sentinel lymph node biopsy.
- Risk of recurrence, prior primary melanoma, family history of melanoma, atypical moles, and patient/physician concern should influence follow-up schedule.

Source: National Comprehensive Cancer Network 2014.[132]

The NCCN recommendations for follow-up for all patients regardless of stage of melanoma can be found above. The NCCN also recommends a skin and lymph node exam for patients with stage IIB to IV melanoma every 3 to 6 months for 2 years, then every 3 to 12 months for 3 years, then annually as clinically necessary.[132] It is important to consider performing a chest X-ray, computed tomography (CT), and/or positron emission tomography (PET)/CT scan every 4 to 12 months to screen for recurrent/metastatic disease, and possibly more frequently in patients who are at higher risk.[132] Since there is a 13% risk of stage IIIC melanoma patients to have brain metastasis,[167] an annual brain magnetic resonance imaging (MRI) can be considered.[132] Routine radiologic screening for asymptomatic recurrent/metastasis is not recommended after 5 years.[132]

1.5.3 Family History of Melanoma

A single first-degree relative with melanoma nearly doubles one's risk for developing melanoma.[126] A positive family history has been associated with younger age of diagnosis of melanoma with 68.6% being diagnosed at 45 years of age or younger.[169] Patients with a family history of melanoma are more likely to have multiple atypical nevi.[169,170] Screening those with a known family history have produced thinner melanomas.[171,172,173,174] A study suggested patients with a family history of melanoma would benefit from targeted dermatologic care.[169] This is in accord with a literature review that found 27% of the reviewed guidelines recommended targeted monitoring.[175]

1.5.4 Familial Atypical Multiple Mole Melanoma Syndrome

The median age of melanoma incidence in patients with familial atypical multiple mole melanoma syndrome (FAMMS) that carry the CDK2NA mutation has been reported to be between 33 and 45,[176,177] but cases of melanoma have also been reported in early teens and twenties.[178] Screening for melanoma patients with FAMMS should begin at age 10 with a baseline full-body exam including oral mucosa and genital area.[179,180,181,182] This screening should also be offered to all first- and some second-degree relatives.[183] It has been suggested FAMMS patients be examined by a health care provider every 6 months to ensure nevi stability.[183] After this is established, patients should be educated on the performance and importance of SSE, and subsequent visits can be performed annually or as needed.[183]

1.5.5 Genetic Testing

FAMMS is a autosomal dominant with variable expressivity and penetrance that typically presents as more than 50 moles.[183] Typical germline mutations of the CDKN2A gene are missense or nonsense mutations in p16(INK4), P15 (INK4b), or p18(INK4c).[183] The Melanoma Genetics Consortium (GenoMEL) has issued statements that genetic testing for CDK2NA is premature citing varying penetrance and family members with a negative genetic test are still at higher risk than general population giving them a false security.[182] Instead, it is recommended that first-degree relatives of individuals at high risk be engaged in the same programs of melanoma prevention and surveillance irrespective of the results of any genetic testing.[182]

1.5.6 Nevoid Basal Cell Carcinoma Syndrome

Patients with nevoid basal cell carcinoma syndrome (NBCCS) usually develop BCCs in the third decade of life with a median age of 25.[184] At the age of 20, the cumulative incidence of BCC is 14% in males and 12% in females. By 50 years of age, 77% of females and 80% of males have been diagnosed with BCC.[185] Approximately 90% of Caucasians with NBCCS develop BCCs, compared to only 40% of African Americans. It has been suggested patients have annual skin examinations.[184]

Genetic Testing

NBCCS is an autosomal dominant disorder.[184] It is estimated that 70 to 80% of mutations are inherited from a parent, while the remaining 20 to 30% are new mutations.[184] Evans and Farndon cited the need for surveillance for complications of NBCCS, such as medulloblastoma in children and jaw cysts and BCCs in adults.[184] Genetic testing for at-risk relatives, including children, may also be appropriate.[184]

1.5.7 Xeroderma Pigmentosum

Xeroderma pigmentosum (XP) is an example of how both genetic and environmental interactions influence the course of disease.[186] XP patients develop AKs at an early age.[187] If XP is diagnosed at 20 years of age or earlier, there is a 10,000-fold increased risk for developing NMSC on sun-exposed sites, and greater than 2,000-fold increased risk for developing cutaneous melanoma.[187] The median onset of NMSC is 9 years of age, and the median age for cutaneous melanoma is 22.[187] Both BCC and SCC can grow quickly and behave aggressively.[188] Complete skin examination with clinical color photographs of the entire skin surface and close-ups (including a ruler) of individual lesions is the suggested management plan.[187] Depending on severity of skin disease, frequent skin examinations approximately every 3 to 12 months are recommended.[186] In addition to regular skin examinations, periodic routine eye and neurologic examinations and audiograms are included in the management plan.[187] Patients or parents should be instructed on morphology of BCC, SCC, and abnormal pigmented lesions in order to perform frequent skin exams.[186]

Genetic Testing

XP is an autosomal recessive mutation of nucleotide excision repair.[187] The diagnosis of XP is based on clinical findings and family history.[187] Functional testing to screen cells for abnormalities in DNA repair is the preferred laboratory diagnostic method.[187] XP patients with XP-A, B, D, F, and G mutations experience severe sunburn after minimal sun exposure.[186] Carrier testing for at-risk individuals and prenatal diagnosis are available.[187]

1.5.8 Consolidation of Medications

Adverse drug reactions reported to the Norwegian Medicine Control Authority from 1970 to 1994 reported photo-induced drug eruptions represented 8% of cutaneous adverse events.[189] The proposed mechanism involves a systemic/cutaneous drug or its metabolites present in the skin and exposed to UV light.[190] Photosensitive reactions are classified as either the more common phototoxic response or the less common photoallergic reactions.[191] Phototoxic eruptions are not immune mediated and occur in all individuals with high doses of exposure of the culprit drug and radiation at the appropriate wavelengths.[190] Intensity of responses are dependent on the dose of the photosensitizer and sunlight.[191] Photoallergic reactions are immune mediated and do not occur in all individuals exposed to the drug and radiation.[190] There have been case reports of patients on known photosensitive drugs for a prolonged period that develop cancer. McCarthy et al report a patient with chronic granulomatous disease on long-term voriconazole that led to multifocal facial SCC.[192] Individuals are more prone to developing SCCs while on photosensitizing drugs and being immunosuppressed.[193,194,195] Miller et al reported two patients on long-term voriconazole that developed five in situ melanomas.[196] A review of 1,380 patients treated with psoralen plus UV-A phototherapy (PUVA) found an increased risk of melanoma in patients receiving more than 250 treatments with the most pronounced risk occurring 15 years from initial treatment.[197] It is important to be mindful of the increased risk of skin cancer long-term therapy with photosensitive drugs poses. ▶ Table 1.7 was modified from Moore and contains common photosensitive drugs.[191]

Table 1.7 Drugs with reported photosensitivity

Diuretic agents	Antimicrobials
Hydrochlorothiazide, furosemide (frusemide), chlorothiazide, bendroflumethiazide, benzthiazide, cyclothiazide, hydroflumethiazide, methyclothiazide, trichlormethiazide, polythiazide, amiloride, ethacrynic acid, triamterene, spironolactone, acetazolamide, metolazone, quinethazone	Demeclocycline, nalidixic acid, sulfamethoxazole, sulfasalazine, ciprofloxacin, enoxacin, lomefloxacin, ofloxacin, norfloxacin, oxytetracycline, tetracycline, doxycycline, methacycline, minocycline, trimethoprim, isoniazid, sulfamethizole, gentamicin, clofazimine, griseofulvin, nitrofurantoin
Nonsteroidal anti-inflammatory drugs	Antipsychotic drugs
Naproxen, ketoprofen, suprofen, tiaprofenic acid, piroxicam, diflunisal, diclofenac, mefenamic acid, nabumetone, sulindac, phenylbutazone, indomethacin, ibuprofen	Chlorpromazine, trifluoperazine, prochlorperazine, thioridazine, chlorprothixene, promethazine, perphenazine, fluphenazine, promazine, haloperidol, thiothixene, triflupromazine, trimeprazine
Antidepressants	Cardiovascular drugs
Amitriptyline, trimipramine, nortriptyline, protriptyline, desipramine, amoxapine, imipramine, doxepin	Amiodarone, nifedipine, quinidine, captopril, enalapril, fosinopril, ramipril, disopyramide, hydralazine, clofibrate, simvastatin
Antimalarials	Hypoglycemics
Chloroquine, quinine, pyrimethamine, mefloquine	Glibenclamide (glyburide), tolbutamide, glipizide, tolazamide, chlorpropamide, acetohexamide
Antihistamines	Cytotoxic drugs
Cyproheptadine, diphenhydramine, brompheniramine, triprolidine, loratadine	Fluorouracil, vinblastine, dacarbazine, procarbazine, methotrexate
Anticonvulsants	Hormones
Carbamazepine, lamotrigine, phenobarbital (phenobarbitone), phenytoin	Corticosteroids, estrogens, progesterones, spironolactone
Systemic dermatological agents	Miscellaneous
Isotretinoin, methoxsalen	Gold salts, azathioprine, hematoporphyrin

Note: Drugs are listed by therapeutic class and generic name. The drugs are listed within each grouping in approximate order of frequency of incidence of reports.

Source: Modified from Moore 2002.[191]

1.6 High-Risk Groups

1.6.1 Outdoor Workers

Outdoor workers have been identified as at-risk group for the development of NMSC due to the nature of their work and high levels of UV exposure.[198] The term "outdoor worker" typically includes individuals who work outdoors for 3 or more hours on a usual workday.[199] Sunburn rates among construction workers has been estimated to be 50 to 80%.[200] Not only do individuals who work outside spend more time in the sun at work, but several studies also show they spend a significant amount of time outside during nonwork hours.[201,202] Studies using dosimetry methods to objectively quantify UV radiation exposure demonstrate that outdoor workers receive higher than recommended doses.[203,204,205,206] Two separate meta-analyses have shown a clear association between occupational UV exposure and increased risk of developing SCC[207] and BCC.[208] The association between occupational UV exposure and melanoma is less clear.[209] A systematic review of 29 published case-control studies revealed a significant positive risk for intermittent sun exposure and a significantly reduced risk for heavy occupational exposure.[129] These findings are supported by a meta-analysis of 41 published studies that demonstrated a positive association for intermittent exposure and an inverse association with high continuous sun exposure and melanoma.[210] Some believe there is sufficient evidence to consider skin cancer as an "occupational disease."[198]

Occupational sun exposure can be minimized or avoided by following recommended sun-protective strategies such as wearing wide-brimmed hats, long-sleeved shirts and pants, sunglasses, regular sunscreen use, seeking shade, and rescheduling work tasks that are during peak UV time (10 a.m.–3 p.m.).[199] Studies have shown low uptake of sun-protective strategies among outdoor workers.[206,211,212] A systematic review of 34 cross-sectional and interventional studies reported that many outdoor workers never or only rarely wore long-sleeved shirt (50–80%), sun-protective headgear (30–80%), and sunscreen (30–100%).[200] It has been shown that employees working under mandatory sun protection policy have fewer solar keratoses and less self-reported skin cancer excisions compared to employees under voluntary sun protection policy.[202] Several methods and interventions have been shown to increase the application of sun protection. Randomized trials incorporating education and awareness about skin cancer protection demonstrated long-term efficacy of workplace-based interventions. The first trial used a UV photograph and/or video about skin cancer that resulted in a significant increase in sun protection behavior for 12 months.[213] Another trial incorporated communication strategies in the Go Sun Smart Health Communication Campaign for ski area employees that led to improved sunscreen and protective clothing use.[214] The third trial involved the SunWise program and the provision of hats and sunscreen for postal workers that also led to improved sunscreen and protective clothing use.[215] Provision of personal protective equipment and education has also been shown to increase sun protection in Israeli workers.[216] Other environmental considerations such as a workplace culture that values sun protection[217,218] and social norms[219] have shown a positive association with sun-safety behaviors.

1.6.2 Pilots

Flight personnel have been reported to have an increased incidence of skin cancer.[220] Aircraft windows block UV radiation and measurements within the cockpit at high cruise altitudes reveal only minimal exposure,[221] but flight personnel are regularly exposed to cosmic radiation that is composed of mainly gamma and neutron radiation.[222] This type of radiation can easily penetrate the body and has been linked to multiple types of cancer ranging from melanoma to brain cancer.[220] Annual radiation dose estimates vary depending on several occupational factors. With factors, such as the worker's job (cockpit or cabin crew), type of flights (long or short haul), and number of hours flown, it is estimated that flight personnel receive an annual radiation dose between 0.2 and 9.1 mSv/y.[223] This is higher than the average annual dose of most nuclear workers, radiologic technologists, and industrial radiographers.[224] It has been estimated that airline pilots are exposed to 2 to 6 mSv/y of ionizing radiation, and approximately 1 mSv of background gamma radiation.[222] A review of cosmic radiation exposure and cancer risk revealed a risk estimate of 1.6 to 2.5 for developing NMSC among airline crew members.[220] The review also reported a risk estimate for developing melanoma ranging from 1.8 to 10.2 in airline pilots and 0.4 to 3.7 in flight attendants. Although higher incidence of skin cancer has been reported, several confounding factors make a clear association challenging.[220] This unclear association makes an approach to skin cancer prevention in this group difficult.

1.6.3 Tanning Beds

Indoor tanning has been labeled as a class I carcinogen by the International Agency for Research on Cancer.[225] One minute in the average indoor tanning machine is estimated to be twice as carcinogenic as 1 minute in the midday Mediterranean sun.[226] Individuals who have used indoor tanning under the age of 25 are at a higher risk for NMSC.[227] The National Health Interview Survey found indoor tanners tended to be non-Hispanic white females, and of those females 62% were 25 or younger.[228] The United States attributable risk fraction was estimated to be 8.2% for SCC and 3.7% for BCC corresponding to approximately 170,000 cases of NMSC associated with indoor tanning.[227] In 2014, estimates of NMSC linked with tanning beds rose to 419,000.[229] A single indoor tanning session has been associated with an increased risk of 67% and 29% for SCC and BCC, respectively.[229] Six tanning sessions per year in a high school and college-aged individual increases the risk developing BCC by 73%.[230] It is estimated that of melanoma cases in patients 18 to 29 years, 765 are linked to tanning bed use.[231] Nearly 25% of early-onset BCC could have been avoided if individuals never tanned indoors.[232] Approximately 3,438 cases of melanoma in Europe can be attributed to tanning bed use.[144] About 10,000 cases of melanoma are linked to indoor tanning in the United States, Europe, and Australia.[229] In a systematic review and meta-analysis, first tanning bed use before the age of 35 was associated with a relative risk of 1.87 for developing melanoma.[144] The review also reported a dose response of 1.8% increased risk of melanoma for each additional indoor tanning session per year.[144] Just one tanning session can increase the user's risk of developing melanoma by 20% and each additional session during the same years increases the risk by another 25.[144] According to the Youth Risk Behavior Surveillance System, 13% of all high school students, 21% of high school girls, 32% of girls in the 12th grade, and 29% of white high school girls use indoor tanning beds.[233] States including California, Hawaii, Illinois, Louisiana, Minnesota, Nevada, Oregon, Texas, Vermont, and Washington have passed laws against indoor tanning by minors.[234] It has also been reported that newer tanning beds are not safer than older models,[235] and since September 2014, the Food and Drug Administration required tanning beds to carry a class II (moderate- to high-risk) warning.[236]

1.7 Sun Protection Methods

The International Agency for Research and Cancer has classified UV radiation as a carcinogen.[237] Survey results from the Center of Disease Control demonstrated that although protective behaviors such as sunscreen use, shade use, and wearing long clothing to the ankles have increased in recent years, sunburn prevalence remains high, with 50.1% of all adults and 65.6% of whites aged 18 to 29 years reporting at least one sunburn in a 1-year period.[238] A survey review showed the highest incidence of sunburns were among men, non-Hispanic whites, young adults, and high-income groups, while women and older adults took more precautions.[10] Sunburns are more common among persons aged 18 to 29 years compared with older adults.[238] It is estimated that less than 40% of adolescents use sun protection.[10] Female adolescents have been reported to use sunscreen more readily, in a wider range of situations, and reapply sunscreen more often when compared to adolescent males.[239] In addition, more female adolescents were found to receive encouragement to use sunscreen from their mothers and peers.[239] As stated previously in the chapter, approximately 60% of parents apply sunscreen.[10] Despite the more sensitive nature of infant and toddler skin, there is evidence suggesting not only that the skin's barrier protection remains immature throughout at least the first 2 years of life, but also that accumulation of UV radiation-induced changes in the skin may begin as early as the first summer of life.[240] A survey of 4,000 elementary students in Florida demonstrated that 51.3% of non-Hispanic white students reported use of SPF 15 or greater sunscreen "most of the time or always" compared with 35.3% of Hispanic and 13.4% of non-Hispanic black students.[241] According to the National Ambulatory Medical Care Survey, children were the population that received the fewest mentions of sunscreen during their appointment.[6] In this section, basic sun protection methods will be discussed, which includes sunscreen, plant phenols, SPF clothing, hats, and sunglasses.

1.7.1 Sunscreen

Sunscreen is one of the most common methods of sun protection used by Americans.[238] The amount of UV radiation required to produce a sunburn with sunscreen applied to the skin in relation to the amount required to produce a sunburn on unprotected skin is known as SPF.[3] As the SPF increases, the amount of protection increases.[3] SPF 30 sunscreen absorbs 96.7% of the erythemogenic UV rays, whereas a SPF 60 sunscreen absorbs 98.3%, which is to say that a sunscreen of SPF 60 prevents almost twice the erythemogenic UV rays from reaching the skin compared to an SPF 30 sunscreen.[242] Most people only use 25 to 50% of the recommended 2 mg/cm^2 of sunscreen, resulting in less sun protection.[243]

Sunscreen is composed of organic and inorganic filters. Organic filters are aromatic compounds that work by absorbing UV light, and inorganic filters can absorb, reflect, and scatter UV light.[244] These filters absorb energy and electrons jump to an excited state, and on return to ground state, release their energy in the form of heat or light in longer wavelength.[245,246,247]

Para-aminobenzoic acid (PABA) derivatives, cinnamates, benzophenones, and octocrylene are examples of organic filters that have been described to cause photoallergy.[248] Approximately less than 1% of allergic contact dermatitis reactions in North America are from sunscreens, but it is the most common cause of photoallergy.[249] The first UV filter available in the United States was p-Aminobenzoic acid,[244] but it also has the potential to cause photoallergy, contact dermatitis, and stain clothes.[250] A cross-sectional analysis of 23,908 patients found the top three most frequent allergens in sunscreens were benzophenone-3 (70.2% for 10% concentration, 64.4% for 3% concentration), DL-alpha-tocopherol (4.8%), and fragrance mix I (4%).[251]

Titanium dioxide (TiO_2) and zinc oxide (ZnO) are frequently employed in sunscreens as inorganic physical sun blockers.[252] Early generations of TiO_2 and ZnO contained larger particles with higher refractive indices, resulting in a thick, white coat with poor particle dispersion and comedogenic potential.[253] Recently, manufacturers have modified these minerals to micro and nano sizes,[244] which scatter less visible light and have more transparent films with improved cosmetic appearance.[254] As TiO_2 is more effective in UVB and ZnO in the UVA range, the combination of these particles assures a broadband UV protection.[252] Compared to organic filters, inorganic filters are less susceptible to degradation from UV exposure and have a lower potential of causing allergic reactions.[253] ▶ Table 1.8 has the approved sunscreen ingredients and their approximate UV coverage.[255]

Sunscreens are meant to protect against the adverse effects of UV-B (290–320 nm) and UV-A (320–400 nm) radiation.[252] UV-A and UV-B are both immunosuppressive.[256] UV-A can penetrate deeper into the skin reaching the dermis.[244] High-energy UV-B rays can create covalent bonds between pyrimidine bases causing direct DNA damage.[257,258] Both UV-A and UV-B can cause indirect damage resulting in the formation of reactive oxygen species, oxidative DNA damage, and activation of

Table 1.8 Approved sunscreen ingredients with absorption range

Type	Absorption range[a] (shaded area)		
	UV-B (290–320 nm)	UV-A2 (320–340 nm)	UV-A1 (340–400 nm)
Chemical sunscreens (organic compounds)			
Cinoxate Ensulizole Homosalate Octinoxate Octisalate Octocrylene Padimate O Para-aminobenzoic acid (PABA) Trolamine	✓		
Dioxybenzone Oxybenzone Sulisobenzone	✓	✓	
Ecamsule Meradimate		✓	
Avobenzone[b]			✓
Physical sunscreens (inorganic compounds)			
Titanium dioxide	✓	✓	
Zinc oxide	✓	✓	✓

Source: Modified from Joe et al 2012.[255]

[a]The ranges are approximations; each sunscreen may not block the entire range of ultraviolet (UV) radiation listed.

[b]Combined with octocrylene to ensure stability.

inflammatory cytokines.[259,260,261] Eventually, these insults can result in sunburns, pigment darkening, premature aging, and photocarcinogenesis.[262,263,264] UV-B sunscreen failed to protect from solar-simulated radiation-induced immunosuppression, whereas a broad-spectrum sunscreen with the same SPF and a higher protection in the UV-A range significantly reduced local UV-induced immunosuppression.[265] A greater average immune protection with UV-A/UV-B sunscreens was seen in 211 volunteers using contact sensitivity as a model.[266] The amount of UV-A protection is also important in preventing local immunosuppression as demonstrated by a study that demonstrated a UV-A protection factor of 14 produced no local immunosuppression, whereas a UV-A protection factor of 6 failed to prevent local immunosuppression.[265] Also, sunscreens with UV-A absorbers have been shown to significantly reduce the formation of pyrimidine dimers and p53 accumulation.[267]

Sunscreen should be used daily throughout the year since 80% of UV light passes through cloud cover, and approximately 25 and 80% is reflected by sand and snow, respectively.[255] Sunscreen should also be applied 15 to 30 minutes before sun exposure, applying it to common areas of NMSC such as the face, ears, hands, arms, and lips.[255] In addition, current recommendations also state that sunscreen should be reapplied every 2 hours and after swimming, sweating, and toweling off.[3]

Health Benefits

When broad-spectrum sunscreen with an SPF of 15 or greater is used as directed with other sun protection measures, sunburns can be prevented with decreased risk of early skin aging and skin cancer (melanoma and SCCs).[268,269,270,271,272] Since 2011, sunscreens that are broad-spectrum SPF ≥ 15 can now include this statement: "If used as directed with other sun protection measures, decreases the risk of skin cancer and early skin aging caused by the sun."[273] Also in 2011 sunscreens that are not broad spectrum and have an SPF of less than 15 have the following statement: "Spending time in the sun increases your risk of skin cancer and early aging."[273] Even suberythemal doses of UV light have been shown to increase thymine dimers, p53 expression, and loss of Langerhans cells.[274] A broad-spectrum sunscreen with an SPF of 8 was shown to reduce these effects as well as decrease the number and size of melanocytes and lower the lysozyme-to-elastin ratio.[275] It is estimated that daily broad-spectrum SPF 15 or greater sunscreen use in a 5-year period could prevent 11 BCCs, 24 SCCs, and 838 AKs along with saving $88,203.[276]

Photoaging

Photoaging is a complex and progressive process that is exacerbated by UV exposure, and sunscreens are considered to be the most effective method of prevention.[244] A randomized, double-blind, placebo-controlled trial of 53 adults with previously diagnosed skin cancer or AKs or both demonstrated that participants that applied UV-A/UV-B sunscreen for 24 months had less solar elastosis on biopsy.[277] Application of a broad-spectrum sunscreen for 6 weeks in 12 French volunteers was shown to minimize or prevent epidermal thickening, decreased procollagen expression, and higher lysozyme-to-elastin ratio.[275] The Nambour Skin Cancer Prevention Trial assigned microtopography grades to participants' left dorsal hands after using a sunscreen of SPF 16. A unit increase in a microtopography grade is associated with deterioration of skin texture, increased visible blood vessels, increased comedones on the face, and increased risk of developing AKs and NMSC.[16,278,279] Results showed daily sunscreen use reduced the likelihood of having higher microtopography grades and also decreased the risk of developing AKs and skin cancer.[272]

Prevention of AKs

AKs have been associated with high-dose cumulative UV exposure.[280] A randomized controlled trial gave participants a broad-spectrum SPF 17 sunscreen to be applied daily, and over a 7-month period the sunscreen group showed reduced emergence of new lesions, decreased total AKs, and greater remission rates in a dose-dependent manner.[281] Daily use of a broad-spectrum SPF 16 sunscreen led to a 24% reduction in AK development.[282]

Prevention of Squamous Cell Carcinoma

SCC has also been associated with high-dose cumulative UV exposure.[280] In a 4.5 year span, application of a broad-spectrum SPF 16 sunscreen 3 to 4 days a week showed a 40% reduction in the development of SCC.[283] After an 8-year follow-up, daily sunscreen users continued to have a 40% lower incidence rate of SCC.[271]

Prevention of Melanoma

Melanoma results from a multifactorial process, and UV exposure has been identified as a modifiable risk factor.[268] Dennis et al demonstrated that high-dose intermittent sun exposure associated with sunburns has a lifetime relative risk of 1.6 in all age groups.[284] Even though UV exposure has been established as a risk factor, evidence to support sunscreen as a preventative method has been ambiguous and controversial.[285,286] A slight decrease in new nevi in children with freckles using a broad-spectrum SPF 30 sunscreen was shown in a randomized controlled trial.[287] However, sunscreen was associated with more nevi compared to the use of clothing in a European study of white school-age children.[288] Physical barriers and sunscreens can partially prevent UV-B effects on nevi, but sunscreens were not quite as effective as physical barriers in the prevention of inflammatory changes induced by UV-B light.[289] A meta-analysis of cohort and case-control studies from 1966 to 2003 revealed there was no protective or harmful association with melanoma and sunscreen use.[290] One study showed a 50% reduction in new primary melanomas and a 73% reduction in invasive melanoma after a 5-year trial period of daily broad-spectrum SPF 16 sunscreen use and a 10-year follow-up.[268] A limitation to this study is the intervention sites excluded the trunk and lower extremities, and the entire body was analyzed for melanomas.[291]

Sunscreens and Basal Cell Carcinoma

Sun exposure has been identified as a risk factor for BCC,[1] but only about two-thirds of BCCs develop on sun-exposed areas.[292] Eight years after the initial trial of daily broad-spectrum SPF 16 sunscreen, van der Pols et al found a 25% reduction in BCC incidence in the sunscreen group that was found to be statistically insignificant.[271] This may be attributed to the latency period described by Situm et al, which suggested that BCC has a latency period of more than 20 years from the time of UV damage to clinical onset.[292]

1.7.2 Green Tea

The health benefits of green tea are attributed to the presence of polyphenols. The most effective and major polyphenol is epigallocatechin-3-gallate (EGCG).[293] There have been studies that have shown polyphenols possess antioxidant, anti-inflammatory, and anticarcinogenic activities in several in vitro and in vivo systems.[294,295] A significant reduction in UV-B–induced DNA damage was shown with topical green tea phenols (GTP) on mouse skin.[296,297] Similarly, topical treatment of human skin with GTPs prior to UV exposure resulted in a dose-dependent repair of cyclobutane pyrimidine dimers.[298] Topical application of green tea or white tea extracts has been shown to provide human skin protection from solar-simulated UV light.[299] Oral GTP[300] and topical EGCG[301] lead to significant reduction in tumor incidence, tumor multiplicity, and tumor size in mice.

1.7.3 Protective Clothing

In the Surgeon General's Call to Action to Prevent Skin Cancer, it is recommended that long-sleeved shirts and long pants and skirts been worn to provide maximal UV protection.[3] The Surgeon General also states that tightly woven fabric and darker colors may also provide more protection. Fabric porosity, type, color, weight, and thickness influence UV protection.[302] A UV-protection factor of over 500 was assigned to jeans, tracksuits, sweatshirts, pullovers, and tights.[303] The investigators also suggested layering of fabrics increases the protective effect. The application of UV absorbers into fabrics significantly improves the UV protection factor.[302] Wet cotton fabrics and polyester with TiO_2 showed significantly decreased UV protection compared to their dry counterparts, whereas in wet modal with TiO_2 and polyester crepe with TiO_2, the UV protection was significantly increased compared to their dry counterparts.[304]

1.7.4 Hats

The Surgeon General recommends wide-brimmed hats made of tightly woven fabric that shade the face, ears, and back of the neck over straw hats or other porous fabrics.[3] This study suggests darker hats may provide better protection. The American Cancer Society recommends wide-brimmed hats with a nonreflective underside or a shade cape.[305]

1.7.5 Sunglasses

Sunglasses are important for the skin around the eye, as well as the eyes themselves.[305] The American Cancer Society describes the ideal sunglasses as blocking 99 to 100% of UV-A and UV-B rays, and sunglasses labeled as "cosmetic" only block about 70% of UV rays.[305] Invisible chemicals that provide UV protection can be applied to the lenses, so it is important to check labels looking "Meets ANSI UV requirements."[305] Large-framed sunglasses with a wraparound frame are ideal and provide protection from light coming from multiple directions.[305] Play sunglasses for children are not sufficient.[305]

1.7.6 Seek Shade

UV light is the strongest between 10 a.m. and 4 p.m.[305] The strength of UV light depends on the time of year and other factors.[305] The Surgeon General warns shade does not block all UV radiation given it does not protect against scattered UV rays.[3] Different surfaces have different reflectivity. Snow can reflect 80 to 90%[306] of UV radiation, sand 20 to 30%,[306] water 5 to 7%,[306] concrete 14 to 17%,[307] and grass 1 to 2%.[307] Windows usually block most UV-B rays, but allow a small portion of UV-A rays.[305]

1.8 Conclusion

Skin cancer is a rising concern[2] and economic burden,[3] making action toward its prevention necessary. Dermatologists play a central role in promoting and preventing skin cancer. In order to maximize skin cancer prevention, a multifaceted approach is best. Raising public awareness and increasing patient education efforts on sun-protective measures, early detection, and treatment of precancers and early forms of skin cancer are key to skin cancer prevention and successful management.

References

[1] Rogers HW, Weinstock MA, Harris AR, et al. Incidence estimate of nonmelanoma skin cancer in the United States, 2006. Arch Dermatol. 2010; 146 (3):283–287

[2] American Cancer Society. Cancer Facts & Figures 2014. 2014 [accessed September 4, 2014]. http://www.cancer.org/acs/groups/content/@research/documents/webcontent/acspc-042151.pdf

[3] U.S. Department of Health and Human Services. The Surgeon General's Call to Action to Prevent Skin Cancer. Washington, DC: U.S. Department of Health and Human Services, Office of the Surgeon General; 2014

[4] Tung R, Vidimos A. Nonmelanoma Skin Cancer. [accessed September 4, 2014]. http://www.clevelandclinicmeded.com/medicalpubs/diseasemanagement/dermatology/nonmelanoma-skin-cancer/

[5] U.S. Preventive Services Task Force. U.S. Preventive Services Task Force Procedure Manual. 2008. August 2011 [accessed September 9, 2014]. http://www.uspreventiveservicestaskforce.org/uspstf08/methods/procmanual1.htm

[6] Akamine KL, Gustafson CJ, Davis SA, Levender MM, Feldman SR. Trends in sunscreen recommendation among US physicians. JAMA Dermatol. 2014; 150(1):51–55

[7] Cheng MY, Moreau JF, McGuire ST, Ho J, Ferris LK. Melanoma depth in patients with an established dermatologist. J Am Acad Dermatol. 2014; 70(5):841–846

[8] American Academy of Dermatology. Basic Dermatology Curriculum. [accessed September 5, 2014]. http://aad.org/education/basic-dermatology-curriculum

[9] U.S. Preventive Services Task Force. Behavioral Counseling to Prevent Skin Cancer: U.S. Preventive Services Task Force recommendation statement website. 2012 [accessed September 5, 2014]. http://www.uspreventiveservicestaskforce.org/uspstf11/skincancouns/skincancounsrs.htm

[10] Buller DB, Cokkinides V, Hall HI, et al. Prevalence of sunburn, sun protection, and indoor tanning behaviors among Americans: review from national surveys and case studies of 3 states. J Am Acad Dermatol. 2011; 65(5) Suppl 1: S114–S123

[11] University of Pennsylvania. Welcome to Pool Cool. 2010 [accessed September 9, 2014]. http://www.med.upenn.edu/poolcool/

[12] Aitken JF, Janda M, Elwood M, Youl PH, Ring IT, Lowe JB. Clinical outcomes from skin screening clinics within a community-based melanoma screening program. J Am Acad Dermatol. 2006; 54(1):105–114

[13] Aitken JF, Youl PH, Janda M, Lowe JB, Ring IT, Elwood M. Increase in skin cancer screening during a community-based randomized intervention trial. Int J Cancer. 2006; 118(4):1010–1016

[14] Marks R. Two decades of the public health approach to skin cancer control in Australia: why, how and where are we now? Australas J Dermatol. 1999; 40(1):1–5

[15] English DR, Armstrong BK, Kricker A, Winter MG, Heenan PJ, Randell PL. Demographic characteristics, pigmentary and cutaneous risk factors for

squamous cell carcinoma of the skin: a case-control study. Int J Cancer. 1998; 76(5):628–634
[16] Kricker A, et al. Pigmentary and cutaneous risk factors for non-melanocytic skin cancer–a case-control study. Int J Cancer. 1991; 48(5):650–662
[17] World Health Organization. Sun Protection in Schools: an Educational Package to Protect Children from Ultraviolet Radiation. 2003 [accessed September 5, 2014]. http://www.who.int/uv/publications/en/sunprot-schools.pdf
[18] Crosby RA, Santelli JS, DiCliemente RJ. Adolescents at risk: a generation in jeopardy. In: Adolescent Health: Understanding and Preventing Risk Behaviors. San Francisco, CA: Jossey-Bass; 2009:3–27
[19] Loescher LJ, Emerson J, Taylor A, Christensen DH, McKinney M. Educating preschoolers about sun safety. Am J Public Health. 1995; 85(7):939–943
[20] Buller MK, Kane IL, Martin RC, et al. Randomized trial evaluating computer-based sun safety education for children in elementary school. J Cancer Educ. 2008; 23(2) in2:74–79
[21] Arizona Department of Health Services. SunWise Skin Cancer Prevention School Program. [accessed September 5, 2014]. http://www.azdhs.gov/phs/sunwise/
[22] Geller A, Rutsch L, Kenausis K, Zhang Z. Evaluation of the SunWise School Program. J Sch Nurs. 2003; 19(2):93–99
[23] Kyle JW, Hammitt JK, Lim HW, et al. Economic evaluation of the US Environmental Protection Agency's SunWise program: sun protection education for young children. Pediatrics. 2008; 121(5):e1074–e1084
[24] Gupta AK, Paquet M, Villanueva E, Brintnell W. Interventions for actinic keratoses. Cochrane Database Syst Rev. 2012; 12:CD004415
[25] Warino L, Tusa M, Camacho F, Teuschler H, Fleischer AB, Jr, Feldman SR. Frequency and cost of actinic keratosis treatment. Dermatol Surg. 2006; 32 (8):1045–1049
[26] Criscione VD, Weinstock MA, Naylor MF, Luque C, Eide MJ, Bingham SF, Department of Veteran Affairs Topical Tretinoin Chemoprevention Trial Group. Actinic keratoses: natural history and risk of malignant transformation in the Veterans Affairs Topical Tretinoin Chemoprevention Trial. Cancer. 2009; 115(11):2523–2530
[27] Dodson JM, DeSpain J, Hewett JE, Clark DP. Malignant potential of actinic keratoses and the controversy over treatment. A patient-oriented perspective. Arch Dermatol. 1991; 127(7):1029–1031
[28] Suchniak JM, Baer S, Goldberg LH. High rate of malignant transformation in hyperkeratotic actinic keratoses. J Am Acad Dermatol. 1997; 37(3, Pt 1):392–394
[29] Goldberg LH, Kaplan B, Vergilis-Kalner I, Landau J. Liquid nitrogen: temperature control in the treatment of actinic keratosis. Dermatol Surg. 2010; 36 (12):1956–1961
[30] Thai KE, Fergin P, Freeman M, et al. A prospective study of the use of cryosurgery for the treatment of actinic keratoses. Int J Dermatol. 2004; 43(9):687–692
[31] Krawtchenko N, Roewert-Huber J, Ulrich M, Mann I, Sterry W, Stockfleth E. A randomised study of topical 5% imiquimod vs. topical 5-fluorouracil vs. cryosurgery in immunocompetent patients with actinic keratoses: a comparison of clinical and histological outcomes including 1-year follow-up. Br J Dermatol. 2007; 157 Suppl 2:34–40
[32] Lubritz RR, Smolewski SA. Cryosurgery cure rate of actinic keratoses. J Am Acad Dermatol. 1982; 7(5):631–632
[33] Patel G, Armstrong AW, Eisen DB. Efficacy of photodynamic therapy vs other interventions in randomized clinical trials for the treatment of actinic keratoses: a systematic review and meta-analysis. JAMA Dermatol. 2014; 150 (12):1281–1288
[34] Szeimies RM, Stockfleth E, Popp G, et al. Long-term follow-up of photodynamic therapy with a self-adhesive 5-aminolaevulinic acid patch: 12 months data. Br J Dermatol. 2010; 162(2):410–414
[35] Gupta AK, Davey V, Mcphail H. Evaluation of the effectiveness of imiquimod and 5-fluorouracil for the treatment of actinic keratosis: critical review and meta-analysis of efficacy studies. J Cutan Med Surg. 2005; 9(5):209–214
[36] Ceilley RI. Mechanisms of action of topical 5-fluorouracil: review and implications for the treatment of dermatological disorders. J Dermatolog Treat. 2012; 23(2):83–89
[37] Askew DA, Mickan SM, Soyer HP, Wilkinson D. Effectiveness of 5-fluorouracil treatment for actinic keratosis: a systematic review of randomized controlled trials. Int J Dermatol. 2009; 48(5):453–463
[38] Adamson DJ, Frew D, Tatoud R, Wolf CR, Palmer CN. Diclofenac antagonizes peroxisome proliferator-activated receptor-gamma signaling. Mol Pharmacol. 2002; 61(1):7–12
[39] Alam CA, Seed MP, Willoughby DA. Angiostasis and vascular regression in chronic granulomatous inflammation induced by diclofenac in combination with hyaluronan in mice. J Pharm Pharmacol. 1995; 47(5):407–411
[40] Lu X, Xie W, Reed D, Bradshaw WS, Simmons DL. Nonsteroidal antiinflammatory drugs cause apoptosis and induce cyclooxygenases in chicken embryo fibroblasts. Proc Natl Acad Sci U S A. 1995; 92(17):7961–7965
[41] Seed MP, Brown JR, Freemantle CN, et al. The inhibition of colon-26 adenocarcinoma development and angiogenesis by topical diclofenac in 2.5% hyaluronan. Cancer Res. 1997; 57(9):1625–1629
[42] Jarvis B, Figgitt DP. Topical 3% diclofenac in 2.5% hyaluronic acid gel: a review of its use in patients with actinic keratoses. Am J Clin Dermatol. 2003; 4 (3):203–213
[43] Ulrich C, Hackethal M, Ulrich M, et al. Treatment of multiple actinic keratoses with topical diclofenac 3% gel in organ transplant recipients: a series of six cases. Br J Dermatol. 2007; 156 Suppl 3:40–42
[44] Akarsu S, Aktan S, Atahan A, Koç P, Özkan S. Comparison of topical 3% diclofenac sodium gel and 5% imiquimod cream for the treatment of actinic keratoses. Clin Exp Dermatol. 2011; 36(5):479–484
[45] Vidal D. Topical imiquimod: mechanism of action and clinical applications. Mini Rev Med Chem. 2006; 6(5):499–503
[46] Korman N, Moy R, Ling M, et al. Dosing with 5% imiquimod cream 3 times per week for the treatment of actinic keratosis: results of two phase 3, randomized, double-blind, parallel-group, vehicle-controlled trials. Arch Dermatol. 2005; 141(4):467–473
[47] Hadley G, Derry S, Moore RA. Imiquimod for actinic keratosis: systematic review and meta-analysis. J Invest Dermatol. 2006; 126(6):1251–1255
[48] Szeimies RM, Karrer S, Radakovic-Fijan S, et al. Photodynamic therapy using topical methyl 5-aminolevulinate compared with cryotherapy for actinic keratosis: a prospective, randomized study. J Am Acad Dermatol. 2002; 47 (2):258–262
[49] Lee PK, Harwell WB, Loven KH, et al. Long-term clinical outcomes following treatment of actinic keratosis with imiquimod 5% cream. Dermatol Surg. 2005; 31(6):659–664
[50] Lebwohl M, Dinehart S, Whiting D, et al. Imiquimod 5% cream for the treatment of actinic keratosis: results from two phase III, randomized, double-blind, parallel group, vehicle-controlled trials. J Am Acad Dermatol. 2004; 50 (5):714–721
[51] Swanson N, Abramovits W, Berman B, Kulp J, Rigel DS, Levy S. Imiquimod 2.5% and 3.75% for the treatment of actinic keratoses: results of two placebo-controlled studies of daily application to the face and balding scalp for two 2-week cycles. J Am Acad Dermatol. 2010; 62(4):582–590
[52] Hauschild A, Stockfleth E, Popp G, et al. Optimization of photodynamic therapy with a novel self-adhesive 5-aminolaevulinic acid patch: results of two randomized controlled phase III studies. Br J Dermatol. 2009; 160(5):1066–1074
[53] Lawrence N, Cox SE, Cockerell CJ, Freeman RG, Cruz PD, Jr. A comparison of the efficacy and safety of Jessner's solution and 35% trichloroacetic acid vs 5% fluorouracil in the treatment of widespread facial actinic keratoses. Arch Dermatol. 1995; 131(2):176–181
[54] Hantash BM, Stewart DB, Cooper ZA, Rehmus WE, Koch RJ, Swetter SM. Facial resurfacing for nonmelanoma skin cancer prophylaxis. Arch Dermatol. 2006; 142(8):976–982
[55] Monheit GD, Chastain MA. Chemical peels. Facial Plast Surg Clin North Am. 2001; 9(2):239–255, viii
[56] Zakopoulou N, Kontochristopoulos G. Superficial chemical peels. J Cosmet Dermatol. 2006; 5(3):246–253
[57] Tse Y, Ostad A, Lee HS, et al. A clinical and histologic evaluation of two medium-depth peels. Glycolic acid versus Jessner's trichloroacetic acid. Dermatol Surg. 1996; 22(9):781–786
[58] Jiang SB, Levine VJ, Nehal KS, Baldassano M, Kamino H, Ashinoff RA. Er:YAG laser for the treatment of actinic keratoses. Dermatol Surg. 2000; 26 (5):437–440
[59] Ostertag JU, Quaedvlieg PJ, Neumann MH, Krekels GA. Recurrence rates and long-term follow-up after laser resurfacing as a treatment for widespread actinic keratoses on the face and scalp. Dermatol Surg. 2006; 32(2):261–267
[60] Iyer S, Friedli A, Bowes L, Kricorian G, Fitzpatrick RE. Full face laser resurfacing: therapy and prophylaxis for actinic keratoses and non-melanoma skin cancer. Lasers Surg Med. 2004; 34(2):114–119
[61] Rendon MI, Berson DS, Cohen JL, Roberts WE, Starker I, Wang B. Evidence and considerations in the application of chemical peels in skin disorders and aesthetic resurfacing. J Clin Aesthet Dermatol. 2010; 3(7):32–43
[62] Abdel-Daim M, Funasaka Y, Kamo T, et al. Effect of chemical peeling on photocarcinogenesis. J Dermatol. 2010; 37(10):864–872

[63] Scola N, Terras S, Georgas D, et al. A randomized, half-side comparative study of aminolaevulinate photodynamic therapy vs. CO(2) laser ablation in immunocompetent patients with multiple actinic keratoses. Br J Dermatol. 2012; 167(6):1366–1373
[64] Rubach BW, Schoenrock LD. Histological and clinical evaluation of facial resurfacing using a carbon dioxide laser with the computer pattern generator. Arch Otolaryngol Head Neck Surg. 1997; 123(9):929–934
[65] Massey RA, Eliezri YD. A case report of laser resurfacing as a skin cancer prophylaxis. Dermatol Surg. 1999; 25(6):513–516
[66] Orringer JS, Johnson TM, Kang S, et al. Effect of carbon dioxide laser resurfacing on epidermal p53 immunostaining in photodamaged skin. Arch Dermatol. 2004; 140(9):1073–1077
[67] Ostertag JU, Quaedvlieg PJ, van der Geer S, et al. A clinical comparison and long-term follow-up of topical 5-fluorouracil versus laser resurfacing in the treatment of widespread actinic keratoses. Lasers Surg Med. 2006; 38 (8):731–739
[68] An KP, Athar M, Tang X, et al. Cyclooxygenase-2 expression in murine and human nonmelanoma skin cancers: implications for therapeutic approaches. Photochem Photobiol. 2002; 76(1):73–80
[69] Einspahr JG, Bowden GT, Alberts DS, et al. Cross-validation of murine UV signal transduction pathways in human skin. Photochem Photobiol. 2008; 84 (2):463–476
[70] Fischer SM, Lo HH, Gordon GB, et al. Chemopreventive activity of celecoxib, a specific cyclooxygenase-2 inhibitor, and indomethacin against ultraviolet light-induced skin carcinogenesis. Mol Carcinog. 1999; 25(4):231–240
[71] Rundhaug JE, Mikulec C, Pavone A, Fischer SM. A role for cyclooxygenase-2 in ultraviolet light-induced skin carcinogenesis. Mol Carcinog. 2007; 46 (8):692–698
[72] Pentland AP, Schoggins JW, Scott GA, Khan KN, Han R. Reduction of UV-induced skin tumors in hairless mice by selective COX-2 inhibition. Carcinogenesis. 1999; 20(10):1939–1944
[73] Buckman SY, Gresham A, Hale P, et al. COX-2 expression is induced by UVB exposure in human skin: implications for the development of skin cancer. Carcinogenesis. 1998; 19(5):723–729
[74] Butler GJ, Neale R, Green AC, Pandeya N, Whiteman DC. Nonsteroidal anti-inflammatory drugs and the risk of actinic keratoses and squamous cell cancers of the skin. J Am Acad Dermatol. 2005; 53(6):966–972
[75] Grau MV, Baron JA, Langholz B, et al. Effect of NSAIDs on the recurrence of nonmelanoma skin cancer. Int J Cancer. 2006; 119(3):682–686
[76] Elmets CA, Ledet JJ, Athar M. Cyclooxygenases: mediators of UV-induced skin cancer and potential targets for prevention. J Invest Dermatol. 2014; 134(10):2497–2502
[77] Rodriguez-Burford C, Tu JH, Mercurio M, et al. Selective cyclooxygenase-2 inhibition produces heterogeneous erythema response to ultraviolet irradiation. J Invest Dermatol. 2005; 125(6):1317–1320
[78] Penning TD, Talley JJ, Bertenshaw SR, et al. Synthesis and biological evaluation of the 1,5-diarylpyrazole class of cyclooxygenase-2 inhibitors: identification of 4-[5-(4-methylphenyl)-3-(trifluoromethyl)-1H-pyrazol-1-yl]benze nesulfonamide (SC-58635, celecoxib). J Med Chem. 1997; 40(9):1347–1365
[79] Elmets CA, Viner JL, Pentland AP, et al. Chemoprevention of nonmelanoma skin cancer with celecoxib: a randomized, double-blind, placebo-controlled trial. J Natl Cancer Inst. 2010; 102(24):1835–1844
[80] Tang JY, Aszterbaum M, Athar M, et al. Basal cell carcinoma chemoprevention with nonsteroidal anti-inflammatory drugs in genetically predisposed PTCH1 + /- humans and mice. Cancer Prev Res (Phila). 2010; 3(1):25–34
[81] Bath-Hextall F, Leonardi-Bee J, Somchand N, Webster A, Delitt J, Perkins W. Interventions for preventing non-melanoma skin cancers in high-risk groups. Cochrane Database Syst Rev. 2007(4):CD005414
[82] Buettner GR. The pecking order of free radicals and antioxidants: lipid peroxidation, alpha-tocopherol, and ascorbate. Arch Biochem Biophys. 1993; 300(2):535–543
[83] Pence BC, Delver E, Dunn DM. Effects of dietary selenium on UVB-induced skin carcinogenesis and epidermal antioxidant status. J Invest Dermatol. 1994; 102(5):759–761
[84] van der Pols JC, Heinen MM, Hughes MC, Ibiebele TI, Marks GC, Green AC. Serum antioxidants and skin cancer risk: an 8-year community-based follow-up study. Cancer Epidemiol Biomarkers Prev. 2009; 18 (4):1167–1173
[85] Clark LC, Combs GF, Jr, Turnbull BW, et al. Nutritional Prevention of Cancer Study Group. Effects of selenium supplementation for cancer prevention in patients with carcinoma of the skin. A randomized controlled trial. JAMA. 1996; 276(24):1957–1963
[86] Fuller CJ, Faulkner H, Bendich A, Parker RS, Roe DA. Effect of beta-carotene supplementation on photosuppression of delayed-type hypersensitivity in normal young men. Am J Clin Nutr. 1992; 56(4):684–690
[87] Greenberg ER, Baron JA, Stukel TA, et al. The Skin Cancer Prevention Study Group. A clinical trial of beta carotene to prevent basal-cell and squamous-cell cancers of the skin. N Engl J Med. 1990; 323(12):789–795
[88] Moon TE, Levine N, Cartmel B, et al. Southwest Skin Cancer Prevention Study Group. Effect of retinol in preventing squamous cell skin cancer in moderate-risk subjects: a randomized, double-blind, controlled trial. Cancer Epidemiol Biomarkers Prev. 1997; 6(11):949–956
[89] Black HS. Influence of dietary factors on actinically-induced skin cancer. Mutat Res. 1998; 422(1):185–190
[90] Black HS. Role of dietary factors in UV-carcinogenesis. Cancer Bull. 1993; 45:232–237
[91] Black HS, Thornby JI, Wolf JE, Jr, et al. Evidence that a low-fat diet reduces the occurrence of non-melanoma skin cancer. Int J Cancer. 1995; 62(2):165–169
[92] Jaax S, Scott LW, Wolf JE, Jr, Thornby JI, Black HS. General guidelines for a low-fat diet effective in the management and prevention of nonmelanoma skin cancer. Nutr Cancer. 1997; 27(2):150–156
[93] Euvrard S, Kanitakis J, Claudy A. Skin cancers after organ transplantation. N Engl J Med. 2003; 348(17):1681–1691
[94] Hartevelt MM, Bavinck JN, Kootte AM, Vermeer BJ, Vandenbroucke JP. Incidence of skin cancer after renal transplantation in The Netherlands. Transplantation. 1990; 49(3):506–509
[95] Webb MC, Compton F, Andrews PA, Koffman CG. Skin tumours posttransplantation: a retrospective analysis of 28 years' experience at a single centre. Transplant Proc. 1997; 29(1–2):828–830
[96] Winkelhorst JT, Brokelman WJ, Tiggeler RG, Wobbes T. Incidence and clinical course of de-novo malignancies in renal allograft recipients. Eur J Surg Oncol. 2001; 27(4):409–413
[97] Bouwes Bavinck JN, Hardie DR, Green A, et al. The risk of skin cancer in renal transplant recipients in Queensland, Australia. A follow-up study. Transplantation. 1996; 61(5):715–721
[98] Jensen P, Hansen S, Møller B, et al. Skin cancer in kidney and heart transplant recipients and different long-term immunosuppressive therapy regimens. J Am Acad Dermatol. 1999; 40(2, Pt 1):177–186
[99] Euvrard S, Kanitakis J, Pouteil-Noble C, et al. Comparative epidemiologic study of premalignant and malignant epithelial cutaneous lesions developing after kidney and heart transplantation. J Am Acad Dermatol. 1995; 33(2, Pt 1):222–229
[100] Ducloux D, Carron PL, Rebibou JM, et al. CD4 lymphocytopenia as a risk factor for skin cancers in renal transplant recipients. Transplantation. 1998; 65 (9):1270–1272
[101] Euvrard S, Kanitakis J, Pouteil-Noble C, et al. Aggressive squamous cell carcinomas in organ transplant recipients. Transplant Proc. 1995; 27 (2):1767–1768
[102] Adamson R, Obispo E, Dychter S, et al. High incidence and clinical course of aggressive skin cancer in heart transplant patients: a single-center study. Transplant Proc. 1998; 30(4):1124–1126
[103] Pollard JD, Hanasono MM, Mikulec AA, Le QT, Terris DJ. Head and neck cancer in cardiothoracic transplant recipients. Laryngoscope. 2000; 110 (8):1257–1261
[104] Veness MJ, Quinn DI, Ong CS, et al. Aggressive cutaneous malignancies following cardiothoracic transplantation: the Australian experience. Cancer. 1999; 85(8):1758–1764
[105] Ong CS, Keogh AM, Kossard S, Macdonald PS, Spratt PM. Skin cancer in Australian heart transplant recipients. J Am Acad Dermatol. 1999; 40(1):27–34
[106] Lippman SM, Kessler JF, Meyskens FL, Jr. Retinoids as preventive and therapeutic anticancer agents (Part I). Cancer Treat Rep. 1987; 71 (4):391–405
[107] Kovach BT, Sams HH, Stasko T. Systemic strategies for chemoprevention of skin cancers in transplant recipients. Clin Transplant. 2005; 19(6):726–734
[108] George R, Weightman W, Russ GR, Bannister KM, Mathew TH. Acitretin for chemoprevention of non-melanoma skin cancers in renal transplant recipients. Australas J Dermatol. 2002; 43(4):269–273
[109] Bavinck JN, Tieben LM, Van der Woude FJ, et al. Prevention of skin cancer and reduction of keratotic skin lesions during acitretin therapy in renal transplant recipients: a double-blind, placebo-controlled study. J Clin Oncol. 1995; 13(8):1933–1938
[110] McKenna DB, Murphy GM. Skin cancer chemoprophylaxis in renal transplant recipients: 5 years of experience using low-dose acitretin. Br J Dermatol. 1999; 140(4):656–660

[111] Harwood CA, Leedham-Green M, Leigh IM, Proby CM. Low-dose retinoids in the prevention of cutaneous squamous cell carcinomas in organ transplant recipients: a 16-year retrospective study. Arch Dermatol. 2005; 141(4):456–464

[112] Chen K, Craig JC, Shumack S. Oral retinoids for the prevention of skin cancers in solid organ transplant recipients: a systematic review of randomized controlled trials. Br J Dermatol. 2005; 152(3):518–523

[113] de Sévaux RG, Smit JV, de Jong EM, van de Kerkhof PC, Hoitsma AJ. Acitretin treatment of premalignant and malignant skin disorders in renal transplant recipients: clinical effects of a randomized trial comparing two doses of acitretin. J Am Acad Dermatol. 2003; 49(3):407–412

[114] DiGiovanna JJ, Sollitto RB, Abangan DL, Steinberg SM, Reynolds JC. Osteoporosis is a toxic effect of long-term etretinate therapy. Arch Dermatol. 1995; 131(11):1263–1267

[115] DiGiovanna JJ. Isotretinoin effects on bone. J Am Acad Dermatol. 2001; 45 (5):S176–S182

[116] Breslow A. Thickness, cross-sectional areas and depth of invasion in the prognosis of cutaneous melanoma. Ann Surg. 1970; 172(5):902–908

[117] Lowe GC, Saavedra A, Reed KB, et al. Increasing incidence of melanoma among middle-aged adults: an epidemiologic study in Olmsted County, Minnesota. Mayo Clin Proc. 2014; 89(1):52–59

[118] Wolff T, Tai E, Miller T. Screening for skin cancer: an update of the evidence for the U.S. Preventive Services Task Force. Ann Intern Med. 2009; 150 (3):194–198

[119] Goggins WB, Tsao H. A population-based analysis of risk factors for a second primary cutaneous melanoma among melanoma survivors. Cancer. 2003; 97 (3):639–643

[120] Dummer R, Panizzon R, Bloch PH, Burg G, Task Force Skin Cancer. Updated Swiss guidelines for the treatment and follow-up of cutaneous melanoma. Dermatology. 2005; 210(1):39–44

[121] Tucker MA, Fraser MC, Goldstein AM, Elder DE, Guerry D, IV, Organic SM. Risk of melanoma and other cancers in melanoma-prone families. J Invest Dermatol. 1993; 100(3):350S–355S

[122] Tucker MA, Halpern A, Holly EA, et al. Clinically recognized dysplastic nevi. A central risk factor for cutaneous melanoma. JAMA. 1997; 277 (18):1439–1444

[123] Kelly JW, Yeatman JM, Regalia C, Mason G, Henham AP. A high incidence of melanoma found in patients with multiple dysplastic naevi by photographic surveillance. Med J Aust. 1997; 167(4):191–194

[124] Bataille V, Bishop JA, Sasieni P, et al. Risk of cutaneous melanoma in relation to the numbers, types and sites of naevi: a case-control study. Br J Cancer. 1996; 73(12):1605–1611

[125] Nikolaou VA, Sypsa V, Stefanaki I, et al. Risk associations of melanoma in a Southern European population: results of a case/control study. Cancer Causes Control. 2008; 19(7):671–679

[126] Gandini S, Sera F, Cattaruzza MS, et al. Meta-analysis of risk factors for cutaneous melanoma: III. Family history, actinic damage and phenotypic factors. Eur J Cancer. 2005; 41(14):2040–2059

[127] Bower CP, Lear JT, Bygrave S, Etherington D, Harvey I, Archer CB. Basal cell carcinoma and risk of subsequent malignancies: a cancer registry-based study in southwest England. J Am Acad Dermatol. 2000; 42(6):988–991

[128] Hemminki K, Dong C. Subsequent cancers after in situ and invasive squamous cell carcinoma of the skin. Arch Dermatol. 2000; 136(5):647–651

[129] Elwood JM, Jopson J. Melanoma and sun exposure: an overview of published studies. Int J Cancer. 1997; 73(2):198–203

[130] Ting W, Schultz K, Cac NN, Peterson M, Walling HW. Tanning bed exposure increases the risk of malignant melanoma. Int J Dermatol. 2007; 46 (12):1253–1257

[131] National Comprehensive Cancer Network. Basal Cell and Squamous Cell Skin Cancers (Version 2.2014). NCCN Clinical Practice Guidelines in Oncology (NCCN Guidelines). 2014 [accessed September 23, 2014]. http://www.nccn.org/professionals/physician_gls/pdf/nmsc.pdf

[132] National Comprehensive Cancer Network. Melanoma (Version 4.2014). NCCN Clinical Practive Guidelines in Oncology (NCCN Guidelines). 2014 [accessed September 23, 2014]. http://www.nccn.org/professionals/physician_gls/pdf/melanoma.pdf

[133] Brady MS, Oliveria SA, Christos PJ, et al. Patterns of detection in patients with cutaneous melanoma. Cancer. 2000; 89(2):342–347

[134] Carli P, De Giorgi V, Palli D, et al. Italian Multidisciplinary Group on Melanoma. Dermatologist detection and skin self-examination are associated with thinner melanomas: results from a survey of the Italian Multidisciplinary Group on Melanoma. Arch Dermatol. 2003; 139 (5):607–612

[135] Epstein DS, Lange JR, Gruber SB, Mofid M, Koch SE. Is physician detection associated with thinner melanomas? JAMA. 1999; 281(7):640–643

[136] Schwartz JL, Wang TS, Hamilton TA, Lowe L, Sondak VK, Johnson TM. Thin primary cutaneous melanomas: associated detection patterns, lesion characteristics, and patient characteristics. Cancer. 2002; 95(7):1562–1568

[137] Körner A, Coroiu A, Martins C, Wang B. Predictors of skin self-examination before and after a melanoma diagnosis: the role of medical advice and patient's level of education. Int Arch Med. 2013; 6(1):8

[138] Berwick M, Begg CB, Fine JA, Roush GC, Barnhill RL. Screening for cutaneous melanoma by skin self-examination. J Natl Cancer Inst. 1996; 88(1):17–23

[139] Moore Dalal K, Zhou Q, Panageas KS, Brady MS, Jaques DP, Coit DG. Methods of detection of first recurrence in patients with stage I/II primary cutaneous melanoma after sentinel lymph node biopsy. Ann Surg Oncol. 2008; 15 (8):2206–2214

[140] Hamidi R, Peng D, Cockburn M. Efficacy of skin self-examination for the early detection of melanoma. Int J Dermatol. 2010; 49(2):126–134

[141] Girardi S, Gaudy C, Gouvernet J, Teston J, Richard MA, Grob JJ. Superiority of a cognitive education with photographs over ABCD criteria in the education of the general population to the early detection of melanoma: a randomized study. Int J Cancer. 2006; 118(9):2276–2280

[142] American Academy of Dermatology. DETECT Skin Cancer: Body Mole Map. 2013 [accessed September 16, 2014]. http://www.aad.org/File%20Library/Global%20navigation/For%20the%20public/SPOT/Body_Mole_Map_2013.pdf

[143] Goodson AG, Grossman D. Strategies for early melanoma detection: approaches to the patient with nevi. J Am Acad Dermatol. 2009; 60(5):719–735, quiz 736–738

[144] Boniol M, Autier P, Boyle P, Gandini S. Cutaneous melanoma attributable to sunbed use: systematic review and meta-analysis. BMJ. 2012; 345:e4757

[145] Torrens R, Swan BA. Promoting prevention and early recognition of malignant melanoma. Dermatol Nurs. 2009; 21(3):115–122, quiz 123

[146] Scottish Intercollegiate Guidelines Network. Cutaneous Melanoma: a national clinical guideline. 2003. February 2004 [accessed September 25, 2014]. http://www.sign.ac.uk/guidelines/fulltext/72/section2.html

[147] Holly EA, Kelly JW, Shpall SN, Chiu SH. Number of melanocytic nevi as a major risk factor for malignant melanoma. J Am Acad Dermatol. 1987; 17 (3):459–468

[148] Marks R, Dorevitch AP, Mason G. Do all melanomas come from "moles"? A study of the histological association between melanocytic naevi and melanoma. Australas J Dermatol. 1990; 31(2):77–80

[149] Bevona C, Goggins W, Quinn T, Fullerton J, Tsao H. Cutaneous melanomas associated with nevi. Arch Dermatol. 2003; 139(12):1620–1624, discussion 1624

[150] Chiu V, Won E, Malik M, Weinstock MA. The use of mole-mapping diagrams to increase skin self-examination accuracy. J Am Acad Dermatol. 2006; 55 (2):245–250

[151] Oliveria SA, Chau D, Christos PJ, Charles CA, Mushlin AI, Halpern AC. Diagnostic accuracy of patients in performing skin self-examination and the impact of photography. Arch Dermatol. 2004; 140(1):57–62

[152] Weinstock MA, Nguyen FQ, Martin RA. Enhancing skin self-examination with imaging: evaluation of a mole-mapping program. J Cutan Med Surg. 2004; 8(1):1–5

[153] MacKie RM, English J, Aitchison TC, Fitzsimons CP, Wilson P. The number and distribution of benign pigmented moles (melanocytic naevi) in a healthy British population. Br J Dermatol. 1985; 113(2):167–174

[154] Balch CM, Mihm MC, Soong S, Gershenwald JE. The Revised Melanoma Staging System and the Impact of Mitotic Rate. The Melanoma Letter, A Publication of the Skin Cancer Foundation. 2010; 28(3):1–6

[155] Moore BA, Weber RS, Prieto V, et al. Lymph node metastases from cutaneous squamous cell carcinoma of the head and neck. Laryngoscope. 2005; 115 (9):1561–1567

[156] Mullen JT, Feng L, Xing Y, et al. Invasive squamous cell carcinoma of the skin: defining a high-risk group. Ann Surg Oncol. 2006; 13(7):902–909

[157] Robinson JK. Follow-up and prevention (basal cell carcinoma). In: Miller SJ, Maloney ME, eds. Cutaneous Oncology: Pathophysiology, Diagnosis, and Management. Malden, MA: Blackwell Science; 1998:695–698

[158] Marcil I, Stern RS. Risk of developing a subsequent nonmelanoma skin cancer in patients with a history of nonmelanoma skin cancer: a critical review of the literature and meta-analysis. Arch Dermatol. 2000; 136 (12):1524–1530

[159] Chen J, Ruczinski I, Jorgensen TJ, et al. Nonmelanoma skin cancer and risk for subsequent malignancy. J Natl Cancer Inst. 2008; 100(17):1215–1222

[160] Shin DM, Maloney ME, Lippman SM. Follow-up and prevention (squamous cell carcinoma). In: Miller SJ, Maloney ME, eds. Cutaneous Oncology:

Pathophysiology, diagnosis, and management. Malden, MA: Blackwell Science; 1998:565–570

[161] Nieweg OE, Kroon BB. The conundrum of follow-up: should it be abandoned? Surg Oncol Clin N Am. 2006; 15(2):319–330

[162] McCarthy WH, Shaw HM, Thompson JF, Milton GW. Time and frequency of recurrence of cutaneous stage I malignant melanoma with guidelines for follow-up study. Surg Gynecol Obstet. 1988; 166(6):497–502

[163] Martini L, Brandani P, Chiarugi C, Reali UM. First recurrence analysis of 840 cutaneous melanomas: a proposal for a follow-up schedule. Tumori. 1994; 80(3):188–197

[164] van der Leest RJ, van Steenbergen LN, Hollestein LM, et al. Conditional survival of malignant melanoma in The Netherlands: 1994–2008. Eur J Cancer. 2014; 50(3):602–610

[165] Pflugfelder A, Kochs C, Blum A, et al. German Dermatological Society, DermatologicCooperative Oncology Group. Malignant melanoma S3-guideline "diagnosis, therapy and follow-up of melanoma.". J Dtsch Dermatol Ges. 2013; 11 Suppl 6:1–116, 1–126

[166] Francken AB, Accortt NA, Shaw HM, et al. Follow-up schedules after treatment for malignant melanoma. Br J Surg. 2008; 95(11):1401–1407

[167] Romano E, Scordo M, Dusza SW, Coit DG, Chapman PB. Site and timing of first relapse in stage III melanoma patients: implications for follow-up guidelines. J Clin Oncol. 2010; 28(18):3042–3047

[168] Francken AB, Shaw HM, Accortt NA, Soong SJ, Hoekstra HJ, Thompson JF. Detection of first relapse in cutaneous melanoma patients: implications for the formulation of evidence-based follow-up guidelines. Ann Surg Oncol. 2007; 14(6):1924–1933

[169] Fisher NM, Schaffer JV, Berwick M, Bolognia JL. Breslow depth of cutaneous melanoma: impact of factors related to surveillance of the skin, including prior skin biopsies and family history of melanoma. J Am Acad Dermatol. 2005; 53(3):393–406

[170] Grange F, Chompret A, Guilloud-Bataille M, et al. Comparison between familial and nonfamilial melanoma in France. Arch Dermatol. 1995; 131 (10):1154–1159

[171] Lucchina LC, Barnhill RL, Duke DM, Sober AJ. Familial cutaneous melanoma. Melanoma Res. 1995; 5(6):413–418

[172] Greene MH, Clark WH, Jr, Tucker MA, Kraemer KH, Elder DE, Fraser MC. High risk of malignant melanoma in melanoma-prone families with dysplastic nevi. Ann Intern Med. 1985; 102(4):458–465

[173] Masri GD, Clark WH, Jr, Guerry D, IV, Halpern A, Thompson CJ, Elder DE. Screening and surveillance of patients at high risk for malignant melanoma result in detection of earlier disease. J Am Acad Dermatol. 1990; 22(6, Pt 1):1042–1048

[174] Carey WP, Jr, Thompson CJ, Synnestvedt M, et al. Dysplastic nevi as a melanoma risk factor in patients with familial melanoma. Cancer. 1994; 74 (12):3118–3125

[175] Watts CG, et al. Clinical practice guidelines for identification, screening and follow-up of individuals at high risk of primary cutaneous melanoma: a systematic review. Br J Dermatol. 2015; 172(1):33–47

[176] Lynch HT, Fusaro RM. Pancreatic cancer and the familial atypical multiple mole melanoma (FAMMM) syndrome. Pancreas. 1991; 6(2):127–131

[177] Bartsch DK, Sina-Frey M, Lang S, et al. CDKN2A germline mutations in familial pancreatic cancer. Ann Surg. 2002; 236(6):730–737

[178] Lynch HT, Frichot BC, III, Lynch JF. Familial atypical multiple mole-melanoma syndrome. J Med Genet. 1978; 15(5):352–356

[179] Lynch HT, Brand RE, Hogg D, et al. Phenotypic variation in eight extended CDKN2A germline mutation familial atypical multiple mole melanoma-pancreatic carcinoma-prone families: the familial atypical mole melanoma-pancreatic carcinoma syndrome. Cancer. 2002; 94(1):84–96

[180] Goldstein AM, Struewing JP, Chidambaram A, Fraser MC, Tucker MA. Genotype-phenotype relationships in U.S. melanoma-prone families with CDKN2A and CDK4 mutations. J Natl Cancer Inst. 2000; 92(12):1006–1010

[181] Czajkowski R, Placek W, Drewa G, Czajkowska A, Uchańska G. FAMMM syndrome: pathogenesis and management. Dermatol Surg. 2004; 30(2)(,)(Pt 2):291–296

[182] Kefford RF, Newton Bishop JA, Bergman W, Tucker MA. Counseling and DNA testing for individuals perceived to be genetically predisposed to melanoma: a consensus statement of the Melanoma Genetics Consortium. J Clin Oncol. 1999; 17(10):3245–3251

[183] Mize DE, Bishop M, Resse E, Sluzevich J. Familial atypical multiple mole melanoma syndrome. In: Riegert-Johnson DL, Boardman LA, Hefferon T, et al., eds. Cancer Syndromes. Bethesda, MD: National Center for Biotechnology Information; 2009

[184] Evans DG, Farndon PA. Nevoid basal cell carcinoma syndrome. In: Pagon RA, Adam MP, Ardinger HH, et al., eds. GeneReviews. Seattle, WA: University of Washington; 2002

[185] Jones EA, Sajid MI, Shenton A, Evans DG. Basal cell carcinomas in gorlin syndrome: a review of 202 patients. J Skin Cancer. 2011; 2011:217378

[186] Tamura D, DiGiovanna JJ, Kraemer KH. Xeroderma pigmentosum. In: Lebwohl MG, Heymann WR, Berth-Jones J, Coulson I, eds. Treatment of Skin Disease: Comprehensive Therapeutic Strategies. London, UK: Elsevier; 2010:789–792

[187] Kraemer KH, DiGiovanna JJ. Xeroderma Pigmentosum. In: Pagon RA, Bird TD, Dolan CR, et al., eds. GeneReviews. Seattle, WA: University of Washington; 2003

[188] Lasso JM, Yordanov YP, Pinilla C, Shef A. Invasive basal cell carcinoma in a xeroderma pigmentosum patient: facing secondary and tertiary aggressive recurrences. J Craniofac Surg. 2014; 25(4):e336–e338

[189] Selvaag E. Clinical drug photosensitivity. A retrospective analysis of reports to the Norwegian Adverse Drug Reactions Committee from the years 1970–1994. Photodermatol Photoimmunol Photomed. 1997; 13(1–2):21–23

[190] Drucker AM, Rosen CF. Drug-induced photosensitivity: culprit drugs, management and prevention. Drug Saf. 2011; 34(10):821–837

[191] Moore DE. Drug-induced cutaneous photosensitivity: incidence, mechanism, prevention and management. Drug Saf. 2002; 25(5):345–372

[192] McCarthy KL, Playford EG, Looke DF, Whitby M. Severe photosensitivity causing multifocal squamous cell carcinomas secondary to prolonged voriconazole therapy. Clin Infect Dis. 2007; 44(5):e55–e56

[193] Vanacker A, Fabré G, Van Dorpe J, Peetermans WE, Maes B. Aggressive cutaneous squamous cell carcinoma associated with prolonged voriconazole therapy in a renal transplant patient. Am J Transplant. 2008; 8 (4):877–880

[194] Brunel AS, Fraisse T, Lechiche C, Pinzani V, Mauboussin JM, Sotto A. Multifocal squamous cell carcinomas in an HIV-infected patient with a long-term voriconazole therapy. AIDS. 2008; 22(7):905–906

[195] Cowen EW, Nguyen JC, Miller DD, et al. Chronic phototoxicity and aggressive squamous cell carcinoma of the skin in children and adults during treatment with voriconazole. J Am Acad Dermatol. 2010; 62(1):31–37

[196] Miller DD, Cowen EW, Nguyen JC, McCalmont TH, Fox LP. Melanoma associated with long-term voriconazole therapy: a new manifestation of chronic photosensitivity. Arch Dermatol. 2010; 146(3):300–304

[197] Stern RS, Nichols KT, Väkevä LH. Malignant melanoma in patients treated for psoriasis with methoxsalen (psoralen) and ultraviolet A radiation (PUVA). The PUVA Follow-Up Study. N Engl J Med. 1997; 336(15):1041–1045

[198] Diepgen TL, Fartasch M, Drexler H, Schmitt J. Occupational skin cancer induced by ultraviolet radiation and its prevention. Br J Dermatol. 2012; 167 Suppl 2:76–84

[199] Horsham C, Auster J, Sendall MC, et al. Interventions to decrease skin cancer risk in outdoor workers: update to a 2007 systematic review. BMC Res Notes. 2014; 7:10

[200] Reinau D, Weiss M, Meier CR, Diepgen TL, Surber C. Outdoor workers' sun-related knowledge, attitudes and protective behaviours: a systematic review of cross-sectional and interventional studies. Br J Dermatol. 2013; 168 (5):928–940

[201] Lewis EC, Mayer JA, Slymen D. Postal workers' occupational and leisure-time sun safety behaviors (United States). Cancer Causes Control. 2006; 17 (2):181–186

[202] Woolley T, Lowe J, Raasch B, Glasby M, Buettner PG. Workplace sun protection policies and employees' sun-related skin damage. Am J Health Behav. 2008; 32(2):201–208

[203] Antoine M, Pierre-Edouard S, Jean-Luc B, David V. Effective exposure to solar UV in building workers: influence of local and individual factors. J Expo Sci Environ Epidemiol. 2007; 17(1):58–68

[204] Hammond V, Reeder AI, Gray A. Patterns of real-time occupational ultraviolet radiation exposure among a sample of outdoor workers in New Zealand. Public Health. 2009; 123(2):182–187

[205] Siani AM, Casale GR, Sisto R, Colosimo A, Lang CA, Kimlin MG. Occupational exposures to solar ultraviolet radiation of vineyard workers in Tuscany (Italy). Photochem Photobiol. 2011; 87(4):925–934

[206] Gies P, Wright J. Measured solar ultraviolet radiation exposures of outdoor workers in Queensland in the building and construction industry. Photochem Photobiol. 2003; 78(4):342–348

[207] Schmitt J, Diepgen T, Bauer A. Occupational exposure to non-artificial UV-light and non-melanocytic skin cancer - a systematic review concerning a new occupational disease. J Dtsch Dermatol Ges. 2010; 8 (4):250–263, 250–264

[208] Bauer A, Diepgen TL, Schmitt J. Is occupational solar ultraviolet irradiation a relevant risk factor for basal cell carcinoma? A systematic review and meta-analysis of the epidemiological literature. Br J Dermatol. 2011; 165(3):612–625
[209] Young C. Solar ultraviolet radiation and skin cancer. Occup Med (Lond). 2009; 59(2):82–88
[210] Gandini S, Sera F, Cattaruzza MS, et al. Meta-analysis of risk factors for cutaneous melanoma: II. Sun exposure. Eur J Cancer. 2005; 41(1):45–60
[211] Glanz K, Buller DB, Saraiya M. Reducing ultraviolet radiation exposure among outdoor workers: state of the evidence and recommendations. Environ Health. 2007; 6:22
[212] Madgwick P, Houdmont J, Randall R. Sun safety measures among construction workers in Britain. Occup Med (Lond). 2011; 61(6):430–433
[213] Stock ML, Gerrard M, Gibbons FX, et al. Sun protection intervention for highway workers: long-term efficacy of UV photography and skin cancer information on men's protective cognitions and behavior. Ann Behav Med. 2009; 38(3):225–236
[214] Anderson PA, Buller DB, Voeks JH, et al. Testing the long-term effects of the Go Sun Smart Worksite Health Communication Campaign: a group-randomized experimental study. J Commun. 2008; 58(3):447–471
[215] Mayer JA, Slymen DJ, Clapp EJ, et al. Promoting sun safety among US Postal Service letter carriers: impact of a 2-year intervention. Am J Public Health. 2007; 97(3):559–565
[216] Azizi E, Flint P, Sadetzki S, et al. A graded work site intervention program to improve sun protection and skin cancer awareness in outdoor workers in Israel. Cancer Causes Control. 2000; 11(6):513–521
[217] Hammond V, Reeder AI, Gray AR, Bell ML. Are workers or their workplaces the key to occupational sun protection? Health Promot J Austr. 2008; 19 (2):97–101
[218] McCool JP, Reeder AI, Robinson EM, Petrie KJ, Gorman DF. Outdoor workers' perceptions of the risks of excess sun-exposure. J Occup Health. 2009; 51 (5):404–411
[219] Hall DM, McCarty F, Elliott T, Glanz K. Lifeguards' sun protection habits and sunburns: association with sun-safe environments and skin cancer prevention program participation. Arch Dermatol. 2009; 145(2):139–144
[220] Sigurdson AJ, Ron E. Cosmic radiation exposure and cancer risk among flight crew. Cancer Invest. 2004; 22(5):743–761
[221] Diffey BL, Roscoe AH. Exposure to solar ultraviolet radiation in flight. Aviat Space Environ Med. 1990; 61(11):1032–1035
[222] Pukkala E, Aspholm R, Auvinen A, et al. Incidence of cancer among Nordic airline pilots over five decades: occupational cohort study. BMJ. 2002; 325 (7364):567
[223] Friedberg W, Faulkner DN, Snyder L, Darden EB, Jr, O'Brien K. Galactic cosmic radiation exposure and associated health risks for air carrier crewmembers. Aviat Space Environ Med. 1989; 60(11):1104–1108
[224] United Nations Scientific Committee on the Effects of Atomic Radiation. Sources and Effects of Ionizing Radiation: 2000 Report to the General Assembly with Scientific Annexes. New York, NY: United Nations; 2000
[225] El Ghissassi F, Baan R, Straif K, et al. WHO International Agency for Research on Cancer Monograph Working Group. A review of human carcinogens–part D: radiation. Lancet Oncol. 2009; 10(8):751–752
[226] Tierney P, Ferguson J, Ibbotson S, Dawe R, Eadie E, Moseley H. Nine out of 10 sunbeds in England emit ultraviolet radiation levels that exceed current safety limits. Br J Dermatol. 2013; 168(3):602–608
[227] Wehner MR, Shive ML, Chren MM, Han J, Qureshi AA, Linos E. Indoor tanning and non-melanoma skin cancer: systematic review and meta-analysis. BMJ. 2012; 345:e5909
[228] Centers for Disease Control and Prevention. National Health Interview Survey. 2010 [accessed November 1, 2014]. http://www.cdc.gov/nchs/nhis.htm
[229] Wehner MR, Chren MM, Nameth D, et al. International prevalence of indoor tanning: a systematic review and meta-analysis. JAMA Dermatol. 2014; 150 (4):390–400
[230] Zhang M, Qureshi AA, Geller AC, Frazier L, Hunter DJ, Han J. Use of tanning beds and incidence of skin cancer. J Clin Oncol. 2012; 30(14):1588–1593
[231] Lazovich D, Vogel RI, Berwick M, Weinstock MA, Anderson KE, Warshaw EM. Indoor tanning and risk of melanoma: a case-control study in a highly exposed population. Cancer Epidemiol Biomarkers Prev. 2010; 19(6):1557–1568
[232] Ferrucci LM, Cartmel B, Molinaro AM, Leffell DJ, Bale AE, Mayne ST. Indoor tanning and risk of early-onset basal cell carcinoma. J Am Acad Dermatol. 2012; 67(4):552–562
[233] Centers for Disease Control and Prevention. Youth Risk Behavior Surveillance System. 2013. July 9, 2014 [accessed November 1, 2014]; Available from: http://www.cdc.gov/HealthyYouth/yrbs/index.htm
[234] Centers for Disease Control and Prevention. Indoor Tanning is Not Safe. 2014. July 15, 2014 [accessed November 1, 2014]. http://www.cdc.gov/cancer/skin/basic_info/indoor_tanning.htm
[235] Colantonio S, Bracken MB, Beecker J. The association of indoor tanning and melanoma in adults: systematic review and meta-analysis. J Am Acad Dermatol. 2014; 70(5):847–57.e1, 18
[236] Ogden N. General and Plastic Surgery Devices: Reclassification of Ultraviolet Lamps for Tanning, Henceforth To Be Known as Sunlamp Products and Ultraviolet Lamps Intended for Use in Sunlamp Products. 2014 [accessed November 1, 2014]. https://www.federalregister.gov/articles/2014/06/02/2014-12546/general-and-plastic-surgery-devices-reclassification-of-ultraviolet-lamps-for-tanning-henceforth-to
[237] International Agency for Research on Cancer. Agents Classified by the IARC Monographs, Volumes 1–100. 2012. July 25, 2014 [accessed October 9, 2014]. http://monographs.iarc.fr/ENG/Classification/ClassificationsAlphaOrder.pdf
[238] Centers for Disease Control and Prevention (CDC). Sunburn and sun protective behaviors among adults aged 18–29 years–United States, 2000–2010. MMWR Morb Mortal Wkly Rep. 2012; 61(18):317–322
[239] Abroms L, Jorgensen CM, Southwell BG, Geller AC, Emmons KM. Gender differences in young adults' beliefs about sunscreen use. Health Educ Behav. 2003; 30(1):29–43
[240] Paller AS, Hawk JL, Honig P, et al. New insights about infant and toddler skin: implications for sun protection. Pediatrics. 2011; 128(1):92–102
[241] Rouhani P, Parmet Y, Bessell AG, Peay T, Weiss A, Kirsner RS. Knowledge, attitudes, and behaviors of elementary school students regarding sun exposure and skin cancer. Pediatr Dermatol. 2009; 26(5):529–535
[242] Osterwalder U, Herzog B. Sun protection factors: world wide confusion. Br J Dermatol. 2009; 161 Suppl 3:13–24
[243] Neale R, Williams G, Green A. Application patterns among participants randomized to daily sunscreen use in a skin cancer prevention trial. Arch Dermatol. 2002; 138(10):1319–1325
[244] Mancebo SE, Hu JY, Wang SQ. Sunscreens: a review of health benefits, regulations, and controversies. Dermatol Clin. 2014; 32(3):427–438, x
[245] Gantz GM, Sumner WG. Stable ultraviolet light absorbers. Text Res J. 1957; 27(3):244–251
[246] Knox JM, Guin J, Cockerell EG. Benzophenones; ultraviolet light absorbing agents. J Invest Dermatol. 1957; 29(6):435–444
[247] Kanof NB. Protection of the skin against the harmful effects of sunlight. AMA Arch Derm. 1956; 74(1):46–49
[248] Bens G. Sunscreens. Adv Exp Med Biol. 2014; 810:429–463
[249] Scheuer E, Warshaw E. Sunscreen allergy: a review of epidemiology, clinical characteristics, and responsible allergens. Dermatitis. 2006; 17(1):3–11
[250] Celleno L, Calzavara-Pinton P, Sala R, Arisi MC, Bussoletti C. Photobiology, photodermatology and sunscreens: a comprehensive overview. Part 2: topical and systemic photoprotection. G Ital Dermatol Venereol. 2013; 148 (1):107–133
[251] Warshaw EM, Wang MZ, Maibach HI, et al. Patch test reactions associated with sunscreen products and the importance of testing to an expanded series: retrospective analysis of North American Contact Dermatitis Group data, 2001 to 2010. Dermatitis. 2013; 24(4):176–182
[252] Smijs TG, Pavel S. Titanium dioxide and zinc oxide nanoparticles in sunscreens: focus on their safety and effectiveness. Nanotechnol Sci Appl. 2011; 4:95–112
[253] Wang SQ, Balagula Y, Osterwalder U. Photoprotection: a review of the current and future technologies. Dermatol Ther (Heidelb). 2010; 23(1):31–47
[254] Mitchnick MA, Fairhurst D, Pinnell SR. Microfine zinc oxide (Z-cote) as a photostable UVA/UVB sunblock agent. J Am Acad Dermatol. 1999; 40 (1):85–90
[255] Jou PC, Feldman RJ, Tomecki KJ. UV protection and sunscreens: what to tell patients. Cleve Clin J Med. 2012; 79(6):427–436
[256] Damian DL, Matthews YJ, Phan TA, Halliday GM. An action spectrum for ultraviolet radiation-induced immunosuppression in humans. Br J Dermatol. 2011; 164(3):657–659
[257] Ravanat JL, Douki T, Cadet J. Direct and indirect effects of UV radiation on DNA and its components. J Photochem Photobiol B. 2001; 63(1–3):88–102
[258] Budden T, Bowden NA. The role of altered nucleotide excision repair and UVB-induced DNA damage in melanomagenesis. Int J Mol Sci. 2013; 14 (1):1132–1151
[259] Djavaheri-Mergny M, Mergny JL, Bertrand F, et al. Ultraviolet-A induces activation of AP-1 in cultured human keratinocytes. FEBS Lett. 1996; 384(1):92–96
[260] Darr D, Fridovich I. Free radicals in cutaneous biology. J Invest Dermatol. 1994; 102(5):671–675

[261] Rünger TM, Kappes UP. Mechanisms of mutation formation with long-wave ultraviolet light (UVA). Photodermatol Photoimmunol Photomed. 2008; 24 (1):2–10
[262] Moyal D, Fourtanier A. Acute and chronic effects of UV on skin. In: Rigel DS, Weiss RA, Lim HW, eds. Photoaging. New York, NY: Marcel Dekker, Inc; 2004:15–32
[263] Gil EM, Kim TH. UV-induced immune suppression and sunscreen. Photodermatol Photoimmunol Photomed. 2000; 16(3):101–110
[264] Sklar LR, Almutawa F, Lim HW, Hamzavi I. Effects of ultraviolet radiation, visible light, and infrared radiation on erythema and pigmentation: a review. Photochem Photobiol Sci. 2013; 12(1):54–64
[265] Moyal DD, Fourtanier AM. Broad-spectrum sunscreens provide better protection from solar ultraviolet-simulated radiation and natural sunlight-induced immunosuppression in human beings. J Am Acad Dermatol. 2008; 58(5) Suppl 2:S149–S154
[266] Baron ED, Fourtanier A, Compan D, Medaisko C, Cooper KD, Stevens SR. High ultraviolet A protection affords greater immune protection confirming that ultraviolet A contributes to photoimmunosuppression in humans. J Invest Dermatol. 2003; 121(4):869–875
[267] Fourtanier A, Moyal D, Seité S. Sunscreens containing the broad-spectrum UVA absorber, Mexoryl SX, prevent the cutaneous detrimental effects of UV exposure: a review of clinical study results. Photodermatol Photoimmunol Photomed. 2008; 24(4):164–174
[268] Green AC, Williams GM, Logan V, Strutton GM. Reduced melanoma after regular sunscreen use: randomized trial follow-up. J Clin Oncol. 2011; 29 (3):257–263
[269] Cancer IARo. IARC Handbook on Cancer Prevention. Volume 5: Sunscreens. Lyon, France: International Agency for Research on Cancer, World Health Organization; 2001
[270] Chesnut C, Kim J. Is there truly no benefit with sunscreen use and Basal cell carcinoma? A critical review of the literature and the application of new sunscreen labeling rules to real-world sunscreen practices. J Skin Cancer. 2012; 2012:480985
[271] van der Pols JC, Williams GM, Pandeya N, Logan V, Green AC. Prolonged prevention of squamous cell carcinoma of the skin by regular sunscreen use. Cancer Epidemiol Biomarkers Prev. 2006; 15(12):2546–2548
[272] Hughes MC, Williams GM, Baker P, Green AC. Sunscreen and prevention of skin aging: a randomized trial. Ann Intern Med. 2013; 158(11):781–790
[273] U.S. Food and Drug Association. FDA Press Release. FDA announces changes to better inform consumers about sunscreen: new rules give consumers more information to help reduce risk of skin cancer, early aging. [accessed October 10, 2014]. http://www.fda.gov/NewsEvents/Newsroom/PressAnnouncements/ucm258940.htm
[274] Young AR, Orchard GE, Harrison GI, Klock JL. The detrimental effects of daily sub-erythemal exposure on human skin in vivo can be prevented by a daily-care broad-spectrum sunscreen. J Invest Dermatol. 2007; 127(4):975–978
[275] Seité S, Fourtanier AM. The benefit of daily photoprotection. J Am Acad Dermatol. 2008; 58(5) Suppl 2:S160–S166
[276] Gordon LG, Scuffham PA, van der Pols JC, McBride P, Williams GM, Green AC. Regular sunscreen use is a cost-effective approach to skin cancer prevention in subtropical settings. J Invest Dermatol. 2009; 129(12):2766–2771
[277] Boyd AS, Naylor M, Cameron GS, Pearse AD, Gaskell SA, Neldner KH. The effects of chronic sunscreen use on the histologic changes of dermatoheliosis. J Am Acad Dermatol. 1995; 33(6):941–946
[278] Green AC, Hughes MC, McBride P, Fourtanier A. Factors associated with premature skin aging (photoaging) before the age of 55: a population-based study. Dermatology. 2011; 222(1):74–80
[279] Holman CD, Armstrong BK, Evans PR, et al. Relationship of solar keratosis and history of skin cancer to objective measures of actinic skin damage. Br J Dermatol. 1984; 110(2):129–138
[280] de Gruijl FR. Photobiology of photocarcinogenesis. Photochem Photobiol. 1996; 63(4):372–375
[281] Thompson SC, Jolley D, Marks R. Reduction of solar keratoses by regular sunscreen use. N Engl J Med. 1993; 329(16):1147–1151
[282] Darlington S, Williams G, Neale R, Frost C, Green A. A randomized controlled trial to assess sunscreen application and beta carotene supplementation in the prevention of solar keratoses. Arch Dermatol. 2003; 139(4):451–455
[283] Green A, Williams G, Neale R, et al. Daily sunscreen application and betacarotene supplementation in prevention of basal-cell and squamous-cell carcinomas of the skin: a randomised controlled trial. Lancet. 1999; 354 (9180):723–729
[284] Dennis LK, Vanbeek MJ, Beane Freeman LE, Smith BJ, Dawson DV, Coughlin JA. Sunburns and risk of cutaneous melanoma: does age matter? A comprehensive meta-analysis. Ann Epidemiol. 2008; 18(8):614–627
[285] Green AC, Williams GM. Point: sunscreen use is a safe and effective approach to skin cancer prevention. Cancer Epidemiol Biomarkers Prev. 2007; 16(10):1921–1922
[286] Berwick M. Counterpoint: sunscreen use is a safe and effective approach to skin cancer prevention. Cancer Epidemiol Biomarkers Prev. 2007; 16 (10):1923–1924
[287] Gallagher RP, Rivers JK, Lee TK, Bajdik CD, McLean DI, Coldman AJ. Broad-spectrum sunscreen use and the development of new nevi in white children: a randomized controlled trial. JAMA. 2000; 283(22):2955–2960
[288] Autier P, Doré JF, Cattaruzza MS, et al. European Organization for Research and Treatment of Cancer Melanoma Cooperative Group. Sunscreen use, wearing clothes, and number of nevi in 6- to 7-year-old European children. J Natl Cancer Inst. 1998; 90(24):1873–1880
[289] Carrera C, Puig-Butillè JA, Aguilera P, et al. Impact of sunscreens on preventing UVR-induced effects in nevi: in vivo study comparing protection using a physical barrier vs sunscreen. JAMA Dermatol. 2013; 149(7):803–813
[290] Dennis LK, Beane Freeman LE, VanBeek MJ. Sunscreen use and the risk for melanoma: a quantitative review. Ann Intern Med. 2003; 139(12):966–978
[291] Goldenhersh MA, Koslowsky M. Increased melanoma after regular sunscreen use? J Clin Oncol. 2011; 29(18):e557–e558, author reply e859
[292] Situm M, Buljan M, Bulat V, Lugović Mihić L, Bolanca Z, Simić D. The role of UV radiation in the development of basal cell carcinoma. Coll Antropol. 2008; 32 Suppl 2:167–170
[293] Katiyar SK. Green tea prevents non-melanoma skin cancer by enhancing DNA repair. Arch Biochem Biophys. 2011; 508(2):152–158
[294] Baliga MS, Katiyar SK. Chemoprevention of photocarcinogenesis by selected dietary botanicals. Photochem Photobiol Sci. 2006; 5(2):243–253
[295] Katiyar S, Elmets CA, Katiyar SK. Green tea and skin cancer: photoimmunology, angiogenesis and DNA repair. J Nutr Biochem. 2007; 18(5):287–296
[296] Chatterjee ML, Agarwal R, Mukhtar H. Ultraviolet B radiation-induced DNA lesions in mouse epidermis: an assessment using a novel 32P-postlabelling technique. Biochem Biophys Res Commun. 1996; 229(2):590–595
[297] Katiyar SK, Elmets CA, Agarwal R, Mukhtar H. Protection against ultraviolet-B radiation-induced local and systemic suppression of contact hypersensitivity and edema responses in C3 H/HeN mice by green tea polyphenols. Photochem Photobiol. 1995; 62(5):855–861
[298] Katiyar SK, Perez A, Mukhtar H. Green tea polyphenol treatment to human skin prevents formation of ultraviolet light B-induced pyrimidine dimers in DNA. Clin Cancer Res. 2000; 6(10):3864–3869
[299] Camouse MM, Domingo DS, Swain FR, et al. Topical application of green and white tea extracts provides protection from solar-simulated ultraviolet light in human skin. Exp Dermatol. 2009; 18(6):522–526
[300] Mantena SK, Meeran SM, Elmets CA, Katiyar SK. Orally administered green tea polyphenols prevent ultraviolet radiation-induced skin cancer in mice through activation of cytotoxic T cells and inhibition of angiogenesis in tumors. J Nutr. 2005; 135(12):2871–2877
[301] Mittal A, Piyathilake C, Hara Y, Katiyar SK. Exceptionally high protection of photocarcinogenesis by topical application of (–)-epigallocatechin-3-gallate in hydrophilic cream in SKH-1 hairless mouse model: relationship to inhibition of UVB-induced global DNA hypomethylation. Neoplasia. 2003; 5(6):555–565
[302] Gambichler T, Altmeyer P, Hoffmann K. Role of clothes in sun protection. Recent Results Cancer Res. 2002; 160:15–25
[303] Ghazi S, Couteau C, Paparis E, Coiffard LJ. Interest of external photoprotection by means of clothing and sunscreen products in young children. J Eur Acad Dermatol Venereol. 2012; 26(8):1026–1030
[304] Gambichler T, Hatch KL, Avermaete A, Altmeyer P, Hoffmann K. Influence of wetness on the ultraviolet protection factor (UPF) of textiles: in vitro and in vivo measurements. Photodermatol Photoimmunol Photomed. 2002; 18 (1):29–35
[305] American Cancer Society. How do I protect myself from UV rays? 2013 [accessed October 10, 2014]. http://www.cancer.org/cancer/cancercauses/sunanduvexposure/skincancerpreventionandearlydetection/skin-cancer-prevention-and-early-detection-u-v-protection
[306] Kinney JP, Long CS. The Ultraviolet Index: a useful tool. Dermatol Online J. 2000; 6(1):2
[307] Rosenthal FS, Phoon C, Bakalian AE, Taylor HR. The ocular dose of ultraviolet radiation to outdoor workers. Invest Ophthalmol Vis Sci. 1988; 29 (4):649–656

2 Clinical Detection of Skin Cancer

Michael Schowalter, Allison Vidimos, and Philip L. Bailin

Skin cancer is a broad term that encompasses all malignant entities of the skin from common carcinomas of the surface epithelium to rare tumors involving skin adnexal structures or appendages such as sweat ducts, sebaceous glands, or hair follicles. This chapter will focus on the clinical detection of commonly encountered skin cancers.

2.1 Basal Cell Carcinoma

2.1.1 Introduction

In practice, cutaneous malignancy is commonly broken down into the melanoma and nonmelanoma skin cancers (NMSC). NMSC represents the largest category of malignancies in the United States, occurring on the order of 3.5 million times per year in approximately 2.2 million patients.[1] NMSC can be further subdivided into basal cell carcinoma (BCC) and squamous cell carcinoma (SCC). BCCs make up the majority of NMSC and are the most common skin cancer in the United States as well as globally. BCC is a malignancy of the basal keratinocyte. Most tumors are sporadic, but patients with certain hereditary disorders are at an increased risk of developing numerous BCCs. BCC represents a large group with numerous subtypes, and as such the presentation and clinical detection of individual tumors varies and will be discussed separately.

2.1.2 History and Physical Exam

Sporadic BCCs are tumors primarily produced by ultraviolet (UV) radiation. As such, tumors concentrate to areas of high sunlight exposure. Careful examination of the head, face, neck, arms, and dorsal hands should be conducted. Specifically on the head, areas of higher UV exposure include nose, scalp, eyelids, ears, and lips. Clinicians should ask historically about new growths or persistent ones that may bleed or scab unprovoked. BCCs are variably painful or itchy. Thorough history includes questioning the nature of past UV radiation exposure such as tanning bed use, intense sun exposure leading to blistering sun burns, or therapeutic UV radiation such as psoralen and ultraviolet A radiation (PUVA). In patients with personal and family history of numerous BCCs, appropriate evaluation for genetic syndromes should be conducted. Patients with Gorlin's syndrome or BCC nevus syndrome (BCCNS) carry germline mutations in the *PTCH1* gene, vastly increasing their susceptibility to the tumors. A review of medical history and medications for evidence of iatrogenic immunosuppression is essential.

2.1.3 Nodular Basal Cell Carcinoma

Nodular or "classic" BCC is the most commonly encountered type, comprising 60 to 80% of all BCC. Nodular BCC appears as pink or red papules concentrated mainly to the head and neck. These papules may have a pearly, waxy, or translucent appearance. Many have grossly apparent telangiectasias coursing through the lesion. Tumor borders may be rolled forming a central area of depression (▶ Fig. 2.1). Nodular BCCs are an indolent subtype that slowly enlarge and may ultimately ulcerate and bleed unprovoked, which leads to the formation of an adherent crust overlying the lesion. Typically, nodular BCCs are not painful lesions unless neglected, large, and ulcerated.

2.1.4 Superficial Basal Cell Carcinoma

Superficial BCC is the next most common subtype, making up approximately 15 to 20% of diagnosed BCCs. This subtype classically involves trunk and extremities, and tumor characteristics are distinct from other BCC subtypes. Lesions are characterized as slow growing, flat, or minimally elevated pink to red scaly plaques, and may be quite subtle (▶ Fig. 2.2). The tumor may focally have superficial erosions or ulcerations with formation of crust. Borders are well defined and may be raised from the adjoining normal skin. These tumors may mimic inflammatory skin conditions such as atopic dermatitis, tinea infections, or psoriasis. Clinicians should be wary of dismissing superficial BCC as a nonmalignant entity in those patients with no prior history of inflammatory skin conditions or when lesions appear in atypical locations such as upper back or extremities distant from joints. These tumors are similarly not painful or pruritic, which may help differentiate these tumors from inflammatory skin conditions. Superficial BCCs are more common in men than in women.

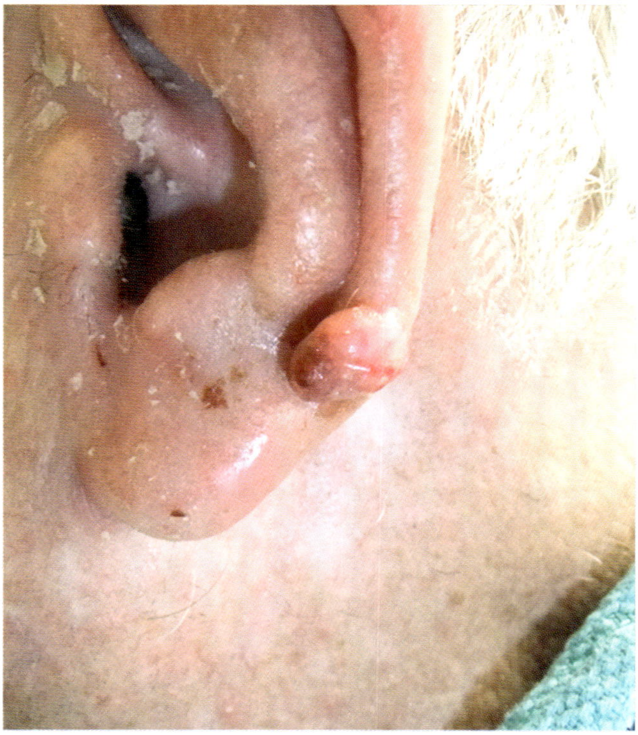

Fig. 2.1 Nodular basal cell carcinoma. Characteristic pearly or translucent appearance, rolled borders, focal ulceration, and overlying crust on the left ear of an elderly, fair-skinned man.

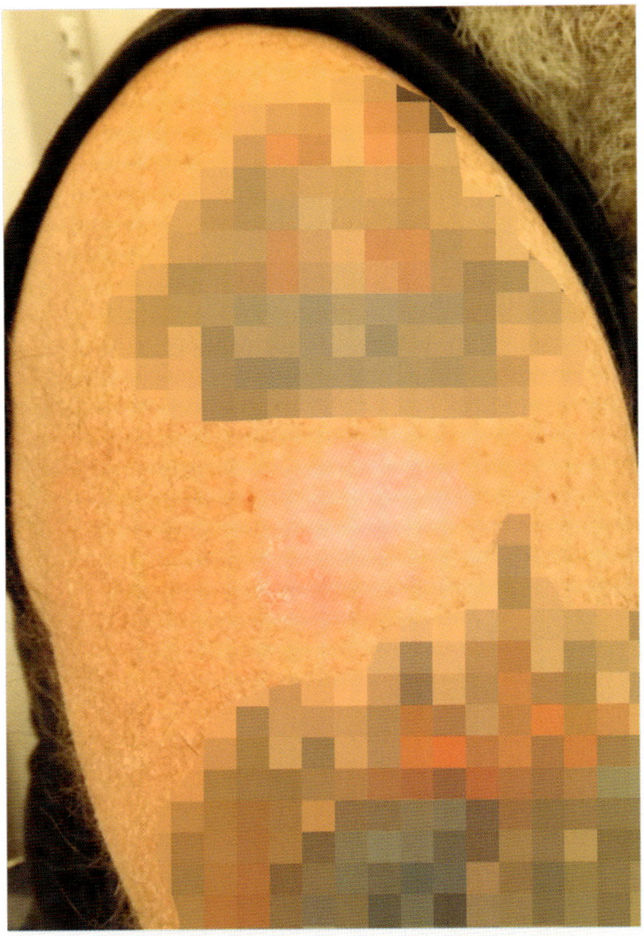

Fig. 2.2 Superficial basal cell carcinoma. Slowly expanding pink scaly plaque with subtle roll to peripheral borders.

2.1.5 Pigmented Variants

Pigmented BCCs are a variant of nodular and superficial BCC in which there is variably retained melanin in the malignant basal cell population (▶ Fig. 2.3). These variants are common in patients with skin of color. Tumors otherwise retain their primary characteristics. These entities may represent a pitfall in clinical diagnosis of skin cancer and as such should be considered when evaluating pigmented lesions.

2.1.6 Morpheaform and Infiltrative Basal Cell Carcinoma

Morpheaform and infiltrative BCCs are rare, clinically similar entities with aggressive pathological patterns that will be discussed together. These entities make up approximately 5 to 10% of all BCCs. Morpheaform BCCs occur most commonly in areas of intense UV exposure, such as head and neck. They present as skin-colored, white, or, less commonly, pink atrophic plaques. Lesions rarely ulcerate unlike most BCC. These tumors may clinically appear as smooth and shiny plaques and feel indurated when palpated. As such, they are commonly confused for scars (▶ Fig. 2.4). Pain and itching may accompany this subtype of BCC, given there is a greater tendency for deep invasion into subcutaneous fat and muscle as well as perineural invasion.

2.2 Squamous Cell Carcinoma

2.2.1 Introduction

SCC is the second most common skin malignancy worldwide. SCC is a malignancy of the squamous keratinocyte epithelium. Tumors are sporadic or may be part of genetic conditions such as xeroderma pigmentosum (XP), oculocutaneous albinism

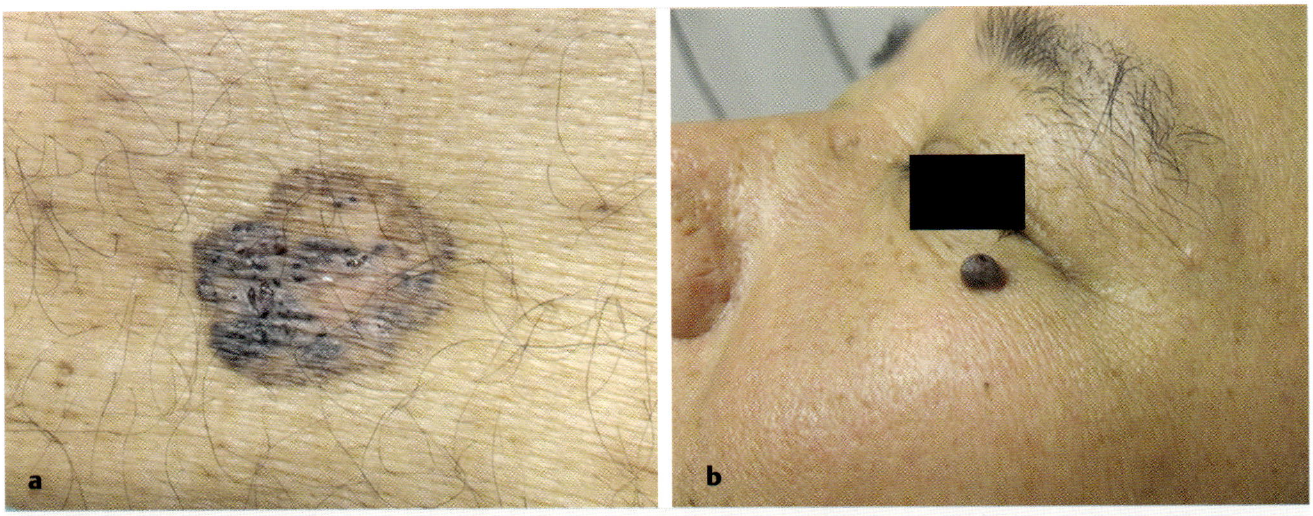

Fig. 2.3 **(a)** Pigmented variant of superficial basal cell carcinoma in a patient of middle-eastern descent. **(b)** Pigmented variant of nodular basal cell carcinoma on the inferior orbital rim in a middle-aged Chinese male.

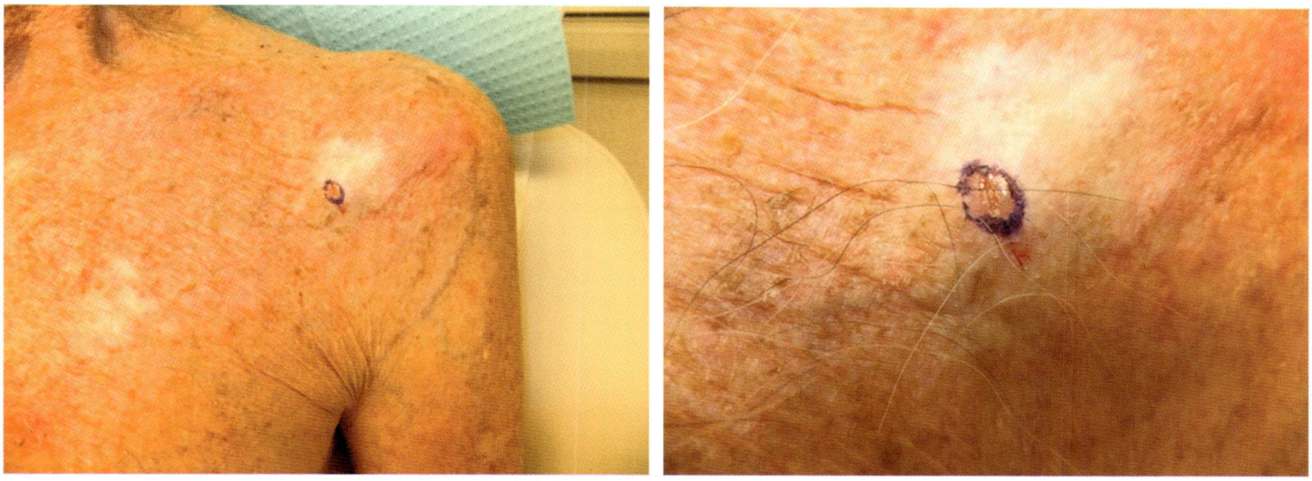

Fig. 2.4 Infiltrative basal cell carcinoma clinically resembling a scar.

(OCA), and epidermodysplasia verruciformis (EV). SCCs are linked to UV exposure, whether natural or occupational. Other risk factors include human papillomavirus (HPV) infection, chronic immune suppression, ionizing radiation, scarring, chronic sinus tract formation, chronic ulcerations, and chemical carcinogenic exposures. In general, patients who have sporadic or UV-induced SCCs do much better than their counterparts who develop the malignancy in chronic wounds, scars, or as a result of immunosuppression. Invasive SCC, defined as tumor that has invaded below the skin basement membrane, can arise within an existing SCC in situ (SCCis) or arise de novo. Various clinical presentations of SCC, including SCCis, will be discussed.

2.2.2 History and Physical Exam

SCCs are induced by both chronic UV exposure and chronic inflammation in the setting of scars and nonhealing wounds. Physicians should be vigilant with the patient with general signs of chronic UV exposure, including numerous solar lentigines, fine facial wrinkling, skin atrophy, telangiectasias, and Favre–Racouchot changes. A subtype, the Marjolin's ulcer, is an ulcerating SCC in sites of past trauma such as burns. As with BCC, a careful examination of areas exposed to UV radiation including head and neck, dorsal hands, and arms should be conducted. Again, a history should concentrate on possible sources for immune suppression, as well as a history of personal or family history of past SCC.

2.2.3 Squamous Cell Carcinoma In Situ

Actinic Keratoses

While some controversy exists over the exact characterization of actinic keratoses (AKs) with regard to malignant potential, AKs, also known as solar keratoses, are generally felt to be a form of low-grade squamous dysplasia. Studies have shown that AKs transform into invasive SCC on the order of 0.025 to 20% per year.[2] It is estimated that a quarter of the population in the northern hemisphere has at least one of these lesions. Clinically, AKs present in a number of different forms. Generally, they are ill-defined, pink to erythematous papules with overlying scale. They are small, with the majority being less than 1 cm in size (▶ Fig. 2.5a). Variants of AKs are named based on clinical appearance: pigmented, hyperkeratotic (or hyperplastic), and verrucous. When exuberantly hyperkeratotic, an AK may be referred to as a cutaneous horn (▶ Fig. 2.5b). AKs have a rough, scaly, or sandpaperlike texture when palpated. AKs are generally diagnosed in the broader clinical context of more widespread UV or actinic damage. Differential diagnosis for AKs includes inflammatory dermatoses of the head and neck, such as seborrheic dermatitis and contact dermatitis. Neoplasms such as Bowen's disease, superficial BCC, and melanoma in situ may mimic AK.

Actinic Cheilitis

Actinic cheilitis (AC) is a clinical variant of AK involving the lips. The characteristic pink or red scaly plaques may simulate chapped or dry lips (▶ Fig. 2.6). The normally well-demarcated vermilion border of the lip may be obscured or blurred. The lower lips are more extensively involved due to increased UV exposure. There is also increased risk for AC in patients who smoke or chew tobacco products.

Bowen's Disease

A distinct form of SCCis, Bowen's disease has distinct clinical and histopathologic presentation. Similar to AK, Bowen's disease may present on sun-exposed skin and mucosa of the head and neck. Bowen's disease may also present in oral or anal mucosa, as well as on the genitals. Clinical appearance is that of a red, well-defined scaly papule or plaque with distinct borders. Bowen's disease lesions may slowly grow both in height and in diameter over time. They may also take on a verrucous or fissured appearance. Differential diagnosis again includes inflammatory conditions, as well as neoplasms mentioned for AK. Mucosal Bowen's may mimic oral candidiasis or oral blistering conditions such as pemphigus or pemphigoid. Bowen's disease on the vaginal mucosa may mimic uncomplicated vaginitis.

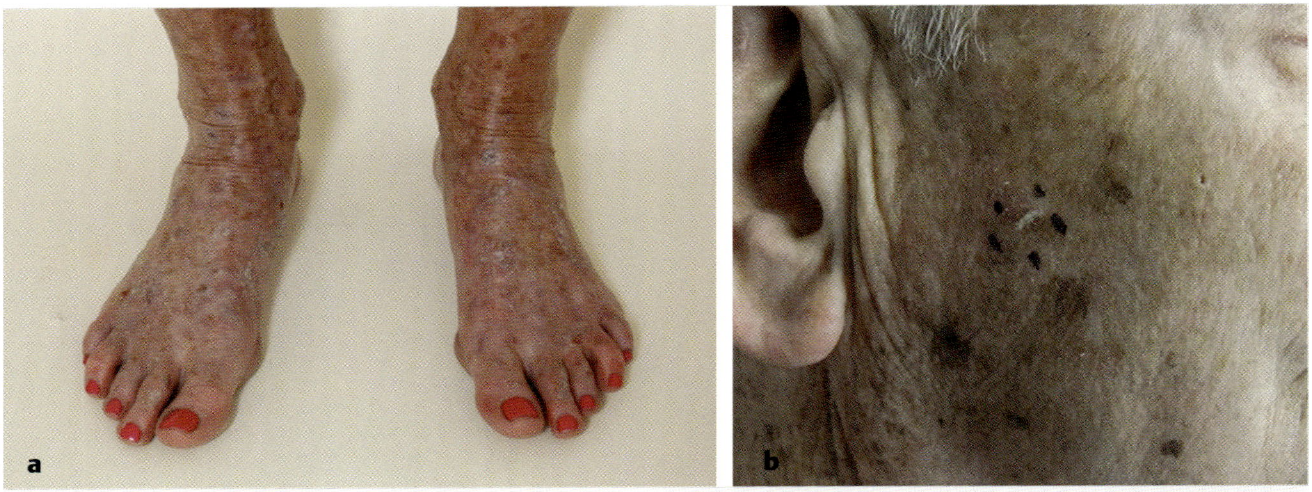

Fig. 2.5 (a) Multiple actinic keratoses in a middle-aged female with remote history of arsenic exposure. (b) Cutaneous horn.

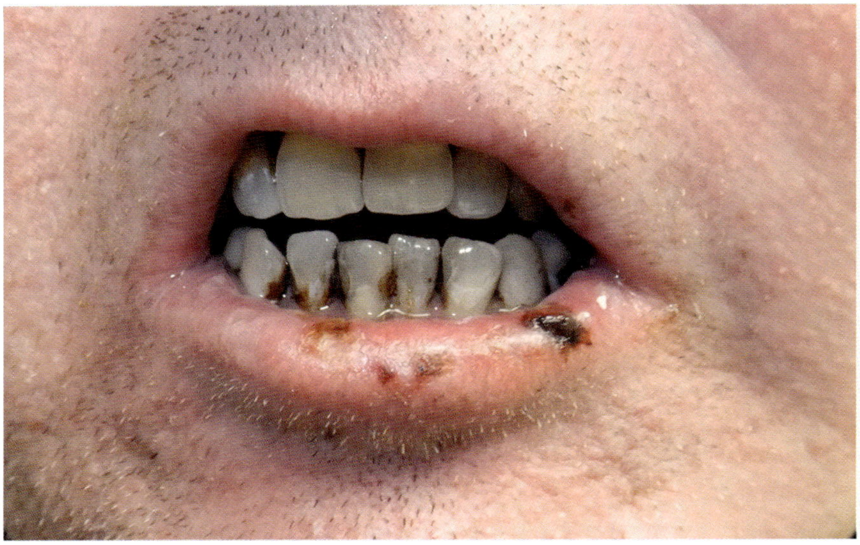

Fig. 2.6 Actinic cheilitis involving the lower lip in a patient with remote history of tobacco use, ultraviolet exposure, and use of a photosensitizing azole antifungal medication.

Erythroplasia of Queyrat

Similar to Bowen's disease, erythroplasia of queyrat represents a raised red plaque of the penis, most commonly the glans penis in uncircumcised men.

Oral Leukoplakia

A form of oral SCCis, oral leukoplakia clinically manifests as a white patch or plaque in the mouth that cannot be scrubbed or rubbed off. The most common area of occurrence is the buccal mucosa along the lateral surfaces of the oral cavity, but can involve any mucosal surface including the tongue (▶ Fig. 2.7). Oral leukoplakia may take on a verrucous appearance, a harbinger for greater propensity for progression to SCC. This entity must be distinguished from benign mucosal conditions such as oral candidiasis, syphilis, or morsicatio buccarum—maceration and irritation of the buccal mucosa due to repeated chewing or biting.

2.2.4 Squamous Cell Carcinoma

Squamous Cell Carcinoma Arising from Squamous Cell Carcinoma In Situ

Most commonly, SCC is associated and contiguous with SCCis that has progressed and invaded over time with lack of treatment. Again, the most common areas affected are those exposed chronically to UV radiation over years, including head and neck, dorsal forearms, and hands. In sunbathers and females, anterior legs including shins are also commonly affected. Middle-aged to elderly men are the highest represented demographic group. Cutaneous SCC may take on a variety of clinical appearances; clinically distinct subtypes will be discussed separately. In general, SCC manifests as a well-defined plaque, larger in size than typical AK or SCCis. Plaques are thicker and may have prominent erosions or ulcerations (▶ Fig. 2.8). There may be focal areas of increased scale or hyperkeratosis, resulting in an exophytic appearance. The lesions may have exudate or be superficially impetiginized, resulting in an adherent scale crust. SCC may take on unusual or distinct clinical appearances due to the past treatments or partial treatments, duration since onset, location of tumor, or host immune system.

Keratoacanthoma

Keratoacanthoma (KA) is a clinically distinct entity, representing a histopathologically well-differentiated form of SCC. KA occurs most commonly in middle-aged to elderly fair-skinned individuals on sites of heavy UV damage. These tumors have a natural history characterized by approximately 1 month of rapid growth from onset, a period of stability without growth that can last 3 to 6 months, and lastly a period of spontaneous involution that takes place over 1 to 2 subsequent months. KAs clinically appear as dome-shaped red or pink papules, or nodules with a central keratinaceous plug (▸ Fig. 2.9). Patients often report that the lesion suddenly appeared.

There are several distinct subtypes of KA based on clinical appearance, location, or number of lesions. Subungual KAs develop on nail beds and may cause significant pain due to rapid growth. Mucosal KAs arise on any mucosal surface, and

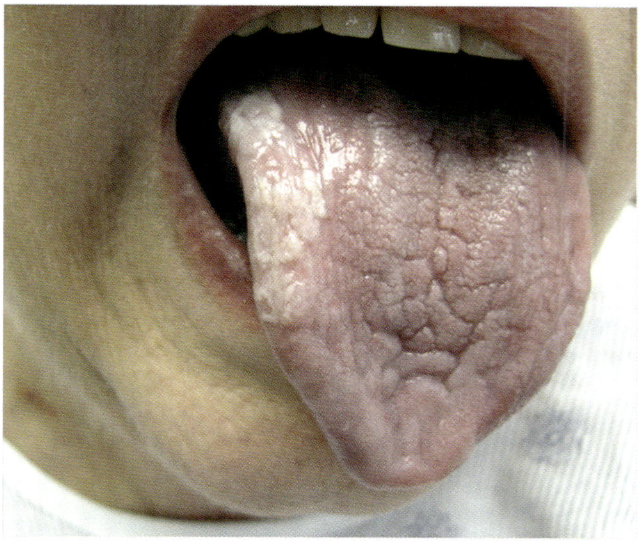

Fig. 2.7 Oral leukoplakia involving the lateral tongue.

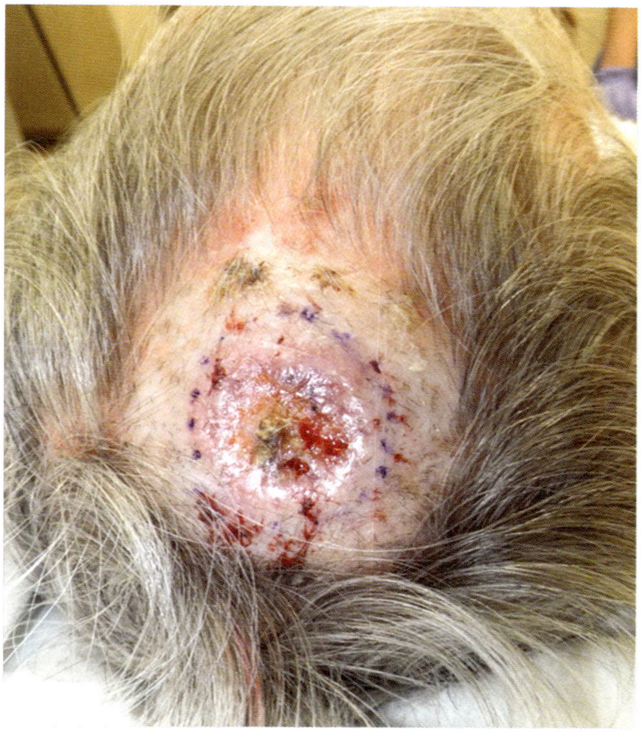

Fig. 2.8 Large ulcerated and bleeding squamous cell carcinoma of the scalp.

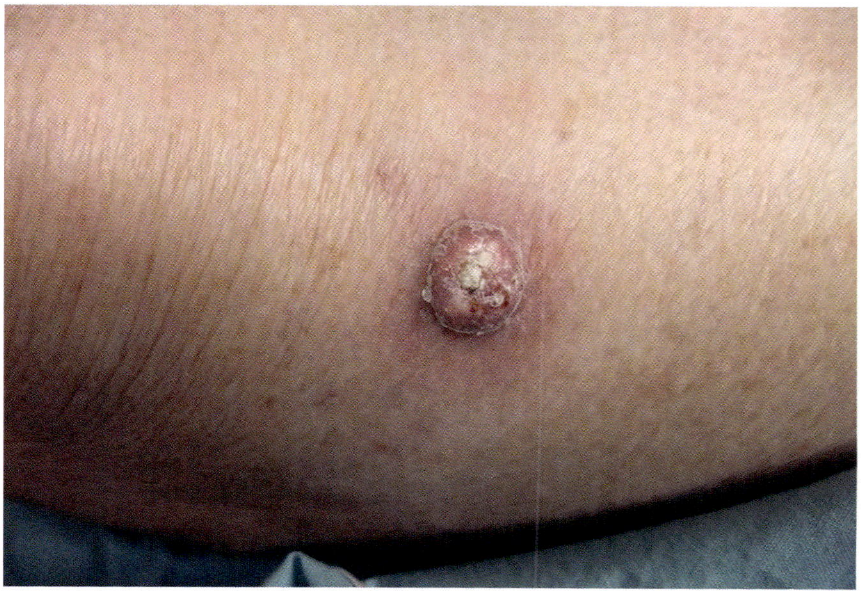

Fig. 2.9 Pink papule on the scalp with central keratin plug. Consistent pathologically with keratoacanthoma.

may occur in syndromes with multiple KAs. Giant KAs are similar in morphology, but larger in size than typical KA. Ranging from 2 to more than 15 cm, these variants have a predilection for the nose, eyelids, and face.[3] While they may spontaneously involute as typical KAs, they may be locally and permanently disfiguring. Keratoacanthoma centrifugum marginatum (KCM) are similarly large, growing sometimes greater than 15 or 20 cm, but have spontaneous central involution. Clinically, this presents as an expanding erythematous rim with central clearing. These variants are less likely to spontaneously resolve than typical or giant KA.[4]

Generalized eruptive keratoacathomas of Grzybowski is a rare syndrome characterized by abrupt occurrence of numerous KAs over many body surface areas, including mucosal surfaces. Hundreds to thousands of pruritic, variably sized lesions may develop over a short period of time.[5] Multiple KAs may present as part of multiple self-healing squamous epithelioma (MSSE) also known as Ferguson–Smith disease, an autosomal dominant disorder involving the transforming growth factor beta receptor 1 (*TGFBR1*) gene.

Verrucous Squamous Cell Carcinoma

Verrucous SCC is considered a low-grade variant of SCC that commonly affects the oral mucosa, feet, and genitalia. These tumors are very slow growing and have a characteristic papillomatous or warty exterior. Though slow growing, these tumors may be locally destructive and disfiguring (▶ Fig. 2.10a). HPV and carcinogen exposure are thought to be driving forces behind this malignancy, rather than UV radiation. Depending on the anatomical locale at presentation, different terms can be used to describe these tumors. Verrucous SCC of the oral cavity is also known as oral florid papillomatosis, while that of the anogenital region is known as a Buschke–Lowenstein tumor (▶ Fig. 2.10b). The later subtype may be associated with verrucous SCC of the urethra or bladder. When pre-

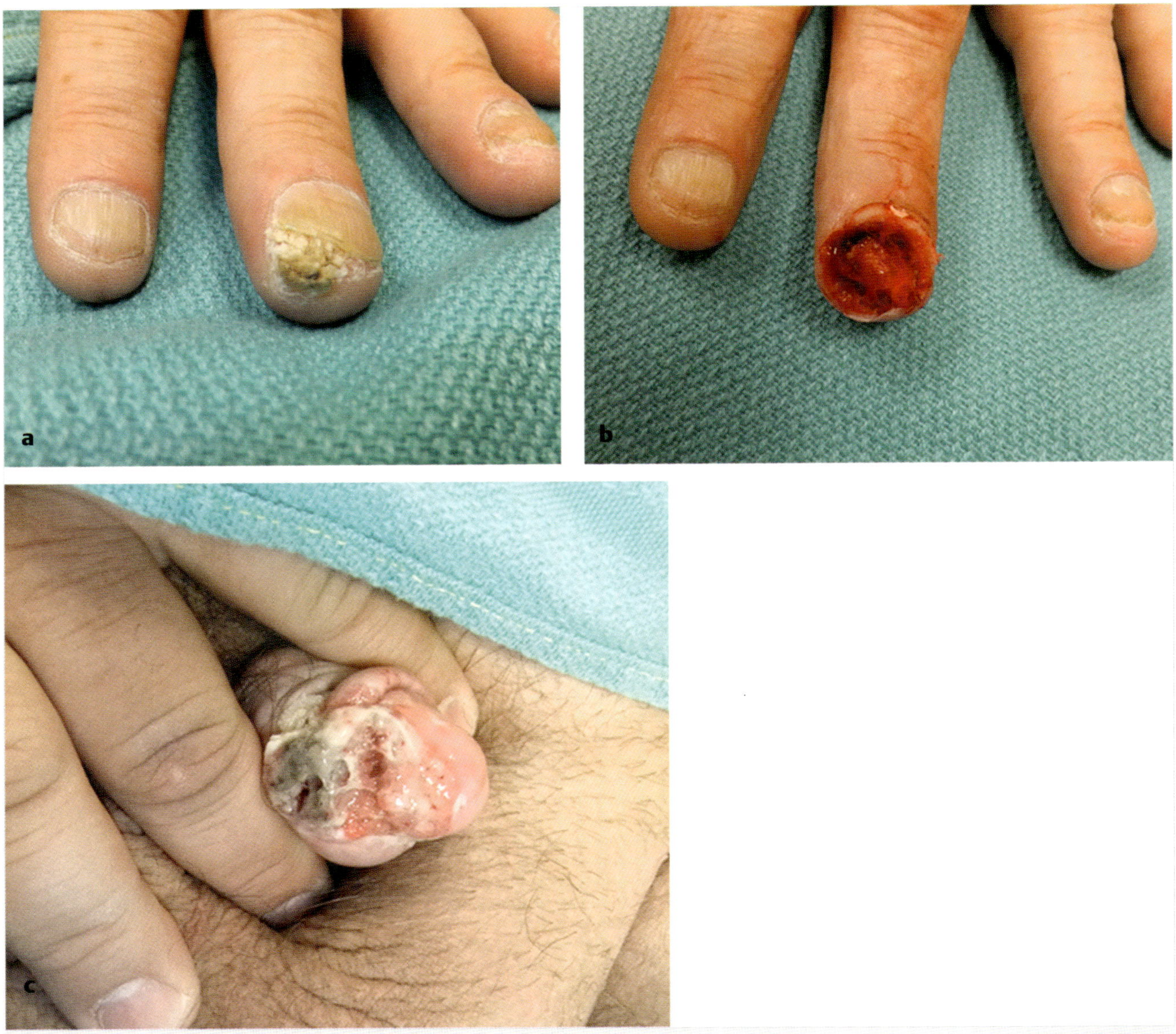

Fig. 2.10 **(a)** Verrucal squamous cell carcinoma (SCC) of the subungual fingertip. **(b)** Photograph after complete resection via Mohs micrographic surgery demonstrates the locally destructive nature of the lesion. **(c)** Verrucal SCC of the penis.

senting on the palms or soles, the term epithelioma cuniculatum is used.

2.3 Melanoma

2.3.1 Melanoma In Situ

Almost all melanomas begin as melanoma in situ, with epidermal proliferation of malignant melanocytes that eventually invade past the epidermal basement membrane into the dermis. Melanoma in situ can clinically present in a number of different ways and be clinically indistinguishable from banal nevi.

Lentigo Maligna

Lentigo maligna (LM) is a specific type of melanoma in situ that commonly occurs on the head and neck of elderly Caucasian individuals. LM clinically presents as a brown, tan, or multicolored pigmented macule or patch that grows slowly over time (▶ Fig. 2.11a). Clinical diagnosis is often difficult or impossible to make in elderly individuals with years of sun damage and numerous obscuring lentigines, seborrheic keratoses, and AKs. Clues that a particular lesion may signify an LM include the following: irregular borders, lesion asymmetry, and radial growth over time. LM is notorious for having malignant extension beyond the visible borders of the tumor. In these circumstances, histologic "skip areas" are seen, further complicating the clinical characterization of LM. A lesion may develop other colors as part of its natural progression, and exhibit black, blue, pink, red, or white hues. Lesions may keep their brown or tan color, but exhibit uneven darkening through the lesion. LM is flat without surface change, which helps to distinguish it from an actinic or solar keratosis. However, a pigmented nodule within a larger LM is typically a harbinger for progression to lentigo maligna melanoma (LMM). Of note, LM is sometimes associated with desmoplastic melanoma, which will be discussed later.

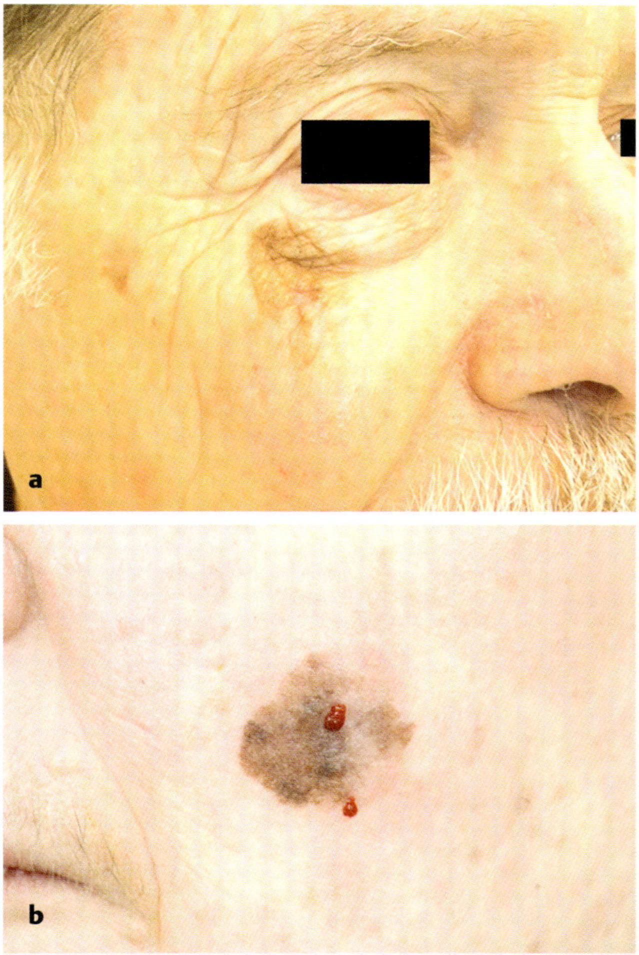

Fig. 2.11 (a) Lentigo maligna involving the face of an elderly male. (b) Lentigo maligna melanoma with exophytic red nodules.

2.3.2 Lentigo Maligna Melanoma

LMM represents the invasive counterpart to the LM. Common clinical features include a brown to black nodule that develops within a broad tan or brown LM that has been slowing growing for months to years as described earlier (▶ Fig. 2.11b). There may be ulceration or bleeding present.

2.3.3 Superficial Spreading Melanoma

Superficial spreading melanoma (SSM) is the most common form of invasive melanoma, despite an increasing incidence of LMM.[6] This tumor subtype is found in adults of any age, with median in the sixth decade of life—though incidence continues to rise in younger age groups.[7,8] These tumors are commonly found on the trunk, back, and lower extremities. Classically, the mnemonic device ABCDE (A-asymmetry, B-borders, C-colors, D-diameter, and E-evolving/enlarging)—often used as a clinical tool for detection of all melanoma—is especially effective in SMM. When compared to banal pigmented lesions, SMM show marked asymmetry, scalloped or irregular borders, multiple colors including red, blue, and black, and usually have size greater than 5 mm (▶ Fig. 2.12). These lesions evolve over time, and may ultimately ulcerate, bleed, and become painful. There is loss of normal skin marking or dermatoglyphics as the lesion expands. The appearance of a scar incorporated into the lesion

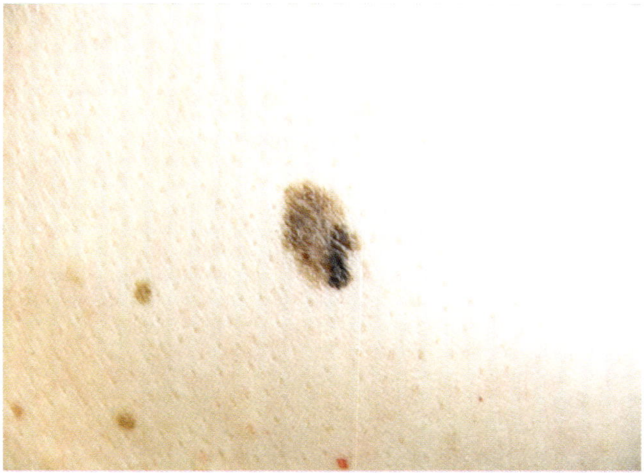

Fig. 2.12 Superficial spreading melanoma.

is sometimes present and histologically represents tumor regression.

2.3.4 Nodular Melanoma

Nodular melanoma makes up approximately 15 to 20% of melanoma diagnoses. Tumors arise on areas of increased UV radiation exposure including head and neck and upper extremities. Nodular melanomas are darkly or variably pigmented smooth or papillomatous nodules that may demonstrate erosion, ulceration, or spontaneous bleeding at late stages (▶ Fig. 2.13).

2.3.5 Acral Melanoma

Acral melanoma or acral lentiginous melanoma (ALM) is a subtype commonly encountered on acral site or within the nail unit. ALM is the most common type of melanoma in patients with skin of color such as those of Asian, African American, or Caribbean decent. Men and women are equally afflicted with ALM, and patients commonly present in middle age. Clinically, tumors may present as darkening of the skin under or surrounding the nail. Hutchinson's sign—which is a dark-brown or black discoloration in the proximal nail fold at the end of a linear black streak through the nail—may be an indicator of melanoma in the nail matrix (▶ Fig. 2.14). As with all melanomas, these tumors may grow in size, change color, and ultimately ulcerate and bleed. Differential diagnosis for these lesions includes pyogenic granuloma, glomus tumor, subungual hematoma, talon noir, tinea nigra, and Kaposi's sarcoma.

2.3.6 Mucosal Melanoma

Melanoma may present on any mucosal surface. Physicians should consider mucosal melanoma for any pigmented lesion on mucosal surface, especially when demonstrating exophytic growth, ulceration, or bleeding.

2.3.7 Desmoplastic and Amelanotic Melanoma

While different histologically, desmoplastic and amelanotic melanoma are clinically similar entities. These lesions present as flesh-toned, pink, or white papules. Desmoplastic melanoma

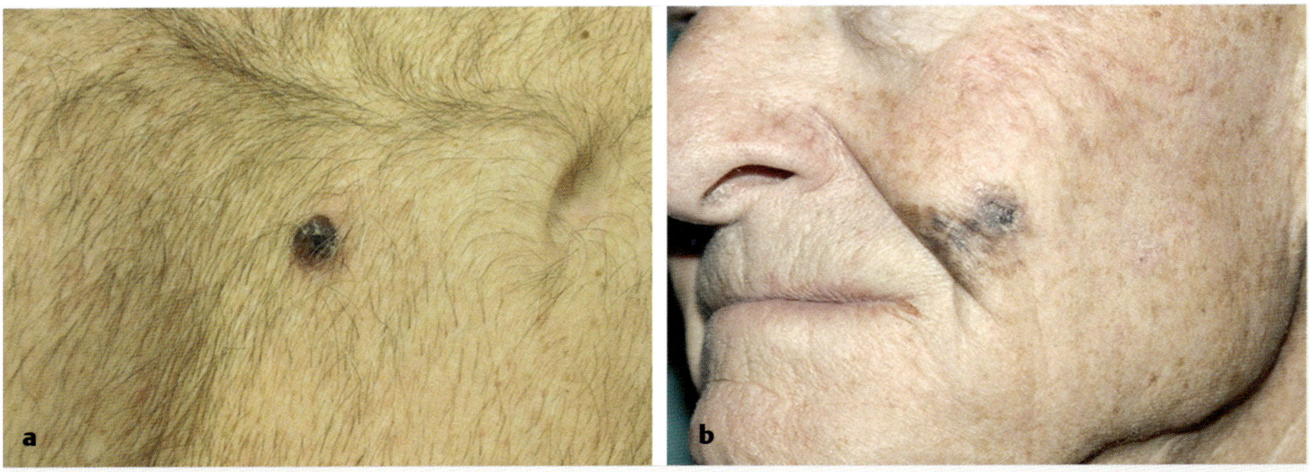

Fig. 2.13 (a, b) Nodular melanoma.

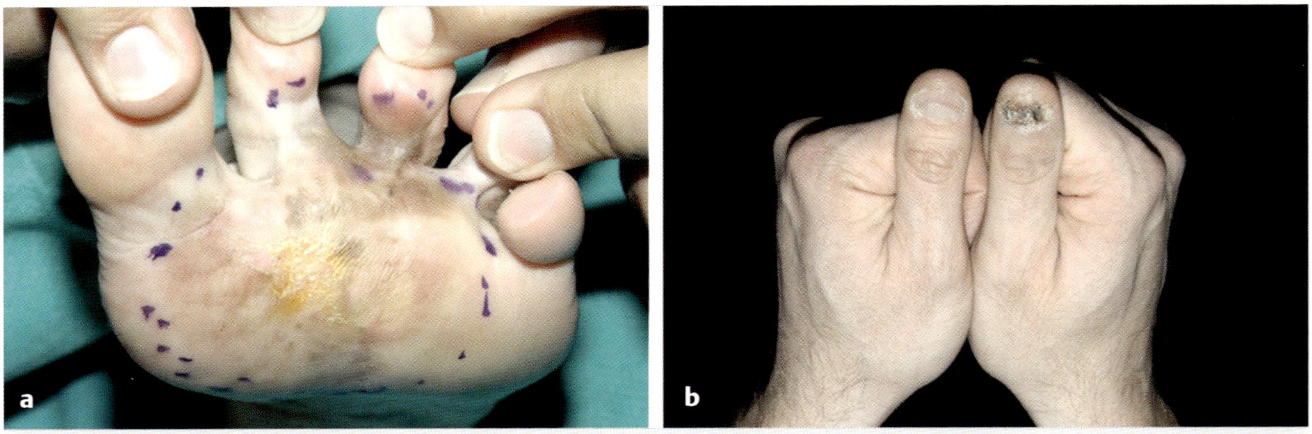

Fig. 2.14 (a, b) Acral melanoma.

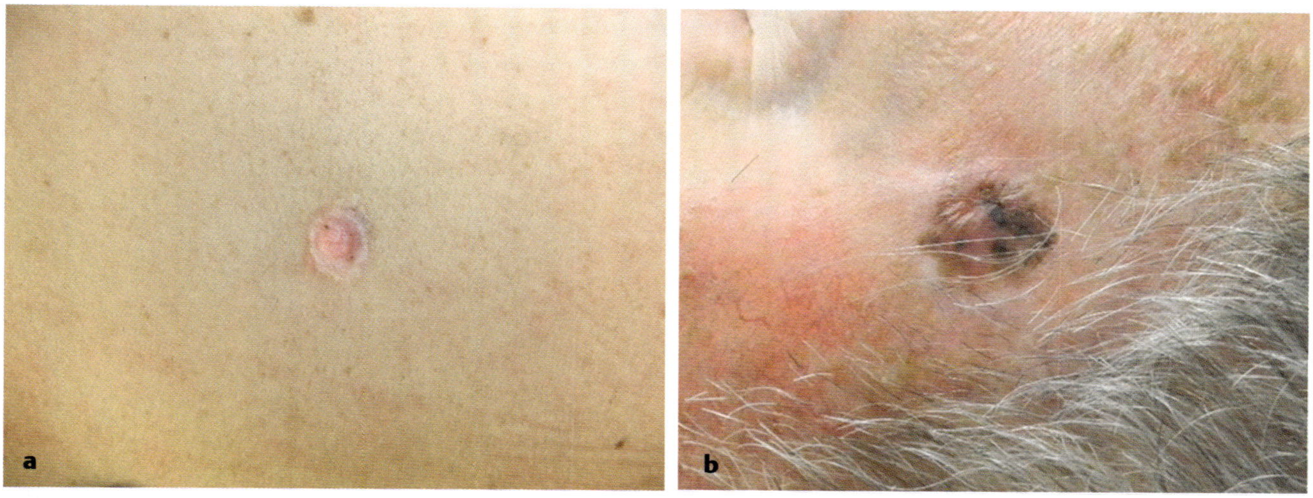

Fig. 2.15 (a) Desmoplastic melanoma. (b) Firm shiny plaque consistent with desmoplastic melanoma extending from lentigo maligna.

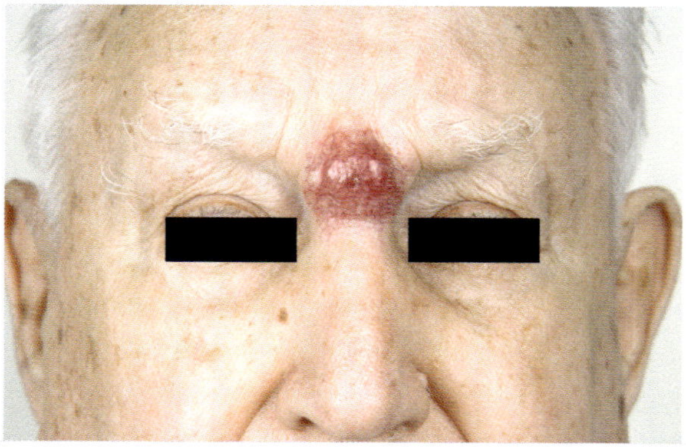

Fig. 2.16 Merkel cell carcinoma of the forehead.

is commonly found on head and neck, and has been described in close proximity to LM. Amelanotic melanoma is the most common subtype found in patients with albinism (▶ Fig. 2.15).

2.4 Merkel Cell Carcinoma

Merkel cell carcinoma (MCC) is a rare form of skin cancer thought to be derived from dermal or epidermal Merkel cells. MCCs occur most commonly in elderly fair-skinned individuals with median age of onset 65 years with a slight male predominance. Many cases are caused by Merkel cell polyomavirus (MCV). They have a predilection for UV-exposed areas on the head and neck, face, and upper extremities. Clinically, these tumors appear as shiny, firm dark-red to violaceous dermal nodules (▶ Fig. 2.16). MCCs are usually asymptomatic. Tumors are generally symmetric and dome-shaped. To aid in diagnosis, the acronym "AEIOU" has been offered to identify key clinical features: asymptomatic, expanding rapidly, immune suppression, older than 50 years of age, and UV damaged.[9] MCC is an aggressive form of skin cancer that has tendency to locally recur and/or metastasize. MCC occurs in greater frequency in older patients, with median age of onset 65 years.

2.5 Dermatofibrosarcoma Protuberans

Dermatofibrosarcoma protuberans (DFSP) is the malignant counterpart to benign dermatofibroma. These rare cutaneous malignancies present mainly on the trunk and proximal extremities as elevated, firm, skin-toned to red nodules or plaques (▶ Fig. 2.17). They tend to grow slowly with time and may ulcerate or bleed. These tumors tend to become painful in their later stages due to tumor invasion into nerve fibers.

2.6 Types of Biopsy Techniques, Rational, Pitfalls

2.6.1 General Principles

Skin biopsies of suspected neoplasms are conducted for several reasons. First and foremost, a skin biopsy is obtained to provide histologic diagnostic evidence regarding a neoplasm of uncertain significance. Skin biopsies can provide important prognostic evidence as well. For example, punch biopsies help determine the depth of an invasive melanoma for staging purposes. Biopsies might also be conducted with a therapeutic or curative intent if sufficient tissue is taken and margins are rendered negative by a pathologist. Specific methodologies for biopsy will be discussed individually, and should be tailored to conditions such as lesion type, location on body, concern for cosmesis, and type of skin involved.

Before a biopsy is performed, it is important to conduct a thorough history and physical examination. A discussion of risks and benefits should also be conducted, and consent obtained. Skin should be cleansed with isopropyl alcohol, chlorhexidine, or povidone iodine. Skin should then be anesthetized with an injectable local anesthetic, such as lidocaine 1%.

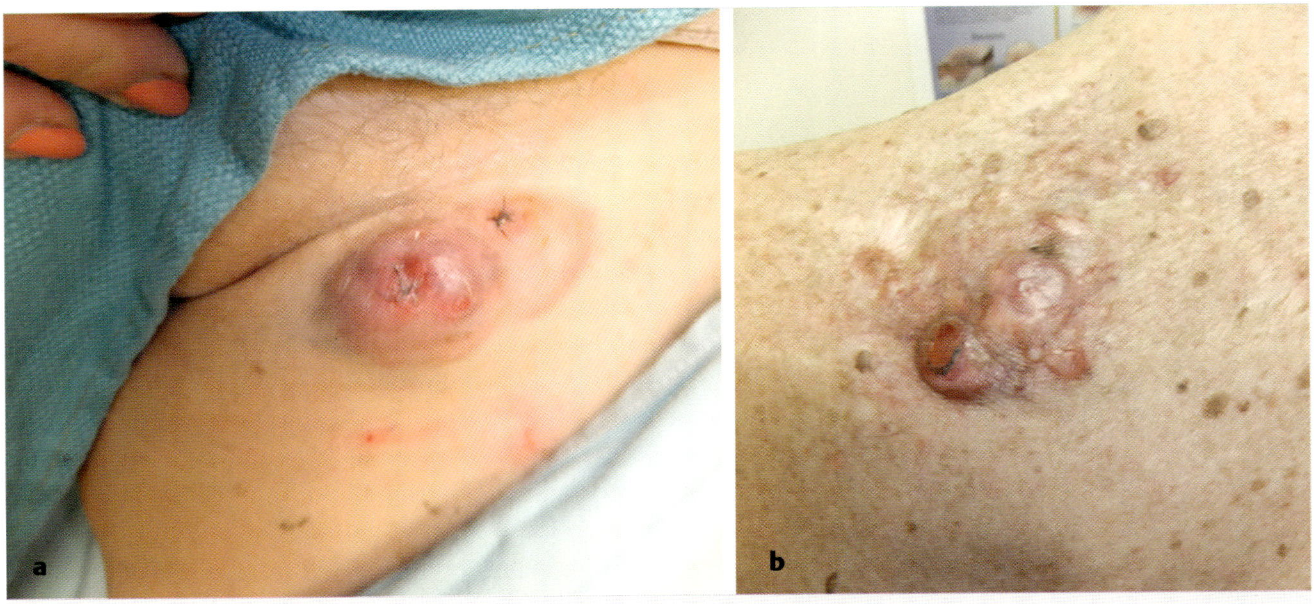

Fig. 2.17 (a) Dermatofibrosarcoma protuberans (DFSP) involving the groin fold. (b) Another DFSP.

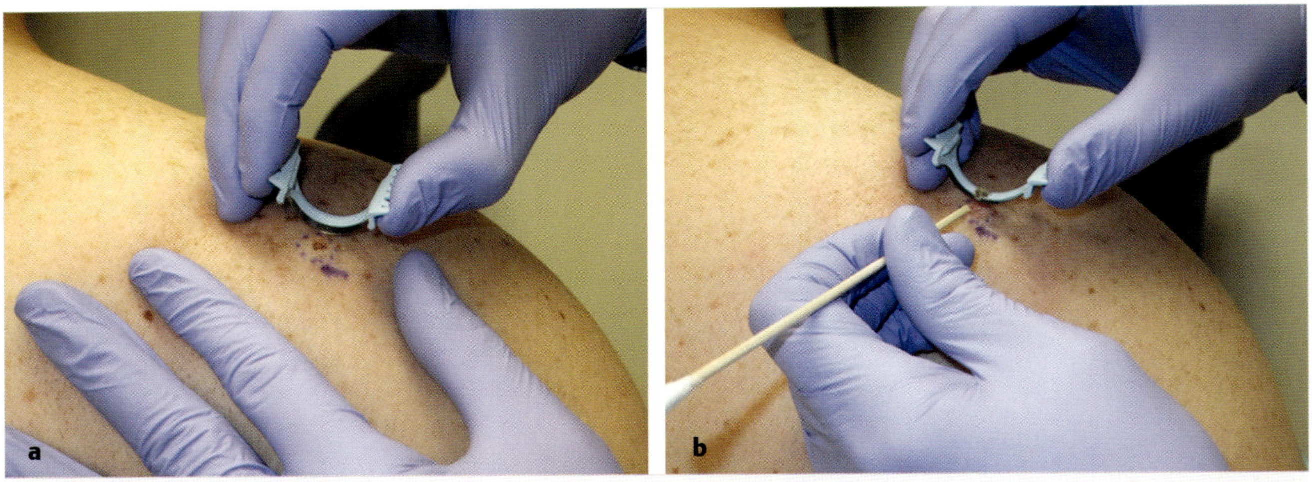

Fig. 2.18 Demonstration of shave biopsy.

2.6.2 Shave Biopsy

A shave biopsy is conducted with a Dermablade, No. 10 or 15 blade. Anesthetic is injected subcutaneously, such that it creates a wheal in the dermis. While stretching the skin, the blade is used to saw through the lesion (▶ Fig. 2.18). Forceps may be used to aid retrieval of the specimen. A hemostatic agent such as aluminum chloride 20% should be applied along with gentle pressure after the procedure. Shave biopsy is preferred for exophytic growths such as SCC, BCC, and KA. For LM, a broad shave or several small "scouting" shaves are preferred to other biopsy techniques. This technique is minimally invasive, requires no sutures, and can be performed quickly in the office. Cosmesis is generally acceptable. Common side effects of this procedure include oval to round scar at site of procedure, postprocedure hyperpigmentation, and possibly cutaneous depression.

2.6.3 Scoop Shave

A "scoop shave" is utilized for lesions that may extend deeper into the dermis or subcutis. A Dermablade may be preferred due to the innate pliability of the instrument. One or more sutures for hemostasis may need to be placed based on depth of the shave.

2.6.4 Punch Biopsy

The punch biopsy technique allows for histologic visualization of all levels of skin from epidermis to subcutaneous fat. As such, punch biopsy is the preferred technique for inflammatory dermatoses. The punch biopsy technique for neoplasms is typically utilized when the depth of tumor invasion is required for diagnostic or prognostic purposes. Punch or excisional biopsy is the technique of choice for lesions suspected to be melanoma. As depth at diagnosis is key to tumor staging and prognosis, these factors cannot be ascertained from a previously shave-biopsied lesion. This technique may also be used with curative intent, if a sufficient size of punch is used to provide curative margins around the lesion of interest. This is known as punch excision. Punch instruments come in a number of sizes. Smaller punches of 1- to 3-mm diameter can be used without the use of sutures. Generally speaking, punch biopsies of 4-mm or greater diameter should be closed with one or more interrupted sutures for adequate hemostasis and cosmesis.

After selecting an appropriately sized instrument, the skin should be made taut by stretching in a direction perpendicular to relaxed skin tension lines. When done properly, an oval-shaped skin defect will form after the procedure, allowing for easy closure. Using a twisting motion between index finger and thumb, the punch is drilled perpendicularly into the skin. Forceps and scissors are used to cut the specimen from attached underlying subcutaneous fat.

Pitfalls of the punch biopsy technique include insufficient epidermal sampling from a small biopsy (2 or 3 mm), and creation of histologic artifact if the skin is crushed with forceps during transfer. To avoid insufficient sampling, several "scouting punches" are often conducted in a larger lesion (i.e., melanoma) to properly sample the neoplasm for both diagnosis and determination of the accurate depth of lesion. Patients should be warned that a small linear scar will likely result from the procedure.

2.6.5 Excisional Biopsy

Excisional biopsies may be utilized to remove a suspected skin cancer in toto. For lesions with strong clinical suspicion for malignancy, or for those lesions too large to remove via punch biopsy, an excisional technique may be useful. Standard margins for excisional biopsy of pigmented lesions are 1 to 3 mm for lesions less than 2 cm. These margins are favored in order to minimally disrupt local skin lymphatic networks in the event that a sentinel lymph node biopsy procedure is needed for those lesions ultimately diagnosed as melanoma.

2.7 Role of Dermoscopy

Dermoscopy or amplified surface microscopy—the microscopic examination of cutaneous neoplasms in vivo—can increase diagnostic sensitivity and specificity in the hands of trained clinicians. A handheld, lightweight dermatoscope illuminates and magnifies skin surface 10 to 20 times the naked eye. When combined with immersion fluids, the upper layer of the skin can be rendered translucent, allowing for better visualization of targeted lesions from epidermis to upper dermis. Newer dermatoscopes equipped with polarized light accomplish the same visualization without immersion fluids. Dermoscopy has been used to more closely describe a broad range of cutaneous neoplasms. We will focus on the technique's utility for classifying pigmented lesions and briefly describe criteria for other common cutaneous malignancy such as BCC. When used in the proper clinical context, dermoscopy improves accuracy and sensitivity for diagnosis of melanoma and BCC over the naked-eye examinations, decreasing needless biopsies.[10] Dermoscopy is often combined with whole-body digital photography or one of a number of advanced diagnostic machines for high-risk patients, a technique that has been demonstrated to increase the detection of melanoma.[11]

2.7.1 Pigmented Neoplasms

Pigmented lesions can microscopically demonstrate a range of unique features such as pigment networks and pseudonetworks, globules, streaks, and parallel pattern. Standardization of the evaluation of pigmented lesions using dermoscopy was accomplished at the Consensus Net Meeting on Dermoscopy, held in 2001 in Rome (for detailed information, see www.dermoscopy.org).[12] This meeting established a consensus two-step algorithm for classification of clinically pigmented lesions using dermoscopy. The first step differentiates lesions between melanocytic and nonmelanocytic pigmented lesions. The following structures were identified as belonging to melanocytic lesions: pigment network or pseudonetwork, aggregated globules, streaks, homogeneous blue pigmentation, or parallel pattern on palms and soles. If none of these features are identified, the lesions should be evaluated for a number of features corresponding to a diagnosis of nonmelanocytic confounder such as seborrheic keratosis, vascular lesion, or pigmented BCC.

After determining that a lesion is likely melanocytic, the consensus classification method guides the clinician to grade the lesion as benign or malignant. Of the many algorithms for grading pigmented lesions, the four most commonly used methods described are pattern analysis described by Pehamberger et al, ABCD rule of dermatoscopy described by Stolz et al, the 7-point checklist by Argenziano et al, and Menzie's method, of course each with modifications and exceptions.[13,14] We will detail the most basic method, pattern analysis.

Pattern analysis relies on the use of discrete elements to formulate a diagnosis (▸ Table 2.1). Elements analyzed include pigment network, diffuse pigmentation, depigmentation, brown globules, black dots, radial streaming, pseudopods, gray-blue veil, and negative pigment network. Melanoma is characterized by irregular networked or diffuse pigment, irregular areas of depigmentation, brown globules, and black dots that are varied in size and irregularly distributed (▸ Fig. 2.19). Melanoma shows radial streaming, pseudopods, and blue-gray veil (▸ Fig. 2.20, ▸ Fig. 2.21, ▸ Fig. 2.22).[15]

2.7.2 Basal Cell Carcinoma

Characteristics of BCC include arborizing vessels, leaflike areas, pigmented (blue-gray, brown-gray) ovoid nests, blue-gray globules, ulceration, and spoke wheel–like areas (▸ Fig. 2.23). Ovoid nests and globules of pigment without definable pigment network are common for BCCs (▸ Fig. 2.24). Spoke wheel–like areas are areas of pigment radiating from a central hub.[16]

2.7.3 Confounders

Confounders such as seborrheic keratoses show milialike cysts and comedolike openings, hairpin blood vessels, sharp demarcation of border, networklike structures, and fingerprintlike structures (▸ Fig. 2.25). Angiomata demonstrate red, blue, or black uniform lacunae (▸ Fig. 2.26). Banal nevi and solar lentigines display regular pigment networks, regular borders, black dots over grids of pigment network, brown-black globules at center, and homogeneous colors (▶ Fig. 2.27).

2.8 Use of Artificial Intelligence Machines

Artificial intelligence (AI) machines are emerging as clinical tools to aid in the detection of skin cancer, primarily melanoma. The current consensus gold standard for diagnosis of melanoma is examination of skin lesion(s) by a trained dermatologist followed by pathological examination of a biopsy of the skin specimen.[17] Most skin examinations are conducted using the naked eye. Clinicians are tasked with finding aberrant pigmented lesions among a plethora of banal nevi. The goal of new AI machines is to improve biopsy decision-making and ultimately find more cutaneous malignancies.

Table 2.1 Pattern analysis of pigmented lesions

	Compound nevus (benign)	Junctional nevus (benign)	Superficial spreading melanoma	Lentigo maligna melanoma	Nodular melanoma
General appearance	Orderly	Orderly, uniform	Polymorphous	Polymorphous	Polymorphous or uniform
Surface	Smooth; hyperkeratotic	Skin surface preserved or smooth, no scale	Skin surface not preserved; may be elevated; irregular	Preserved surface; flat	Not preserved, nodular, smooth, or hyperkeratotic
Pigment pattern	Regular pigment network, blurred; even and regular brown globules; central in tense uniform pigmentation; black dots at center of lesion may occur	Regular pigment network at periphery; uniform and regularly spaced brown globules; central uniform pigmentation; black dots in center of lesion may occur	Irregular, prominent pigment network; brown and black globules of uneven size; intensely colored patches; black dots at periphery; areas of uniform pigment blue-gray to brown in color	Highly irregular; prominent pigment network; loss of pigment network in nodular areas	Usually uniform pigment; at periphery a thin rim of prominent and irregular pigment; uniform black dots at periphery gray, blue, brown, or black in color
Border	Regular, simple outline; network thins at periphery	Regular, pigment network thins at periphery	Pigment network irregular; stops abruptly at edge; pseudopods and radial streaming present	Pigment network stops abruptly at edge; pseudopods and radial streaming present	Pigment network irregular, stops abruptly; pseudopods either blue or black; radial streaming present
Depigmentation or hypopigmentation	Regular; well defined	Usually absent	Bizarre and irregular with pink or white areas	White and pink areas of depigmentation with irregular outline	White and pink areas with irregular outline; often speckled with black and blue dots

Source: Adapted from Pehamberger et al.[13]

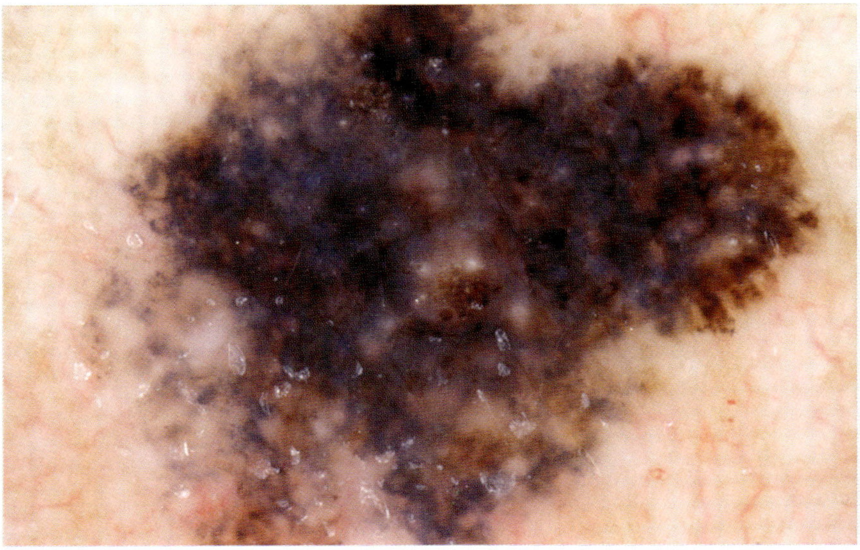

Fig. 2.19 Melanoma in situ (Mis) demonstrating irregular pigment network, areas of diffuse pigmentation, and irregular areas of depigmentation. (Dermatoscopic images are courtesy of Dr. Jeffrey Meffert.)

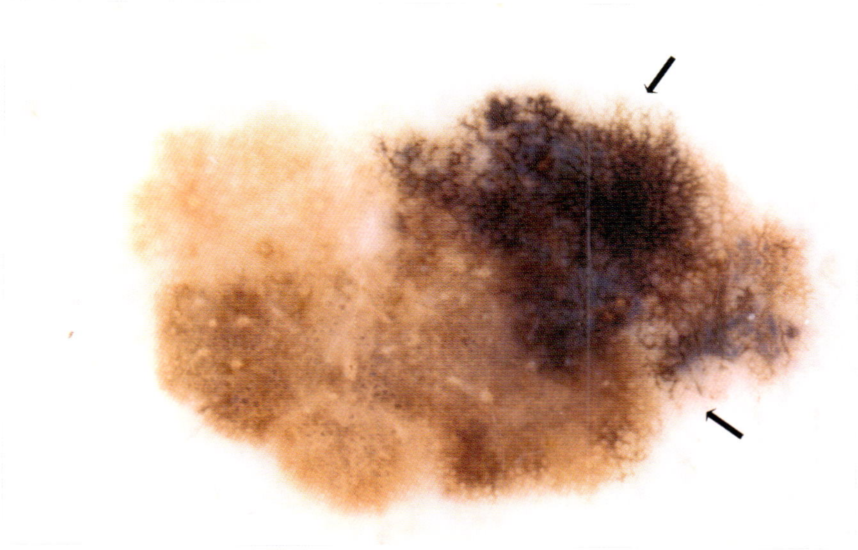

Fig. 2.20 Invasive melanoma arising in a nevus. Arrows demonstrate areas of radial streaming. Also note prominent blue-gray veil through the more heavily pigmented portion of the lesion.

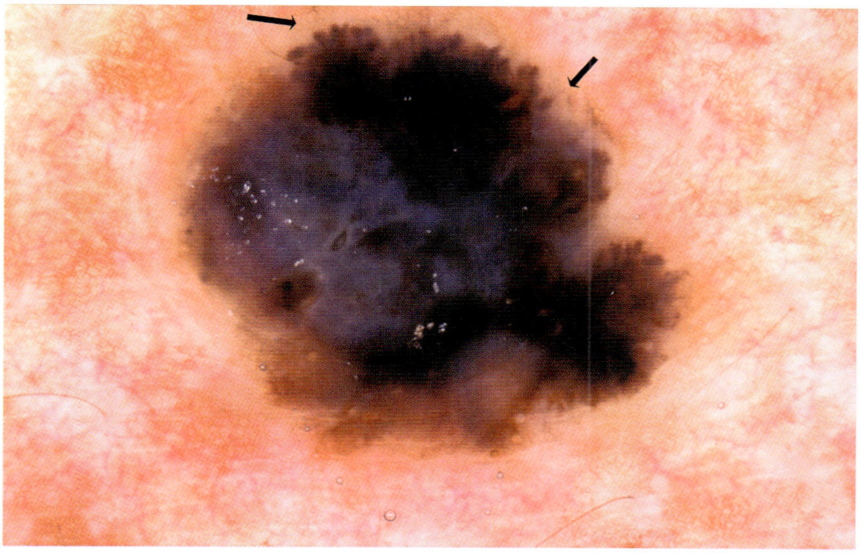

Fig. 2.21 Invasive melanoma demonstrating prominent blue-gray veil. Arrows demonstrate pseudopods at periphery.

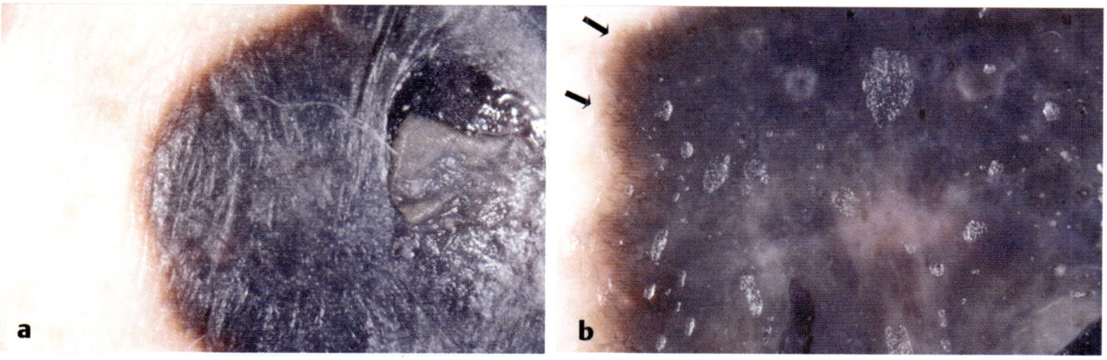

Fig. 2.22 **(a)** Large, ulcerated nodular melanoma. **(b)** Dermatoscopic image demonstrating blue-gray veil, diffuse pigmentation, and irregular central depigmentation. Arrows demonstrate radial streaming.

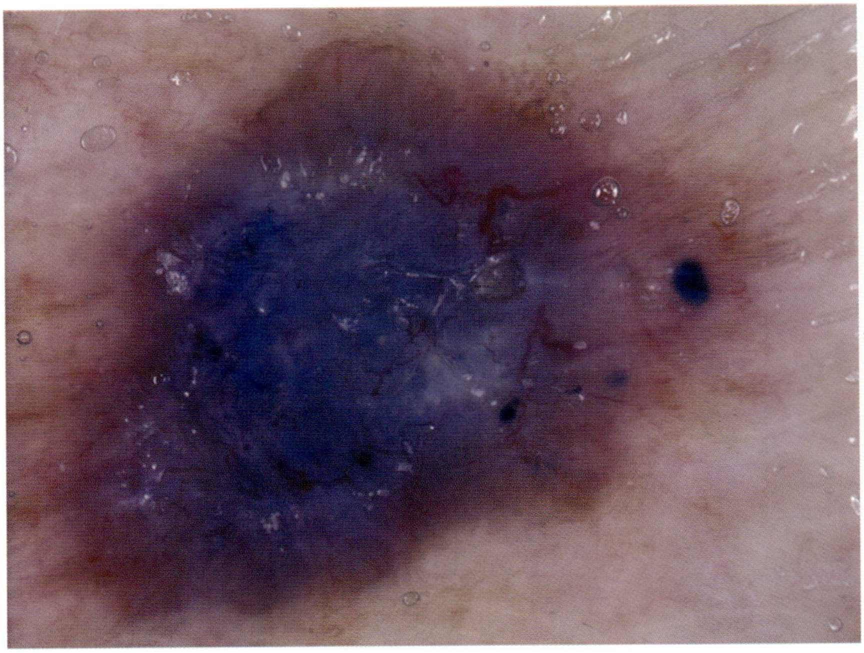

Fig. 2.23 Pigmented nodular basal cell carcinoma. The lesion demonstrates arborizing telangiectasia and large blue ovoid nests.

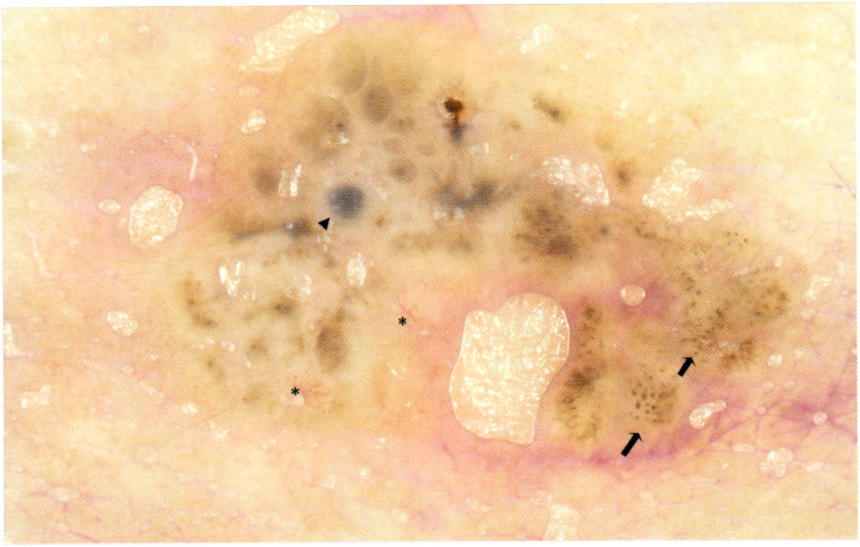

Fig. 2.24 Pigmented nodular basal cell carcinoma. Arrows point to multiple blue-gray globules, arrowhead to large blue-gray ovoid nest, asterisks to arborizing telangiectasias.

2.8.1 MelaFind

MelaFind (MELA Sciences, Inc., Irvington, NY) is a user-friendly handheld imaging device designed to aid in the diagnosis of melanoma among atypical melanocytic lesions, that is, those that have one or more clinical or historical characteristics of melanoma. The device received premarket approval by the Food and Drug Administration in November 2011, as a pigmented lesion biopsy tool. It is available for physicians trained in the clinical diagnosis of skin cancer who have completed the MelaFind training program. MelaFind utilizes 10 spectral bands of light, from 430 to 950 nm (blue to near-infrared) to analyze pigmented lesions in vivo. Images captured with the handheld device are analyzed by software for lesion symmetry, color variation, perimeter changes, texture changes, and wavelet maxima. MelaFind software algorithms are proprietary, having been developed with use of clinical and histopathological data from nearly 9,000 biopsied lesions from 7,000 test patients. MelaFind differs from other novel AI diagnostic tools in that it ultimately provides a "lesions score" and makes a recommendation for or against biopsy for the operator.

Not all lesions are considered suitable for MelaFind, and several restrictions are described. It can be used for lesions between 2 and 22 mm that are accessible to the handheld component of the machine and at least 1 cm away from the eye. Target lesions must be pigmented; MelaFind is not suitable for evaluation of amelanotic or skin-toned nevi. Skin must be intact without ulceration, bleeding, scale crust, ink markings, or foreign matter. Lastly, several anatomic sites are off-limits, including palmar, plantar, mucosal, and subungual regions. Lesions should always be evaluated with MelaFind in the context of a full-body skin examination.

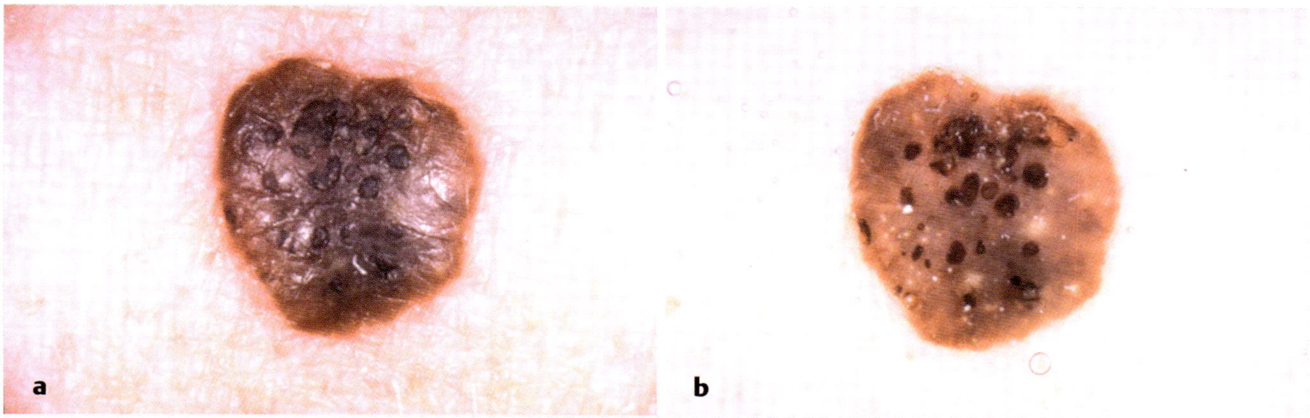

Fig. 2.25 (a, b) Seborrheic keratosis. This waxy, brown, "stuck-on" lesion displays many milialike cysts and comedolike openings throughout lesion.

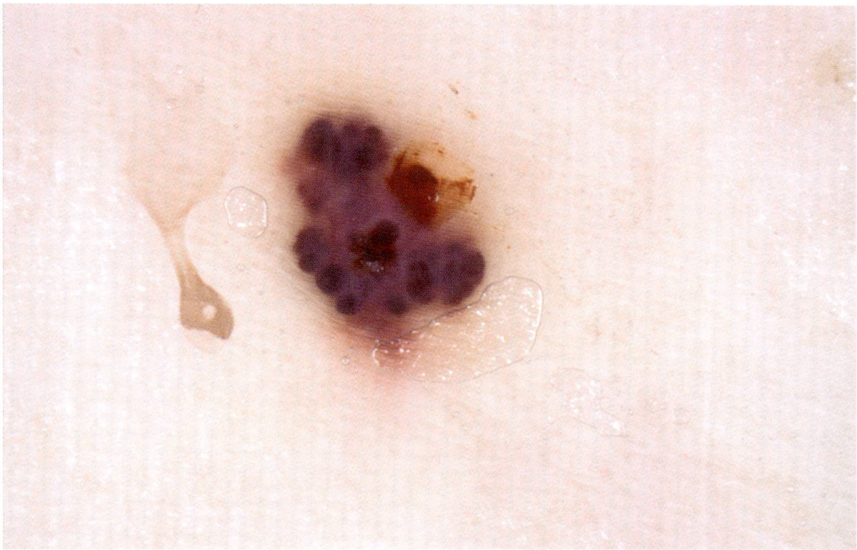

Fig. 2.26 Cherry angioma, made up of uniform red and violaceous lacunae.

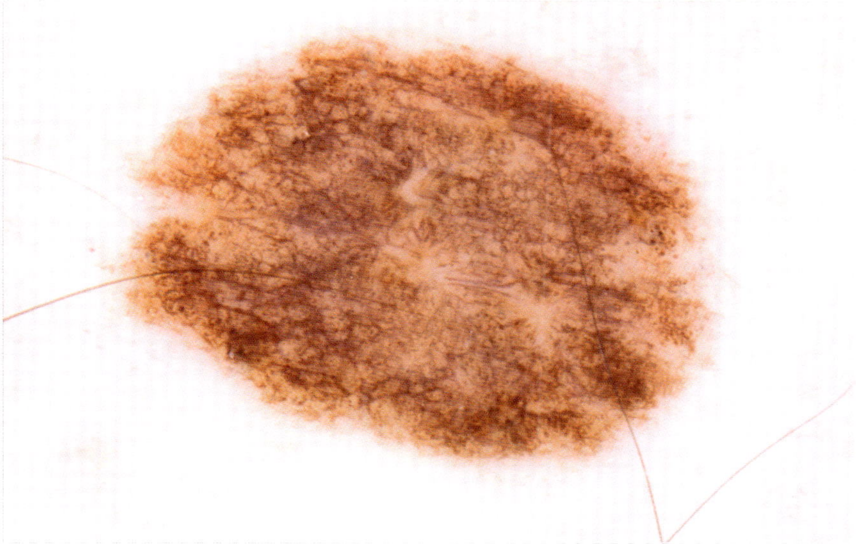

Fig. 2.27 Banal compound nevus showing regular pigment network, uniform color. Pigment network stops abruptly at periphery of lesion.

Clinical trial data have confirmed the utility of MelaFind to aid detection of melanoma. The pivotal trial examined MelaFind use at seven different sites within the United States on 1,831 lesions from 1,383 patients.[18] In the study, MelaFind showed sensitivity of 98.4% and specificity of 9.9% for detection of melanoma. This was compared with values of 78% sensitivity and 3.7% specificity for clinician standard examinations with or without the aid of a dermatoscope. The biopsy ratio (i.e., the number of normal or benign lesions biopsied for detected melanoma or high-grade dysplastic nevus) was 7.6. This is compared to varied reports of biopsy ratio for unaided clinicians from 1:5 to 1:500, and similar to those values reported for experienced dermatologists with demoscopy.[19,20] MelaFind has the potential to enable clinicians to detect more melanoma while sparing more benign lesions, limiting unneeded procedures and potentially decreasing overall health care costs.

2.8.2 Confocal Microscopy and Other Nonstandard Assays and Techniques

Confocal Scanning Laser Microscopy

Confocal scanning laser microscopy (CSLM) is yet another noninvasive imaging tool garnering increased attention in both the clinical and research setting. CSLM captures in vivo horizontal images of skin from epidermis to papillary dermis in real time. CSLM works by focusing a laser beam at a point on the skin. Light is reflected back through an aperture on the device. There are two modes, reflectance and fluorescence. In the clinical setting, CSLM utilizes the reflectance mode, which takes advantage of the inherent variability in reflectance patterns of various skin organelles and appendages. Melanin granules have high refractive index. This allows visualization of the concentration and uniformity of melanin concentration and melanocytes.[21] Hemoglobin can also be visualized, allowing for interpretation of blood flow. Reflectance confocal microscopy (RCM) uses a near-infrared 830-nm laser, which provides an imaging depth of 250 to 300 µm in normal skin, allowing visualization into the superficial dermis.

Clinical trials show that CSLM has excellent sensitivity (88.15–97.5%) and specificity (83–99%) for determining melanoma or melanoma in situ from benign melanocytic lesions when utilized by a trained operator.[22,23,24] While automated models are in development, CSLM still relies on clinician interpretation of image output in order to make a decision to biopsy.

SIAscope

Similar to MelaFind, spectrophotometric intracutaneous analysis (SIA) utilizes images captured using a range of radiation from 400 to 1,000 nm to aid in the clinical diagnosis of melanoma. The clinical device is aptly named the SIAscope (Biocompatibles, Farnham, Surrey). SIAscope is used by centering the handset on a pigmented lesion of maximum size of 24 mm. Eight narrowband images are obtained of skin lesions in vivo, and software analyzes cutaneous chromophores such as melanin, blood, and collagen within the papillary dermis. Information can be gathered regarding the position of melanin relative to the dermoepidermal junction, that is, allowing a clinician to assess melanocyte invasion in real time. Images obtained by SIAscope are returned to clinical as SIAgraphs, which contain detailed information of dermal components for clinicians.[25]

Clinical trials demonstrate that siascopy may aid in clinical detection of melanoma when one or more characteristic patterned features are identified. For example, identification of dermal melanin, blood displacement with blush (defined as central blood displacement with peripheral blood increase compared to surrounding normal skin), and lesion size greater than or equal to 6 mm along predicted diagnosis of melanoma with an 82.7% sensitivity and 80.1 sensitivity.[25] Presence of deep dermal melanin, used as a single feature, predicted diagnosis of melanoma with 96.2% sensitivity and 56.8% specificity in a test set of 348 pigmented lesions.

2.9 Common Look-Alikes

2.9.1 Seborrheic Keratoses

Over one-half of all adult patients will have at least one seborrheic keratosis (SK), a benign lesion commonly described as a waxy-brown, "stuck-on," or "barnaclelike" hyperkeratotic papule (▶ Fig. 2.28). SKs have a predilection for the trunk, but may be ubiquitous. Lesions are symmetric, and often oval-shaped, as they stretch along skin tension lines. Variants include flatter macular seborrheic keratoses of the face and head, stucco keratoses—multiple SKs of the lower limbs, and dermatosis papulosa nigra—a more heavily pigmented variant in darker skinned individuals. Seborrheic keratoses should be clinically recognized, and biopsy or excision avoided. Differential diagnosis includes pigmented lesions or common warts.

2.9.2 Lentigo

Lentigo or lentigo simplex represents a tan or light-brown macule on sun-exposed areas such as face, dorsal hands, and forearms. Pigment is usually even, and borders are sharp (▶ Fig. 2.29). These lesions represent acquired melanocytic

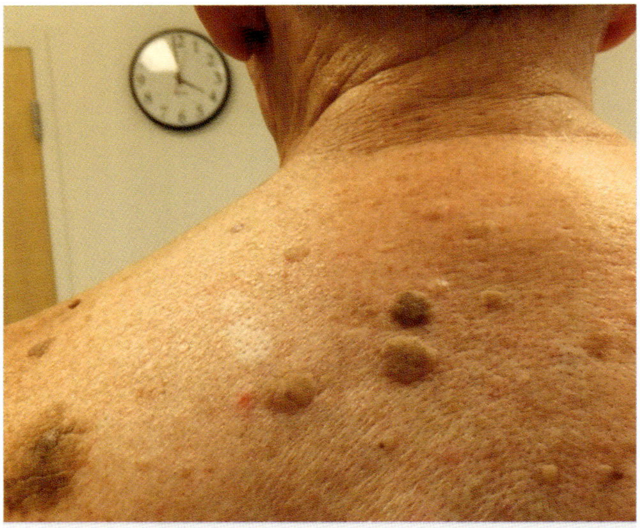

Fig. 2.28 Numerous seborrheic keratoses across the upper back of an elderly male.

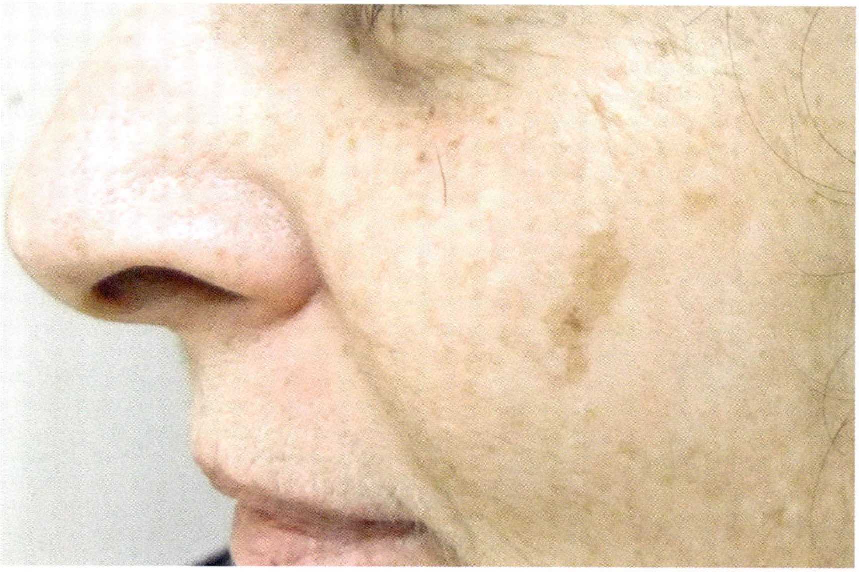

Fig. 2.29 Multiple prominent facial lentigines.

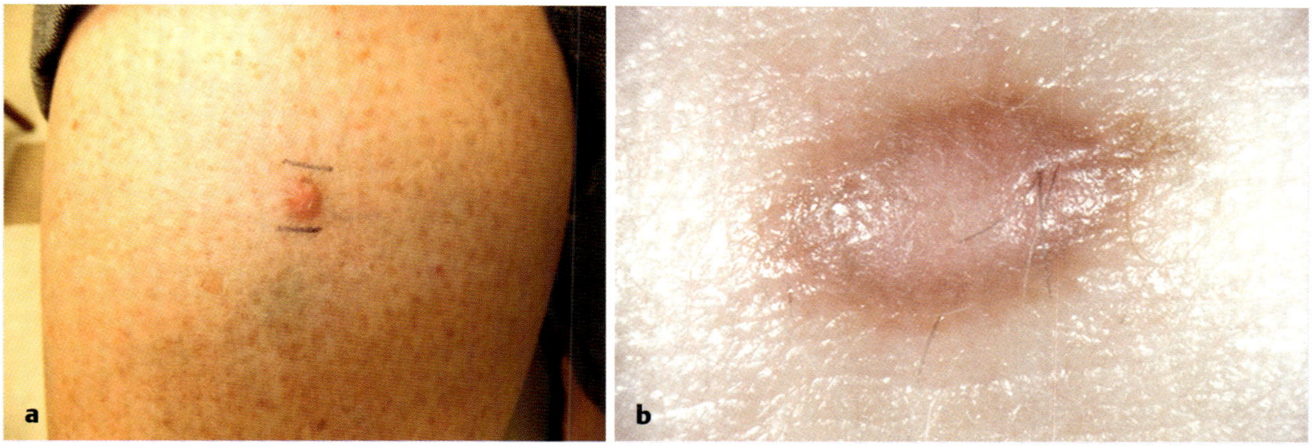

Fig. 2.30 (a, b) Dermatofibroma. Two examples of shiny brown or pink papules commonly on the lower extremities of females.

hyperplasia. Patients are typically over 30 years of age, fair-skinned, and have background UV damage.

2.9.3 Dermatofibroma

A dermatofibroma (DF) is a small (< 1 cm) symmetric papule or nodule usually found on the lower extremities of females. DFs may appear brown or pink with color accentuated on the periphery of the lesion (▸ Fig. 2.30). When manually pinched, DFs have a characteristic central depression; this is known as the "dimple sign." These lesions may itch or sting given that they are made of proliferating fibroblasts and may encompass cutaneous nerves. DFs are thought to be the result of local minor trauma induced by acts such as shaving. These lesions are benign with no malignant potential.

2.9.4 Acrochordon

More commonly known as skin tags, acrochorda are commonly seen in patients over the age of 40 in areas of skin friction such as the groin, axilla, or neck crease (▸ Fig. 2.31).

2.9.5 Sebaceous Hyperplasia

Sebaceous hyperplasia manifests as a small waxy or greasy yellow papule, usually on the central face. These lesions are small, commonly less than 5 mm in size. Lesions may have slight central dell or depression (▸ Fig. 2.32). They may be grouped (▸ Fig. 2.33). Lesions of sebaceous hyperplasia are commonly confused for BCC.

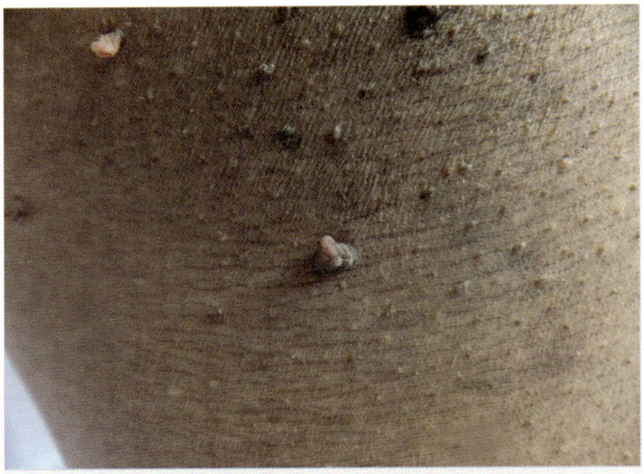

Fig. 2.31 Multiple acrochorda in the right axillary vault of a middle-aged African American male.

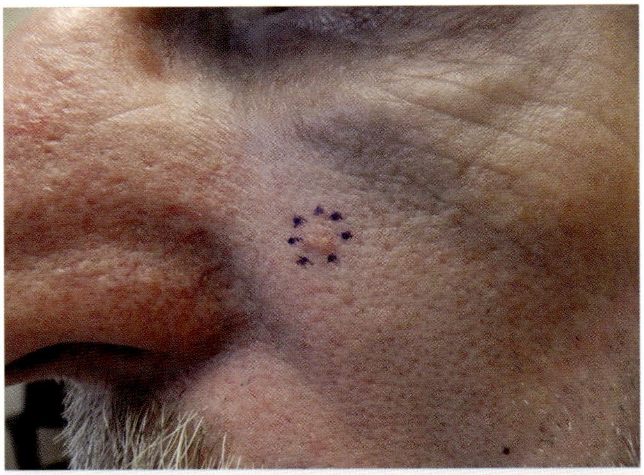

Fig. 2.32 Sebaceous hyperplasia. Lesions are commonly yellow or pink and display a central dell or depression.

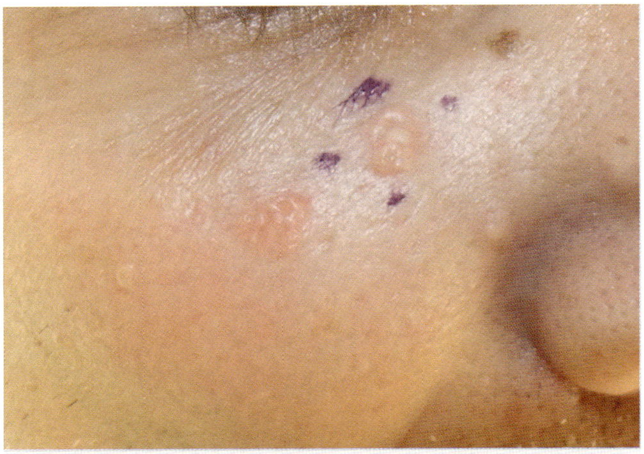

Fig. 2.33 Grouped sebaceous hyperplasia.

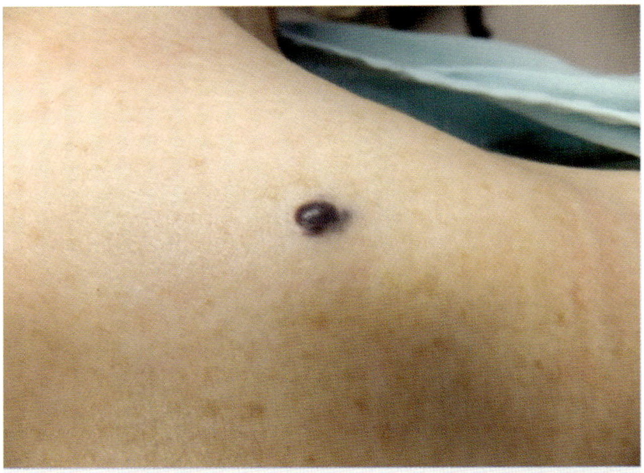

Fig. 2.34 Thrombosed angioma.

2.9.6 Cherry Angioma

Angiomata represent small bright red papules commonly of the trunk. Thrombosed angiomata appear purple (▶ Fig. 2.34). Patients with one or more cherry angioma commonly have a strong family history of such lesions. These lesions will blanch when pressure is applied with a transparent glass slide.

2.9.7 Pyogenic Granuloma

A pyogenic granuloma is a rapidly growing red to purple papule that grows commonly in the head and neck, extremities, or oral mucosa (▶ Fig. 2.35). These lesions commonly bleed. Pyogenic granulomas are common in young adults, and overrepresented in pregnant females.

2.9.8 Erosive Pustular Dermatitis of Scalp

There are many chronic inflammatory conditions of the skin that may mimic malignancy. Erosive pustular dermatitis of the scalp develops as enlarging erosive and ulcerative plaques with associated pus and scale crust (▶ Fig. 2.36). Patients are typically older, may have associated solar damage, and can be mistaken for impetiginized SCC or multiple AKs of the scalp.

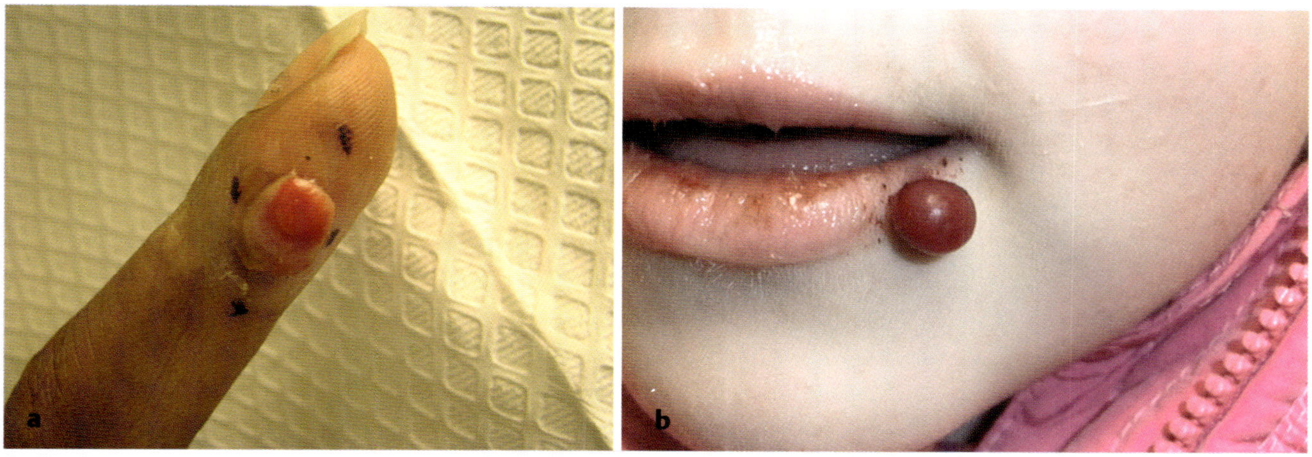

Fig. 2.35 **(a)** Pyogenic granuloma arising on a distal digit.**(b)** Large pyogenic granuloma near the lateral oral commissure of an infant.

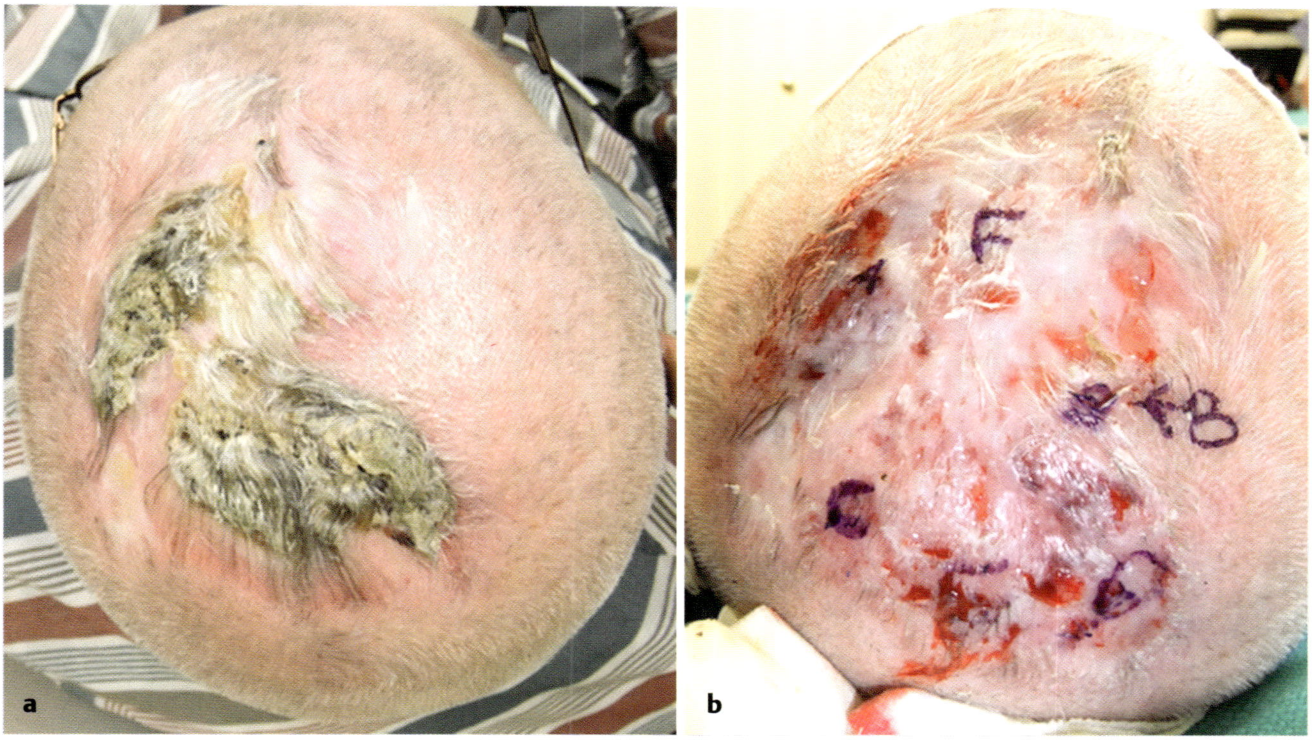

Fig. 2.36 **(a)** Erosive pustular dermatosis of the scalp with overlying scale crust. **(b)** After removal of scale crust.

References

[1] Rogers HW, Weinstock MA, Harris AR, et al. Incidence estimate of nonmelanoma skin cancer in the United States, 2006. Arch Dermatol. 2010; 146 (3):283–287

[2] Quaedvlieg PJ, Tirsi E, Thissen MR, Krekels GA. Actinic keratosis: how to differentiate the good from the bad ones? Eur J Dermatol. 2006; 16 (4):335–339

[3] Browne F, O'Connell M, Merchant W, Potts E, Fenn C, Stables G. Spontaneous resolution of a giant keratoacanthoma penetrating through the nose. Clin Exp Dermatol. 2011; 36(4):369–371

[4] El-Khayat RH, McGrath C, Walsh MY, Ferguson M, Hoey SE. Spontaneous resolution of keratoacanthoma centrifugum marginatum. Clin Exp Dermatol. 2014; 39(7):854–856

[5] Nofal A, Assaf M, Ghonemy S, Nofal E, Yosef A. Generalized eruptive keratoacanthoma: a diagnostic and therapeutic challenge. Int J Dermatol. 2015; 54 (2):160–167

[6] Swetter SM, Boldrick JC, Jung SY, Egbert BM, Harvell JD. Increasing incidence of lentigo maligna melanoma subtypes: northern California and national trends 1990–2000. J Invest Dermatol. 2005; 125(4):685–691

[7] Garbe C, Leiter U. Melanoma epidemiology and trends. Clin Dermatol. 2009; 27(1):3–9

[8] Bradford PT, Anderson WF, Purdue MP, Goldstein AM, Tucker MA. Rising melanoma incidence rates of the trunk among younger women in the United States. Cancer Epidemiol Biomarkers Prev. 2010; 19(9):2401–2406

[9] Heath M, Jaimes N, Lemos B, et al. Clinical characteristics of Merkel cell carcinoma at diagnosis in 195 patients: the AEIOU features. J Am Acad Dermatol. 2008; 58(3):375–381

[10] Carli P, de Giorgi V, Chiarugi A, et al. Addition of dermoscopy to conventional naked-eye examination in melanoma screening: a randomized study. J Am Acad Dermatol. 2004; 50(5):683–689

[11] Wang SQ, Kopf AW, Koenig K, Polsky D, Nudel K, Bart RS. Detection of melanomas in patients followed up with total cutaneous examinations, total cutaneous photography, and dermoscopy. J Am Acad Dermatol. 2004; 50(1):15–20

[12] Argenziano G, Soyer HP, Chimenti S, et al. Dermoscopy of pigmented skin lesions: results of a consensus meeting via the Internet. J Am Acad Dermatol. 2003; 48(5):679–693

[13] Pehamberger H, Steiner A, Wolff K. In vivo epiluminescence microscopy of pigmented skin lesions. I. Pattern analysis of pigmented skin lesions. J Am Acad Dermatol. 1987; 17(4):571–583

[14] Braun RP, Rabinovitz HS, Oliviero M, Kopf AW, Saurat JH. Dermoscopy of pigmented skin lesions. J Am Acad Dermatol. 2005; 52(1):109–121

[15] Pehamberger H, Binder M, Steiner A, Wolff K. In vivo epiluminescence microscopy: improvement of early diagnosis of melanoma. J Invest Dermatol. 1993; 100(3):356S–362S

[16] Longo C, Lallas A, Kyrgidis A, et al. Classifying distinct basal cell carcinoma subtype by means of dermatoscopy and reflectance confocal microscopy. J Am Acad Dermatol. 2014; 71(4):716–724.e1

[17] Patel JK, Konda S, Perez OA, Amini S, Elgart G, Berman B. Newer technologies/techniques and tools in the diagnosis of melanoma. Eur J Dermatol. 2008; 18 (6):617–631

[18] Monheit G, Cognetta AB, Ferris L, et al. The performance of MelaFind: a prospective multicenter study. Arch Dermatol. 2011; 147(2):188–194

[19] Kupetsky EA, Ferris LK. The diagnostic evaluation of MelaFind multi-spectral objective computer vision system. Expert Opin Med Diagn. 2013; 7(4):405–411

[20] Terushkin V, Warycha M, Levy M, Kopf AW, Cohen DE, Polsky D. Analysis of the benign to malignant ratio of lesions biopsied by a general dermatologist before and after the adoption of dermoscopy. Arch Dermatol. 2010; 146 (3):343–344

[21] Meyer LE, Otberg N, Sterry W, Lademann J. In vivo confocal scanning laser microscopy: comparison of the reflectance and fluorescence mode by imaging human skin. J Biomed Opt. 2006; 11(4):044012

[22] Gerger A, Koller S, Kern T, et al. Diagnostic applicability of in vivo confocal laser scanning microscopy in melanocytic skin tumors. J Invest Dermatol. 2005; 124(3):493–498

[23] Gerger A, Hofmann-Wellenhof R, Langsenlehner U, et al. In vivo confocal laser scanning microscopy of melanocytic skin tumours: diagnostic applicability using unselected tumour images. Br J Dermatol. 2008; 158(2):329–333

[24] Langley RG, Walsh N, Sutherland AE, et al. The diagnostic accuracy of in vivo confocal scanning laser microscopy compared to dermoscopy of benign and malignant melanocytic lesions: a prospective study. Dermatology. 2007; 215 (4):365–372

[25] Moncrieff M, Cotton S, Claridge E, Hall P. Spectrophotometric intracutaneous analysis: a new technique for imaging pigmented skin lesions. Br J Dermatol. 2002; 146(3):448–457

3 Treatment of Squamous and Basal Cell Carcinoma of the Skin

Rogerio I. Neves and Morgan Brgoch

3.1 Introduction

Basal cell and squamous cell skin cancers, collectively known as nonmelanoma skin cancers (NMSCs), are the most common cancer in the United States. An estimated 5 million cases of NMSC are diagnosed annually; this exceeds the incidence of all other cancers combined.[1,2] In the United States alone, the diagnosis and treatment of NMSCs has increased dramatically with a growth rate of 77% over the past two decades. The average annual number of adults treated for skin cancer increased from 3.4 million in 2002–2006 to 4.9 million in 2007–2011. During this period, the average annual total cost for skin cancer increased from $3.6 billion to $8.1 billion, representing an increase of 126.2%, while the average annual total cost for all other cancers increased by 25.1%. During 2007–2011, nearly 5 million adults were treated for skin cancer annually, with average treatment costs of $8.1 billion each year, about $4.8 billion for NMSCs and $3.3 billion for melanoma.[2,3] While surveillance and diagnosis has continued to improve, the incidence of this common malignancy also appears to be rising rapidly.[4]

Basal cell carcinomas (BCCs) are roughly four to five times more common than squamous cell carcinomas (SCCs). More than 2.8 million new cases of BCC are diagnosed each year in the United States alone, and are estimated to result in more than 3,000 deaths.[5,6,7] Although rarely metastatic, BCC and SCC can produce substantial local invasion and destruction along with disfigurement and may involve extensive areas of underlying soft tissue, cartilage, and bone.

Cutaneous squamous cell carcinoma (cSCC) is the second most common NMSC worldwide. While most of these lesions can be successfully managed with excision, there is a subset of lesions that metastasize, leading to severe morbidity and mortality. While small, the number of cSCCs that metastasize has been compared to the metastatic rate of renal and oropharyngeal carcinomas.[8]

The skin is a complex organ made up of multiple cell types and many of these cell types can undergo malignant transformation at various points in their differentiation, leading to tumors with distinct histology and dramatically different biological behaviors, such as SCC and BCC. The outer layer or epidermis is made primarily of keratinocytes but has several other minor cell populations. The bottom layer is formed of basal keratinocytes abutting the basement membrane. The basement membrane is formed from products of keratinocytes and dermal fibroblasts, such as collagen and laminin, and is an important anatomical and functional structure. As the basal keratinocytes divide and differentiate, they lose contact with the basement membrane and form the spinous cell layer, the granular cell layer, and the keratinized outer layer or stratum corneum.

The true cytologic origin of BCC remains in question; however, BCC and basal cell keratinocytes share many histologic similarities. Alternatively, the outer root sheath cells of the hair follicle have also been proposed as the cell of origin for BCC.[9,10] This is suggested by the fact that BCCs occur predominantly on hair-bearing skin. BCCs rarely metastasize but can invade tissue locally or regionally, with a potential for perineural invasion and rapid spread. A tendency for superficial necrosis in the center in the lesion has resulted in the characteristic name "rodent ulcer," frequently used to describe such growths.

Similarly, debate remains about the origin of SCC; however, the leading hypothesis illustrates the derivation of cutaneous SCC from epidermal stem cells associated with the hair follicles.[11] A variety of tissues, such as lung and uterine cervix, also give rise to SCC, with varying characteristics depending on the tissue source. SCC derived from different anatomic locations can have moderately differing aggressiveness and expected clinical course; for example, SCC from glabrous (smooth, hairless) skin frequently has a lower metastatic rate than SCC arising from the vermillion border of the lip or from scars.[12]

Estimates of the incidence of BCC are imprecise, given there is currently no central registry that collects data on BCC occurrence. Lower estimates cited by The American Cancer Society estimates that more than 2 million NMSCs were treated in the United States in 2006. However, a population-based study estimated a higher number of lesions, reporting that approximately 3.5 million NMSCs were treated in the United States during the same year.[1] Additionally, several incidence-based mathematical models support a higher prevalence of NMSC in the United States.[13] According to the model, approximately 13 million white non-Hispanic individuals living in the United States in 2007 may have had a personal history of at least one NMSC.

Individuals with a history of BCC are at increased risk for subsequent lesions. Approximately 40% of patients who have had one BCC will develop another lesion within 5 years.[14,15] Multiple epidemiologic observations provide insights into the etiology of BCC. Namely, BCC is particularly common in Caucasians and very uncommon in blacks and other dark-skinned populations. In white populations in the United States, the incidence of BCC has increased by more than 10% per year, and the lifetime risk of developing a BCC is estimated at 30%.[16,17,18] An increasing incidence has also been noted in other countries, such as Canada, Finland, and Australia,[19,20,21] with evidence of increasing incidence of aggressive-growth histologic subtypes.[22]

There is notable geographic variation in incidence, likely secondary to environmental exposures and protection strategies. States closer to the equator, such as Hawaii and California, have an incidence of BCC at least twice that of the Midwestern United States.[23,24,25] There are also prominent global variations in incidence. Northern European countries, such as Finland, have an incidence one-fourth that of the Midwestern United States versus Australia where rates are 40 times that of Finland.[19,26]

Men have a 30% higher incidence than women and also a higher incidence of superficial type BCC.[19,23,27,28] The incidence of BCC increases with age; persons aged 55 to 75 have about a 100-fold higher incidence of BCC than those younger than 20.[29]

Although an aging population with higher life expectancies may account for part of the increasing incidence of BCC, the incidence of BCC among Americans younger than 40 also appears to be increasing, particularly among women.[4]

In the United States, the average age of onset of cutaneous SCC is 65 years;[30] however, there are increasing reports of patients as young as 20 to 30 years of age in regions of higher ultraviolet (UV) exposure such as Florida and southern California. There is a predilection for males, but the incidence of SCC originating on the legs is greater in females. Factors that increase the risk for SCC include Fitzpatrick skin types I and II, outdoor occupations such as farming and construction work, and exposure to human papillomavirus (HPV) types 16, 18, and 31.[31]

Exposure to UV radiation and sunlight is the greatest risk factor, as illustrated in studies showing a direct correlation between psoralen plus ultraviolet A light (PUVA) exposure and the incidence of SCC.[32,33,34,35] In this study, the relative risk for developing SCC in patients with 350 to 450 PUVA treatments compared with less than 50 treatments was 6.01.[13,34] Treatment with PUVA increases the risk for SCC by two mechanisms, which refer to, respectively, its mutagenic effects and its immunosuppressive effects.

Overall, SCC is uncommon in dark-skinned individuals, but it remains the most common cutaneous cancer in African-Americans. In such individuals, the cancer usually occurs in areas that are not sun exposed.[36] Darkly pigmented skin possesses greater amounts of melanin in the epidermis, which partially protects against the carcinogenic effects of UV light. As a result, sun exposure is a less common etiology. As in the overall population, SCC in darker skin is often preceded by the development of actinic keratosis (AK).[37,38]

BCC is a common skin cancer arising from the basal layer of epidermis and its appendages. These tumors have been referred to as "epitheliomas" because of their low metastatic potential. However, the term carcinoma is appropriate, since they are locally invasive, aggressive, and destructive of skin and the surrounding structures including bone.

3.2 Risk Factors for Basal Cell Carcinoma

3.2.1 Ultraviolet Radiation

Sun exposure is the most important environmental cause of BCC, and most risk factors relate directly to a person's sun exposure habits or susceptibility to solar radiation. These risk factors include having fair skin, light-colored eyes, red hair, northern European ancestry, older age, childhood freckling, and an increased number of past sunburns.[39,40,41]

The type, quantity, and timing of sun exposure associated with an increased risk of BCC are not clearly defined. Childhood sun exposure appears to be more important than exposure during adult life.[40,42] In a Canadian case control study that included 226 men with BCC and 406 age-matched controls, the development of BCC was strongly correlated with childhood and adolescent sun exposure but not cumulative or recent sun exposure.[42] In other studies, however, adult sun exposure also was a risk factor for BCC.[41] It has been estimated that aggressive sun protection before the age of 18 years could reduce the number of NMSCs by almost 80%.[43] Several trials provide evidence that sunscreen use decreases the incidence of SCCs and that there are no adverse effects from sunscreen use.[44,45] However, a randomized trial evaluating the effects of sunscreen and the antioxidant beta carotene over a 4-year period found that those using topical sunscreen had a 40% reduction in SCCs but no decrease in BCCs.[46]

The frequency and intensity of sun exposure may also be important. Solar exposure in intermittent, intense increments increases the risk of BCC more than a similar dose delivered more continuously over the same period of time.[47] Evidence in renal transplant recipients provides additional support to the concept that acute or intermittent sun exposure increases the risk of BCC.[48] Additionally, indirect support for an important role for sun exposure is derived from a large, nested case-control study of female nurses.[49] In the study, a contributory role of extensive sun exposure was suggested by the finding that women in the highest quartile for baseline serum vitamin D levels were at greater risk for the subsequent development of BCC than women in the lowest quartile (odds ratio [OR] 2.07; 95% confidence interval [CI]: 1.52–2.80). The authors proposed that the plasma vitamin D level was a potential indicator of the degree of long-term sun exposure.

3.2.2 Tanning Beds

The use of tanning beds may increase the risk for early development of BCC.[50,51,52,53,54] A cohort study of approximately 73,000 female nurses found that women who used tanning beds more than six times per year during high school or college were more likely to develop BCC than women who did not use tanning booths during these time periods (adjusted hazard ratio 1.73; 95% CI: 1.52–1.98).[55] A contribution of UV light exposure from indoor tanning to BCC is also suggested by the results of a 2012 meta-analysis of observational studies.[53] Subjects with a history of any tanning bed use were more likely to develop BCC than those who had never used tanning beds (relative risk 1.29; 95% CI: 1.08–1.53). The relative risk for BCC for individuals who began tanning prior to age 25 was 1.40 (95% CI: 1.29–1.52). A subsequent population-based case-control study, including approximately 650 cases of BCC and 450 controls, found that tanning bed users had a 60% increased risk of developing a BCC at or before the age of 50 years (OR 1.6; 95% CI: 1.3–2.1).[54] The risk was doubled for those reporting a first use of tanning devices before the age of 20.

3.2.3 Chronic Arsenic Exposure

Superficial multicentric BCC occurs 30 to 40 years after chronic exposure of arsenic, which may occur as a result of ingesting contaminated drinking water, seafood, or medications.[56,57,58,59]

3.2.4 Ionizing Radiation

Superficial therapeutic ionizing radiation, as for facial acne, psoriasis, or tinea capitis, increases the risk of NMSC, including BCC.[60,61] The latency period for development of BCCs is estimated to be approximately 20 years, and lesions are limited to sites with radiation exposure. Due to the advent of other effective therapies, the use of ionizing radiation for the treatment of inflammatory skin conditions has declined.

Ionizing radiation used to treat childhood cancers also increases the risk for the subsequent development of BCC. This was illustrated in a study of 776 subjects documenting an approximately 10-fold higher rate of BCC than was expected in this population.[62] All of the BCCs were located within the radiation field. In addition, a case–control study of 199 patients with a history of both childhood cancer and BCC and 597 controls with a history of childhood cancer without BCC found a linear dose–response relationship between the radiation dose and risk for BCC. An increase in risk was detected among patients who received at least 1 Gy of radiation to the skin, and patients who received 35 Gy or more were 40 times more likely to develop BCC than those who were not treated with radiation (OR 39.8; 95% CI: 8.6–185). The treatment of other noncutaneous disorders with radiation therapy (RT) has also been associated with the appearance of BCC.[60,63,64]

Studies of survivors of the atomic bomb explosions in Japan support the role of exposure to ionizing radiation in the development of BCC. In a retrospective study of bomb survivors, the incidence of subsequent BCC increased with proximity to the hypocenter of the explosion.[65]

3.2.5 Therapeutic Exposure

Therapeutic exposure to PUVA for cutaneous disorders such as psoriasis increases the risk of NMSC, particularly SCC.[66,67] The risk of BCC in patients treated with PUVA is lower than the risk for cutaneous SCC. In a 30-year prospective cohort study documenting the incidence of NMSC in patients given PUVA for psoriasis, the increase in risk for BCC was modest compared with cutaneous SCC.[68]

3.2.6 Photosensitizing Drugs

The association of BCC with UV light exposure has led to questions about the impact of photosensitizing drugs on development of BCC. An association between prior use of photosensitizing tetracyclines or diuretics and increased risk for BCC has been documented in several observational studies.[69,70] In addition, an American population-based case–control study of 1,567 adults with BCC and 1,906 controls found a minor increase in risk for multiple BCC (OR 1.4; 95% CI: 1–2.1) and BCC before the age of 51 (OR 1.5; 95% CI: 1.1–2.1) among participants who recalled use of a photosensitizing medication.[69] Additional studies are necessary to clarify the relationship between photosensitizing drugs and BCC.

3.2.7 Immunosuppression

Chronic immunosuppression (as occurs with solid organ transplantation and with human immunodeficiency virus [HIV] infection) may increase risk for the development of BCC, although the increase in risk is less than that observed for SCC.[71] The risk for BCC after solid organ transplantation appears to increase linearly over time, whereas the risk for SCC rises exponentially.[72,73] The increased risk for skin cancer in organ transplant recipients is attributed to chronic exposure to immunosuppressive agents. The specific impact of systemic glucocorticoid therapy on BCC risk is uncertain; studies performed in patients without a history of organ transplantation conflict on whether systemic glucocorticoid therapy significantly increases risk for BCC.[73,74,75]

Support for an increased risk for BCC among HIV-positive individuals was demonstrated in a retrospective cohort study of HIV-positive ($n = 6{,}560$) and HIV-negative ($n = 36{,}821$) non-Hispanic white patients. The study found that patients with HIV infection were approximately twice as likely to develop BCC than patients without HIV infection (adjusted rate ratio 2.1; 95% CI: 1.8–2.3).[76,77]

3.2.8 Previous Personal History of Nonmelanoma Skin Cancer

A personal history of BCC or SCC is strongly associated with subsequent BCC or SCC.[15] There is an approximate 20% increased risk of a subsequent lesion within the first year after a skin cancer has been diagnosed.[15,78,79] The mean age of occurrence for these NMSCs is the mid-60 s.[14,15] In addition, several studies have found that individuals with a history of skin cancer have an increased risk of a subsequent diagnosis of a noncutaneous cancer.[80,81,82,83,84] In the absence of other risk factors or evidence of a defined cancer susceptibility syndrome, as discussed below, skin cancer patients are encouraged to follow screening recommendations for the general population for sites other than the skin.

Genetic variation may play a role in susceptibility to BCC. Some gene sequence variants that are affiliated with increased risk of BCC also correlate with light skin pigmentation.[85] In addition, genome-wide association studies have identified genetic variants (see below) that may influence BCC risk through other pathways, such as an effect on the growth or differentiation of basal layers of the epidermis or an effect on the P53 tumor suppressor gene or hedgehog pathways.[86,87,88,89,90,91,92]

Genes that affect the immune response may also impact susceptibility to BCC. Cytotoxic lymphocyte-associated antigen-4 (*CTLA-4*) is expressed on regulatory T cells and is involved in UV-induced immune tolerance. In a case–control study, genetic variation at the *CTLA-4* locus influenced the risk of BCC, particularly among patients with a higher number of severe sunburns.[93]

The most significant genetic components for BCC are the *PTCH1* and *PTCH2* genes. *PTCH1* mutations in the gene coding for the transmembrane receptor protein *PTCH1*, or *PTCH*, are associated with basal cell nevus syndrome (BCNS) and sporadic cutaneous BCCs. *PTCH1*, the human homolog of the Drosophila segment polarity gene patched (ptc), is an integral component of the hedgehog signaling pathway, which serves many developmental (appendage development, embryonic segmentation, neural tube differentiation) and regulatory (maintenance of stem cells) roles.[94,95]

In the resting state, the transmembrane receptor protein *PTCH1* acts catalytically to suppress the seven-transmembrane protein Smoothened (SMO), preventing further downstream signal transduction.[96,97] Stoichiometric binding of the hedgehog ligand to *PTCH1* releases inhibition of SMO, with resultant activation of transcription factors (*GLI1, GLI2*), cell proliferation genes (*cyclin D, cyclin E, myc*), and regulators of angiogenesis.[97, 98] Thus, the balance of *PTCH1* (inhibition) and SMO (activation) manages the essential regulatory downstream hedgehog signal transduction pathway. Loss-of-function mutations of *PTCH1* or gain-of-function mutations of SMO tip this balance toward constitutive activation, a key event in potential neoplastic transformation.

Demonstration of allelic loss on chromosome 9q22 in both sporadic and familial BCCs suggested the potential presence of an associated tumor suppressor gene.[99,100] Further investigation identified a mutation in *PTCH1* that localized to the area of allelic loss.[101] Up to 30% of sporadic BCCs demonstrate *PTCH1* mutations.[102] In addition to BCC, medulloblastoma and rhabdomyosarcoma, along with other tumors, have been associated with *PTCH1* mutations. All three malignancies are associated with BCNS, and most people with clinical features of BCNS demonstrate *PTCH1* mutations, predominantly truncation in type.[103]

Truncating mutations in *PTCH2*, a homolog of *PTCH1* mapping to chromosome 1p32.1–32.3, have been demonstrated in both BCC and medulloblastoma.[104,105] *PTCH2* displays 57% homology to *PTCH1*, differing in the conformation of the hydrophilic region between transmembrane portions 6 and 7, and the absence of C-terminal extension.[106] While the exact role of *PTCH2* remains unclear, there is evidence to support its involvement in the hedgehog signaling pathway.[104]

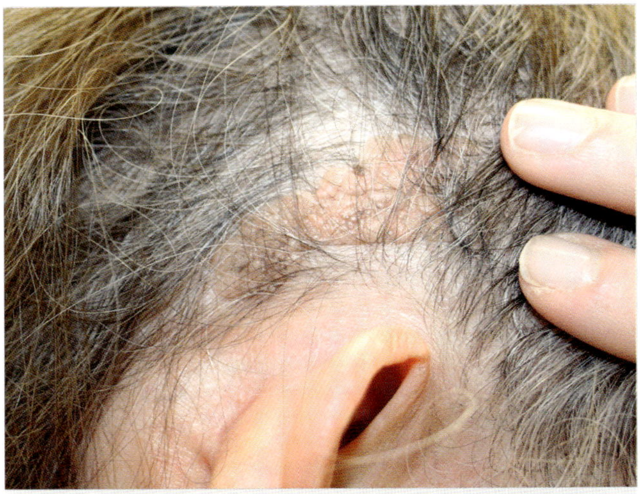

Fig. 3.2 Nevus sebaceous (NS). The diagnosis of NS is usually based upon the clinical presentation. In most cases, NS is apparent at birth and presents as a well-defined, thin, yellow-orange or tan, oval, round, or linear plaque. Sometimes lesions are not noticed until later in childhood or after puberty. A biopsy for histopathologic confirmation may be warranted if the diagnosis is uncertain. The definitive treatment of NS is full-thickness excision. The decision to excise should be made in individual patients, based upon age, extension, and location of the lesion, and patient's or parents' concern about the cosmetic appearance and/or risk of malignancy.

3.2.9 Nevus Sebaceous

Nevus sebaceous (▶ Fig. 3.1, ▶ Fig. 3.2, ▶ Fig. 3.3) is an uncommon congenital hamartoma of the skin composed of epidermal, follicular, sebaceous, and apocrine elements. BCC may develop within nevus sebaceous, though this occurrence is rare. BCCs are the most commonly reported malignant neoplasm occurring in roughly 0.5 to 7% of sebaceous nevi.[107,108] In a retrospective study of 596 nevus sebaceous excisions from adults and

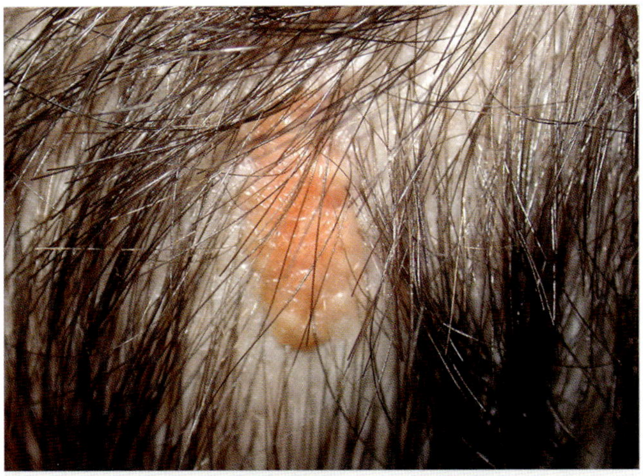

Fig. 3.1 Nevus sebaceous (NS). In infancy and childhood, NS remains mostly unchanged, due to the quiescence of sebaceous glands. At puberty, under hormonal influences, lesions thicken and become verrucous or nodular. Rapid, circumscribed enlargement or ulceration should arouse suspicion for malignant transformation.

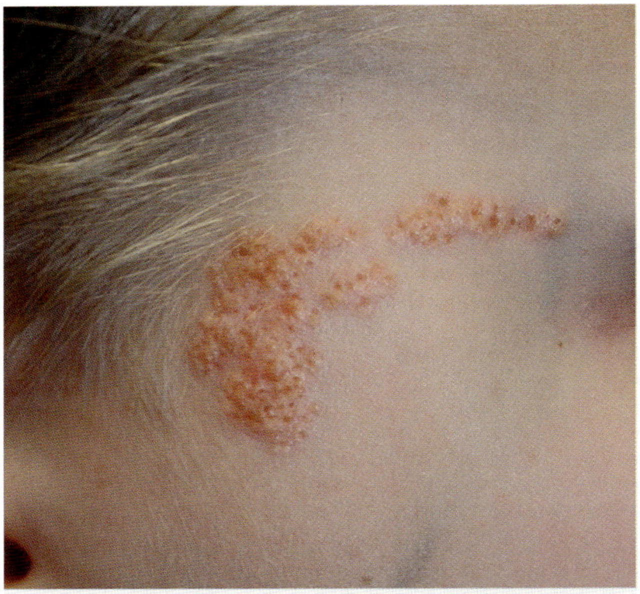

Fig. 3.3 Nevus sebaceous (NS). A variety of benign and malignant epithelial neoplasms may arise within NS. Benign tumors include trichoblastoma, syringocystadenoma papilliferum, trichilemmoma, sebaceoma, nodular hidradenoma, hidrocystoma, and eccrine poroma. Malignant neoplasms include basal cell carcinoma, apocrine carcinoma, trichilemmal carcinoma, sebaceous carcinoma, microcystic adnexal carcinoma, porocarcinoma, and squamous cell carcinoma. The exact incidence and the lifetime risk of malignancy arising in NS are unknown. The risk of malignancy increases with age, but basal cell carcinomas have been reported also in children.

children, BCC was detected in specimens from five adults (0.8%).[109] A separate review of 631 children with 651 lesions of nevus sebaceous found that BCC may also develop within nevus sebaceous in children; BCC was found in excisional specimens from five patients (0.8%).[107]

3.2.10 Inherited Disorders

While most arise sporadically, BCC is also associated with several clinical syndromes including Bazex syndrome, Gorlin's syndrome (BCNS), and highly UV-sensitive conditions such as xeroderma pigmentosum (XP). Constitutive activation of the sonic hedgehog signaling pathway is thought to play a significant role in the majority of BCC pathogenesis.[110,111] Bazex syndrome is characterized by multiple BCCs and follicular atrophoderma.[112] Rombo syndrome presents with atrophoderma vermiculatum and vellus hair cysts with milia-like appearance.[113] Patients with XP are at increased risk for BCC as well as SSCs and melanomas. The incidence of these malignancies for individuals with XP under the age of 20 is approximately 2,000 times that seen in the general population.[114,115,116]

3.2.11 Family History

Individuals with BCCs and/or SCCs report a higher frequency of these cancers in their family members than do controls. The importance of this finding is unclear. Apart from defined genetic disorders with an increased risk of BCC, a positive family history of any skin cancer is a strong predictor of the development of BCC.

3.2.12 Nevoid BCC Syndrome (Gorlin's Syndrome)

Nevoid BCC syndrome is also known as the Gorlin–Goltz syndrome and is inherited in an autosomal dominant manner; however, approximately 30–50% of cases represent sporadic mutations.[117,118,119] Its prevalence has been estimated at approximately 1 in 56,000 and manifests in young adulthood.[120] In most cases, the abnormality is due to a mutation in the patched gene (*PTCH*) of chromosome 9 q22–q31, thereby resulting in upregulated proliferation.[119,121,122]

Currently, no genetic test has been developed for widespread use, and diagnosis remains based on clinical criteria. The diagnosis may be established with documentation of two major criteria or one major and two minor criteria[123,124] (▸ Table 3.1).

Table 3.1 Major and minor diagnostic criteria for diagnosis of nevoid basal cell carcinoma syndrome (NBCCS)

Major criteria	Minor criteria
Multiple (> 2) BCCs at any age or one BCC less than 20 y or > 10 BCCs	Congenital skeletal defects: bifid, fused, splayed, or missing rib, or bifid, wedged, or used vertebra
Histologically proven odontogenic keratocyst or a polyostotic bone cyst	Cardiac or ovarian fibroma
Palmar or plantar pits (3 or more)	Medulloblastoma
Ectopic calcification: bilamellar or early (< 20 y) calcification of the falx cerebri	Large head with occipitofrontal circumference > 97th percentile, with frontal bossing
Family history of basal cell nevus syndrome	Congenital malformation: cleft lip and/or palate, polydactyly, congenital eye defect such as cataract, microphthalmos or coloboma

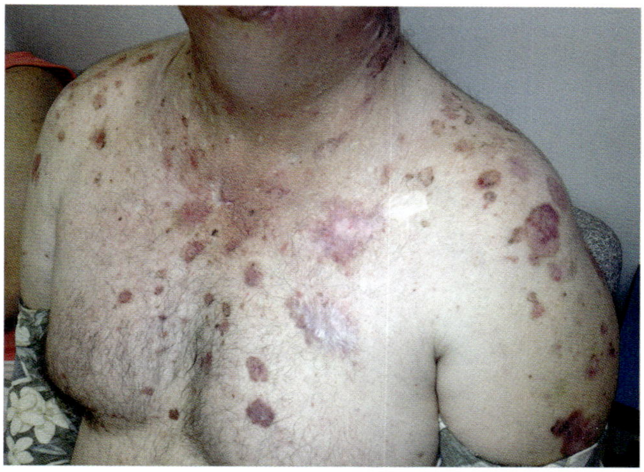

Fig. 3.4 Gorlin's syndrome. People with Gorlin's syndrome need education about the syndrome, and may need counseling and support because coping with the multiple BCCs and multiple surgeries is often difficult. Genetic counseling is advised for prospective parents, since one parent with Gorlin's syndrome have 50% chance that their child will also be affected.

3.3 Clinical Features

The clinical features of nevoid BCC syndrome include the presence of numerous BCCs with a higher prevalence of nodular, superficial, and infundibulocystic types (▸ Fig. 3.4). Patients may also have cysts of the skin (steatocystomas) and bone, particularly the mandible (▸ Fig. 3.5) and maxilla (odontogenic keratocysts).[118,123] Also present are skeletal anomalies including spinal and rib deformities, excessive ossification of cranial bones and falx cerebri with concurrent frontal bossing and bridging of the sella turcica.[118,123,125] Palmoplantar pits (▸ Fig. 3.6 and ▸ Fig. 3.7) may appear during the second decade of life in addition to psychiatric or neurologic dysfunction including schizophrenia, mental retardation, and cerebellar degeneration.[126,127] In the absence of distinct criteria, clinical suspicion of Gorlin's syndrome may be indicated for any patient with multiple histologically proven BCCs arising at a young age. Morbidity and premature mortality in nevoid basal cell carcinoma syndrome (NBCCS) are primarily related to the development of skin cancers and other tumors associated with the syndrome.

The BCNS (NBCCS Gorlin's syndrome) is a rare, autosomal dominant disorder due to germline mutations of the human patched gene (PTCH). The histologic appearance of the BCCs in BCNS does not differ from those seen in sporadic cases. The

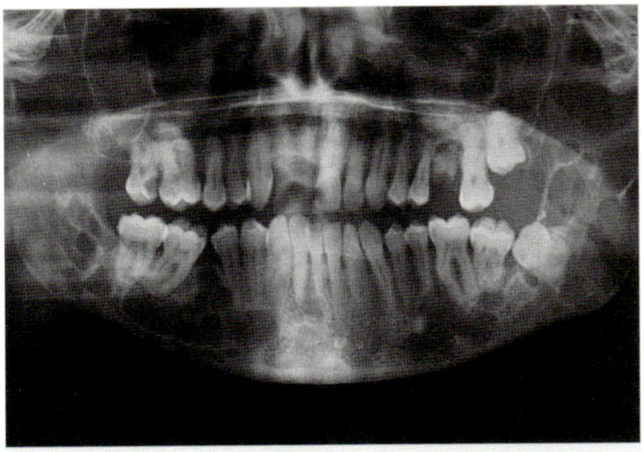

Fig. 3.5 Mandibular cysts of Gorlin's syndrome. When patients with Gorlin's syndrome have mandible tumors, they are characterized as keratocystic odontogenic tumors. Above is a Panorex example.

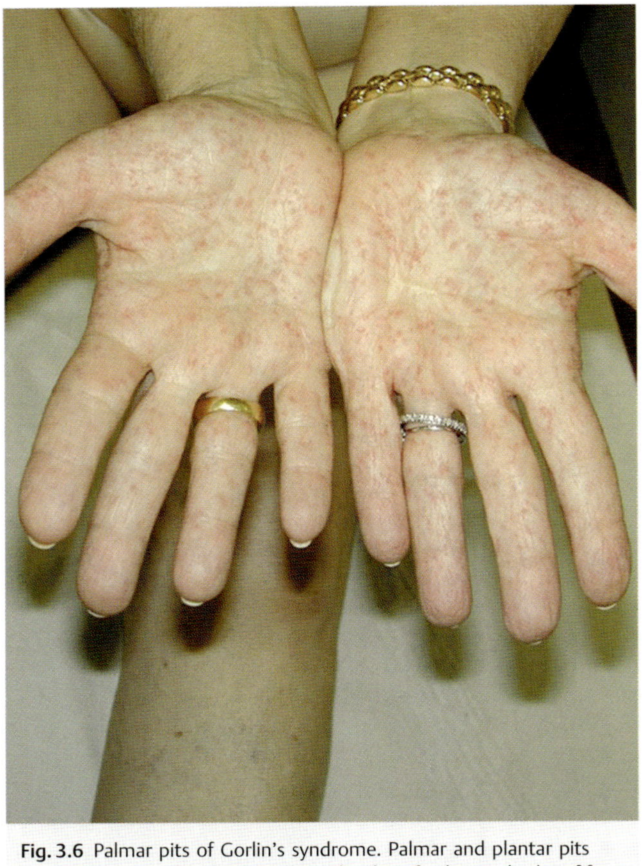

Fig. 3.6 Palmar pits of Gorlin's syndrome. Palmar and plantar pits appear as punctiform depressions in the skin of palms and soles of feet. These changes are caused by a partial or complete absence of the stratum corneum. They are usually asymmetric, flesh-, pink- or red-colored, and range from 2 to 3 mm in diameter and 1 to 3 mm in depth. In Gorlin's syndrome, pits appear in 30 to 65% of patients by the age of 10 years and in 85% of patients over the age of 20 years.

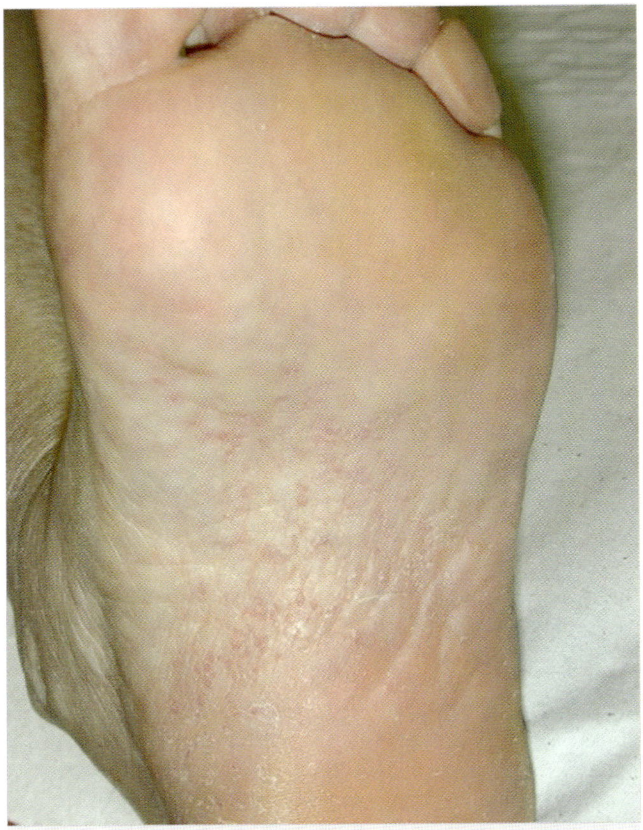

Fig. 3.7 Plantar pits of Gorlin's syndrome.

diagnosis should be suspected in patients who present with multiple BCCs, especially when these occur at an early age and are located on the trunk. These patients require aggressive approaches to therapy and frequently are disfigured from surgical treatments by the third decade of life. Affected patients have distinct clinical features and predilection for multiple tumors, especially multiple BCCs, usually by age 35.[99] Clinical features often include macrocephaly, hypertelorism, bifid ribs, palmar and plantar pitting, osseous cysts (of the mandible), and medulloblastoma (3–5%).[99,128]

3.4 Prevention of Basal Cell Carcinoma

The primary approach to the prevention of BCCs is protection from UV radiation exposure. The various techniques to minimize solar exposure are discussed elsewhere. Data on the prevention of BCC through additional drugs or therapies are controversial.[129,130,131,132] The results of an 11-month randomized trial of 240 patients with actinically damaged skin suggested that celecoxib may be beneficial for chemoprevention. In this trial, patients treated with celecoxib (200 mg twice daily for 9 months) developed fewer BCCs than patients who were given placebo (adjusted rate ratio 0.40; 95% CI: 0.18–0.93).[133] In contrast, a Danish population-based case–control study failed to find an association between the use of celecoxib or other prescription nonsteroidal anti-inflammatory drugs (NSAIDs) and overall risk for BCC.[134] Another population-based case–control study did not find an association between the use of any NSAIDs and the overall risk of BCC.[135] In subgroup analyses, a modest risk reduction was observed among long-term users of ibuprofen (OR 0.85; 95% CI: 0.77–0.94), and risk was further reduced among mono-users (OR 0.61; 95% CI: 0.48–0.78).[135]

The Australian Oral Nicotinamide to Reduce Actinic Cancer (ONTRAC) trial preliminarily showed that nicotinamide, a form of vitamin B3, significantly reduced the rates of new cutaneous malignancies in people at high risk of the disease.[136] Taken as a twice-daily pill, nicotinamide reduced the incidence of new nonmelanoma skin cancers (NMSCs) by 23%. AK was reduced in the nicotinamide group by 11% at 3 months and by 20% at 9 months of usage. Researchers believe that nicotinamide thus helps replenish cellular energy after sunlight exposure, giving cells the energy boost they need to repair deoxyribonucleic acid (DNA) damage and prevent immune suppression.[136]

3.5 Clinical Presentation

Approximately 70% of BCCs occur on the face, consistent with the etiologic role of solar radiation. Fifteen percent present on the trunk, and only rarely is BCC diagnosed on areas like the penis, vulva, or perianal skin. Clinically, BCCs appear as pearly and telangiectatic papules or nodules with or without ulceration, or as indurated, erythematous, or ulcerated patches with a discrete papular border, and may be pigmented. BCCs display different morphological growth patterns: superficial or multifocal, nodular, micronodular, infiltrating, sclerosing (sclerodermiform), or morpheaform.

The diversity in the phenotypic appearance of BCCs indicates that the cell of origin may be a stem or progenitor cell. Moreover, these observations raise the question as to whether BCC is a monoclonal tumor or whether it is the result of field cancerization. Studies investigating clonal patterns of X chromosome inactivation suggest that the majority of BCCs do represent monoclonal tumors and that anatomically distinct BCCs may sometimes share the same cellular origin.[137]

About 30% of BCCs are superficial BCCs. For unclear reasons, men have a higher incidence of superficial BCC, in particular, than women. Superficial BCCs most commonly occur on the trunk, and typically present as slightly scaly, nonfirm macules, patches, or thin plaques light red to pink in color (▶ Fig. 3.8 and ▶ Fig. 3.9). The center of the lesion sometimes exhibits an atrophic appearance and the periphery may be rimmed with fine translucent papules. A shiny quality may be evident when a superficial BCC is illuminated. Occasionally, spotty brown or black pigment as shown in ▶ Fig. 3.10 is present, which may contribute to confusion with melanoma.[138] These lesions are referred to as pigmented BCCs. However, both nodular and superficial BCCs can produce pigment. Superficial BCCs tend to grow slowly, and can vary in size from macules measuring just a few millimeters in diameter to lesions several centimeters in diameter or more if left untreated. Superficial BCCs are usually asymptomatic.[138,139,140]

Nodular BCCs, which represent about 60% of cases, typically present on the face as a pink or flesh-colored papule. As shown in ▶ Fig. 3.11, ▶ Fig. 3.12, ▶ Fig. 3.13, ▶ Fig. 3.14, these lesions usually have a pearly or translucent quality and a telangiectatic vessel is frequently seen within the papule. Ulceration is frequent, and the term "rodent ulcer" refers to these ulcerated nodular BCCs. Nodular BCCs in particular may resemble adnexal

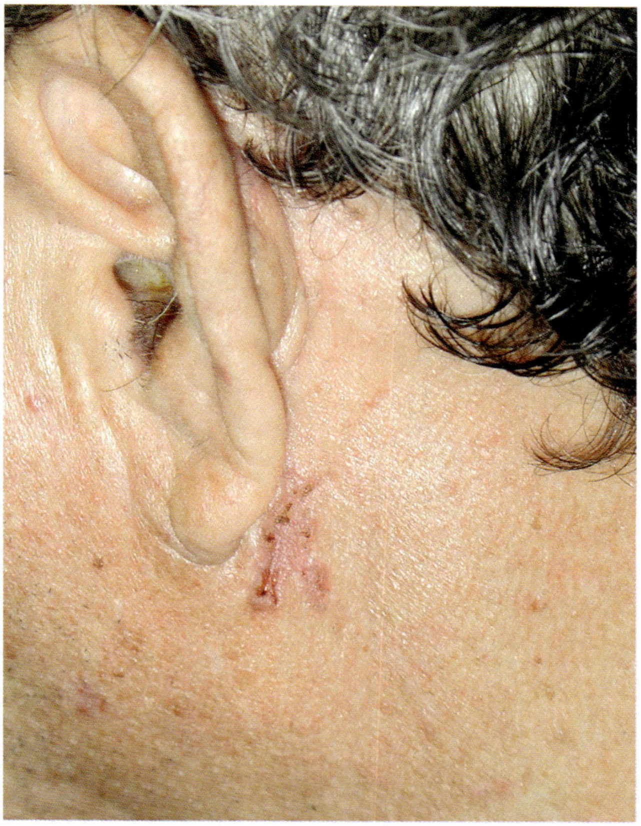

Fig. 3.8 Superficial basal cell carcinoma (BCC). Superficial BCCs are usually asymptomatic. They present as a flaky erythematous lesions with irregular borders that are slightly elevated.

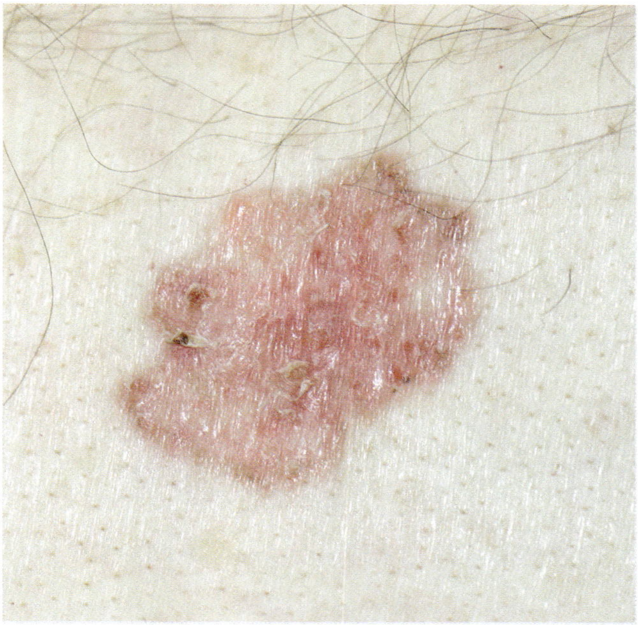

Fig. 3.9 Superficial basal cell carcinoma (BCC). These often grow slowly but can grow to several centimeters in size if neglected.

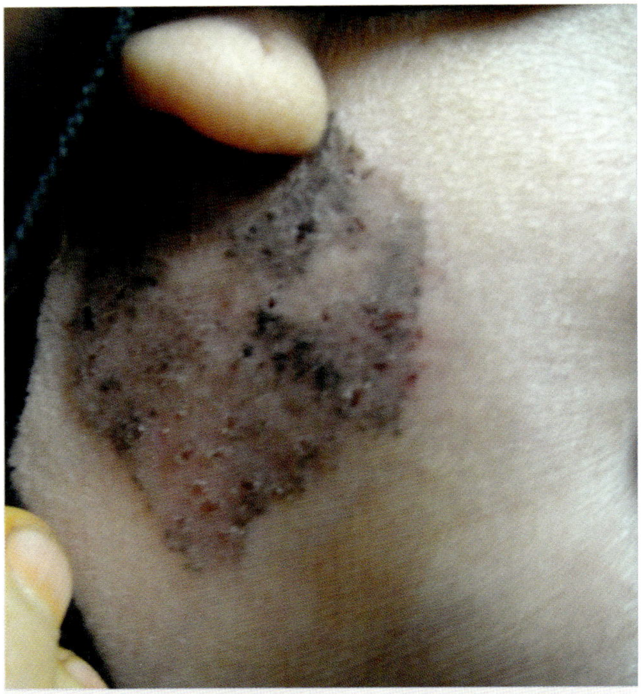

Fig. 3.10 Pigmented superficial basal cell carcinoma (BCC). It may also be pigmented or resembling a benign inflammatory process, especially psoriasis, seborrheic eczema, or nummular dermatitis.

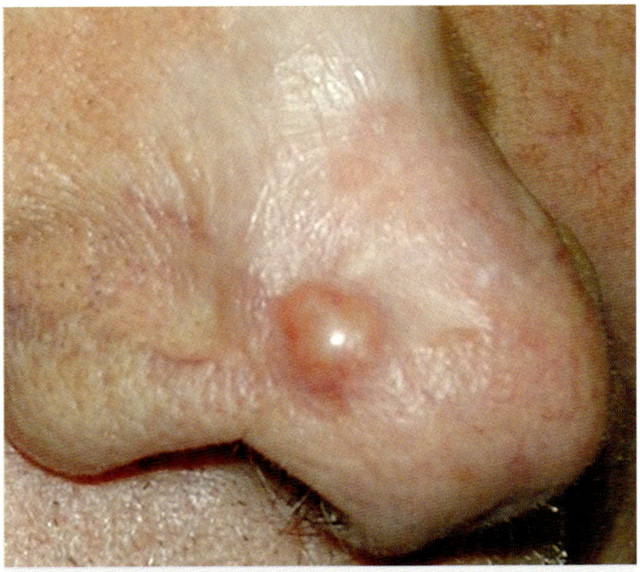

Fig. 3.11 Nodular basal cell carcinoma (BCC). The nodular type of basal BCC presents as a pink papule often with pearly borders and fine telangiectasias.

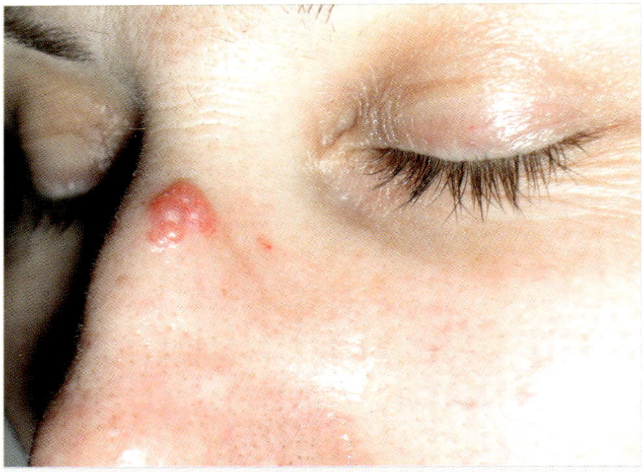

Fig. 3.12 Nodular basal cell carcinoma (BCC).

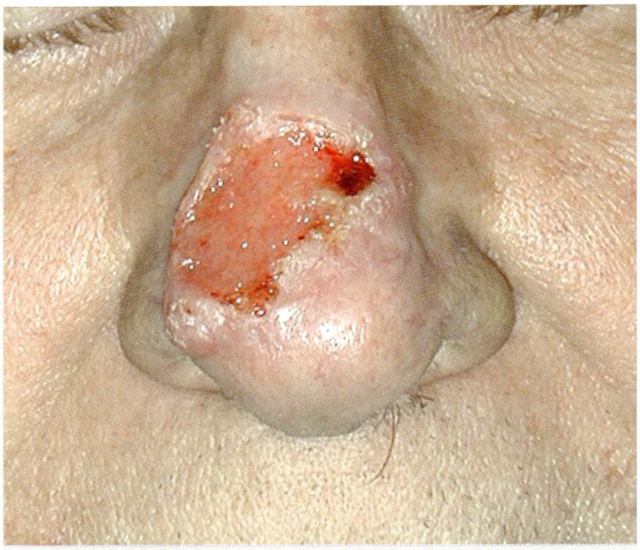

Fig. 3.13 Ulcerated nodular basal cell carcinoma (BCC). BCC grows over time. With increase in size, it can ulcerate.

tumors or, in some regions, SCC, as these BCCs demonstrate a variety of types of differentiation including basosquamous or metatypical, cystic, adenoid, pigmented, and infundibulocystic differentiation.[141,142]

Micronodular BCC manifests a plaque-like indurated lesion with a poorly demarcated contour (▶ Fig. 3.15).[143,144] Lesions invade deeply in the dermis and so have an increased incidence of recurrence.[145,146,147] Micronodular BCC manifests tumor nests with roughly the same shape and contour as nodular BCC, but which are nonetheless smaller and widely dispersed in an often asymmetric distribution extending deeper into the dermis and/or subcutis, as shown in ▶ Fig. 3.16.

Morpheaform (sclerodermiform) or sclerosing BCCs constitute 5 to 10% of BCCs. These lesions are typically smooth, flesh-colored, or very lightly erythematous papules or plaques that are frequently atrophic resembling scleroderma or "scar-like"; they usually have a firm or indurated quality with ill-defined borders. Some authors group morpheaform, infiltrative, and micronodular as "aggressive-growth" BCC, because they behave similarly.[22] Infiltrative and micronodular subtypes are less

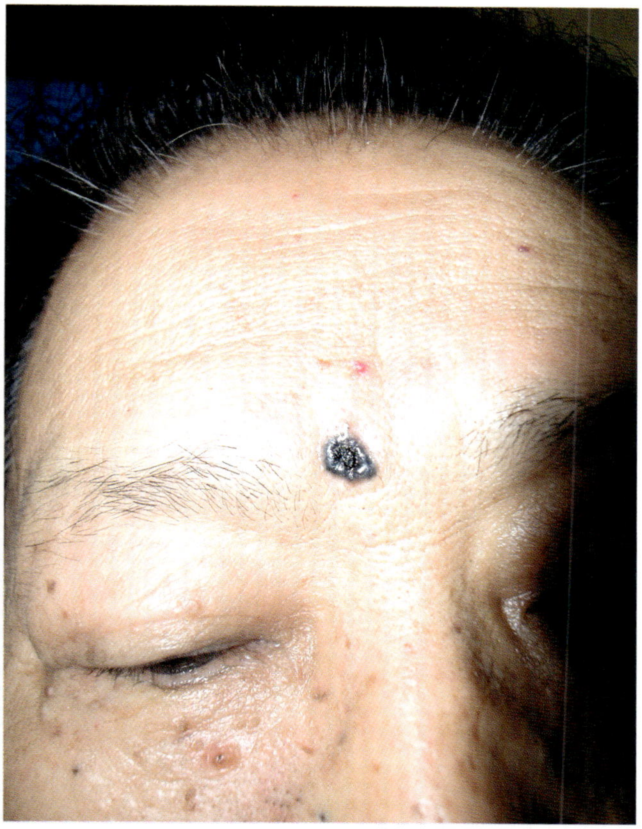

Fig. 3.14 Pigmented nodular basal cell carcinoma (BCC). BCC may also be pigmented, and sometimes it is easy to confuse it with a malignant melanoma. Pigment may be present in different concentrations in pigmented BCC.

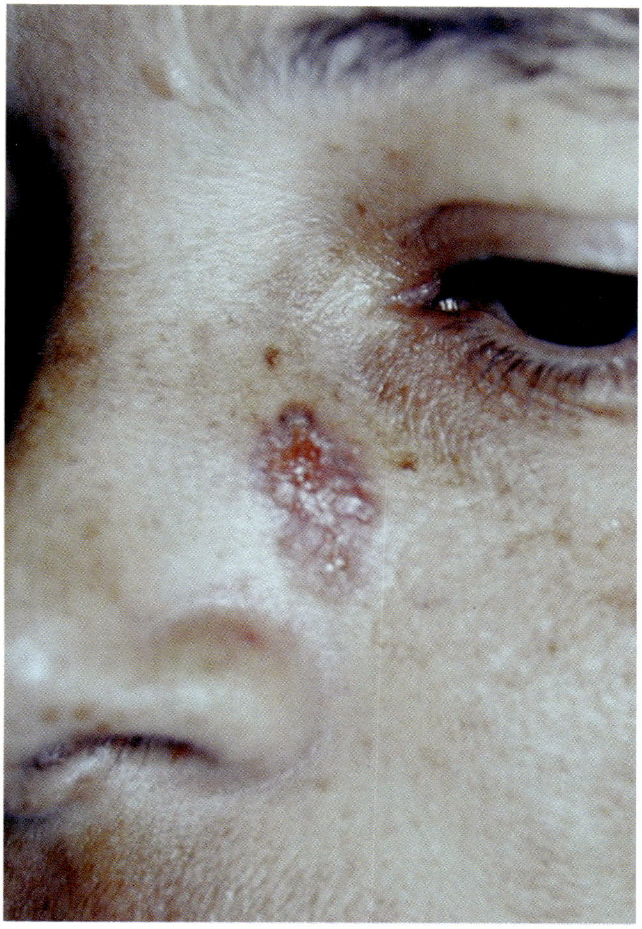

Fig. 3.15 Micronodular basal cell carcinoma (BCC). Micronodular BCCs present as multiple small aggregated nodules. These can invade deeper into the skin and be more aggressive.

common than the morpheaform BCC (▶ Fig. 3.17, ▶ Fig. 3.18, ▶ Fig. 3.19).

Several other BCC subtypes have been described and have a mixed histology and features of more than one histologic subtype (▶ Fig. 3.20 and ▶ Fig. 3.21). BCCs may show a variety of specific cell lineage differentiation features that do not impact prognosis. These include, but are not restricted, to keratotic BCC, infundibulocystic BCC, follicular BCC, which shows collision features with pilomatricoma, pleomorphic BCC, BCC with eccrine differentiation, BCC with sebaceous differentiation, the fibroepithelioma of Pinkus, and the BCC with myoepithelial differentiation. Basosquamous cell carcinoma is an additional subtype often noted to have a potential for invasion similar to SCC.

Clinicians familiar with the clinical manifestations of BCC are often able to make the diagnosis based upon clinical examination. Dermoscopy, shown in ▶ Fig. 3.22 and ▶ Fig. 3.23, is also an important diagnostic tool that every physician who works with skin cancer should be familiar with. Although biopsies are required for a definitive diagnosis, dermoscopy may be used to aid in the clinical evaluation of lesions that are suspicious for BCC.[148,149] Common dermatoscopic features of BCC include "arborizing" blood vessels (discrete, thickened, red blood vessels that branch like a tree) and blue-gray ovoid nests. Pigmented BCCs often demonstrate brown leaf-like structures on dermatoscopic examination, which represent heavily pigmented aggregates of tumor cells.[149]

A skin biopsy is usually performed to provide histologic confirmation of the diagnosis. In cases for which the clinical diagnosis of BCC appears certain and the tumor lacks clinical features associated with a high risk for tumor recurrence, clinicians experienced in the diagnosis of BCC sometimes choose to perform the definitive treatment without previous biopsy. However, the decision not to perform a biopsy prior to definitive treatment is not without risk. Because the histologic features of a tumor provide additional information on the risk for tumor recurrence following treatment, not performing a biopsy prior to definitive treatment may result in a failure to detect a tumor with aggressive histologic features that might be best managed with a different approach to therapy. The misdiagnosis of a different tumor as BCC (amelanotic melanoma, Merkel cell carcinoma) is an additional risk of deferring a biopsy, mostly for those who use destruction methods like curettage and electrodesiccation instead of excision biopsy. To reduce the risk for patient mismanagement, one should always perform a

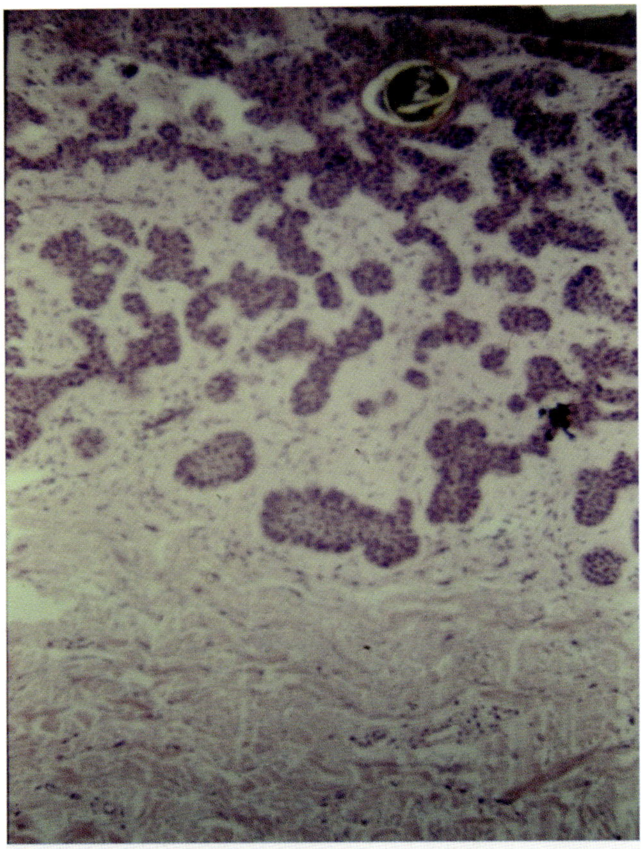

Fig. 3.16 Micronodular basal cell carcinoma (BCC) histopathology. Characteristic feature of small cell nests scattered through the tissue without surrounding stroma.

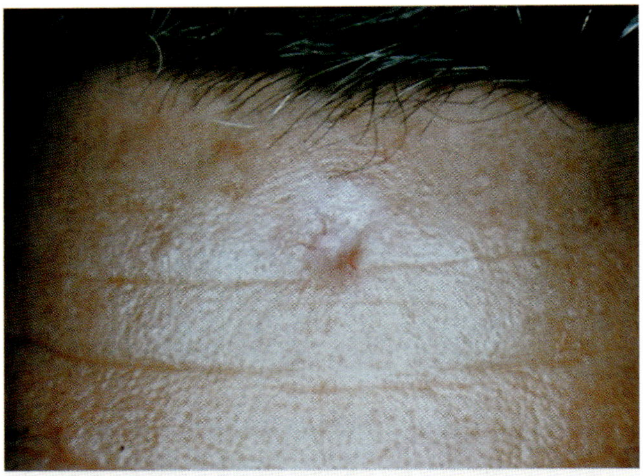

Fig. 3.17 Morpheaform basal cell carcinomas (BCCs) are typically smooth, flesh- or ivory-colored, or very lightly erythematous papules or plaques that are frequently atrophic and sometimes with telangiectasias.

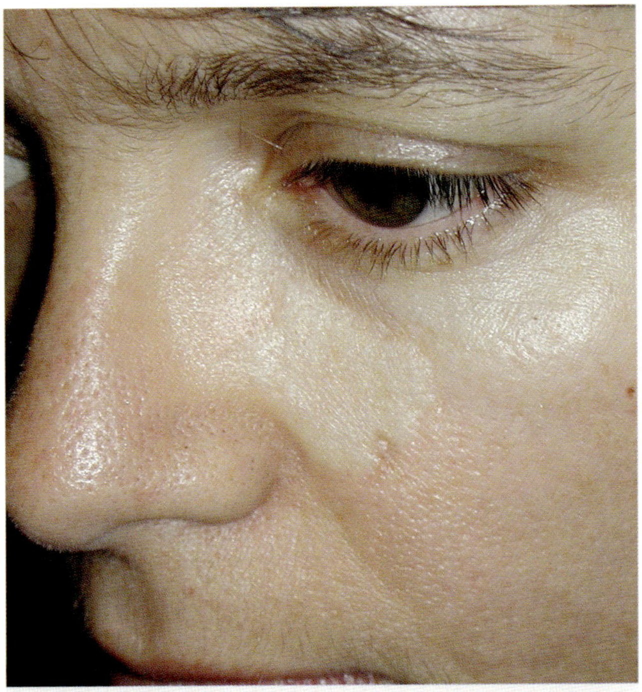

Fig. 3.18 Morpheaform basal cell carcinoma. They usually are firm or indurated with ill-defined borders and may resemble scleroderma.

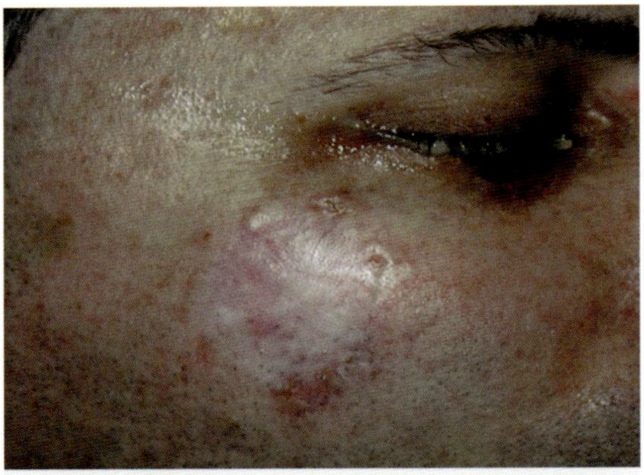

Fig. 3.19 Morpheaform basal cell carcinoma.

biopsy when the diagnosis is uncertain or the lesion exhibits features atypical for BCC, the patient lacks a prior history of BCC, or the lesion exhibits clinical features suggestive of a BCC with a high risk for recurrence.

Shave biopsies, punch biopsies, and excisional biopsies may all be used for the initial tissue sampling for diagnosis of BCC. Although shave and punch biopsies are frequently performed for diagnosis due to the simplicity of these procedures, clinicians should be aware that biopsies that remove only a portion of the lesion do not provide an accurate assessment of the histologic subtype of a tumor.[150,151,152,153] With punch biopsies, an aggressive histologic subtype may be missed in nearly 20% of cases.[150,151] A retrospective study in which the majority of biopsy procedures were shave biopsies (230 shave biopsies and

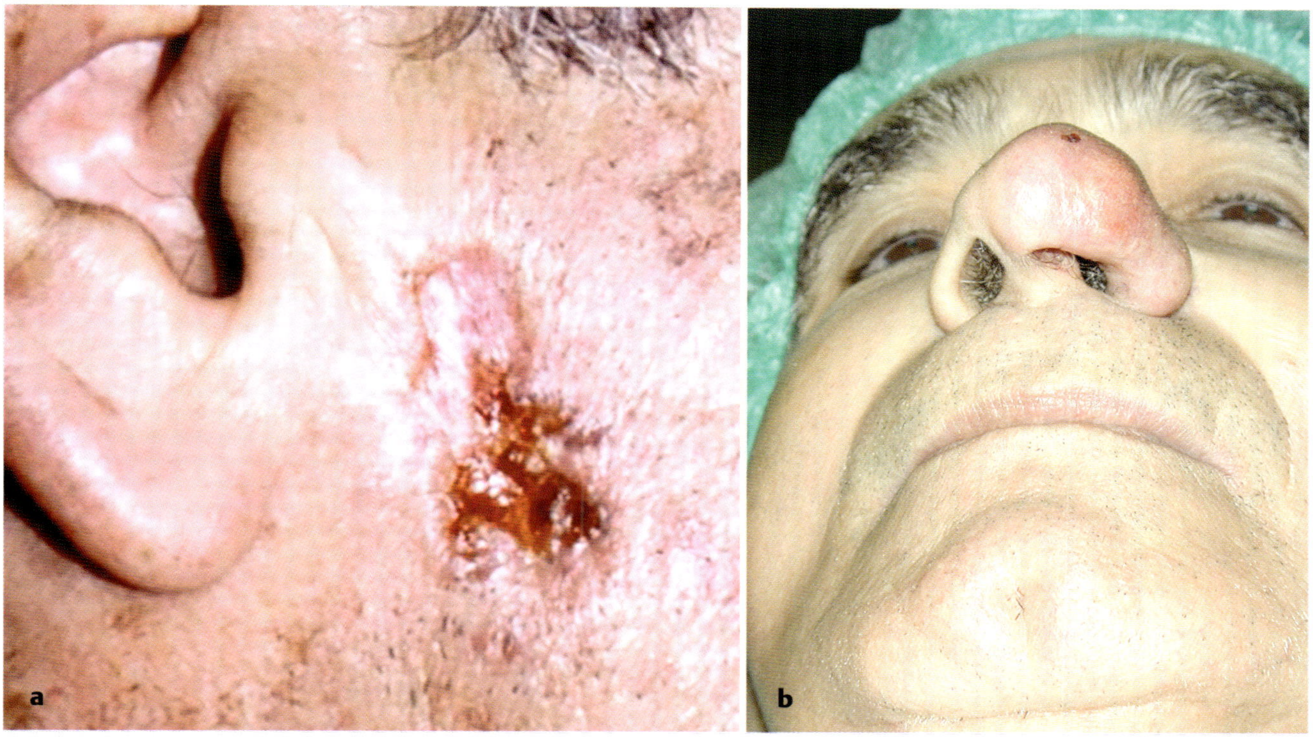

Fig. 3.20 **(a)** Adenoid cystic basal cell carcinoma (BCC). Raised nodule with a thin rim of skin at the periphery. It showed a central ulcer with crusting and irregular rolled borders. **(b)** BCC with adenoid differentiation of the nose requiring surgical excision.

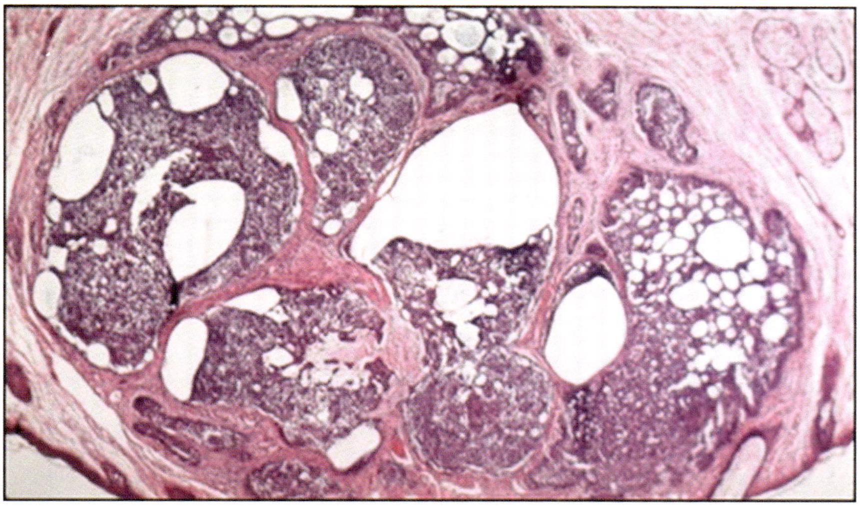

Fig. 3.21 Histopathology adenoid cystic basal cell carcinoma. Histological picture showing a predominant adenoid pattern with thin strands of basaloid cells in a reticulate arrangement, with many tubules and cystically dilated spaces containing mucin.

27 punch biopsies) found that an aggressive histologic subtype was missed in 7% of cases.[152]

The differential diagnosis varies with the pathologic subtype of BCC with nodular, superficial, or morpheaform having various presentations. Early nodular variants with little ulceration clinically may be identical to benign growths such as dermal nevi, small epidermal inclusion cysts, or even sebaceous hyperplasia. A single lesion of molluscum contagiosum has a similar appearance, as does amelanotic melanoma. Larger lesions with central ulceration can appear cup shaped. These can resemble SCC, keratoacanthomas. Superficial BCCs may be confused with inflammatory disorders of the skin such as nummular eczema or psoriasis; therefore, superficial BCC should be considered when a lesion presumed to be inflammatory fails to respond to topical corticosteroids. Morpheaform BCCs frequently appear in or adjacent to a scar or other site of trauma. The induration of the lesion simulates localized scleroderma. Additionally, pigmented nodular or superficial BCCs may resemble melanoma or, less likely, a benign nevus.

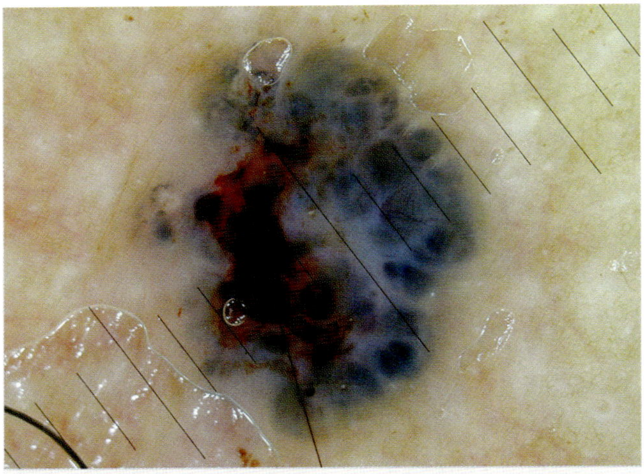

Fig. 3.22 Dermoscopy of pigmented basal cell carcinoma showing blue ovoid nests, structureless areas, and ulceration.

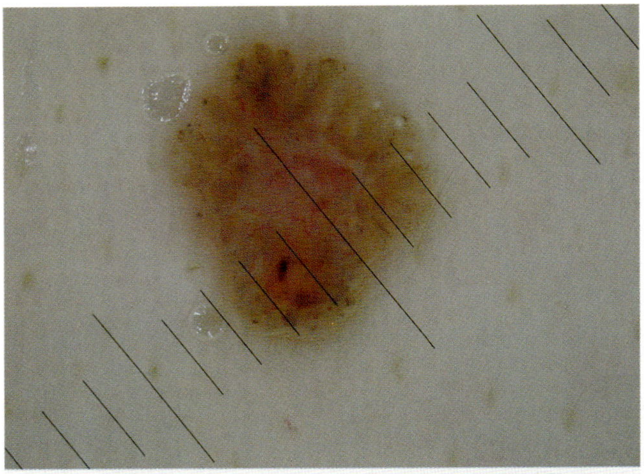

Fig. 3.23 Dermoscopy basal cell carcinoma showing typical absence of pigment network with pinkish color, asymmetrical arborizing vessels, milia formation, and leaflike areas on the periphery of the lesion.

3.6 Biopsy Techniques

Multiple biopsy techniques exist and should be implemented judiciously to each individual patient circumstance. The technique should ideally produce the information necessary for diagnosis and possible staging while maintaining subsequent options for follow-up procedures and long-term care. Disregard to potential follow-up procedures could hinder successful excision, adequate margins, or cosmesis. For example, failure to properly orient the long axis of an incisional or excisional biopsy with respect to future resection could complicate the eventual closure and limit reconstructive options.[154]

3.6.1 Incisional Biopsy

The incisional biopsy is typically indicated in large lesions in which excision would cause a large defect area, unable to be managed with primary closure. It may also be used in cosmetically sensitive areas before final pathologic diagnosis can be obtained, and a plan for definitive closure/reconstruction can be obtained. The clinician should also attempt to excise a small margin of tissue with the specimen to aid the pathologist in comparing the normal to the abnormal tissue.

3.6.2 Excisional Biopsy

This is the preferred method in relatively small lesions where primary closure and a good cosmetic outcome can be achieved. The advantages of excisional biopsy also include the ability to provide the pathologist with the native architecture, orientation, depth, and appearance of surrounding tissues. In general, margins of 1 to 2 mm are usually sufficient for the primary excision and initial diagnosis, with special attention to excise below the base of the lesion to determine potential Breslow thickness. Furthermore, postoperative margin assessment (POMA) may be requested to ensure adequate excision or diagnose a positive margin that may be missed with traditional pathology sections.[155]

3.6.3 Punch Biopsy

This is a relatively simple method of obtaining a sample of tissue from a cutaneous lesion. Multiple punches and propriety devices are available including the Tru-Cut needle to obtain a core of tissue from an unknown mass in the skin and/or subcutaneous tissues. The diameter of the punch may be determined by the provider to ensure adequate tissue is sent for pathology.

3.6.4 Shave Biopsy

Shave biopsy is the most common technique used by dermatologists and primary care physicians. The defect site is usually managed by allowing it to heal via secondary intention with adequate scar outcomes. While advantageous in regard to ease of use, cost, and minimal complications, this technique may fail to determine the depth of the tumor margin, and thereby preventing proper staging of the lesion.

3.6.5 Fine-Needle Aspiration Biopsy

This is usually reserved for metastatic lesions that may be easily seen or palpated in the skin or subcutaneous tissue. It is performed by making multiple passes with a hollow-bore needle into the lesion while applying suction on the syringe. The harvested tissue is then placed directly onto a slide for further fixation and analysis.[156]

3.7 Approach to Treatment

3.7.1 Topical Therapies

Topical therapies include 5-fluorouracil (5-FU) and imiquimod and must be applied for several weeks to maximize potential benefit. In general, both induce mild to moderate inflammatory reactions at the sites of application.[157]

Topical 5-Fluorouracil

5-FU exerts its affects through interference of DNA synthesis by inhibiting thymidylate synthase, therefore rapidly proliferating cells are most sensitive to its cytotoxic effect. Topical 5-FU is available in a variety of strengths and formulations; the 5% cream or solution is used for the treatment of BCC applied twice daily for at least 3 to 6 weeks; however, treatment may continue until reaching the desired clinical response.[157]

Treatment with topical 5-FU should be restricted to superficial BCCs in noncritical locations.[157] Various relatively small studies have documented cure rates of up to 95% using 5-FU cream in patients with carefully selected superficial BCCs, although lower cure rates are reported by others.[157,158] Treatment of nonsuperficial, recurrent, or other high-risk BCCs with 5-FU results in low cure rates and is generally inadvisable.[159,160,161] In particular, nodular and aggressive BCCs are generally considered contraindications to topical 5-FU given that superficial treatment may give the false impression of a cure despite persistent dermal disease.

Topical 5-FU causes a brisk inflammatory reaction in the treated sites, which is an indication of activity. Prior to treatment, patients should be thoroughly educated on anticipated side effects, including undesired cosmetic effects, pain, erythema, edema, erosions, and ulceration with potential drainage. Therapy may be discontinued if the inflammation is not tolerated. Alternatively, tolerance may be improved through reduction of drug concentration, application of an emollient or application of an intermediate-potency topical steroid.[159,160,161] Special care should be taken when applying 5-FU to areas near the eyes, lips, and nose as well as avoiding intense sun exposure during treatment.

Following discontinuation of topical 5-FU therapy, healing generally takes place over the ensuing 2 weeks or more. The residual erythema and occasional hyperpigmentation usually fade with time. In general, long-term favorable cosmetic results are obtained with observation. Other unusual side effects include persistent telangiectasias, pigmentary changes, and hypertrophic scarring in high-risk areas.

3.7.2 Imiquimod

Imiquimod 5% cream is an immune response modifier (Toll-like receptor 7 agonist) approved for treatment of superficial BCCs in low-risk sites. Imiquimod is thought to promote apoptosis in skin cancer cells by circumventing the antiapoptotic mechanisms deployed by tumor cells or by stimulating monocytes/macrophages and dendritic cells to produce cytokines that stimulate cell-mediated immunity.[162,163,164]

The efficacy of imiquimod for superficial BCC has been documented in multicenter randomized trials that compared imiquimod 5% cream (applied once daily five or seven times per week for 6 weeks) in a total of 724 patients with superficial BCC.[164] Twelve weeks after treatment, the histologic clearance rates for the 5- and 7-day imiquimod treatment groups were 82 and 79%, respectively, compared with 3% in the control group. The severity of erythema, erosion, and scabbing/crusting was associated with higher clearance rates; however, long-term follow-up was not reported. This was corroborated in a randomized trial that assessed the response of superficial BCC to 6 weeks of daily therapy with imiquimod 5% cream.[165] Twelve weeks after treatment, histologic clearance rates in the imiquimod and vehicle groups were 80 and 6%, respectively.[165]

Although imiquimod's efficacy has been established, clinicians should be aware that the likelihood of treatment success is higher with surgical excision (SE). A trial of 257 patients with superficial BCC and 244 patients with nodular BCC were randomly assigned to treatment with imiquimod 5% cream (once daily for 6 weeks for superficial BCC and once daily for 12 weeks for nodular BCC) or SE with a 4-mm margin found that patients treated with SE were significantly less likely to experience treatment failure or tumor recurrence within 3 years.[166] Among the patients with superficial BCC, clinical cure rates from SE and imiquimod were 98 and 85%, respectively.[166] Patient satisfaction with the cosmetic appearance of sites of imiquimod treatment and SE was also similar at 6 months and 3 years after treatment.[166]

The thickness of a superficial BCC may influence the likelihood of response to imiquimod therapy. A retrospective study of 127 biopsy specimens from superficial BCCs that were subsequently treated with imiquimod (applied 5 days per week for 6 weeks) found that while 11 of 19 tumors (58%) > 0.4 mm deep recurred after treatment, none of 108 tumors ≤ 0.4 mm deep recurred (mean follow-up 34 months, range 3–91 months).[167] If these findings are supported by future investigations, the depth of superficial BCC may become a consideration in the selection of imiquimod treatment.

The few randomized trials that have evaluated the use of imiquimod as an adjunctive therapy for nodular BCC prior to SE have yielded conflicting findings.[168,169] In a randomized trial of 70 patients with nodular BCC on the face, 4 weeks of imiquimod treatment prior to Mohs surgery was associated with reductions in tumor size and surgical defect size. However, a smaller randomized trial failed to find a statistically significant benefit of imiquimod therapy.[168] There is also a theoretical concern that pretreatment with imiquimod could contribute to false negative surgical margins by inducing noncontiguous areas of residual tumor.[170]

In general, imiquimod is used for the treatment of primary superficial BCCs in low-risk sites where recurrence is unlikely to be accompanied by substantial morbidity. Because of concern for consistent patient adherence to the longer treatment period suggested for nodular BCC and the availability of more effective treatment,[166] imiquimod is not routinely used for the treatment of nodular BCC. Imiquimod is reserved for the treatment of nonsuperficial BCCs only in those patients who are poor surgical candidates or who have limited life expectancies. The selection of imiquimod over a surgical procedure for superficial BCC usually stems from patient-specific factors such as patient preference to avoid surgery.[166]

The standard regimen for imiquimod treatment of superficial BCC is application of imiquimod to the BCC once daily 5 days per week for 6 weeks. If the irritation becomes too severe, the patient may take 2 to 3 days off and then resume treatment. Local skin irritation is an expected side effect of imiquimod therapy. Patients may experience itching, weeping, redness, soreness, bleeding, and/or pain within the treated area.[166] In addition, hypopigmentation may develop after therapy.[166,171]

3.8 Photodynamic Therapy

Photodynamic therapy (PDT) utilizes both light and porphyrins to cause tumor destruction. PDT is applied to the lesion, which results in a higher concentration of the porphyrins within the cancerous cells, and the ability to focus light on the involved area. Although PDT has been approved for the treatment of BCC in many European countries, U.S. Food and Drug Administration (FDA) approval has not been granted for the treatment of BCC.

To perform PDT, a photosensitizing porphyrin such as 5-aminolevulinic acid (ALA) or methyl aminolevulinate (MAL) is applied topically to the lesion.[172,173] Although the porphyrin porfimer can be administered systemically, systemic therapy can be associated with prolonged photosensitivity.[172,173] Several hours after topical application of the porphyrin, the area is exposed to visible light. The light penetrates the skin and is selectively absorbed by the photosensitizer, which generates reactive oxygen species. This in turn can cause lipid peroxidation, protein crosslinking, increased membrane permeability, and ultimately cell death. In addition to direct effects on tumor cells, PDT can damage blood vessels, resulting in impaired blood flow, and can stimulate a vigorous local inflammatory reaction that may contribute to tumor destruction.[174]

Response to PDT has been variable. Superficial lesions appear to be most responsive to therapy with response rates ranging from 72 to 100%.[175,176,177,178] Three randomized controlled trials (RCTs) with long-term follow-up have compared various PDT protocols against simple SE for sBCC and primary nBCC. All demonstrated statistically superior clearance rates with SE over PDT.[179] Side effects from topical PDT include photosensitivity, pain, erythema, edema, ulceration, and temporary pigmentary change at the treated site. Healing is usually complete within 2 weeks and there is low probability of scarring.

3.9 Radiation Therapy

Radiation therapy (RT) is an option for the treatment of BCCs in patients who are poor candidates for surgical intervention or in patients with positive surgical margins. RT is usually administered in a fractionated schedule to limit treatment-related side effects; however, it requires multiple sessions and strict compliance (▶ Table 3.2). RT results in relative sparing of cosmetically and functional tissues, its noninvasive and painless nature, and its utility for many patients who are not candidates for surgical intervention or for whom it is difficult to attain histologic clearance. Unlike SE, RT does not provide histologic control of the tumor margin. Most large series report overall 5-year cure rates of 91 to 93% for previously untreated BCCs, with rates as high as 96% for smaller BCCs at low risk for recurrence.[180,181,182] For patients with recurrent BCCs, the reported cure rates are generally reported between 86 and 91%.[180,181,182,183] BCCs that recur following RT may behave more aggressively than those recurring after surgical procedures, with higher rates of second recurrence and distant metastasis.[184]

Short-term cutaneous side effects of RT include erythema and edema, scaling, vesicles, bullae, erosions, ulceration, pain, and occasionally infection. Healing generally occurs within 3 to 4 weeks following the final treatment, but symptoms may persist for months in severe cases. Other less common short-term side effects include a "comedo reaction," which is a benign condition characterized by the appearance of large, open comedones at the periphery of the treated areas.

Table 3.2 Radiation therapy regimens for basal cell carcinoma

Tumor diameter	Margin	Electron beam radiation therapy
< 2 cm	1–1.5 cm	64 Gy in 32 fractions over 6–6.4 wk
		55 Gy in 20 fractions over 4 wk
		50 Gy in 15 fractions over 3 wk
		35 Gy in 5 fractions over 5 d
> 2 cm	1.5–2 cm	66 Gy in 33 fractions over 6–6.6 wk
		55 Gy in 20 fractions over 4 wk
Postoperative adjuvant Therapy		50 Gy in 20 fractions over 4 wk
		60 Gy in 30 fractions over 6 wk

Delayed effects of radiation within the treatment field include permanent alopecia that usually occurs within the treatment field. Patients should be advised of this prior to treatment, and pretreatment counseling is essential. Chronic radiation dermatitis generally appears months to years following therapy and is characterized by permanently mottled areas of hypopigmentation and hyperpigmentation, a dry, hyperkeratotic, atrophic, shiny epidermis, telangiectasias, and dermal fibrosis. Severe dermal and subcutaneous fibrosis is an uncommon consequence of RT for cutaneous malignancies.

Delayed radiation necrosis may develop months to years following RT, and is marked by spontaneous breakdown of the skin within the treatment field, with erythema, erosions or ulcerations, crusting, and discomfort. Radiation necrosis is usually precipitated by trauma, infection, or exposure to cold or sunshine, and is secondary to poor vascularity and atrophy of the previously irradiated area. Irradiation of cartilaginous and bony structures such as the ear and nose may result in chondroradionecrosis or osteoradionecrosis, although this is uncommon using modern techniques.[185]

Risk factors for secondary cancers after RT include higher radiation doses, larger radiation fields, sun-exposed sites, fair skin, and early age of radiation exposure. Increased fractionation with a smaller dose per fraction reduces this risk. Although some investigators think that the risk of radiation-induced cutaneous malignancy is much smaller using modern treatment protocols, RT continues to be avoided in young people and in those with genetic susceptibility to radiation-induced malignancies.[186] Incidental radiation exposure to other tissues can also result in delayed complications, such as cataracts, infertility, and thyroid cancer. These are uncommon events that should be avoided with proper shielding during therapy.

3.10 Intralesional Therapy

Intralesional therapies (interferons, 5-FU, or bleomycin) are used infrequently for the management of BCC; however, these therapies may have a place in modern regimens.[187,188] A systematic review of open label studies, case series, and the few randomized trials that have investigated the efficacy of intralesional interferon for BCC found overall cure rates for interferon beta, interferon alfa-2a, and interferon alfa-2b of 63, 68, and 76%, respectively.[187] Data are limited on the use of intralesional 5-FU and bleomycin; however, the results of a few case reports and small case series suggest that these therapies may be highly effective for BCC.[189,190,191,192] Adverse effects of intralesional interferon, 5-FU, and bleomycin include local pain, erythema, necrosis, and ulceration.[187] Systemic side effects are less likely with intralesional injection than with systemic administration, but may also occur. Risks of interferon therapy include fever, malaise, headaches, myalgias, cytopenia, hepatotoxicity, and nephrotoxicity. Pulmonary toxicity, cutaneous sclerosis, and Raynaud phenomenon have been associated with bleomycin. Gastrointestinal distress and cytopenias are potential adverse effects of 5-FU. Evidence is limited on the long-term efficacy of intralesional therapies for BCC.

3.11 Targeted Therapy for BCC Including LABCC and MBCC and Hedgehog Pathway

BCCs that are extensive or invade below the dermis and potentially vital structures are difficult to surgically clear without significant morbidity. Many of these may become locally advanced or metastasize. Although low, estimates of the metastatic rate of BCC ranged from 0.0029 to 0.55%.[193] In another report, the population-based case mortality rate from BCC was approximately 0.05%.[194] Men develop metastatic disease more frequently than women, although the reason for this is unknown. Metastatic lesions usually result from primary, deeply invasive, or large lesions with an area of greater than 10 cm.[2,193] The most common sites for metastasis include the regional lymph nodes, lungs, bones, skin, and liver.[195]

BCCs that metastasize to either local or distant lymph nodes or distant organs would best be addressed through systemic therapy. Together, these locally advanced or metastatic BCCs comprise a disease group termed "locally advanced BCCs" (LABCCs). While accurate estimates of the incidence of LABCCs are difficult to obtain, in part due to the lack of widespread use of a staging system by dermatologists and lack of uniform reporting requirements for NMSCs, LABCCs are thought to represent roughly 1 to 10% of all BCCs, with metastatic BCCs accounting for 0.0028 to 0.5%.[196,197,198] From our clinical experience, patients presenting with LABCCs appear to fall into two categories: those who present with LABCC due to delay in accessing medical attention or those who have BCCs that are intrinsically aggressive, are refractory, or recur after treatment. Included in this group are those patients with chronic immunosuppression following organ transplant and some patients with Gorlin's syndrome. Therapeutic options for such patients are limited.[199,200]

The Hedgehog pathway was initially identified as a critical developmental regulator of embryonic segment polarity in *Drosophila* in 1980.[201] This and related developmental work in fly body patterning was recognized by the Nobel Prize in Physiology and Medicine in 1995. Vertebrate homologs of the *Drosophila* Hedgehog ligand were first reported in 1993, and definition of central components of the mammalian signaling pathway followed in the late 1990s and early 2000s.[202] The first definitive linkage of mutation in this pathway to cancer, that is, to development of BCC, was made in 1996.[101,203]

Hedgehog signaling regulates embryonic development ensuring that tissues reach their correct location, size, and cellular content. The Hedgehog pathway normally remains inactive in adult tissues; however, reactivation of this pathway results in malignant transformation and tumorigenesis.[204,205] More than 90% of all BCCs have identified abnormal Hedgehog pathway signaling. There are two classic mechanisms of Hedgehog pathway reactivation: mutation-driven signaling (ligand independent) and abnormal signaling in the tumor microenvironment (ligand dependent).[94] In mutation-driven signaling, tumor cells harbor mutations in key components of the Hedgehog pathway allowing for independent activation of the biomolecular system and subsequent stimulation of unregulated proliferation.[206] In ligand-dependent activation, tumor cells overexpress Hedgehog ligands that activate surrounding stromal cells leading to uncontrolled growth.[207] Mutations in two major receptor proteins, Patched-1 (PTCH1) and Smoothened (SMO), may result in abnormal activation of the Hedgehog pathway and are the focus of proposed interventions.

As shown in ▶ Fig. 3.24, Hedgehog pathway activation occurs via binding of an extracellular Hedgehog ligand (Shh) to PTCH1, a transmembrane receptor. Once bound, PTCH1 is internalized and degraded, allowing for release of a the transmembrane protein SMO from the inhibitory effect of PTCH1.[111] SMO can then move from the intracellular compartment to the cell membrane of the cilium and activate the GLI family of transcription factors. Activated GLI factors enter the nucleus and initiate the transcription of target genes.[111] The majority of sporadic BCCs contain mutations that result in inactivation of PTCH1, with subsequent constitutional activation of SMO.[208] Inhibition of SMO activation, either through appropriate PTCH hindrance or through new SMO inhibitors such as vismodegib (Erivedge, Genentech), prevents unregulated proliferation.

Basal cell carcinoma (BCC), medulloblastoma, rhabdomyosarcoma, and other human tumors are associated with mutations that activate the proto-oncogene Smoothened (SMO) or that inactivate the tumor suppressor Patched (PTCH). Smoothened and Patched mediate the cellular response to the Hedgehog (Hh) secreted protein signal, and oncogenic mutations affecting these proteins cause excess activity of the Hh response pathway.

The story of how the first inhibitor of the Hh pathway, cyclopamine, was discovered is one of the most fascinating in biomedicine. In the late 1950s, pregnant ewes were found to produce one-eyed offspring, or extreme holoprosencephaly[199,209](▶ Fig. 3.25).

In the 1970s, the active agent inducing these changes, cyclopamine, was isolated and its structural formula identified. Subsequent studies in the 1990s in chick embryos demonstrated cyclopamine's ability to induce holoprosencephaly and to bind

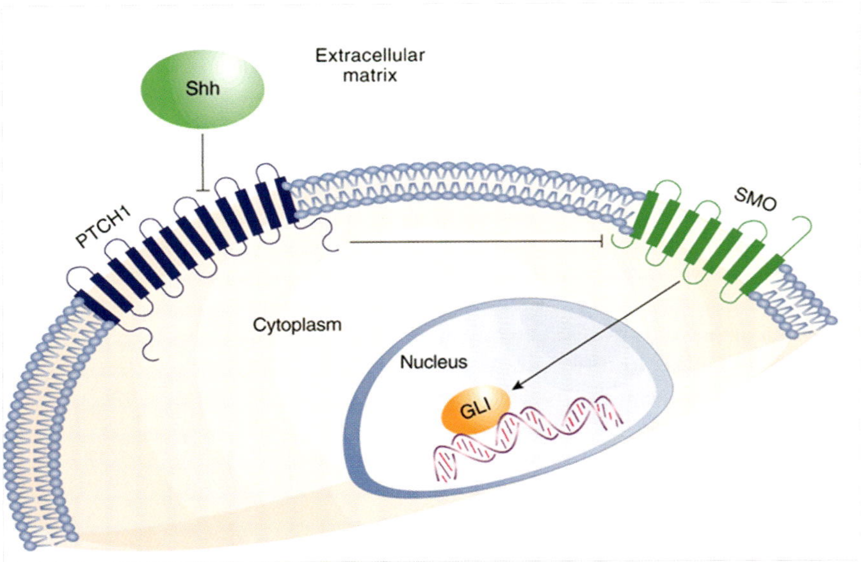

Fig. 3.24 Simplified schematic of common mutations in the Hedgehog signaling pathway leading to basal cell carcinoma from pathway activation. (Reprinted with permission from Sheridan C. Genentech obtains proof of concept for hedgehog inhibition. Nat Biotechnol 2009;27:968–969.)

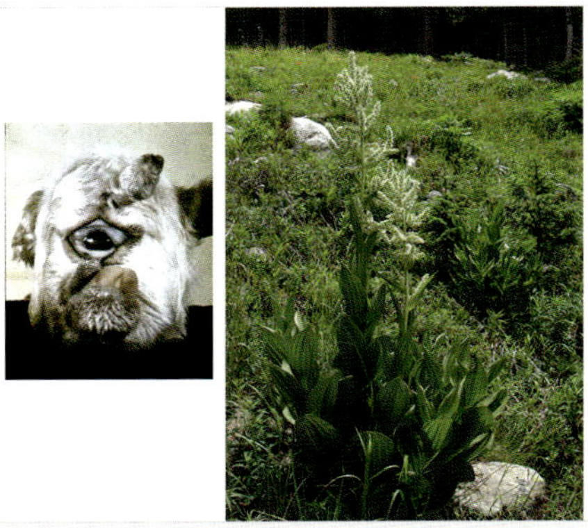

Fig. 3.25 In the decade after World War II, Idaho farmers noticed that a random batch of their lambs was being born with strange birth defects. The creatures had underdeveloped brains and a single eye planted, Cyclops-like, in the middle of their foreheads. In 1957, they called in scientists that worked for 11 years to solve the mystery: corn lilies. When the animals moved to higher ground during droughts, they snacked on the flowers. The lilies, it turned out, contained a poison, later dubbed cyclopamine that stunted developing lamb embryos. The adult mothers remained unharmed. The case of the cyclopamine and the one-eyed Idaho lambs remained a freakish chemistry footnote for the next three decades.

the transmembrane protein, Smoothened.[210] Subsequently, a number of analogues were developed by modifications to cyclopamine to improve solubility, and oral bioavailability. Collectively, these analogues are called Smoothened inhibitors (SIs), due to their targeting of the Smoothened protein.

In 2000, Taipale et al showed that cyclopamine inhibits the Hh response and was a potential "mechanism-based" therapeutic agent for treatment of some tumors. They showed that cyclopamine or synthetic derivatives with improved potency, block activation of the Hh response pathway, and abnormal cell growth associated with both types of oncogenic mutation. Their results also indicated that cyclopamine could act by influencing the balance between active and inactive forms of SMO.[211,212,213]

This discovery, together with rapidly accumulating evidence implicating the Hh pathway in oncogenesis, led to focused efforts by multiple biotechnology and pharmaceutical companies to develop cyclopamine derivatives with improved pharmacologic properties or to develop agents that effectively outcompeted cyclopamine for binding to the critical cell-surface activator of Hh signaling, the 7-transmembrane G-protein-coupled–like receptor, SMO. Vismodegib is a member of this class: structurally unrelated to cyclopamine but able to bind with high affinity and specificity to SMO, leading to potent suppression of Hh signaling in reporter systems and in a preclinical model of Hh-dependent disease.[214] An Investigational New Drug application for vismodegib was filled with the FDA in September 2006, leading to launch of a first-in-human phase I clinical trial at three U.S. sites in January 2007.

Multiple orally available smoothness inhibitors are currently in human clinical trials against BCCs. The first and only U.S. FDA-approved SI for advanced BCCs (aBCCs) to date is vismodegib, which became commercially available in 2012. The phase II study with 96 aBCC patients leading to FDA approval demonstrated an independently assessed response rate of 30% in patients with metastatic BCC and 43% response rate in LABCC.[215] A subsequent study of 119 aBCC patients showed similar findings.[216] The availability of vismodegib as highly targeted therapy for aBCCs is one of the greatest success stories in translational medicine.

Initial investigation of Vismodegib documented its therapeutic effects in both in vitro studies with downregulation of GLI1 by approximately 90% compared to controls and in ex vivo analysis with reported downregulation of GLI1 by greater than 50% in skin biopsy specimens excised from treated patients.[214,217] A phase 1 trial with vismodegib included 68 patients with solid tumors, of which 33 had aBCC, 8 had pancreatic cancer, 1 had medulloblastoma, in addition to 17 other types. The overall rate of complete or partial response was 58% with specific response of 50% in patients with metastatic BCC and 60% in patients with

LABCC.[217] Despite vast heterogeneity with respect to tumor histology, patient characteristics, and dosing concentrations, vismodegib was generally well tolerated with 8.8% experiencing a grade 4 event (hyponatremia, fatigue, pyelonephritis, presyncope, resectable pancreatic adenocarcinoma, and paranoia with hyperglycemia), and 27.9% of patients experienced a grade 3 event (hyponatremia [10.3%], abdominal pain [7.4%], and fatigue [5.9%]).

A multicenter, nonrandomized phase 2 clinical trial of vismodegib in 104 patients was conducted from February 2009 through November 2010.[215] Of the 33 patients with metastatic BCC, 10 (30%) had a response as judged by independent review, and 15 (45%) had a response as judged by site investigators. In the 63 patients with LABCC, 38 (60%) had at least a partial response as judged by site investigators, with 13 (21%) judged to have a complete response with verification established by the absence of residual disease on biopsy.[218]

An additional phase 2 trial was conducted in 41 patients with basal cell nevus syndrome (BCNS).[219] Vismodegib was associated with a decrease in the number of new and existing surgically eligible BCCs with surgically eligible BCCs occurring at a rate of 2 per year in the vismodegib group compared with 29 per year in the control group ($p < 0.001$). There was also a significantly greater decrease in the size of existing surgically eligible BCCs in patients receiving vismodegib (65% in the vismodegib group vs. 11% in the control group; $p = 0.003$).[218]

Current research and clinical trials focusing on the administration of synthetic SMO inhibitors, or Hh pathway inhibitors, for patients with locally advanced and metastatic basal cell carcinoma (MBCC) are ongoing.[220,221] Clinical trials have shown exceptional decrements in tumor burden as well as resolution of metastatic disease with the drug as the sole treatment modality, thus reducing the need for SE and associated morbidity and mortality.[218] Furthermore, recent case reports have documented the use of vismodegib as a potential neoadjuvant therapy prior to surgical or radiotherapeutic intervention.[216,222,223]

Although ongoing clinical trials for topical and systemic therapies are currently pending, vismodegib remains the only FDA-approved Hh pathway inhibitor approved for the treatment of metastatic and LABCC.[224]

More recently, evolving treatment protocols have led to novel algorithms of treatment under clinical trial settings. Targeted therapy with Hh inhibitors including vismodegib has served as both a viable alternative and adjunct to SE alone in the author's practice. As example we present data of our first consecutive series of 20 patients initially treated from April 2012 to June 2013. All adult patients with locally advanced basal cell carcinoma (LABCC) and/or recurring or MBCC who were not candidates for surgery or RT (due to clinical morbidities or patient's refusal of surgery/RT) received vismodegib 150 mg once a day until disease progression, unacceptable side effects, or discontinuation of treatment at patients' request. The peak plasma concentration of vismodegib is reached 48 hours after oral administration and maintained for 72 hours, formulating the currently recommending schedule of 150-mg PO daily.[217,225] LABCC was defined as at least one lesion 20 mm or more in areas of limited tissue availability (eyelid, ear, nasal ala, etc.); patients that had recurrence after two or more surgical procedures and curative resection was unlikely and surgery was expected to result in substantial morbidity and/or deformity.

Response was defined as a decrease of ≥ 30% in the externally visible or radiographic dimension or complete resolution of ulceration if present at baseline. Radiographic imaging was obtained for all patients with MBCC and for patients with LABCC who had radiographically measurable disease. Objective response of vismodegib on tumor regression and prevention of disease progression was visually and clinically appreciable in almost all treated patients. As of the data-cutoff point 13/20 (65%) patients had complete response (defined as the absence of residual BCC on assessment of a biopsy specimen) and 7/20 (35%) patients had partial response. As of the data-cutoff point, 13 of the 13 patients who had a complete response did not have disease progression (▶ Fig. 3.26 and ▶ Fig. 3.27). One patient was excluded from treatment on his request due to unacceptable side effects (loss of taste and muscle cramps). Most common side effects were loss of taste (100%), muscle spasms (80%), hair loss (50%), weight loss (30%), and fatigue (10%). Once treatment stopped, the side effects subsided. Surgery was performed in the seven patients who had partial response. Minimal residual tumor was identified in five of them and no residual tumor was found in two of the patients.

In ▶ Fig. 3.27a, marked resolution of the tumor with reduction in vertical height and surrounding erythema was evident by day 30 of treatment. By day 120, there were no palpable lesions and the surrounding erythema and induration associated with the metastatic lesion had been greatly diminished. Radiographically, the patient had exceptional regression of tumor burden matching the clinical picture. The chemotherapeutic agent not only benefited the cutaneous manifestations of disease, but also had a profound effect on systemic metastases as shown in ▶ Fig. 3.27b. By day 120, the patient with cutaneous lesions (▶ Fig. 3.27) had radiographic evidence of complete resolution of pulmonary metastases.

In this series of 20 consecutive patients, vismodegib showed encouraging results with objective response rate superior to 90% and provided substantial clinical benefit for the selected patients. However, treatment patterns, clinical outcomes, health care resource use, and definitions of advanced and complex/difficult-to-treat disease are not uniformly adopted in the literature and clinical practice.

Itraconazole, an antifungal agent, has also been identified as a potent inhibitor of the Hh signaling pathway.[226] In a phase II trial including 29 patients with sporadic BCC > 4 mm, 15 patients were treated with 200 mg twice daily for 4 weeks prior to surgery and 4 patients with 100 mg twice daily for 1 to 4 months (mean 2.3 months).[227] Itraconazole reduced tumor size by 24% and promoted re-epithelialization in 8 patients with a total of 57 tumors. Further data from more robust trials are pending; however, itraconazole may play a role in vismodegib-resistant subjects or in BCC prevention.

3.12 Surgical Management

Surgical options for BCCs at low risk for recurrence include electrodesiccation and curettage (ED&C), conventional SE, and

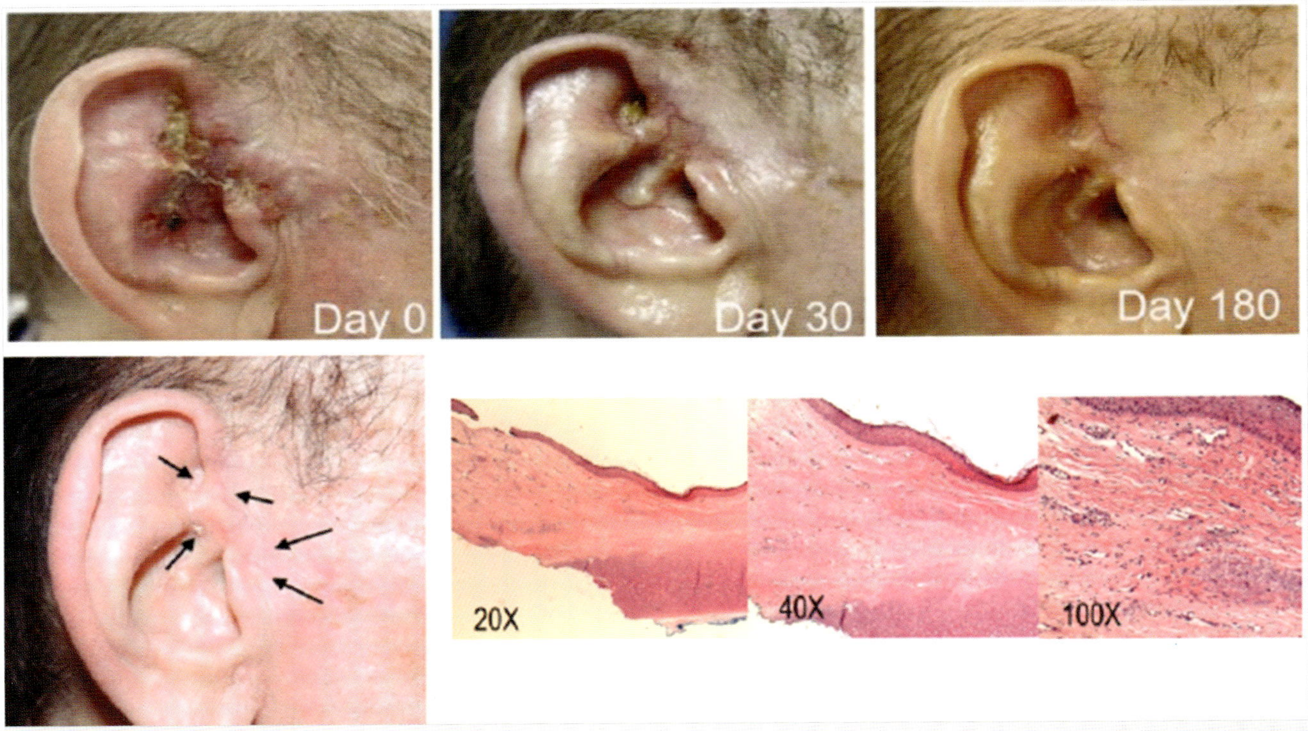

Fig. 3.26 Locally advanced basal cell carcinoma involving the ear. Response after 1 and 4 months of treatment. Biopsy sites after 8 months of treatment and pathology showing absence of tumor in all sites. Patient remains without evidence of disease 1 year after discontinuing treatment.

cryosurgery. Cryosurgery is infrequently used for this indication and ED&C is mainly used by dermatologists and primary care physicians.

3.12.1 Electrodesiccation and Curettage

The procedure of curettage and electrodesiccation is used most often for the treatment of selected small basal cell carcinomas (BCCs) and squamous cell carcinomas (SCCs). It is a deceptively simple procedure that requires proper selection of tumor and a skilled practitioner. Otherwise, the recurrence rate is unacceptably high. The tumor is prepared and anesthetized with a local anesthetic. The curette, an oval instrument with a cutting edge, is used to remove the soft cancerous skin. The tumor margins are determined by "feel," with normal skin having a firm and gritty consistency. After curettage, the base and borders of the wound are electrodesiccated to destroy residual tumor and to provide hemostasis. The wound heals by secondary intention in 2 to 3 weeks.

Although ED&C is a fast and easily performed treatment for BCC, the procedure does not include histologic confirmation of tumor removal and is not appropriate for BCCs with clinical or histologic features that suggest an elevated risk for tumor recurrence. The expected unpleasant cosmetic results of ED&C (a round hypopigmented scar) also should be considered during treatment selection. Curettage and electrodesiccation (C&E) is the process of alternatively scraping away tumor tissue with a curette down to a firm layer of normal dermis and denaturing the area by electrodessication. Up to three cycles may be performed in a session. Although a fast and cost-effective technique for superficial lesions, it does not allow histologic margin assessment. Overall 5-year cure rates reported for BCC and SCC are 92% and 96%, respectively.[228] However, recurrence rates can be high for high-risk locations (21%) and high-risk histologic subtypes (27%).

This technique is deemed effective for low-risk tumors if following distinct criteria. First, this technique should not be used to treat areas with terminal hair growth due to the risk that a tumor extending down follicular structures might not be adequately removed. Second, if the subcutaneous layer is reached during the curettage, SE should be performed. Third, if curettage has been performed based only on the appearance of a low-risk tumor, biopsy results of the tissue taken at the time of curettage should be reviewed to make sure that there are no high-risk pathologic features that would require additional therapy.

3.12.2 Surgical Excision

SE is the gold standard and used for the treatment of both BCCs at low or high risk for recurrence. Data on the efficacy of SE for BCC are primarily limited to retrospective case series and randomized trials.[180,229,230,231,232] Because SE of BCCs with 4 to 5 mm margins has been associated with 5-year cure rates exceeding 95%,[180,229,230,231,233] it remains the most commonly practiced technique. Currently, 4-mm surgical margins are commonly used for the excision of these lesions. The results of a 2010 meta-analysis of published studies on conventionally excised BCCs that excluded studies of previously excised, irradiated lesions, or morpheaform BCCs confirmed that rates of

[138] Kazlouskaya V, Malhotra S, Navarro R, et al. Dermal changes in superficial basal cell carcinoma, melanoma in situ and actinic keratosis and their implications. J Cutan Pathol. 2013; 40(12):1014–1020

[139] Mina MA, Picariello A, Fewkes JL. Superficial basal cell carcinomas of the head and neck. Dermatol Surg. 2013; 39(7):1003–1008

[140] Humphreys TR, Malhotra R, Scharf MJ, Marcus SM, Starkus L, Calegari K. Treatment of superficial basal cell carcinoma and squamous cell carcinoma in situ with a high-energy pulsed carbon dioxide laser. Arch Dermatol. 1998; 134(10):1247–1252

[141] Grando SA, Schofield OM, Skubitz AP, Kist DA, Zelickson BD, Zachary CB. Nodular basal cell carcinoma in vivo vs in vitro. Establishment of pure cell cultures, cytomorphologic characteristics, ultrastructure, immunophenotype, biosynthetic activities, and generation of antisera. Arch Dermatol. 1996; 132(10):1185–1193

[142] Brownell I. Nodular basal cell carcinoma: when in doubt, cut it out. J Drugs Dermatol. 2007; 6(12):1245–1246

[143] Hendrix JD, Jr, Parlette HL. Micronodular basal cell carcinoma. A deceptive histologic subtype with frequent clinically undetected tumor extension. Arch Dermatol. 1996; 132(3):295–298

[144] Crowson AN. Basal cell carcinoma: biology, morphology and clinical implications. Mod Pathol. 2006; 19 Suppl 2:S127–S147

[145] Sexton M, Jones DB, Maloney ME. Histologic pattern analysis of basal cell carcinoma. Study of a series of 1039 consecutive neoplasms. J Am Acad Dermatol. 1990; 23(6, Pt 1):1118–1126

[146] Boyd AS, Rapini RP. Cutaneous collision tumors. An analysis of 69 cases and review of the literature. Am J Dermatopathol. 1994; 16(3):253–257

[147] Boyd AS. Tumors of the epidermis. In: Barnhill R, Crowson AN, eds. Textbook of Dermatopathology. 2nd ed. New York, NY: McGraw-Hill; 2004:575–634

[148] Altamura D, Menzies SW, Argenziano G, et al. Dermatoscopy of basal cell carcinoma: morphologic variability of global and local features and accuracy of diagnosis. J Am Acad Dermatol. 2010; 62(1):67–75

[149] Zalaudek I, Kreusch J, Giacomel J, Ferrara G, Catricalà C, Argenziano G. How to diagnose nonpigmented skin tumors: a review of vascular structures seen with dermoscopy: part II. Nonmelanocytic skin tumors. J Am Acad Dermatol. 2010; 63(3):377–386, quiz 387–388

[150] Wolberink EA, Pasch MC, Zeiler M, van Erp PE, Gerritsen MJ. High discordance between punch biopsy and excision in establishing basal cell carcinoma subtype: analysis of 500 cases. J Eur Acad Dermatol Venereol. 2013; 27 (8):985–989

[151] Mosterd K, Thissen MR, van Marion AM, et al. Correlation between histologic findings on punch biopsy specimens and subsequent excision specimens in recurrent basal cell carcinoma. J Am Acad Dermatol. 2011; 64(2):323–327

[152] Haws AL, Rojano R, Tahan SR, Phung TL. Accuracy of biopsy sampling for subtyping basal cell carcinoma. J Am Acad Dermatol. 2012; 66(1):106–111

[153] Russell EB, Carrington PR, Smoller BR. Basal cell carcinoma: a comparison of shave biopsy versus punch biopsy techniques in subtype diagnosis. J Am Acad Dermatol. 1999; 41(1):69–71

[154] Al-Ghamdi Y. Basal cell carcinoma: shave biopsy versus punch biopsy technique in subtype diagnosis. J Am Acad Dermatol. 2002; 46(4):643–, author reply, 643–644

[155] Breuninger H, Schaumburg-Lever G. Control of excisional margins by conventional histopathological techniques in the treatment of skin tumours. An alternative to Mohs' technique. J Pathol. 1988; 154(2):167–171

[156] Sriskandan N, Manjaly G, Howlett DC. Re: Breeze J, Andi A, Williams MD, Howlett DC. The use of fine needle core biopsy under ultrasound guidance in the diagnosis of a parotid mass [Br. J. Oral Maxillofac. Surg. 2009;47 (1):78–9]. Br J Oral Maxillofac Surg. 2009; 47(6):493–494

[157] Goette DK. Topical chemotherapy with 5-fluorouracil. A review. J Am Acad Dermatol. 1981; 4(6):633–649

[158] Reymann F. Treatment of basal cell carcinoma of the skin with 5-fluorouracil ointment. A 10-year follow-up study. Dermatologica. 1979; 158(5):368–372

[159] Klostermann GF. Basal-cell carcinoma of large dimension. Dermatologica. 1970; 140 Suppl 1:1–, 54

[160] Mohs FE, Jones DL, Bloom RF. Tendency of fluorouracil to conceal deep foci of invasive basal cell carcinoma. Arch Dermatol. 1978; 114(7):1021–1022

[161] Epstein E. Fluorouracil paste treatment of thin basal cell carcinomas. Arch Dermatol. 1985; 121(2):207–213

[162] Schön M, Bong AB, Drewniok C, et al. Tumor-selective induction of apoptosis and the small-molecule immune response modifier imiquimod. J Natl Cancer Inst. 2003; 95(15):1138–1149

[163] Urosevic M, Dummer R, Conrad C, et al. Disease-independent skin recruitment and activation of plasmacytoid predendritic cells following imiquimod treatment. J Natl Cancer Inst. 2005; 97(15):1143–1153

[164] Geisse J, Caro I, Lindholm J, Golitz L, Stampone P, Owens M. Imiquimod 5% cream for the treatment of superficial basal cell carcinoma: results from two phase III, randomized, vehicle-controlled studies. J Am Acad Dermatol. 2004; 50(5):722–733

[165] Schulze HJ, Cribier B, Requena L, et al. Imiquimod 5% cream for the treatment of superficial basal cell carcinoma: results from a randomized vehicle-controlled phase III study in Europe. Br J Dermatol. 2005; 152(5):939–947

[166] Bath-Hextall F, Ozolins M, Armstrong SJ, et al. Surgery versus Imiquimod for Nodular Superficial basal cell carcinoma (SINS) study group. Surgical excision versus imiquimod 5% cream for nodular and superficial basal-cell carcinoma (SINS): a multicentre, non-inferiority, randomised controlled trial. Lancet Oncol. 2014; 15(1):96–105

[167] McKay KM, Sambrano BL, Fox PS, Bassett RL, Chon S, Prieto VG. Thickness of superficial basal cell carcinoma (sBCC) predicts imiquimod efficacy: a proposal for a thickness-based definition of sBCC. Br J Dermatol. 2013; 169 (3):549–554

[168] Butler DF, Parekh PK, Lenis A. Imiquimod 5% cream as adjunctive therapy for primary, solitary, nodular nasal basal cell carcinomas before Mohs micrographic surgery: a randomized, double blind, vehicle-controlled study. Dermatol Surg. 2009; 35(1):24–29

[169] van der Geer S, Martens J, van Roij J, et al. Imiquimod 5% cream as pretreatment of Mohs micrographic surgery for nodular basal cell carcinoma in the face: a prospective randomized controlled study. Br J Dermatol. 2012; 167 (1):110–115

[170] Moehrle M, Breuninger H, Schippert W, Häfner HM. Letter: imiquimod 5% cream as adjunctive therapy for primary, solitary, nodular basal cell carcinomas before Mohs micrographic surgery: a randomized, double-blind, vehicle-controlled study. Dermatol Surg. 2010; 36(3):428–430

[171] Vidal D, Matías-Guiu X, Alomar A. Fifty-five basal cell carcinomas treated with topical imiquimod: outcome at 5-year follow-up. Arch Dermatol. 2007; 143(2):266–268

[172] Foley P. Clinical efficacy of methyl aminolevulinate (Metvix) photodynamic therapy. J Dermatolog Treat. 2003; 14 Suppl 3:15–22

[173] Foley P. Clinical efficacy of methyl aminolaevulinate photodynamic therapy in basal cell carcinoma and solar keratosis. Australas J Dermatol. 2005; 46 Suppl 3:S8–S10, discussion S23–S25

[174] Kalka K, Merk H, Mukhtar H. Photodynamic therapy in dermatology. J Am Acad Dermatol. 2000; 42(3):389–413, quiz 414–416

[175] Fantini F, Greco A, Del Giovane C, et al. Photodynamic therapy for basal cell carcinoma: clinical and pathological determinants of response. J Eur Acad Dermatol Venereol. 2011; 25(8):896–901

[176] Cosgarea R, Susan M, Crisan M, Senila S. Photodynamic therapy using topical 5-aminolaevulinic acid vs. surgery for basal cell carcinoma. J Eur Acad Dermatol Venereol. 2013; 27(8):980–984

[177] Roozeboom MH, Arits AH, Nelemans PJ, Kelleners-Smeets NW. Overall treatment success after treatment of primary superficial basal cell carcinoma: a systematic review and meta-analysis of randomized and nonrandomized trials. Br J Dermatol. 2012; 167(4):733–756

[178] Arits AH, Mosterd K, Essers BA, et al. Photodynamic therapy versus topical imiquimod versus topical fluorouracil for treatment of superficial basal-cell carcinoma: a single blind, non-inferiority, randomised controlled trial. Lancet Oncol. 2013; 14(7):647–654

[179] Clark CM, Furniss M, Mackay-Wiggan JM. Basal cell carcinoma: an evidence-based treatment update. Am J Clin Dermatol. 2014; 15(3):197–216

[180] Silverman MK, Kopf AW, Gladstein AH, Bart RS, Grin CM, Levenstein MJ. Recurrence rates of treated basal cell carcinomas. Part 4: X-ray therapy. J Dermatol Surg Oncol. 1992; 18(7):549–554

[181] Rowe DED, Carroll RJ, Day CL, Jr. Long-term recurrence rates in previously untreated (primary) basal cell carcinoma: implications for patient follow-up. J Dermatol Surg Oncol. 1989; 15(3):315–328

[182] Locke J, Karimpour S, Young G, Lockett MA, Perez CA. Radiotherapy for epithelial skin cancer. Int J Radiat Oncol Biol Phys. 2001; 51(3):748–755

[183] Wilder RB, Shimm DS, Kittelson JM, Rogoff EE, Cassady JR. Recurrent basal cell carcinoma treated with radiation therapy. Arch Dermatol. 1991; 127 (11):1668–1672

[184] Fleming ID, Amonette R, Monaghan T, Fleming MD. Principles of management of basal and squamous cell carcinoma of the skin. Cancer. 1995; 75(2) Suppl:699–704

[185] Petrovich Z, Kuisk H, Langholz B, et al. Treatment of carcinoma of the skin with bone and/or cartilage involvement. Am J Clin Oncol. 1988; 11 (2):110–113

[186] Goldschmidt H, Breneman JC, Breneman DL. Ionizing radiation therapy in dermatology. J Am Acad Dermatol. 1994; 30(2, Pt 1):157–182, quiz 183–186

[187] Kirby JS, Miller CJ. Intralesional chemotherapy for nonmelanoma skin cancer: a practical review. J Am Acad Dermatol. 2010; 63(4):689–702

[188] Good LM, Miller MD, High WA. Intralesional agents in the management of cutaneous malignancy: a review. J Am Acad Dermatol. 2011; 64(2):413–422

[189] Avant WHW, Huff RC. Intradermal 5-fluorouracil in the treatment of basal cell carcinoma of the face. South Med J. 1976; 69(5):561–563

[190] Kurtis B, Rosen T. Treatment of cutaneous neoplasms by intralesional injections of 5-fluorouracil (5-FU). J Dermatol Surg Oncol. 1980; 6(2):122–127

[191] Gyurova MS, Stancheva MZ, Arnaudova MN, Yankova RK. Intralesional bleomycin as alternative therapy in the treatment of multiple basal cell carcinomas. Dermatol Online J. 2006; 12(3):25

[192] Mishima Y, Matunaka M. Effect of bleomycin on benign and malignant cutaneous tumours. Acta Derm Venereol. 1972; 52(3):211–215

[193] von Domarus H, Stevens PJ. Metastatic basal cell carcinoma. Report of five cases and review of 170 cases in the literature. J Am Acad Dermatol. 1984; 10(6):1043–1060

[194] Weinstock MA, Bogaars HA, Ashley M, Litle V, Bilodeau E, Kimmel S. Nonmelanoma skin cancer mortality. A population-based study. Arch Dermatol. 1991; 127(8):1194–1197

[195] Wysong A, Aasi SZ, Tang JY. Update on metastatic basal cell carcinoma: a summary of published cases from 1981 through 2011. JAMA Dermatol. 2013; 149(5):615–616

[196] Danial C, Lingala B, Balise R, et al. Markedly improved overall survival in 10 consecutive patients with metastatic basal cell carcinoma. Br J Dermatol. 2013; 169(3):673–676

[197] Moser S, Borm J, Mihic-Probst D, Jacobsen C, Kruse Gujer AL. Metastatic basal cell carcinoma: report of a case and review of the literature. Oral Surg Oral Med Oral Pathol Oral Radiol. 2014; 117(2):e79–e82

[198] Soleymani AD, Scheinfeld N, Vasil K, Bechtel MA. Metastatic basal cell carcinoma presenting with unilateral upper extremity edema and lymphatic spread. J Am Acad Dermatol. 2008; 59(2) Suppl 1:S1–S3

[199] Mohan SV, Chang AL. Advanced basal cell carcinoma: epidemiology and therapeutic innovations. Curr Dermatol Rep. 2014; 3:40–45

[200] Mohan SV, Chang AL. Precision medicine and precision therapeutics: hedgehog signaling pathway, basal cell carcinoma and beyond. Semin Cutan Med Surg. 2014; 33(2):68–71

[201] Nüsslein-Volhard C, Wieschaus E. Mutations affecting segment number and polarity in Drosophila. Nature. 1980; 287(5785):795–801

[202] Ingham PW, McMahon AP. Hedgehog signaling in animal development: paradigms and principles. Genes Dev. 2001; 15(23):3059–3087

[203] Johnson RL, Rothman AL, Xie J, et al. Human homolog of patched, a candidate gene for the basal cell nevus syndrome. Science. 1996; 272 (5268):1668–1671

[204] Atwood SX, Whitson RJ, Oro AE. "Patch"ing up our tumor signaling knowledge. J Invest Dermatol. 2013; 133(5):1131–1133

[205] Dreier J, Dummer R, Felderer L, Nägeli M, Gobbi S, Kunstfeld R. Emerging drugs and combination strategies for basal cell carcinoma. Expert Opin Emerg Drugs. 2014; 19(3):353–365

[206] Xie J, Bartels CM, Barton SW, Gu D. Targeting hedgehog signaling in cancer: research and clinical developments. OncoTargets Ther. 2013; 6:1425–1435

[207] Lipinski RJ, Gipp JJ, Zhang J, Doles JD, Bushman W. Unique and complimentary activities of the Gli transcription factors in Hedgehog signaling. Exp Cell Res. 2006; 312(11):1925–1938

[208] Reifenberger J, Wolter M, Knobbe CB, et al. Somatic mutations in the PTCH, SMOH, SUFUH and TP53 genes in sporadic basal cell carcinomas. Br J Dermatol. 2005; 152(1):43–51

[209] Keeler RF, Binns W. Teratogenic compounds of Veratrum californicum (Durand). V. Comparison of cyclopian effects of steroidal alkaloids from the plant and structurally related compounds from other sources. Teratology. 1968; 1(1):5–10

[210] Chen JK, Taipale J, Cooper MK, Beachy PA. Inhibition of Hedgehog signaling by direct binding of cyclopamine to Smoothened. Genes Dev. 2002; 16 (21):2743–2748

[211] Taipale J, Chen JK, Cooper MK, et al. Effects of oncogenic mutations in Smoothened and Patched can be reversed by cyclopamine. Nature. 2000; 406(6799):1005–1009

[212] Cooper MK, Porter JA, Young KE, Beachy PA. Teratogen-mediated inhibition of target tissue response to Shh signaling. Science. 1998; 280 (5369):1603–1607

[213] Incardona JP, Gaffield W, Kapur RP, Roelink H. The teratogenic Veratrum alkaloid cyclopamine inhibits sonic hedgehog signal transduction. Development. 1998; 125(18):3553–3562

[214] Robarge KD, Brunton SA, Castanedo GM, et al. GDC-0449-a potent inhibitor of the hedgehog pathway. Bioorg Med Chem Lett. 2009; 19(19):5576–5581

[215] Sekulic A, Migden MR, Oro AE, et al. Efficacy and safety of vismodegib in advanced basal-cell carcinoma. N Engl J Med. 2012; 366(23):2171–2179

[216] Chang AL, Atwood SX, Tartar DM, Oro AE. Surgical excision after neoadjuvant therapy with vismodegib for a locally advanced basal cell carcinoma and resistant basal carcinomas in Gorlin syndrome. JAMA Dermatol. 2013; 149(5):639–641

[217] Lorusso PM, Jimeno A, Dy G, et al. Pharmacokinetic dose-scheduling study of hedgehog pathway inhibitor vismodegib (GDC-0449) in patients with locally advanced or metastatic solid tumors. Clin Cancer Res. 2011; 17(17):5774–5782

[218] Rudin CM. Vismodegib. Clin Cancer Res. 2012; 18(12):3218–3222

[219] Tang JY, Mackay-Wiggan JM, Aszterbaum M, et al. Inhibiting the hedgehog pathway in patients with the basal-cell nevus syndrome. N Engl J Med. 2012; 366(23):2180–2188

[220] Ruiz Salas V, Alegre M, Garcés JR, Puig L. Locally advanced and metastatic basal cell carcinoma: molecular pathways, treatment options and new targeted therapies. Expert Rev Anticancer Ther. 2014; 14(6):741–749

[221] Ruiz-Salas V, Alegre M, López-Ferrer A, Garcés JR. Vismodegib: a review. Actas Dermosifiliogr. 2014; 105(8):744–751

[222] Lallas A, Pyne J, Kyrgidis A, et al. The clinical and dermoscopic features of invasive cutaneous squamous cell carcinoma depend on the histopathological grade of differentiation. Br J Dermatol. 2015; 172(5):1308–1315

[223] Kahana A, Worden FP, Elner VM. Vismodegib as eye-sparing adjuvant treatment for orbital basal cell carcinoma. JAMA Ophthalmol. 2013; 131 (10):1364–1366

[224] Tang JY, Marghoob AA. Emerging treatments and signaling pathway inhibitors. Semin Cutan Med Surg. 2011; 30(4) Suppl:S14–S18

[225] LoRusso PM, Rudin CM, Reddy JC, et al. Phase I trial of hedgehog pathway inhibitor vismodegib (GDC-0449) in patients with refractory, locally advanced or metastatic solid tumors. Clin Cancer Res. 2011; 17 (8):2502–2511

[226] Kim J, Tang JY, Gong R, et al. Itraconazole, a commonly used antifungal that inhibits Hedgehog pathway activity and cancer growth. Cancer Cell. 2010; 17(4):388–399

[227] Kim DJ, Kim J, Spaunhurst K, et al. Open-label, exploratory phase II trial of oral itraconazole for the treatment of basal cell carcinoma. J Clin Oncol. 2014; 32(8):745–751

[228] Samarasinghe V, Madan V. Nonmelanoma skin cancer. J Cutan Aesthet Surg. 2012; 5(1):3–10

[229] Dubin N, Kopf AW. Multivariate risk score for recurrence of cutaneous basal cell carcinomas. Arch Dermatol. 1983; 119(5):373–377

[230] Bart RS, Schrager D, Kopf AW, Bromberg J, Dubin N. Scalpel excision of basal cell carcinomas. Arch Dermatol. 1978; 114(5):739–742

[231] Szeimies RM, Ibbotson S, Murrell DF, et al. Excilight Study Group. A clinical study comparing methyl aminolevulinate photodynamic therapy and surgery in small superficial basal cell carcinoma (8–20 mm), with a 12-month follow-up. J Eur Acad Dermatol Venereol. 2008; 22(11):1302–1311

[232] Berroeta L, Clark C, Dawe RS, Ibbotson SH, Fleming CJ. A randomized study of minimal curettage followed by topical photodynamic therapy compared with surgical excision for low-risk nodular basal cell carcinoma. Br J Dermatol. 2007; 157(2):401–403

[233] Wolf DJ, Zitelli JA. Surgical margins for basal cell carcinoma. Arch Dermatol. 1987; 123(3):340–344

[234] Gulleth Y, Goldberg N, Silverman RP, Gastman BR. What is the best surgical margin for a Basal cell carcinoma: a meta-analysis of the literature. Plast Reconstr Surg. 2010; 126(4):1222–1231

[235] Rowe DE, Carroll RJ, Day CL, Jr. Mohs surgery is the treatment of choice for recurrent (previously treated) basal cell carcinoma. J Dermatol Surg Oncol. 1989; 15(4):424–431

[236] Smeets NW, Krekels GA, Ostertag JU, et al. Surgical excision vs Mohs' micrographic surgery for basal-cell carcinoma of the face: randomised controlled trial. Lancet. 2004; 364(9447):1766–1772

[237] Malik V, Goh KS, Leong S, Tan A, Downey D, O'Donovan D. Risk and outcome analysis of 1832 consecutively excised basal cell carcinomas in a tertiary referral plastic surgery unit. J Plast Reconstr Aesthet Surg. 2010; 63 (12):2057–2063

[238] Palmer VM, Wilson PR. Incompletely excised basal cell carcinoma: residual tumor rates at Mohs re-excision. Dermatol Surg. 2013; 39(5):706–718

[239] Robinson JK, Fisher SG. Recurrent basal cell carcinoma after incomplete resection. Arch Dermatol. 2000; 136(11):1318–1324

[240] Muller FM, Dawe RS, Moseley H, Fleming CJ. Randomized comparison of Mohs micrographic surgery and surgical excision for small nodular basal cell carcinoma: tissue-sparing outcome. Dermatol Surg. 2009; 35 (9):1349–1354
[241] Lane JE, Kent DE. Surgical margins in the treatment of nonmelanoma skin cancer and Mohs micrographic surgery. Curr Surg. 2005; 62(5):518–526
[242] Kuflik EG. Cryosurgery for cutaneous malignancy. An update. Dermatol Surg. 1997; 23(11):1081–1087
[243] Kuflik EG, Gage AA. The five-year cure rate achieved by cryosurgery for skin cancer. J Am Acad Dermatol. 1991; 24(6, Pt 1):1002–1004
[244] Graham GF. Cryosurgery. Clin Plast Surg. 1993; 20(1):131–147
[245] Zacarian SA. Cryosurgery of cutaneous carcinomas. An 18-year study of 3,022 patients with 4,228 carcinomas. J Am Acad Dermatol. 1983; 9 (6):947–956
[246] Biro L, Price E. Cryosurgical management of basal cell carcinoma of the eyelid: a 10-year experience. J Am Acad Dermatol. 1990; 23(2, Pt 1):316–317
[247] Williams LS, Mancuso AA, Mendenhall WM. Perineural spread of cutaneous squamous and basal cell carcinoma: CT and MR detection and its impact on patient management and prognosis. Int J Radiat Oncol Biol Phys. 2001; 49 (4):1061–1069
[248] Moy RL, Eliezri YD, Nuovo GJ, Zitelli JA, Bennett RG, Silverstein S. Human papillomavirus type 16 DNA in periungual squamous cell carcinomas. JAMA. 1989; 261(18):2669–2673
[249] Moy RL, Quan MB. The presence of human papillomavirus type 16 in squamous cell carcinoma of the proximal finger and reconstruction with a bilobed transposition flap. J Dermatol Surg Oncol. 1991; 17(2):171–175
[250] Anwar J, Wrone DA, Kimyai-Asadi A, Alam M. The development of actinic keratosis into invasive squamous cell carcinoma: evidence and evolving classification schemes. Clin Dermatol. 2004; 22(3):189–196
[251] Cantisani C, De Gado F, Ulrich M, et al. Actinic keratosis: review of the literature and new patents. Recent Pat Inflamm Allergy Drug Discov. 2013; 7 (2):168–175
[252] Christensen E, Bofin A, Gudmundsdóttir I, Skogvoll E. Cytological diagnosis of basal cell carcinoma and actinic keratosis, using Papanicolaou and May-Grünwald-Giemsa stained cutaneous tissue smear. Cytopathology. 2008; 19 (5):316–322
[253] Dréno B, Amici JM, Basset-Seguin N, Cribier B, Claudel JP, Richard MA, AKTeam™. Management of actinic keratosis: a practical report and treatment algorithm from AKTeam™ expert clinicians. J Eur Acad Dermatol Venereol. 2014; 28(9):1141–1149
[254] Feldman SR, Fleischer AB, Jr. Progression of actinic keratosis to squamous cell carcinoma revisited: clinical and treatment implications. Cutis. 2011; 87 (4):201–207
[255] Bart RS, Andrade R, Kopf AW. Cutaneous horns. A clinical and histopathologic study. Acta Derm Venereol. 1968; 48(5):507–515
[256] Copcu E, Sivrioglu N, Culhaci N. Cutaneous horns: are these lesions as innocent as they seem to be? World J Surg Oncol. 2004; 2:18
[257] Jones T, Blanco-Guzman M. A cutaneous horn-benign or malignant? J Craniomaxillofac Surg. 2013; 41(2):144–146
[258] Leffell DJ. The scientific basis of skin cancer. J Am Acad Dermatol. 2000; 42 (1, Pt 2):18–22
[259] Thompson SC, Jolley D, Marks R. Reduction of solar keratoses by regular sunscreen use. N Engl J Med. 1993; 329(16):1147–1151
[260] Flohil SC, van der Leest RJ, Dowlatshahi EA, Hofman A, de Vries E, Nijsten T. Prevalence of actinic keratosis and its risk factors in the general population: the Rotterdam Study. J Invest Dermatol. 2013; 133(8):1971–1978
[261] Marks R, Rennie G, Selwood TS. Malignant transformation of solar keratoses to squamous cell carcinoma. Lancet. 1988; 1(8589):795–797
[262] Criscione VD, Weinstock MA, Naylor MF, Luque C, Eide MJ, Bingham SF, Department of Veteran Affairs Topical Tretinoin Chemoprevention Trial Group. Actinic keratoses: natural history and risk of malignant transformation in the Veterans Affairs Topical Tretinoin Chemoprevention Trial. Cancer. 2009; 115(11):2523–2530
[263] Quaedvlieg PJ, Tirsi E, Thissen MR, Krekels GA. Actinic keratosis: how to differentiate the good from the bad ones? Eur J Dermatol. 2006; 16 (4):335–339
[264] Fuchs A, Marmur E. The kinetics of skin cancer: progression of actinic keratosis to squamous cell carcinoma. Dermatol Surg. 2007; 33(9):1099–1101
[265] Accardi R, Gheit T. Cutaneous HPV and skin cancer. Presse Med. 2014; 43(12, Pt 2):e435–e443
[266] Lee JJ, Hong WK, Hittelman WN, et al. Predicting cancer development in oral leukoplakia: ten years of translational research. Clin Cancer Res. 2000; 6 (5):1702–1710
[267] Shiu MN, Chen TH, Chang SH, Hahn LJ. Risk factors for leukoplakia and malignant transformation to oral carcinoma: a leukoplakia cohort in Taiwan. Br J Cancer. 2000; 82(11):1871–1874
[268] Markopoulos A, Albanidou-Farmaki E, Kayavis I. Actinic cheilitis: clinical and pathologic characteristics in 65 cases. Oral Dis. 2004; 10(4):212–216
[269] Jadotte YT, Schwartz RA. Solar cheilosis: an ominous precursor: part I. Diagnostic insights. J Am Acad Dermatol. 2012; 66(2):173–184, quiz 185–186
[270] Vieira RA, Minicucci EM, Marques ME, Marques SA. Actinic cheilitis and squamous cell carcinoma of the lip: clinical, histopathological and immunogenetic aspects. An Bras Dermatol. 2012; 87(1):105–114
[271] Cohen JL. Erbium laser resurfacing for actinic cheilitis. J Drugs Dermatol. 2013; 12(11):1290–1292
[272] Dufresne RG, Jr, Cruz AP, Zeikus P, Perlis C, Jellinek NJ. Dermabrasion for actinic cheilitis. Dermatol Surg. 2008; 34(6):848–850
[273] Smith KJ, Germain M, Yeager J, Skelton H. Topical 5% imiquimod for the therapy of actinic cheilitis. J Am Acad Dermatol. 2002; 47(4):497–501
[274] Sotiriou E, Lallas A, Goussi C, et al. Sequential use of photodynamic therapy and imiquimod 5% cream for the treatment of actinic cheilitis: a 12-month follow-up study. Br J Dermatol. 2011; 165(4):888–892
[275] Yazdani Abyaneh MA, Falto-Aizpurua L, Griffith RD, Nouri K. Photodynamic therapy for actinic cheilitis: a systematic review. Dermatol Surg. 2015; 41 (2):189–198
[276] Ulrich C, Forschner T, Ulrich M, Stockfleth E, Sterry W, Termeer C. Management of actinic cheilitis using diclofenac 3% gel: a report of six cases. Br J Dermatol. 2007; 156 Suppl 3:43–46
[277] Lima GdaS, Silva GF, Gomes AP, de Araújo LM, Salum FG. Diclofenac in hyaluronic acid gel: an alternative treatment for actinic cheilitis. J Appl Oral Sci. 2010; 18(5):533–537
[278] Barry RB, McKenzie J, Berg D, Langtry JA. Direct primary closure without undermining in the repair of vermilionectomy defects of the lower lip. Br J Dermatol. 2012; 167(5):1092–1097
[279] Shah AY, Doherty SD, Rosen T. Actinic cheilitis: a treatment review. Int J Dermatol. 2010; 49(11):1225–1234
[280] Brash DE, Rudolph JA, Simon JA, et al. A role for sunlight in skin cancer: UV-induced p53 mutations in squamous cell carcinoma. Proc Natl Acad Sci U S A. 1991; 88(22):10124–10128
[281] Surdu S. Non-melanoma skin cancer: occupational risk from UV light and arsenic exposure. Rev Environ Health. 2014; 29(3):255–264
[282] Wang H, Xu Y, Shi J, Gao X, Geng L. Photodynamic therapy in the treatment of basal cell carcinoma: a systematic review and meta-analysis. Photodermatol Photoimmunol Photomed. 2015; 31(1):44–53
[283] Wang LS, Handorf EA, Wu H, Liu JC, Perlis CS, Galloway TJ. Surgery and Adjuvant Radiation for High-risk Skin Adnexal Carcinoma of the Head and Neck. Am J Clin Oncol. 2015
[284] Wang X, Shi L, Tu Q, et al. Treating cutaneous squamous cell carcinoma using 5-aminolevulinic acid polylactic-co-glycolic acid nanoparticle-mediated photodynamic therapy in a mouse model. Int J Nanomedicine. 2015; 10:347–355
[285] Pierceall WE, Ananthaswamy HN. Transformation of NIH3T3 cells by transfection with UV-irradiated human c-Ha-ras-1 proto-oncogene DNA. Oncogene. 1991; 6(11):2085–2091
[286] Bukhari MH, Niazi S, Anwar M, Chaudhry NA, Naeem S. Prognostic significance of new immunohistochemistry scoring of p53 protein expression in cutaneous squamous cell carcinoma of mice. Ann N Y Acad Sci. 2008; 1138:1–9
[287] Aldabagh B, Angeles JG, Cardones AR, Arron ST. Cutaneous squamous cell carcinoma and human papillomavirus: is there an association? Dermatol Surg. 2013; 39(1, Pt 1):1–23
[288] Weinstock MA, Fisher DE. Indoor ultraviolet tanning: what the data do and do not show regarding risk of melanoma and keratinocyte malignancies. J Natl Compr Canc Netw. 2010; 8(8):867–872, quiz 873
[289] Partridge ME, Pariser RJ. Ocular and cutaneous squamous cell carcinoma in an African American man with epidermodysplasia verruciformis resulting in blindness and death. J Am Acad Dermatol. 2003; 49(5) Suppl:S262–S264
[290] Dyall-Smith D, Ross JB. Cutaneous malignancies in renal transplant recipients from Nova Scotia, Canada. Australas J Dermatol. 1995; 36(2):79–82
[291] Cohen EB, Komorowski RA, Clowry LJ. Cutaneous complications in renal transplant recipients. Am J Clin Pathol. 1987; 88(1):32–37
[292] Basić-Jukić N, Bubić-Filipi L, Prgomet D, et al. Head and neck malignancies in Croatian renal transplant recipients. Bosn J Basic Med Sci. 2010; 10 Suppl 1: S37–S39
[293] Birkeland SA, Storm HH, Lamm LU, et al. Cancer risk after renal transplantation in the Nordic countries, 1964–1986. Int J Cancer. 1995; 60(2):183–189

[294] Penn I. Occurrence of cancers in immunosuppressed organ transplant recipients. Clin Transpl. 1998; 12:147–158

[295] Smith KJ, Haley H, Hamza S, Skelton HG. Eruptive keratoacanthoma-type squamous cell carcinomas in patients taking sorafenib for the treatment of solid tumors. Dermatol Surg. 2009; 35(11):1766–1770

[296] Smith KJ, Hamza S, Skelton H. The imidazoquinolines and their place in the therapy of cutaneous disease. Expert Opin Pharmacother. 2003; 4 (7):1105–1119

[297] Smith KJ, Hamza S, Skelton H. Topical imidazoquinoline therapy of cutaneous squamous cell carcinoma polarizes lymphoid and monocyte/macrophage populations to a Th1 and M1 cytokine pattern. Clin Exp Dermatol. 2004; 29(5):505–512

[298] Kempf W, Mertz KD, Hofbauer GF, Tinguely M. Skin cancer in organ transplant recipients. Pathobiology. 2013; 80(6):302–309

[299] Martorell-Calatayud A, Sanmartín Jimenez O, Cruz Mojarrieta J, Guillén Barona C. Cutaneous squamous cell carcinoma: defining the high-risk variant. Actas Dermosifiliogr. 2013; 104(5):367–379

[300] Frierson HF, Jr, Cooper PH. Prognostic factors in squamous cell carcinoma of the lower lip. Hum Pathol. 1986; 17(4):346–354

[301] Frierson HF, Jr, Deutsch BD, Levine PA. Clinicopathologic features of cutaneous squamous cell carcinomas of the head and neck in patients with chronic lymphocytic leukemia/small lymphocytic lymphoma. Hum Pathol. 1988; 19 (12):1397–1402

[302] Somos S, Farkas B, Schneider I. Cancer protection in xeroderma pigmentosum variant (XP-V). Anticancer Res. 1999; 19(3B) 3b:2195–2199

[303] Diepgen TL, Mahler V. The epidemiology of skin cancer. Br J Dermatol. 2002; 146 Suppl 61:1–6

[304] Diepgen TL, Drexler H, Schmitt J. [Epidemiology of occupational skin cancer due to UV-irradiation]. Hautarzt. 2012; 63(10):769–777

[305] Behroozan DS, Glaich A, Goldberg LH. Dermatofibrosarcoma protuberans following tanning bed use. J Drugs Dermatol. 2005; 4(6):751–754

[306] Paredes F. [Marjölin ulcer]. Acta Med Port. 1998; 11(2):185–187

[307] Chalya PL, Mabula JB, Rambau P, et al. Marjolin's ulcers at a university teaching hospital in Northwestern Tanzania: a retrospective review of 56 cases. World J Surg Oncol. 2012; 10:38

[308] Challa VR, Deshmane V, Ashwatha Reddy MB. A retrospective study of Marjolin's ulcer over an eleven year period. J Cutan Aesthet Surg. 2014; 7 (3):155–159

[309] Chang JB, Kung TA, Cederna PS. Acute Marjolin's ulcers: a nebulous diagnosis. Ann Plast Surg. 2014; 72(5):515–520

[310] Copcu E. Marjolin's ulcer: a preventable complication of burns? Plast Reconstr Surg. 2009; 124(1):156e–164e

[311] Copcu E, Aktas A, Sişman N, Oztan Y. Thirty-one cases of Marjolin's ulcer. Clin Exp Dermatol. 2003; 28(2):138–141

[312] Esther RJ, Lamps L, Schwartz HS. Marjolin ulcers: secondary carcinomas in chronic wounds. J South Orthop Assoc. 1999; 8(3):181–187

[313] Türegün M, Nişanci M, Güler M. Burn scar carcinoma with longer lag period arising in previously grafted area. Burns. 1997; 23(6):496–497

[314] Cantwell MM, Murray LJ, Catney D, et al. Second primary cancers in patients with skin cancer: a population-based study in Northern Ireland. Br J Cancer. 2009; 100(1):174–177

[315] Hussain SK, Sundquist J, Hemminki K. The effect of having an affected parent or sibling on invasive and in situ skin cancer risk in Sweden. J Invest Dermatol. 2009; 129(9):2142–2147

[316] Hemminki K, Zhang H, Czene K. Familial invasive and in situ squamous cell carcinoma of the skin. Br J Cancer. 2003; 88(9):1375–1380

[317] Lindström LS, Yip B, Lichtenstein P, Pawitan Y, Czene K. Etiology of familial aggregation in melanoma and squamous cell carcinoma of the skin. Cancer Epidemiol Biomarkers Prev. 2007; 16(8):1639–1643

[318] Parikh SA, Patel VA, Ratner D. Advances in the management of cutaneous squamous cell carcinoma. F1000Prime Rep. 2014; 6:70

[319] Metchnikoff C, Mully T, Singer JP, Golden JA, Arron ST. The 7th edition AJCC staging system for cutaneous squamous cell carcinoma accurately predicts risk of recurrence for heart and lung transplant recipients. J Am Acad Dermatol. 2012; 67(5):829–835

[320] Schmults CD. High-risk cutaneous squamous cell carcinoma: identification and management. Adv Dermatol. 2005; 21:133–152

[321] Schmults CD, Karia PS, Carter JB, Han J, Qureshi AA. Factors predictive of recurrence and death from cutaneous squamous cell carcinoma: a 10-year, single-institution cohort study. JAMA Dermatol. 2013; 149(5):541–547

[322] Jambusaria-Pahlajani A, Kanetsky PA, Karia PS, et al. Evaluation of AJCC tumor staging for cutaneous squamous cell carcinoma and a proposed alternative tumor staging system. JAMA Dermatol. 2013; 149(4):402–410

[323] Braathen LR, Morton CA, Basset-Seguin N, et al. International Society for Photodynamic Therapy in Dermatology. Photodynamic therapy for skin field cancerization: an international consensus. J Eur Acad Dermatol Venereol. 2012; 26(9):1063–1066

[324] Caccialanza M, Piccinno R, Grammatica A. Radiotherapy of recurrent basal and squamous cell skin carcinomas: a study of 249 re-treated carcinomas in 229 patients. Eur J Dermatol. 2001; 11(1):25–28

[325] Veness M, Richards S. Role of modern radiotherapy in treating skin cancer. Australas J Dermatol. 2003; 44(3):159–166, quiz 167–168

[326] Al-Othman MO, Mendenhall WM, Amdur RJ. Radiotherapy alone for clinical T4 skin carcinoma of the head and neck with surgery reserved for salvage. Am J Otolaryngol. 2001; 22(6):387–390

[327] Veness MJ, Morgan GJ, Palme CE, Gebski V. Surgery and adjuvant radiotherapy in patients with cutaneous head and neck squamous cell carcinoma metastatic to lymph nodes: combined treatment should be considered best practice. Laryngoscope. 2005; 115(5):870–875

[328] Zwald F. Practice gaps. Immediate curettage and electrodessication following biopsy of suspected basal cell carcinoma at initial visit. JAMA Dermatol. 2013; 149(8):981

[329] Brodland DG, Zitelli JA. Surgical margins for excision of primary cutaneous squamous cell carcinoma. J Am Acad Dermatol. 1992; 27(2, Pt 1):241–248

[330] Narayanan K, Hadid OH, Barnes EA. Mohs micrographic surgery versus surgical excision for periocular basal cell carcinoma. Cochrane Database Syst Rev. 2014; 12(12):CD007041

[331] Chren M-M, Linos E, Torres JS, Stuart SE, Parvataneni R, Boscardin WJ. Tumor recurrence 5 years after treatment of cutaneous basal cell carcinoma and squamous cell carcinoma. J Invest Dermatol. 2013; 133(5):1188–1196

[332] van Loo E, Mosterd K, Krekels GAM, et al. Surgical excision versus Mohs' micrographic surgery for basal cell carcinoma of the face: a randomised clinical trial with 10 year follow-up. Eur J Cancer. 2014; 50(17):3011–3020

[333] Suissa D. Surgery for basal cell carcinoma: study biases. Br J Dermatol. 2005; 152(4):822–823, author reply 823

[334] Mosterd K, Krekels GA, Nieman FH, et al. Surgical excision versus Mohs' micrographic surgery for primary and recurrent basal-cell carcinoma of the face: a prospective randomised controlled trial with 5-years' follow-up. Lancet Oncol. 2008; 9(12):1149–1156

[335] Bouzari N, Olbricht S. Histologic pitfalls in the Mohs technique. Dermatol Clin. 2011; 29(2):261–272, ix

[336] Murphy ME, Brodland DG, Zitelli JA. Errors in the interpretation of Mohs histopathology sections over a 1-year fellowship. Dermatol Surg. 2008; 34 (12):1637–1641

[337] Zachary CB, Rest EB, Furlong SM, Arcedo PN, McGeorge BC, Kist DA. Rapid cytokeratin stains enhance the sensitivity of Mohs micrographic surgery for squamous cell carcinoma. J Dermatol Surg Oncol. 1994; 20(8):530–535

[338] O'Brien CJ, McNeil EB, McMahon JD, Pathak I, Lauer CS, Jackson MA. Significance of clinical stage, extent of surgery, and pathologic findings in metastatic cutaneous squamous carcinoma of the parotid gland. Head Neck. 2002; 24(5):417–422

[339] Reschly MJ, Messina JL, Zaulyanov LL, Cruse W, Fenske NA. Utility of sentinel lymphadenectomy in the management of patients with high-risk cutaneous squamous cell carcinoma. Dermatol Surg. 2003; 29(2):135–140

[340] Reschly MJ, Shenefelt PD. Controversies in skin surgery: electrodessication and curettage versus excision for low-risk, small, well-differentiated squamous cell carcinomas. J Drugs Dermatol. 2010; 9(7):773–776

[341] Ross AS, Schmults CD. Sentinel lymph node biopsy in cutaneous squamous cell carcinoma: a systematic review of the English literature. Dermatol Surg. 2006; 32(11):1309–1321

[342] Bumpous J. Metastatic cutaneous squamous cell carcinoma to the parotid and cervical lymph nodes: treatment and outcomes. Curr Opin Otolaryngol Head Neck Surg. 2009; 17(2):122–125

[343] Schmitt AR, Brewer JD, Bordeaux JS, Baum CL. Staging for cutaneous squamous cell carcinoma as a predictor of sentinel lymph node biopsy results: meta-analysis of American Joint Committee on Cancer criteria and a proposed alternative system. JAMA Dermatol. 2014; 150(1):19–24

[344] Ahmed MM, Moore BA, Schmalbach CE. Utility of head and neck cutaneous squamous cell carcinoma sentinel node biopsy: a systematic review. Otolaryngol Head Neck Surg. 2014; 150(2):180–187

[345] Lippman SM, Meyskens FL, Jr. Treatment of advanced squamous cell carcinoma of the skin with isotretinoin. Ann Intern Med. 1987; 107(4):499–502

[346] Lippman SM, Meyskens FL, Jr. Vitamin A derivatives in the prevention and treatment of human cancer. J Am Coll Nutr. 1988; 7(4):269–284

[347] Lippman SM, Parkinson DR, Itri LM, et al. 13-cis-retinoic acid and interferon alpha-2a: effective combination therapy for advanced squamous cell carcinoma of the skin. J Natl Cancer Inst. 1992; 84(4):235–241

[348] Lippman SM, Shimm DS, Meyskens FL, Jr. Nonsurgical treatments for skin cancer: retinoids and alpha-interferon. J Dermatol Surg Oncol. 1988; 14 (8):862–869

[349] Moore DF, Jr, Pazdur R, Sugarman S, et al. Pilot phase II trial of 13-cis-retinoic acid and interferon-alpha combination therapy for advanced pancreatic adenocarcinoma. Am J Clin Oncol. 1995; 18(6):525–527

[350] Bonner JA, Harari PM, Giralt J, et al. Radiotherapy plus cetuximab for locoregionally advanced head and neck cancer: 5-year survival data from a phase 3 randomised trial, and relation between cetuximab-induced rash and survival. Lancet Oncol. 2010; 11(1):21–28

[351] Brahmer JR, Tykodi SS, Chow LQ, et al. Safety and activity of anti-PD-L1 antibody in patients with advanced cancer. N Engl J Med. 2012; 366 (26):2455–2465

[352] Belai EB, de Oliveira CE, Gasparoto TH, et al. PD-1 blockage delays murine squamous cell carcinoma development. Carcinogenesis. 2014; 35 (2):424–431

[353] Miller SJ, Alam M, Andersen J, et al. Basal cell and squamous cell skin cancers. J Natl Compr Canc Netw. 2010; 8(8):836–864

[354] Johnson TM, Rowe DE, Nelson BR, Swanson NA. Squamous cell carcinoma of the skin (excluding lip and oral mucosa). J Am Acad Dermatol. 1992; 26(3, Pt 2):467–484

[355] Rowe DE, Carroll RJ, Day CL, Jr. Prognostic factors for local recurrence, metastasis, and survival rates in squamous cell carcinoma of the skin, ear, and lip. Implications for treatment modality selection. J Am Acad Dermatol. 1992; 26(6):976–990

[356] LeBoeuf NR, Schmults CD. Update on the management of high-risk squamous cell carcinoma. Semin Cutan Med Surg. 2011; 30(1):26–34

4 Surgical Treatment of Cutaneous Melanoma

Andrea M. Abbott, Matthew P. Doepker, and Vernon K. Sondak

4.1 Epidemiology

Melanoma is currently the fifth most common cancer in the United States, and its incidence is continuing to increase. In 2017, over 87,000 new cases of invasive melanoma will be diagnosed, accounting for about 4.5% of new cancer cases in the United States. Although the 5-year survival rate continues to improve, and is now estimated at 92% for all stages at presentation, about 10,000 deaths from this disease now occur in the United States annually.[1] Because of its relatively early age of onset, melanoma is one of the most devastating malignant diseases in terms of the years of potential life lost per death.[2]

Both environmental and genetic factors increase an individual's risk for developing melanoma (▶ Table 4.1). Caucasian race and fair complexion predispose an individual to developing melanoma, as do mutations in several known—and likely multiple as yet unknown—melanoma susceptibility genes.[3,4] Melanoma affects a broad age range. According to recent cancer statistics, the peak incidence is between the ages of 55 and 74 years, with a median age at time of diagnosis of 64 years.[5] Three-quarters of all cases will occur before age 70, and approximately 20% occur in individuals under 40 years of age. Environmental exposure in the form of ultraviolent radiation is the most well-studied and modifiable etiologic factor in the development of melanoma. Intermittent, high-intensity exposure (e.g., blistering sunburns) contributes most dramatically to the development of melanoma. Dark-skinned individuals may be less likely than fair-skinned individuals to develop melanoma due to the protective effect of eumelanin. Even in individuals with a genetic predisposition, exposure to ultraviolet radiation is the primary factor determining whether an at-risk person actually develops melanoma.[6,7]

Table 4.1 Risk factors influencing the development of cutaneous melanoma

Demographic risk factors	
Race	Caucasian > Hispanic > American Indian/Alaska Native > Asian Pacific Islander > Black
Gender	Male > Female
Age	Median age at diagnosis 62 years old
Phenotypic features	Light hair, light eyes, fair skin, multiple atypical nevi
Environmental risk factors	
Ultraviolet light	Intermittent/intense and chronic cumulative exposure
Cancer history	Melanoma or nonmelanoma skin cancer: threefold relative risk Childhood history of sarcoma, lymphoma, leukemia, or central nervous system: 2.5-fold risk
Immunosuppression	Threefold to fourfold risk after organ transplantation
Socioeconomic status	More likely to have thicker and more aggressive tumors if lower socioeconomic status
Genetic risk factors	
Family history of melanoma	1.7-fold increased relative risk
CDKN2A, CDK4 mutations	Familial melanoma syndrome

Source: Adapted from Sondak VK, Jensen EJ, Margolin KA. Melanoma and other cutaneous malignancies. In: Norton JA, Barie PS, Bollinger RR, et al, eds. 2nd ed. Surgery: Basic Science and Clinical Evidence. York, NY: Springer; 2008.

4.2 Biopsy Techniques and Orientation of Incision

Any patient who presents with a new or abnormal pigmented skin lesion, with increasing size, change in color, or developing irregular borders, should be considered for a biopsy for definitive diagnosis. The approach to biopsy for a suspicious cutaneous lesion often varies depending on the location of the lesion and the preference and training of the physician performing the biopsy. The gold standard for tissue diagnosis when melanoma is suspected is excisional biopsy with a 1 mm to 2 mm margin of normal skin, including some subcutaneous fat (see Chapter 2). This may not be feasible in all cases due to the location of the lesion, and often is more than the minimum necessary for the diagnosis of a benign lesion.[8] Several other biopsy approaches are reasonable to achieve adequate tissue to allow the pathologist to make a diagnosis and assess all relevant histologic features. These techniques include superficial shave biopsy, deep scallop shave biopsy, punch biopsy, incisional biopsy, and the aforementioned excisional biopsy. When any form of partial biopsy is performed, the biopsy should focus on obtaining a sample of the most elevated portion of the lesion to provide the best estimate of tumor thickness. It is ideal to also include a portion of normal skin in the biopsy; however, the main goal should be to obtain the most suspicious and elevated portion of the lesion in the specimen. For lesions that are large or in cosmetically sensitive areas, a punch biopsy that obtains a full-thickness sample is often the best initial diagnostic approach. If a partial biopsy is performed and a portion of the suspicious lesion remains, indicating this on the pathology request helps make the pathologist aware that the lesion was not removed in its entirety, aiding in the diagnostic process.

If a lesion is suspected to be melanoma, cryosurgery and electrodessication should not be performed given they can distort normal tissue planes and do not allow for an adequate histologic evaluation. Partial-thickness shave biopsy of pigmented lesions remains controversial. One of the biggest criticisms of shave biopsy is that partial sampling does not assess the true thickness of a melanoma, if present. Thus, inaccurate microstaging and inappropriate treatment decisions may result.[9,10] A multi-institution, retrospective study evaluated over 600 patients diagnosed via shave biopsy with a melanoma that had a Breslow thickness ≤ 2 mm to determine the accuracy of microstaging in these patients. The results demonstrated that the treatment recommendations for excision margin width or sentinel lymph node biopsy changed based on more extensive residual melanoma in the re-excision specimen in only 2% and 1.3% of patients, respectively.[11] This study supports the use of shave biopsy as a diagnostic tool for patients with pigmented lesions, especially when they are not considered highly suspicious for melanoma. In essence, it is better to have a partial biopsy of a melanoma than no biopsy at all.

The orientation of the biopsy incision is also of importance, in order to facilitate subsequent surgical treatment in the event of a melanoma diagnosis. A punch or shave biopsy will not impact the approach to definitive surgery of a melanoma, but incisional and excisional biopsies should be planned with the potential need for wide excision and/or sentinel node biopsy in mind. Utilizing the principles of Langer's lines may achieve a better cosmetic result for the biopsy scar, but Langer's lines often run in a transverse direction on the extremity, whereas biopsy incisions there should be vertical in orientation. Doing so allows for subsequent wide excision to be done with the greatest chance for primary closure while minimizing the disruption of lymphatics that could impact the accuracy of sentinel node biopsy, if required.

4.3 Margins of Excision

The goal of the initial biopsy is to obtain a diagnosis, but once a diagnosis of melanoma is made, the emphasis shifts to determining the appropriate margins of excision around the biopsy site or residual pigmented lesion. Adequate margins may reduce the risk of local recurrence, while insufficient margins may predispose the patient to a recurrence of disease. A histologically negative margin is always the goal of surgery on the primary melanoma site. The chosen margin should be measured from the edges of the previous biopsy site or any residual pigmentation. Of note, these are "radial" margins, meaning measured in all directions on the skin except downward. The deep margin is the investing fascia of the muscle, which may or may not be included en bloc at the surgeon's discretion. The recommendation for how much of a margin of normal tissue is taken beyond the biopsy site is based on the Breslow thickness of the melanoma as well as the anatomic location of the tumor. Different margin widths may be recommended for melanomas that are in situ, thin (≤ 1 mm), intermediate (1.1–2 mm or 2.1–4 mm), or thick (> 4 mm).

4.3.1 Melanoma in situ

Melanoma in situ is a lesion with a capacity to progress to invasive melanoma and, like invasive melanoma, should be resected with a measured margin of normal skin and with the goal of achieving histologically negative margins. Recommendations from the National Comprehensive Cancer Network (NCCN) are for a 0.5 cm to 1 cm margin; however, no randomized, prospective study has been conducted to definitively answer what margin is truly necessary.[12] In the absence of prospective data, we take into account the location of the lesion and the presence of any residual pigmentation (which might signal the presence of invasive melanoma) in deciding on an appropriate margin of excision for melanoma in situ. In areas with greater tissue laxity, a 1 cm margin may be more easily obtained and is therefore favored, especially when residual pigmentation is present. Conversely, in cosmetically sensitive areas such as the face, neck, hands, and feet, or in locations where the skin is under greater tension, a margin of 0.5 cm is more likely to be used.

4.3.2 Invasive Melanoma: Thin and Intermediate Thickness

The recommended margins of excision for invasive melanoma range from 1 to 2 cm based on the Breslow thickness of the primary tumor. Current NCCN recommendations call for a 1-cm margin for thin melanoma (T1), 1 cm to 2 cm for intermediate melanoma (T2–T3), and 2 cm for thick melanoma (T4).[12] The World Health Organization (WHO) trial, two Swedish Melanoma Study Group Trials, and the Intergroup Melanoma Trial have provided prospective randomized trial data that serve as the basis for current margin width recommendations (▶ Table 4.2). In the WHO trial, over 600 patients with melanomas ≤ 2 mm in thickness were randomized to either a 1 cm or 3 cm margin. There was no statistical difference between the study arms in local recurrence, disease-free survival, or overall survival.[13] This trial concluded 3 cm margins were not necessary for melanomas 2 mm or less in thickness. In particular, the risk of any form of recurrence was very low for melanomas 1-mm thick or thinner even with a 1 cm margin. Hence, a 1 cm margin has become the worldwide standard for excision of invasive melanomas up to 1 mm in thickness, regardless of location of the tumor.

The first Swedish Melanoma Study Group Trial evaluated 989 patients with melanomas 0.8 mm to 2 mm in thickness that were resected with either a 2 cm or 5 cm margin. The study

Table 4.2 The authors' recommendations for surgical management of the primary tumor and regional lymph nodes in clinically localized melanoma

Melanoma thickness	Recommendations regarding margin	Recommendations regarding sentinel lymph node biopsy
Melanoma in situ	0.5–1 cm	Not recommended
< 0.76 mm	1 cm	Not recommended
0.76–0.99 mm (no ulceration and mitotic rate < 1/mm²)	1 cm	SLNB in younger, otherwise healthy patients; nodal observation in older or infirm patients
0.76–0.99 mm (ulcerated or mitotic rate ≥ 1/mm²)	1 cm	SLNB unless contraindicated
≥ 1.0 mm	1–2 cm for 1.0–2.0 mm; 2 cm for > 2.0 mm	SLNB unless contraindicated

Abbreviation: SLNB, sentinel lymph node biopsy.

evaluated overall and recurrence-free survival and found no statistically significant difference between the arms.[14] The authors concluded that 5 cm margins were not necessary for a melanoma 2 mm or less in thickness.

The Intergroup Melanoma Trial evaluated outcomes when margins of 2 cm versus 4 cm were used for patients with a melanoma between 1 mm and 4 mm in thickness. The study evaluated local recurrence as the site of first relapse and at any time, and found no significant difference in outcomes between the two arms. The local recurrence rates as first relapse and at any time for a 2 cm margin (0.4 and 2.1%, respectively) were not significantly different when compared to a resection margin of 4 cm (0.9 and 2.6%, respectively). A trend toward improved overall survival at 10 years was seen in the 4-cm group, 70 versus 77%, but this was not statistically significant.[15]

In the second Swedish Melanoma Study Group Trial, 936 patients with a melanoma greater than 2-mm thick were randomized to margins of either 2 cm or 4 cm. The authors reported no statistically significant differences in local recurrence or overall survival between the two arms.[16]

Haigh et al conducted a meta-analysis and systematic review of three of these trials (WHO, Intergroup Trial, and the first Swedish Melanoma Study Group Trial). When the data were combined, local recurrence, disease-free survival, and mortality were not statistically different between patients with primary cutaneous melanoma up to 4 mm in thickness undergoing excision with 1 cm to 2 cm margins compared to those randomized to 3 cm to 5 cm margins.[17]

Taken together, the data from all of these studies support the recommendation of 1 cm margins for a thin melanoma and 1 cm to 2 cm margins for an intermediate thickness melanoma. Although no randomized trials have directly compared 1 cm versus 2 cm margins for an intermediate thickness melanoma, we use a 2 cm margin for most melanomas that are 2 mm in thickness or greater except in anatomically constrained areas like the face, ears or distal extremities, where only a 1 cm margin can routinely be obtained. For a melanoma between 1.1 mm and 2 mm in thickness, a 1 cm margin is acceptable when the narrower margin allows for primary closure but a 2 cm margin would require skin grafting or significant tissue undermining to achieve closure. We are particularly likely to use a 1 cm margin for melanomas in this thickness range that are nonulcerated, with a relatively low mitotic rate and no evidence of angiolymphatic invasion. We have shown that using a 1 cm margin in this setting was associated with an acceptably low rate of local recurrence.[18]

4.3.3 Thick Melanoma

The NCCN recommends that thick melanomas, defined as tumors greater than 4 in thickness, should be resected with a 2 cm margin.[12] A large, multi-institution retrospective (nonrandomized) study of over 270 patients reviewed outcomes in patients with a thick melanoma who had a resection margin of either 2 cm or greater than 2 cm. Margins wider than 2 cm did not improve outcomes, given that local recurrence, disease-free survival, and overall survival were not significantly different between the two treatment arms after a median follow-up of 27 months.[19]

Thomas et al randomized 900 patients with tumor thickness of 2 mm or greater to excision with either a 1 cm or 3 cm margin. After a median follow-up of 60 months, there was increased locoregional recurrence in the 1 cm arm ($p = 0.05$), but no significant difference in overall survival between the arms. This study prohibited any form of nodal staging, be it elective lymph node dissection or sentinel lymph node biopsy. The absence of nodal evaluation raises an important point when considering the impact of the results of this trial. If lymph node evaluation had been conducted, there is a possibility that there would have been an imbalance in regional nodal disease between the two arms, which may have attributed more to the locoregional recurrence rate than the actual margin of excision. When only local and in-transit recurrences were considered, there were 37 recurrences in the 453 patients on the 1-cm arm (8.2%) versus 25 in the 447 patients on the 3-cm arm (5.6%), a difference that was not statistically significant. But there were 20 more nodal basin recurrences in the 1 cm arm than in the 3-cm arm, reinforcing the possibility that any observed outcome differences were at least partially related to imbalances in the number of stage III patients in each arm rather than an effect of the surgical treatment.[20] While there are no data directly comparing a 2 cm and a 3 cm margin for thick melanoma, whenever a 2 cm margin has been prospectively or retrospectively compared to a wider (4 cm or 5 cm) margin, there has been no evidence of an advantage for the wider margin. Hence, we do not recommend either a 1 cm or a 3 cm margin for a thick melanoma, but rather routinely use a 2 cm margin whenever anatomically feasible, even if it requires a reconstruction to achieve this margin.

4.4 Sentinel Lymph Node Biopsy

While the margin of resection is important for control of local disease, melanoma frequently metastasizes via the lymphatic system, and the regional nodal basins are the most common site of melanoma metastasis. Evaluation of the nodal basin may be indicated at the time of initial wide excision. The sentinel lymph node represents the first lymph node in the lymph node basin directly draining the primary tumor. If the melanoma has metastasized via lymphatic channels, the sentinel lymph node would be the first lymph node to contain tumor deposits. The status of the regional nodes as determined by sentinel lymph node biopsy to determine the presence or absence of metastatic disease has been shown in a prospective randomized trial to be the most important prognostic factor in patients with clinically localized, intermediate-thickness melanoma.[21]

Sentinel lymph node biopsy should be performed in appropriately selected patients with clinically negative regional nodes at the time of wide excision of the primary tumor. A dual localization technique utilizing both injection of radiocolloid and injection of vital blue dye, either isosulfan blue or methylene blue, is most commonly used. The blue dye allows for direct visualization of the lymphatic channel and the sentinel lymph node itself. The use of blue dye alone has allowed the sentinel node to be identified in approximately 85 to 90% of cases, but the combination of both radiocolloid and blue dye increases the success rate to over 99%.[22] We utilize isosulfan blue whenever a vital blue dye is employed, and do not use methylene blue for sentinel node localization at all due to higher reported local complication rates.[23] One-half to 1 mCi of radiocolloid labeled with ^{99m}technetium is injected intradermally, generally 1 to 4 hours before surgery, but if necessary the injection may be performed up to 24 hours prior to surgery.[22] A variety of different radiocolloids are used around the world (e.g., sulfur colloid, tilmanocept, albumin nanocolloid and antimony trisulfide), with little or nothing in the way of head-to-head comparison data to determine which might be superior.[24,25] Whichever and whenever the radiocolloid is injected, planar or computed tomographic lymphoscintigraphy is performed during the hour immediately thereafter in order to delineate the number and general location of the sentinel nodes. After the induction of anesthesia in the operating room, the vital blue dye is injected intradermally around the biopsy site or the primary tumor. A total volume of 0.5 to 1.5 mL is generally sufficient to identify the sentinel lymph nodes. Intraoperatively, a handheld gamma probe helps to direct the trajectory of dissection and guide the surgeon down to the "hot" and usually blue sentinel node(s).

Despite the high rate of accuracy with a dual localization technique, some surgeons do not routinely use blue dye. The choice to use radiocolloid alone may be due to limited availability of vital blue dye, concern that the use of blue dye will stimulate an allergic reaction, or because the patient is pregnant (we do not use blue dye during pregnancy because a maternal allergic reaction could be catastrophic for the fetus).[23,26,27,28,29] In the Multicenter Selective Lymphadenectomy Trial-I (MSLT-1), the incidence of allergic reaction after isosulfan dye injection was only 0.2%,[30] and in our experience the incidence of allergic reactions is even lower than that. Hence, we routinely utilize isosulfan blue dye in nonpregnant patients. One other issue relating to the use of vital blue dye is the presence of a tattoo on the skin in the drainage area of the nodal basin(s) undergoing sentinel node biopsy. Tattoo ink gradually leaches out of the skin site and accumulates in the regional nodes, coloring them enough to be easily seen. If the tattoo contained blue, green, or black ink, pigments within the node can be confused with vital blue dye or even metastatic melanoma.[31] For this reason, we sometimes do not use vital blue dye in cases where a large tattoo is in the same draining basin as the primary melanoma, and focus our attention only on the radioactivity within the nodes.

The morbidity associated with sentinel lymph node biopsy is low, but potential complications include seroma, lymphocele, wound infection, and, in very rare cases, lymphedema.[30,32] The morbidity of sentinel lymph node biopsy has been evaluated in prospective clinical trials. In MSLT-1, the rate of complications for patients undergoing sentinel lymph node biopsy was 10.1%.[30] The Sunbelt Melanoma Trial evaluated complication rates for sentinel lymph node biopsy alone and, for patients with positive sentinel nodes, sentinel lymph node biopsy and completion lymph node dissection. The complication rates were higher in patients undergoing lymph node dissection, while the risk of complications was low for sentinel lymph node biopsy alone (wound infection 1.1%, lymphedema 0.7%, and seroma/hematoma 2.3% for sentinel node biopsy versus 7, 11.7, and 5.9% for sentinel node biopsy followed by lymph node dissection).[33,34]

While the utility of sentinel lymph node biopsy in determining the spread of cancer and providing a prognostic benefit is clear, the role it plays in providing a survival benefit is not. One prospective, randomized trial has addressed this question. In MSLT-1, patients were randomly assigned to undergo either wide excision of the primary tumor with observation of the nodal basin or wide excision with sentinel lymph node biopsy and subsequent completion lymph node dissection if there was a positive sentinel lymph node. Final analysis of the 1,347 patients with intermediate thickness melanoma who were evaluated in the study demonstrated no difference in melanoma-specific survival at 10 years for patients who underwent sentinel lymph node biopsy versus observation. There was, however, an improvement in disease-free survival for patients undergoing sentinel lymph node biopsy. Patients with a positive sentinel lymph node biopsy who then had completion lymph node dissection were found to have an improved distant disease-free survival compared to patients in the observation group who failed in the nodal basin with clinically obvious disease (54.8 versus 35.6%, $p = 0.02$). Melanoma-specific survival at 10 years was also improved in the sentinel lymph node biopsy positive group compared to the observation group of patients who failed in the nodal basin (62.1 versus 41.5%, $p = 0.006$).[30]

The NCCN currently recommends that sentinel lymph node biopsy be discussed and offered to patients with intermediate-thickness melanoma (1–4 mm).[12] Controversy still exists regarding the routine recommendation for sentinel lymph node biopsy in patients with thin melanoma (< 1 mm). The risk of having a positive sentinel lymph node biopsy in a patient with a thin melanoma has been reported in the literature to be around 5%, but there are clearly subsets of patients within the broader group of T1 melanoma cases with a higher or lower risk of a positive sentinel node. Since we and many others use a 5% sentinel node positivity threshold as the level at which to consider the procedure for an otherwise healthy patient, it is important to identify which subsets of patients with T1 melanoma are or are not good candidates for sentinel node biopsy. Studies have demonstrated that the percentage of cases with a positive sentinel node increases when the melanoma is ≥ 0.76 mm in thickness, ulcerated, or mitotically active (mitotic rate ≥ 1/mm^2).[35,36,37] The NCCN, American Society of Clinical Oncology (ASCO), and Society of Surgical Oncology (SSO) all recommend that sentinel lymph node biopsy be considered in patients with melanomas that are 0.76 to 1 mm if the melanoma is ulcerated or the mitotic rate is ≥ 1/mm^2. Sentinel lymph node biopsy, however, should still be considered in appropriately selected patients with thin melanomas in this thickness range (0.76–1 mm) that are not ulcerated or mitotically active.[12,38]

Controversy also exists regarding sentinel lymph node biopsy for patients with clinically node-negative thick melanomas (≥ 4 mm). The final analysis of MSLT-1 evaluated 290 patients with thick melanomas, defined as greater than 3.5 mm. Fifty-seven (33%) out of the 173 patients in the sentinel lymph node biopsy arm had sentinel lymph node metastasis, while 116 (67%) had no evidence of nodal metastasis. Twelve of the 116 sentinel node-negative patients eventually developed nodal disease, bringing the overall incidence of nodal metastasis in the sentinel lymph node biopsy arm to 39.9% (the rate of nodal metastasis in the nodal observation arm was 37.6%). The 10-year disease-free survival rates for the sentinel lymph node biopsy and observation arms were 50.7 and 40.5%, respectively ($p = 0.03$). In those patients with thick melanoma found to have sentinel lymph node metastasis, the 10-year melanoma-specific survival was significantly worse (48%) compared to those without sentinel lymph node metastasis (64.6%, $p = 0.03$).[39,40]

More recently, Yamamoto et al published a single institution, retrospective review of patients seen over a 10-year period with melanoma ≥ 4 mm. The endpoints evaluated included recurrence-free survival and disease-specific survival. Sentinel lymph node biopsy was performed in 412 patients and of those, 161 (39%) had a positive sentinel lymph node. Forty-six other patients presented with clinically palpable disease. Of the 251 patients who had a negative sentinel lymph node biopsy, 14 (6%) recurred in the mapped nodal basin, for a calculated false-negative rate of 12.3%. The median disease-specific survival of 82 months for patients with a negative sentinel lymph node was significantly better than for those with a positive sentinel lymph node (41 months) or for patients with clinically node-positive disease (27 months; $p < 0.0001$). The authors also reported a significant difference in median recurrence-free survival between patients with negative sentinel lymph nodes compared to patients with positive sentinel lymph nodes or clinically palpable disease (32 versus 14 and 7 months, respectively; $p < 0.0001$). The authors concluded sentinel lymph node biopsy should be considered in those with clinically node-negative thick melanoma due to the prognostic information obtained and the acceptably low false-negative rate.[41]

Some surgeons have advocated repeat sentinel lymph node biopsy in the event of local recurrence or development of resectable in-transit disease, assuming a prior sentinel lymph node biopsy was negative.[42,43,44] The technical feasibility of repeat sentinel lymph node biopsy has been evaluated in two separate studies, and the ability to detect a sentinel lymph node using either ^{99m}technetium sulfur colloid alone or in combination with blue dye was reported as 12 of 12 (100%) cases in one study and 32 of 33 (97%) cases in another.[42,45] However, the prognostic significance and staging reliability of finding a "sentinel" lymph node in the context of recurrence is not clear. At present, we do not perform repeat sentinel node biopsy for patients with local or in-transit recurrence, preferring instead to evaluate and follow the nodal basin with serial ultrasonography. If, however, a patient presents with local recurrence without ever having undergone a sentinel node biopsy, we will consider sentinel node biopsy in conjunction with wide excision of the local recurrence site in selected patients.

4.5 Lymphadenectomy

Lymphadenectomy broadly refers to the en bloc removal of all lymph node tissue in a draining nodal basin. The most common initial site of melanoma metastasis involves the regional lymph nodes. Lymph node involvement has been shown to be the most important prognostic factor in otherwise localized melanoma.[38] Prior to the widespread use of sentinel lymph node biopsy, the two options available to manage the draining nodal basin were either an elective lymphadenectomy (i.e., the elective removal of all clinically negative nodes in the draining basin[s]) or a therapeutic lymphadenectomy (i.e., deferring lymphadenectomy until the time of clinically detected nodal basin recurrence; ▸ Table 4.3). Both of these approaches have significant drawbacks. Approximately 16 to 20% of patients with an intermediate-thickness melanoma are expected to have clinically occult nodal metastasis at the time of diagnosis of their primary.[46] This means many patients undergoing elective lymphadenectomy are subjected to unnecessary operative morbidity without any benefit in regional control or improved survival. Conversely, delaying lymph node dissection until clinical recurrence may result in patients recurring with unresectable disease in the regional nodal basin. Even if the disease is resectable at the time of recurrence, prospective randomized trial data suggest that such patients are at increased risk of complications from their lymphadenectomy—including severe lymphedema.[47] They are also more likely to meet criteria for adjuvant radiation,[30,48] which again increases the likelihood of lymphedema. Moreover, the results of the MSLT-1 study demonstrated that patients in the observation arm with intermediate-thickness melanoma who developed nodal recurrence had worse melanoma-specific survival than those who were found to have microscopic disease in the sentinel node and underwent completion lymphadenectomy at the time of diagnosis.[39] Another disadvantage of deferring lymphadenectomy is that a subset of patients who recur in the regional nodes also have evidence of distant metastatic disease at that time. While it may be true that some of these patients were spared the need for a lymphadenectomy that would not have improved their overall outcome, in other cases these patients will develop persistent and often severe problems due to uncontrolled regional disease that systemic treatments do not always completely eliminate. Ultimately, due to the alternative provided by sentinel node biopsy with selective lymphadenectomy for only node-positive cases, both elective and therapeutic lymphadenectomy have been abandoned as the primary strategy for clinically node-negative melanoma cases. Therapeutic lymphadenectomy, however, remains the gold standard in virtually all cases of clinically node-positive melanoma without detectable distant metastases.

Table 4.3 Options for the surgical management of the regional lymph nodes in melanoma

Types of lymph node evaluation	
Sentinel lymph node biopsy	Removal of lymph node(s) that are radioactive and/or have blue dye uptake—the sentinel node is thought to represent the first lymph node in the drainage pattern of the primary tumor
Radical lymphadenectomy	En bloc removal of all lymph node tissue in a draining lymph node basin, for any indication
Elective lymphadenectomy	Radical lymphadenectomy performed without any clinical evidence of lymphadenopathy (by exam or imaging) or histologic evidence of microscopic lymph node evaluation
Completion lymphadenectomy	Radical lymphadenectomy performed in a lymph node basin after a positive sentinel node biopsy
Therapeutic lymphadenectomy	Radical lymphadenectomy performed in a lymph node basin containing clinically detected lymph node involvement

The current standard of care for most clinically node-negative melanomas greater than 0.75 mm thick is to perform a sentinel lymph node biopsy at the time of wide excision, and completion lymphadenectomy for those patients with any positive sentinel lymph nodes.[12,38] Only about 15 to 18% of completion lymphadenectomy specimens contain additional nodes (i.e., nonsentinel nodes) with metastatic disease.[39] The impact of completion lymphadenectomy after positive sentinel lymph node biopsy on survival is being evaluated in MSLT-2, in which patients with a positive sentinel lymph node biopsy were randomized to either undergo completion lymph node dissection or nodal basin observation with serial ultrasounds. The study finished accrual in 2014 and we are awaiting the final results.[39] Until those results are available, the standard of care for sentinel node-positive cases remains completion lymph node dissection. Reports of successful management of the sentinel node-positive basin by observation and serial ultrasonography, combined with the morbidity of lymphadenectomy, have led many patients to choose not to undergo completion lymphadenectomy.[49,50] The preliminary results of a small European randomized trial, showing equivalent 3-year survival outcomes for sentinel node-positive patients whether or not completion lymphadenectomy was carried out, have likely encouraged this trend further.[51] We believe that, until much more mature results of larger studies are available, this conservative approach should only be undertaken by a fully informed patient who is aware of the risk of nodal basin recurrence and willing to return for routine surveillance including nodal ultrasounds. Even with ultrasound surveillance of the nodal basin, up to 50% of nodal recurrences are first detected by the patient, so the patient must also be committed to self-examination and to return promptly if palpable lymphadenopathy develops between scheduled visits.[52]

Significance of In-Transit and Interval Nodes in Melanoma

In most cases, melanoma will drain to the major nodal basins, that is, the cervical, axillary, and ilioinguinal nodal basins.[53] The use of preoperative lymphoscintigraphy as part of the sentinel lymph node biopsy procedure has led to the increased recognition of draining nodes outside of these major nodal basins. Melanoma may metastasize to nodes within minor lymph node basins, which have been classified as epitrochlear, popliteal, and internal mammary,[53] or to nodes described as interval or in transit. These nodes, when identified, can be routinely removed during the sentinel node biopsy procedure.

This terminology can be confusing, and a classification system to help more accurately define these has been proposed by Zager et al. They defined "interval nodes" as any superficial (i.e., outside the chest and abdominal cavity) lymph nodes identified by lymphoscintigraphy, other imaging studies, incidentally at surgery or clinically based on involvement with tumor that are not located within the defined confines of a major or minor nodal basin. In keeping with the common terminology used to describe regional recurrences, they defined "in-transit nodes" as *any* nodes located between the primary cutaneous melanoma and the major basin that is traditionally considered to drain that site.[54] This definition would include any interval and minor basin nodes that would not be removed with a standard lymphadenectomy of the corresponding major basin. The reported rates of minor basin or interval node drainage during sentinel lymph node biopsy procedures have been between 2.1 and 9.8%.[55,56] McMasters et al analyzed the Sunbelt Melanoma Trial database and identified 62 (3.1%) patients with in-transit nodes out of 2,332 patients undergoing sentinel lymph node biopsy, and of those, 13 nodes (21%) were positive for metastatic disease.[57] In 11 of the 13 cases, only the interval nodes, and not the sentinel nodes from the major basin, contained tumor. An additional study by Puleo et al showed 75 (6%) out of 1,172 patients had in-transit nodes identified, and of those 12 (16%) were positive for micrometastatic disease.[58] These results justify an effort to biopsy in-transit nodes, which in both studies seemed to have the same prognostic impact as a positive node in a major basin. An area of controversy deals with the management of the upstream nodal basin after a positive in-transit node. As with the sentinel node-positive major basin itself, we believe there are times when carefully selected patients can be followed without major basin completion lymphadenectomy.

4.6 Immediate versus Delayed Reconstruction of the Primary Site

Reconstructive techniques with rotational or advancement flaps or skin grafts may be necessary after excision of a melanoma in a cosmetically sensitive area or when large margins are required in an area of skin tension that does not allow for primary skin closure such as the scalp, hand, close to joints, etc. In these situations, it is appropriate to ensure that negative margins have been obtained before tissue rearrangement takes place. Once tissue rearrangement occurs, the ability to determine which margin is involved by tumor becomes more difficult and sometimes impossible. Delayed reconstruction is one effective manner by which to allow adequate margin assessment prior to a planned definitive reconstruction. Several methods for margin assessment and temporary closure exist. In general, we prefer either wide excision and temporary graft placement (e.g., AlloDerm skin substitute[59] or homograft skin) or staged marginal excision and subsequent central tumor excision and reconstruction.[60] There are advantages and disadvantages to each strategy and patient selection is paramount to achieving long-term success.

Staged contoured marginal excision and subsequent central tumor excision is the process whereby the margins around the tumor are the only tissue excised at the time of initial operation, and once these margins are determined to be free of melanoma or melanoma in situ, then definitive excision of the entire lesion and appropriate reconstruction are performed. The identification of the margins of the lesion can be augmented intraoperatively by using a Wood's lamp. Then, beginning a distance 0.5 to 1 cm from the defined lesion perimeter depending on whether the preoperative diagnosis is in situ or invasive disease, a small full-thickness strip of skin, usually 2 to 3 mm in width, is either excised in a rectangular fashion around the primary or contoured to follow anticipated lines of reconstruction.[60] The defect is closed, generally with a running suture around the entire perimeter of the marginal excision. The thin strips of tissue are oriented and sent to the pathologist for permanent histopathologic evaluation. The specimens are evaluated with standard hematoxylin and eosin staining, and immunohistochemical stains are employed as necessary. If the margins are all found to be negative for melanoma (invasive or in situ), then the central lesion is excised and the defect reconstructed at that time. Conversely, if any margins are found to be positive for melanoma, then excision of those margins are repeated using a further 0.5 to 1 cm, until negative peripheral margins are obtained and central excision and reconstruction can be undertaken. This technique may be particularly useful in the setting of lentigo maligna (which is melanoma in situ) and lentigo maligna melanoma (invasive melanoma) on the face or dorsum of the hands. The advantage of this approach is that it obviates the potential risk of repeat surgery for positive margins after significant tissue rearrangement or flap reconstruction has been performed. In a series of 127 patients with lentigo maligna of the head and neck, Glazer et al found that a 5 mm margin was adequate for complete excision in only 77% of cases, so immediate reconstruction after a standard wide excision would have been associated with positive margins in roughly a quarter of cases.[60]

Mohs surgery has been used by some dermatologic surgeons to achieve complete excision of melanomas in cosmetically sensitive areas, allowing subsequent reconstruction to take place with the knowledge that the margins of excision are free of tumor. A large prospective study evaluated 1,120 cases of melanoma in situ treated with Mohs surgery. In this study, the minimum surgical margin taken as part of the initial Mohs procedure was 6 mm, with an additional 3 mm of skin taken in each area where a positive margin was encountered. In this study, 98.9% of melanoma in situ cases were cleared with Mohs surgery after two stages, that is, a 9-mm margin, versus only 86% cleared with the first-stage 6-mm margin.[61] A major issue limiting the application of Mohs surgery is the difficulty differentiating atypical but nonmalignant melanocytes from melanoma in situ, particularly in sun-damaged skin, using the frozen section histopathology performed during the Mohs technique. The availability of rapid immunohistochemical staining for frozen section specimens can address this issue. We believe Mohs surgery for melanoma in situ should only be used in settings that have this staging capability and only after an initial defined margin first-stage excision is carried out. That notwithstanding, our preference remains staged marginal excision rather than Mohs surgery for melanoma in situ/lentigo maligna. We do not use Mohs surgery at all for invasive melanoma.

4.7 Special Topics

Certain situations (i.e., based on histopathologic subtype, age of the patient, or other considerations) arise where the standard recommendations for melanoma treatment may be modified. Several such situations are discussed below.

4.7.1 Desmoplastic Melanoma

Desmoplastic melanoma is a rare variant of cutaneous melanoma with an annual incidence rate of 2 per million. Risk factors associated with desmoplastic melanoma include extensive and chronic sun exposure. The majority of desmoplastic melanomas are found on the head and neck and occur in older adults.[62] Desmoplastic melanoma is characterized by malignant spindled melanocytes within a collagenous myxoid stroma. Desmoplastic melanoma is further divided into two histological subtypes: pure and mixed desmoplastic melanoma. Two histology-specific considerations arise in the management of desmoplastic melanoma: when should postoperative radiation to the primary site be added and when should sentinel lymph node biopsy be performed?

Desmoplastic melanoma has been reported to have a higher rate of local recurrence than other histologic types of cutaneous melanoma.[62,63,64] This has led some authors to advocate for adjuvant radiation to the primary site. Guadagnolo et al conducted a retrospective review of 130 patients diagnosed with desmoplastic melanoma (100 pure, 30 mixed). Of those 130, 59 (45%) were treated with surgery alone and 71 (55%) had surgery and adjuvant radiation. Of the patients who underwent surgery alone, 14 (24%) experienced a recurrence, while only 5 (7%) patients who received both surgery and radiation therapy developed a local recurrence ($p = 0.009$).[65] On multivariate analysis, the authors found only a margin negative resection and postoperative radiation to be associated with improved local control.

Strom et al retrospectively reviewed a total of 277 patients over a 21-year period with desmoplastic melanoma who were treated by surgery with or without adjuvant radiation therapy. The primary endpoint was local control, which was defined as freedom from disease recurrence within the radiated field of the primary tumor bed. Of the 277 patients, 113 (40.8%) received adjuvant radiation therapy. The authors reported patients with positive margins benefited the most from adjuvant radiation therapy. Thirty-five patients had positive resection margins; 14% (3/22) of those who received radiation therapy developed a recurrence, while 54% (7/13) who did not receive radiation developed a recurrence ($p = 0.003$). The authors also demonstrated significantly improved local control in patients with negative resection margins and high-risk features, defined as Breslow thickness greater than 4 mm, Clark level V, or a head and neck primary site. The authors concluded radiation therapy may be safely omitted if the margins are negative, the Breslow thickness is less than 4 mm, no perineural invasion is seen, and the tumor is in a non–head and neck location.[63]

Chen et al reported adjuvant radiation to be beneficial in patients with locally recurrent desmoplastic melanoma, and those with gross residual disease, perineural involvement, or after excision with narrow margins.[62] We recommend adjuvant radiation in all cases of desmoplastic melanoma with positive or close margins after wide excision, and in most tumors with perineural invasion or thickness ≥ 4 mm, especially on the head and neck.

The role of sentinel lymph node biopsy in desmoplastic melanoma is controversial. Overall, desmoplastic melanoma has a lower rate of regional nodal metastasis compared to other subtypes of cutaneous melanoma. Desmoplastic melanoma has been reported to have a sentinel lymph node positivity rate of less than 10%.[66] Various studies report conflicting data on the impact of sentinel lymph node biopsy in desmoplastic melanoma on overall survival. Using the Surveillance, Epidemiology, and End Results (SEER) database, Wasif et al found no significant difference in overall survival between sentinel node-negative and node-positive patients.[67] Other studies have reported a threefold increase in the risk of death when the sentinel lymph node is positive.[68] When broken down by subtype, mixed desmoplastic melanoma has been shown to have rates of lymph node metastasis that are comparable to nondesmoplastic cutaneous melanoma, but even pure desmoplastic melanomas may have a sentinel node positivity rate high enough to justify sentinel lymph node biopsy in healthy patients.[69] NCCN guidelines note that the role of sentinel lymph node biopsy remains controversial in pure desmoplastic melanoma, whereas the ASCO/SSO guidelines call for sentinel lymph node biopsy in desmoplastic melanoma.[12,38]

4.7.2 Pediatric Melanoma

The incidence of melanoma arising in children less than 18 years of age is rising in the United States.[70] The cause of this increase is likely to be multifactorial and may stem from an increased global awareness of melanoma, which prompts skin evaluation at an earlier age, the use of tanning beds among teenagers, and advances in pathologic evaluation that have allowed for more accurate diagnosis. The diagnosis of melanoma in the pediatric population can be a challenge because these lesions often lack the characteristic properties typical of adult melanomas (asymmetry, irregular borders, change in color, increase in diameter, etc.).[71] The histopathology of melanoma in this age range can also present a diagnostic challenge even among expert dermatopathologists.[72] Despite the diagnostic challenges, pediatric patients with melanoma tend to have a more favorable prognosis than adult patients with melanoma.[73]

The initial workup for a lesion suspected to be a melanoma in the pediatric patient is essentially the same as in an adult. A full skin exam evaluating the presence of typical and atypical nevi as well as congenital nevi is useful to assist in future skin evaluations. A detailed family history may be useful as some cases have been linked to an inherited melanoma susceptibility gene.

The operative management of pediatric melanoma is similar to adult melanoma.[74] Younger patients tend to have a higher incidence of nodal metastasis but less risk of local recurrence, so a 1-cm margin is commonly employed in children even for thicker lesions. Sentinel lymph node biopsy is generally utilized according to the same standards and principles as in cases of adult melanoma. The decision to pursue completion lymph node dissection after a positive sentinel lymph node biopsy must be done weighing the potential lifelong implications of a node dissection versus the alternative of serial lymph node surveillance with ultrasound. The standard of care recommendation remains a completion lymph node dissection for most pediatric patients with positive sentinel nodes and all patients with palpable nodal involvement.

Although pediatric patients with stage III melanoma have a relatively better prognosis as compared to adults, adjuvant therapy is often recommended.[75] Interferon is relatively well tolerated in younger patients, and the patients and their families are often highly motivated to pursue adjuvant treatment. At our center, pediatric patients treated with interferon commonly receive the standard 1 month of intravenous interferon used in the adult high-dose interferon regimen, but this is followed by 11 months of weekly treatment with pegylated interferon.[76] This hybrid regimen takes advantage of the favorable pharmacokinetic properties of pegylated interferon as a maintenance therapy, while minimizing the number of injections the young patient must endure. Adjuvant radiation is less likely to be recommended in this patient population due to the potential effects on growth and development.

4.8 Conclusion

Surgery in the form of radical wide excision of the primary tumor with appropriate negative margins remains the gold standard of treatment for melanoma. Sentinel lymph node biopsy is recommended as part of the staging workup for patients with intermediate-thickness and thick melanoma without clinical evidence of nodal disease. Controversy still exists regarding the approach to the regional nodal basin for patients with thin melanoma, where the decision to perform a sentinel lymph node biopsy should be individualized. Completion lymph node dissection is recommended for patients with positive sentinel lymph node disease; however, the impact lymphadenectomy has on overall survival remains uncertain. Plastic surgeons often find themselves on the front lines of the surgical management of melanoma and should be familiar with standard recommendations as well as those special situations where modifications to those recommendations might be appropriate.

References

[1] Siegel RL, Miller KD, Jemal A. Cancer statistics, 2017. CA Cancer J Clin. 2017; 67(1):7–30

[2] Guy GP, Ekwueme DU. Years of potential life lost and indirect costs of melanoma and non-melanoma skin cancer: a systematic review of the literature. Pharmacoeconomics. 2011; 29(10):863–874

[3] Gibbs DC, Orlow I, Kanetsky PA, et al. GEM Study Group. Inherited genetic variants associated with occurrence of multiple primary melanoma. Cancer Epidemiol Biomarkers Prev. 2015; 24(6):992–997

[4] Rastrelli M, Tropea S, Rossi CR, Alaibac M. Melanoma: epidemiology, risk factors, pathogenesis, diagnosis and classification. In Vivo. 2014; 28 (6):1005–1011

[5] Howlader N, Noone AM, Krapcho M, Miller D, Bishop K, Kosary CL, Yu M, Ruhl J, Tatalovich Z, Mariotto A, Lewis DR, Chen HS, Feuer EJ, Cronin KA (eds). SEER Cancer Statistics Review, 1975-2014, National Cancer Institute. Bethesda, MD, https://seer.cancer.gov/csr/1975_2014/, based on November 2016 SEER data submission, posted to the SEER web site, April 2017. Accessed May 15, 2017.

[6] Chaudru V, Chompret A, Bressac-de Paillerets B, Spatz A, Avril MF, Demenais F. Influence of genes, nevi, and sun sensitivity on melanoma risk in a family sample unselected by family history and in melanoma-prone families. J Natl Cancer Inst. 2004; 96(10):785–795

[7] Rouzaud F, Kadekaro AL, Abdel-Malek ZA, Hearing VJ. MC1R and the response of melanocytes to ultraviolet radiation. Mutat Res. 2005; 571(1–2):133–152

[8] Farma JM, Kulkarni N, Hsu C. Surgical management of primary and recurrent melanoma. Surg Oncol Clin N Am. 2015; 24(2):239–247

[9] Pflugfelder A, Weide B, Eigentler TK, et al. Incisional biopsy and melanoma prognosis: facts and controversies. Clin Dermatol. 2010; 28(3):316–318

[10] Riker AI, Glass F, Perez I, Cruse CW, Messina J, Sondak VK. Cutaneous melanoma: methods of biopsy and definitive surgical excision. Dermatol Ther (Heidelb). 2005; 18(5):387–393

[11] Zager JS, Hochwald SN, Marzban SS, et al. Shave biopsy is a safe and accurate method for the initial evaluation of melanoma. J Am Coll Surg. 2011; 212 (4):454–460, discussion 460–462

[12] Coit DG, Thompson JA, Igazi A, et al. NCCN Guidelines insights: Melanoma, Version 3. J Natl Compr Canc Netw. 2016; 14(8):945–958

[13] Veronesi U, Cascinelli N, Adamus J, et al. Thin stage I primary cutaneous malignant melanoma. Comparison of excision with margins of 1 or 3 cm. N Engl J Med. 1988; 318(18):1159–1162

[14] Cohn-Cedermark G, Rutqvist LE, Andersson R, et al. Long term results of a randomized study by the Swedish Melanoma Study Group on 2-cm versus 5-cm resection margins for patients with cutaneous melanoma with a tumor thickness of 0.8–2.0 mm. Cancer. 2000; 89(7):1495–1501

[15] Balch CM, Soong SJ, Smith T, et al. Investigators from the Intergroup Melanoma Surgical Trial. Long-term results of a prospective surgical trial comparing 2 cm vs. 4 cm excision margins for 740 patients with 1–4 mm melanomas. Ann Surg Oncol. 2001; 8(2):101–108

[16] Gillgren P, Drzewiecki KT, Niin M, et al. 2-cm versus 4-cm surgical excision margins for primary cutaneous melanoma thicker than 2 mm: a randomised, multicentre trial. Lancet. 2011; 378(9803):1635–1642

[17] Haigh PI, DiFronzo LA, McCready DR. Optimal excision margins for primary cutaneous melanoma: a systematic review and meta-analysis. Can J Surg. 2003; 46(6):419–426

[18] Doepker MP, Thompson ZJ, Fisher KJ, et al. Is a wider margin (2 cm vs. 1 cm) for a 1.01–2.0 mm melanoma necessary? Ann Surg Oncol. 2016; 23 (7):2336–2342

[19] Heaton KM, Sussman JJ, Gershenwald JE, et al. Surgical margins and prognostic factors in patients with thick (> 4 mm) primary melanoma. Ann Surg Oncol. 1998; 5(4):322–328

[20] Thomas JM, Newton-Bishop J, A'Hern R, et al. United Kingdom Melanoma Study Group, British Association of Plastic Surgeons, Scottish Cancer Therapy Network. Excision margins in high-risk malignant melanoma. N Engl J Med. 2004; 350(8):757–766

[21] Ambe CM, Sondak VK. Sentinel lymph node biopsy in melanoma and other cutaneous malignancies. Am J Hematol Oncol. 2014; 10:39

[22] Morton DL, Thompson JF, Essner R, et al. Multicenter Selective Lymphadenectomy Trial Group. Validation of the accuracy of intraoperative lymphatic mapping and sentinel lymphadenectomy for early-stage melanoma: a multicenter trial. Ann Surg. 1999; 230(4):453–463, discussion 463–465

[23] Neves RI, Reynolds BQ, Hazard SW, Saunders B, Mackay DR. Increased postoperative complications with methylene blue versus lymphazurin in sentinel lymph node biopsies for skin cancers. J Surg Oncol. 2011; 103(5):421–425

[24] Sondak VK, King DW, Zager JS, et al. Combined analysis of phase III trials evaluating [99mTc]tilmanocept and vital blue dye for identification of sentinel lymph nodes in clinically node-negative cutaneous melanoma. Ann Surg Oncol. 2013; 20(2):680–688

[25] Wilhelm AJ, Mijnhout GS, Franssen EJ. Radiopharmaceuticals in sentinel lymph-node detection - an overview. Eur J Nucl Med. 1999; 26(4) Suppl: S36–S42

[26] Liu LC, Parrett BM, Jenkins T, et al. Selective sentinel lymph node dissection for melanoma: importance of harvesting nodes with lower radioactive counts without the need for blue dye. Ann Surg Oncol. 2011; 18(10):2919–2924

[27] Liu Y, Truini C, Ariyan S. A randomized study comparing the effectiveness of methylene blue dye with lymphazurin blue dye in sentinel lymph node biopsy for the treatment of cutaneous melanoma. Ann Surg Oncol. 2008; 15 (9):2412–2417

[28] Cragan JD. Teratogen update: methylene blue. Teratology. 1999; 60(1):42–48

[29] Andtbacka RHI, Donaldson MR, Bowles TL, et al. Sentinel lymph node biopsy for melanoma in pregnant women. Ann Surg Oncol. 2013; 20(2):689–696

[30] Morton DL, Cochran AJ, Thompson JF, et al. Multicenter Selective Lymphadenectomy Trial Group. Sentinel node biopsy for early-stage melanoma: accuracy and morbidity in MSLT-I, an international multicenter trial. Ann Surg. 2005; 242(3):302–311, discussion 311–313

[31] Manganoni AM, Sereni E, Pata G, et al. Pigmentation of axillary sentinel nodes from extensive skin tattoo mimics metastatic melanoma: case report. Int J Dermatol. 2014; 53(6):773–776

[32] Baas PC, Schraffordt Koops H, Hoekstra HJ, van Bruggen JJ, van der Weele LT, Oldhoff J. Groin dissection in the treatment of lower-extremity melanoma. Short-term and long-term morbidity. Arch Surg. 1992; 127(3):281–286

[33] McMasters KM, Egger ME, Edwards MJ, et al. Final results of the Sunbelt Melanoma Trial: a multi-institutional prospective randomized phase III study evaluating the role of adjuvant high-dose interferon alfa-2b and completion lymph node dissection for patients staged by sentinel lymph node biopsy. J Clin Oncol. 2016; 34(10):1079–1086

[34] McMasters KM, Noyes RD, Reintgen DS, et al. Sunbelt Melanoma Trial. Lessons learned from the Sunbelt Melanoma Trial. J Surg Oncol. 2004; 86(4):212–223

[35] Han D, Yu D, Zhao X, et al. Sentinel node biopsy is indicated for thin melanomas ≥ 0.76 mm. Ann Surg Oncol. 2012; 19(11):3335–3342

[36] Andtbacka RH, Gershenwald JE. Role of sentinel lymph node biopsy in patients with thin melanoma. J Natl Compr Canc Netw. 2009; 7(3):308–317

[37] Gershenwald JE, Coit DG, Sondak VK, Thompson JF. The challenge of defining guidelines for sentinel lymph node biopsy in patients with thin primary cutaneous melanomas. Ann Surg Oncol. 2012; 19(11):3301–3303

[38] Wong SL, Balch CM, Hurley P, et al. American Society of Clinical Oncology, Society of Surgical Oncology. Sentinel lymph node biopsy for melanoma: American Society of Clinical Oncology and Society of Surgical Oncology joint clinical practice guideline. J Clin Oncol. 2012; 30(23):2912–2918

[39] Morton DL, Thompson JF, Cochran AJ, et al. MSLT Group. Final trial report of sentinel-node biopsy versus nodal observation in melanoma. N Engl J Med. 2014; 370(7):599–609

[40] Doepker MP, Zager JS. Sentinel lymph node mapping in melanoma in the twenty-first century. Surg Oncol Clin N Am. 2015; 24(2):249–260

[41] Yamamoto M, Fisher KJ, Wong JY, et al. Sentinel lymph node biopsy is indicated for patients with thick clinically lymph node-negative melanoma. Cancer. 2015; 121(10):1628–1636

[42] Beasley GM, Speicher P, Sharma K, et al. Efficacy of repeat sentinel lymph node biopsy in patients who develop recurrent melanoma. J Am Coll Surg. 2014; 218(4):686–692

[43] Singletary SE, Tucker SL, Boddie AW, Jr. Multivariate analysis of prognostic factors in regional cutaneous metastases of extremity melanoma. Cancer. 1988; 61(7):1437–1440

[44] van Poll D, Thompson JF, Colman MH, et al. A sentinel node biopsy does not increase the incidence of in-transit metastasis in patients with primary cutaneous melanoma. Ann Surg Oncol. 2005; 12(8):597–608

[45] Coventry BJ, Chatterton B, Whitehead F, James C, Gill PG. Sentinel lymph node dissection and lymphatic mapping for local subcutaneous recurrence in melanoma treatment: longer-term follow-up results. Ann Surg Oncol. 2004; 11 (3) Suppl:203S–207S

[46] Joshua AM. Melanoma prevention: are we doing enough? A Canadian perspective. Curr Oncol. 2012; 19(6):e462–e467

[47] Sondak VK, Sarnaik AA. Minimizing morbidity while preserving outcome after inguinal lymphadenectomy: navigating between scylla and charybdis. Ann Surg Oncol. 2011; 18(4):909–911

[48] Burmeister BH, Henderson MA, Ainslie J, et al. Adjuvant radiotherapy versus observation alone for patients at risk of lymph-node field relapse after therapeutic lymphadenectomy for melanoma: a randomised trial. Lancet Oncol. 2012; 13(6):589–597

[49] Gershenwald JE, Andtbacka RH, Prieto VG, et al. Microscopic tumor burden in sentinel lymph nodes predicts synchronous nonsentinel lymph node involvement in patients with melanoma. J Clin Oncol. 2008; 26(26):4296–4303

[50] Wong SL, Morton DL, Thompson JF, et al. Melanoma patients with positive sentinel nodes who did not undergo completion lymphadenectomy: a multi-institutional study. Ann Surg Oncol. 2006; 13(6):809–816

[51] Leiter U, Stadler R, Mauch C, et al. Complete lymph node dissection versus no dissection in patients with sentinel lymph node biopsy positive melanoma (DeCOG-SLT): a multicentre, randomised, phase 3 trial. Lancet Oncol. 2016; 17(6):757–767

[52] Bamboat ZM, Konstantinidis IT, Kuk D, Ariyan CE, Brady MS, Coit DG. Observation after a positive sentinel lymph node biopsy in patients with melanoma. Ann Surg Oncol. 2014; 21(9):3117–3123

[53] van der Ploeg AP, Haydu LE, Spillane AJ, et al. Outcome following sentinel node biopsy plus wide local excision versus wide local excision only for primary cutaneous melanoma: analysis of 5840 patients treated at a single institution. Ann Surg. 2014; 260(1):149–157

[54] Zager JS, Puleo CA, Sondak VK. What is the significance of the in transit or interval sentinel node in melanoma? Ann Surg Oncol. 2011; 18 (12):3232–3234

[55] Carling T, Pan D, Ariyan S, Narayan D, Truini C. Diagnosis and treatment of interval sentinel lymph nodes in patients with cutaneous melanoma. Plast Reconstr Surg. 2007; 119(3):907–913

[56] Vidal-Sicart S, Pons F, Fuertes S, et al. Is the identification of in-transit sentinel lymph nodes in malignant melanoma patients really necessary? Eur J Nucl Med Mol Imaging. 2004; 31(7):945–949

[57] McMasters KM, Chao C, Wong SL, et al. Sunbelt Melanoma Trial Group. Interval sentinel lymph nodes in melanoma. Arch Surg. 2002; 137(5):543–547, discussion 547–549

[58] Puleo CA, Sondak VK, Cruse CW, Berman CG, Zager JS, Messina JL. Melanoma sentinel node metastases in non-traditional sites. In: Proceedings Fifth Biennial International Sentinel Node Society Conference, November 1–4, 2006:127

[59] Deneve JL, Turaga KK, Marzban SS, et al. Single-institution outcome experience using AlloDerm® as temporary coverage or definitive reconstruction for cutaneous and soft tissue malignancy defects. Am Surg. 2013; 79(5):476–482

[60] Glazer ES, Porubsky CF, Francis JD. Treatment of head and neck melanoma in situ with staged contoured marginal excisions. Ann Plast Surg. 2017. 78(6): 663-667

[61] Kunishige JH, Brodland DG, Zitelli JA. Surgical margins for melanoma in situ. J Am Acad Dermatol. 2012; 66(3):438–444

[62] Chen LL, Jaimes N, Barker CA, Busam KJ, Marghoob AA. Desmoplastic melanoma: a review. J Am Acad Dermatol. 2013; 68(5):825–833

[63] Strom T, Caudell JJ, Han D, et al. Radiotherapy influences local control in patients with desmoplastic melanoma. Cancer. 2014; 120(9):1369–1378

[64] Lens MB, Newton-Bishop JA, Boon AP. Desmoplastic malignant melanoma: a systematic review. Br J Dermatol. 2005; 152(4):673–678

[65] Guadagnolo BA, Prieto V, Weber R, Ross MI, Zagars GK. The role of adjuvant radiotherapy in the local management of desmoplastic melanoma. Cancer. 2014; 120(9):1361–1368

[66] Egger ME, Huber KM, Dunki-Jacobs EM, et al. Incidence of sentinel lymph node involvement in a modern, large series of desmoplastic melanoma. J Am Coll Surg. 2013; 217(1):37–44, discussion 44–45

[67] Wasif N, Gray RJ, Pockaj BA. Desmoplastic melanoma - the step-child in the melanoma family? J Surg Oncol. 2011; 103(2):158–162

[68] Feng Z, Wu X, Chen V, Velie E, Zhang Z. Incidence and survival of desmoplastic melanoma in the United States, 1992–2007. J Cutan Pathol. 2011; 38 (8):616–624

[69] George E, McClain SE, Slingluff CL, Polissar NL, Patterson JW. Subclassification of desmoplastic melanoma: pure and mixed variants have significantly different capacities for lymph node metastasis. J Cutan Pathol. 2009; 36(4):425–432

[70] Wong JR, Harris JK, Rodriguez-Galindo C, Johnson KJ. Incidence of childhood and adolescent melanoma in the United States: 1973–2009. Pediatrics. 2013; 131(5):846–854

[71] Cordoro KM, Gupta D, Frieden IJ, McCalmont T, Kashani-Sabet M. Pediatric melanoma: results of a large cohort study and proposal for modified ABCD detection criteria for children. J Am Acad Dermatol. 2013; 68(6):913–925

[72] Gerami P, Busam K, Cochran A, et al. Histomorphologic assessment and interobserver diagnostic reproducibility of atypical spitzoid melanocytic neoplasms with long-term follow-up. Am J Surg Pathol. 2014; 38(7):934–940

[73] Ferrari A, Bono A, Baldi M, et al. Does melanoma behave differently in younger children than in adults? A retrospective study of 33 cases of childhood melanoma from a single institution. Pediatrics. 2005; 115(3):649–654

[74] Sreeraman Kumar R, Messina JL, Sondak VK, Reed DR. Treating melanoma in adolescents and young adults: challenges and solutions. Clin Oncol Adolescents Young Adults.. 2015; 5:75–86

[75] Sondak VK, Messina JL. Unusual presentations of melanoma: melanoma of unknown primary site, melanoma arising in childhood, and melanoma arising in the eye and on mucosal surfaces. Surg Clin North Am. 2014; 94 (5):1059–1073, ix

[76] Sreeraman Kumar R, Messina JL, Reed D, Navid F, Sondak VK. Pediatric melanoma and atypical melanocytic neoplasms. Cancer Treat Res. 2016; 167:331–369

5 Treatment of Rare Skin Malignancies

Karri Adamson and William W. Dzwierzynski

5.1 Introduction

The skin is the largest organ in the body, and it is not surprising that skin cancer is the most common type of cancer. The skin has a multitude of functions; these include being a protective barrier, a structure of mechanical support, an organ for temperature regulation, a system for excreting toxic substances, an organ for immunologic function, and a sensory organ. While skin cancer usually presents as basal cell and squamous cell cancers or melanoma, cancerous changes can develop in any of the cells that perform the varied functions of the skin. Like the more common skin cancers, most are more common in the Caucasian population, and ultraviolet (UV) exposure is thought to be a risk factor in many of these malignancies. Although these cancers are rare compared to common cutaneous cancers, knowledge of them is important for their treatment.

5.2 Merkel Cell Carcinoma

5.2.1 Background

Friedrich Merkel first described Merkel cells in 1875. These slowly adapting mechanoreceptors are derived from the neural crest and reside in the basal layer of the epidermis. Cyril Toker reported a tumor of these cells in 1972, initially describing it as a trabecular skin carcinoma. Six years later, Tang and Toker discovered dense core granules in some of those tumors, which in the skin are only found in Merkel cells.[1] The name Merkel cell carcinoma was introduced in 1980.

5.2.2 Epidemiology

Merkel cell carcinoma is a rare tumor with an incidence of less than 1/100,000 in the United States. Caucasian men are affected most commonly, at an average age of around 70 years. Caucasian patients account for 94% of cases, with an incidence rate 11.3 times greater than African American patients. Over 75% of cases occur in patients over the age of 64 years, with almost half of the cases affecting patients over the age of 74 years. Men are affected about twice as often as women and are diagnosed at an earlier age. Sun exposure (particularly UVB light) seems to play a role, with the highest incidence in the United States occurring in Hawaii, the state with the highest UVB index. The location of tumors correlates with sun-exposed regions, with the head and neck (most commonly the face) affected most often.[2] Mucosal lesions account for 4.5% of cases. Arsenic and infrared have also been theorized to have a role in the development of Merkel cell carcinoma.[3]

Immunocompromised patients are at greater risk, including those with chronic lymphocytic leukemia, acquired immunodeficiency syndrome, and organ transplant patients. Immunocompromised patients develop Merkel cell carcinoma earlier, with a mean age of 53 in transplant patients, and may have worse outcomes.[4]

The AEIOU mnemonic may be useful for remembering patient demographics. It stands for *A*symptomatic, *E*xpanding, *I*mmunosuppression, *O*lder than 50 years, and *U*ltraviolet exposure in fair-skinned patients.[5]

5.2.3 Diagnosis

Merkel cell carcinoma is difficult to diagnose clinically, lacking distinctive characteristics. The head and neck are most commonly affected, followed by the extremities, and, less commonly, the trunk. It may occur anywhere on the skin or mucosa, and usually presents as a skin toned, red, or purple intradermal nodule that has rapidly grown (▶ Fig. 5.1a, b). The epidermis may be ulcerated. Most tumors are less than 2 cm at the time of diagnosis.[6]

As with most suspicious skin lesions, a biopsy should be performed using punch, incisional, or close-margin excisional technique depending on the lesion location and size. The most common initial clinical suspicion is usually an epidermal cyst,[7]

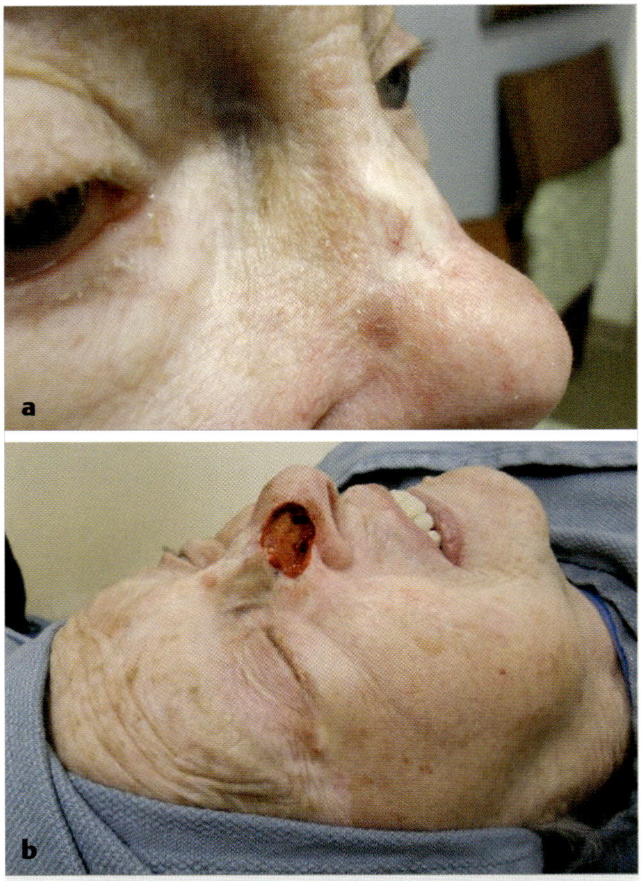

Fig. 5.1 **(a)** A 73-year-old female with 3 months' history of nodule on her nasal sidewall that was confirmed to be Merkel cell carcinoma on biopsy. **(b)** Following excision by Mohs micrographic surgery. The lesion was larger than its clinical appearance.

but the differential diagnosis includes basal cell carcinoma, squamous cell carcinoma, amelanotic melanoma, adnexal tumors, and cutaneous metastases.[3] A dermatopathologist should be requested for analysis of the biopsy. Hematoxylin and eosin (H&E) stains show small, round, blue cells, common in neuroendocrine tumors (▶ Fig. 5.2a, b). Immunohistochemistry must be completed to confirm the diagnosis, since metastatic small cell lung carcinoma (SCLC) can be indistinguishable on H&E. Cytokeratin-20 (CK-20) is found in 89 to 100% in cases of Merkel cell carcinoma, and is uncommonly seen in SCLC (▶ Fig. 5.3). Merkel cell carcinoma stains are positive for neurofilaments in most cases, but SCLC stains are not. Conversely, thyroid transcription factor 1 is positive in most SCLCs, but it is seen rarely in Merkel cell carcinoma.[8] For lesions that test equivocally, additional stains including chromogranin, synaptophysin, CD56, and neuron-specific enolase may be used to evaluate for other diagnoses.[9]

About 5% of Merkel cell carcinomas present in a lymph node with an unknown primary. Half of these are found in cervical nodes and 40% in inguinal nodes, while known primary tumors have positive nodes in the axillary or inguinal region more commonly than in the cervical region.[10] Diagnosis in these cases is made by pathology with the same stains mentioned earlier.

5.2.4 Workup

At the time of diagnosis, two-thirds of patients have local disease, one-quarter have lymph node involvement, and 7% have distant metastases.[11] A thorough review of systems should be obtained, and a complete physical examination including skin evaluation and palpation for lymphadenopathy should be performed. Sixteen to 24% of patients have palpable regional nodes.[7,12] The National Comprehensive Cancer Network (NCCN) recommends imaging studies for patients with clinically positive nodes. Positron emission tomography–computed tomography (PET-CT) is preferred, which is sensitive and specific, but CT or magnetic resonance imaging (MRI) is an option if PET-CT is not available.[9] PET-CT leads to a change in management in one-third of patients. Upstaging is relatively common (22% of total patients), most often with a finding of bone metastases, but downstaging also occurs in 5% of the cases. The PET stage is associated with survival, making it a useful test for prognosis.[13] Another indication for imaging is when small cell carcinoma of the lung with skin metastasis is a possible diagnosis. For example, when a biopsy is suspicious for Merkel cell carcinoma on histology, but is CK-20 negative, the NCCN recommends CT, MRI, or PET-CT to evaluate for a different primary cancer.[9]

5.2.5 Merkel Cell Polyomavirus

In 2008, Feng et al identified a polyomavirus present in 80% of Merkel cell tumors, compared to about 10% of control skin samples. This virus was named Merkel cell polyomavirus (MCV).[14] This virus is a part of normal human flora, and infected patients are asymptomatic. Most people acquire MCV by middle age. The virus is then integrated into the genome.[15] MCV infection and high levels of antibodies against MCV are associated with a higher risk of developing Merkel cell carcinoma; however, these factors are associated with better survival rates.[16]

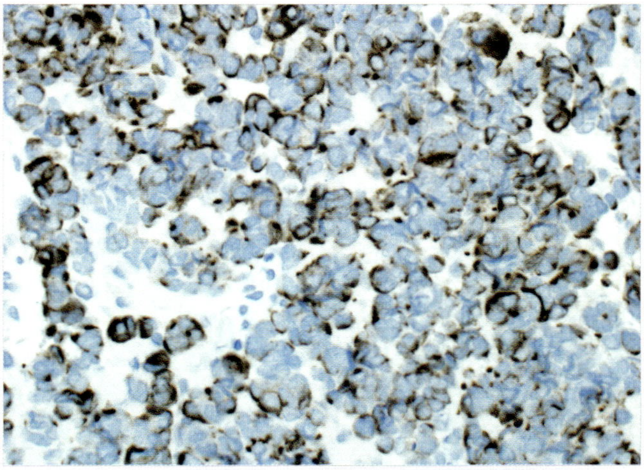

Fig. 5.3 Positive cytokeratin 20 stain, found in nearly all cases of Merkel cell carcinoma.

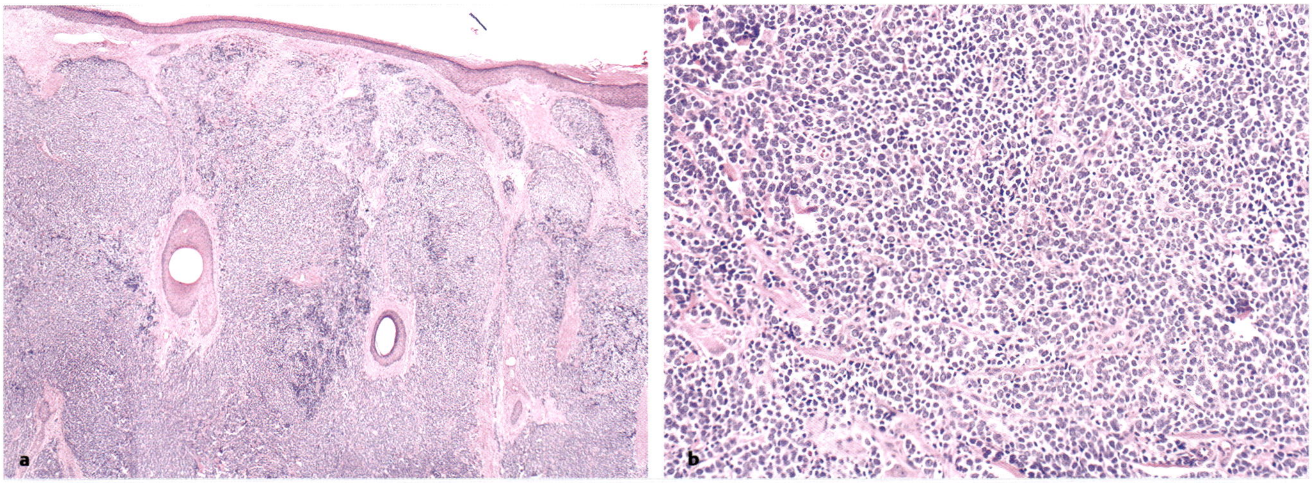

Fig. 5.2 **(a)** Hematoxylin and eosin (H&E) stain of Merkel cell carcinoma shows small round blue cells. **(b)** High-power view.

5.2.6 Staging

The tumor, node, metastasis (TNM) Staging System is used for Merkel cell carcinoma, as described by the American Joint Committee on Cancer. T1 indicates tumors less than or equal to 2 cm, T2 tumors 2 to 5 cm, and T3 tumors over 5 cm. N0 indicates no nodal involvement, and N1 indicates metastases to regional nodes. M0 means no metastases, and M1 means distant metastasis (beyond lymph nodes).[17] Stage 0 tumors are in situ. Stages I and II are local, with stage II including tumors greater than or equal to 2 cm. Stage III indicates nodal involvement, and stage IV tumors have distant metastasis. Distant metastases occur most commonly in the liver, followed by the lungs, bones, and brain.[3]

5.2.7 Surgical Treatment

The NCCN guidelines recommend wide excision with 1- to 2-cm margins, removing the specimen down to fascia. Some studies, however, found no change in local recurrence with 2-cm margins compared to 1 cm, and therefore some authors advocate for 2-cm margins only in cases where the primary tumor is greater than 2 cm.[3,12] Mohs or modified Mohs (Mohs excision, followed by a 0.5- or 1-cm margin after the final section) is also acceptable in areas of cosmetic concern, such as the face. The central portion of the specimen should be sent as a permanent specimen. The wound should be closed with the goal of rapid healing if radiation therapy is planned[9] (▶ Fig. 5.4a, b).

Sentinel lymph node biopsy (SLNB) should be performed in all patients at the time of the wide excision, both for staging and for therapeutic reasons (▶ Fig. 5.4c). Sentinel node status is the most important information for staging (▶ Fig. 5.5). Merkel cell carcinoma spread is generally lymphatic rather than hematogenous. Lymph nodes are commonly involved at the time of diagnosis, even in relatively small and/or superficial tumors with up to 37% having a positive sentinel node.[6,18] In patients without palpable lymphadenopathy, micrometastases are found in 23%.[12] Positive sentinel nodes are more common in tumors that spread below the dermis, and in older patients.[18] Sentinel nodes should be evaluated using the appropriate stains as mentioned earlier. Pathology should also note the amount of tumor burden and whether the tumor spreads beyond the capsule of the lymph node.[9]

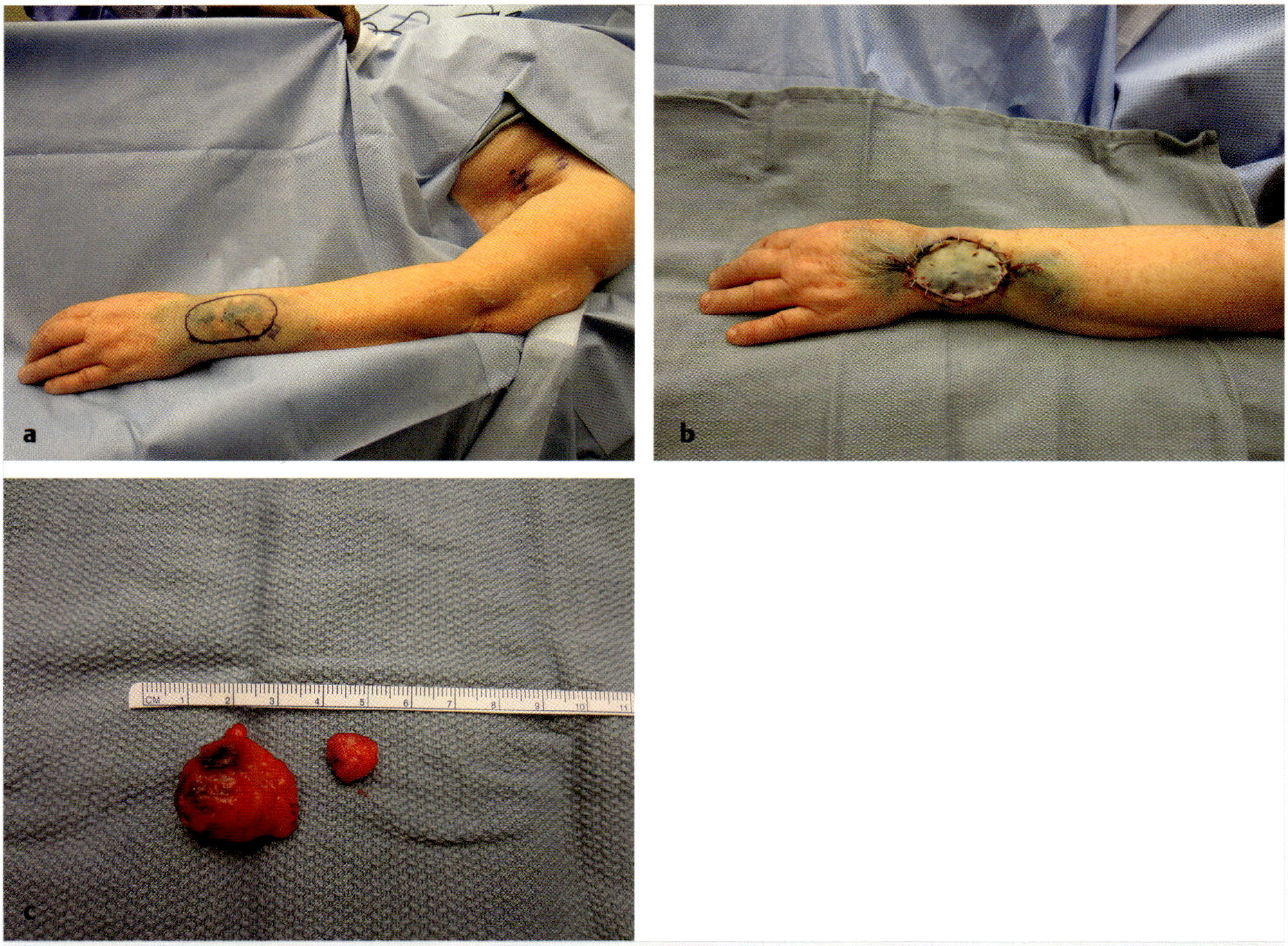

Fig. 5.4 **(a)** Merkel cell carcinoma excision after biopsy. The scar was marked with 2-cm margins and injected with methylene blue for sentinel lymph node biopsy. **(b)** After wide excision down to investing fascia, the wound was covered. **(c)** Sentinel lymph nodes were identified in the axilla. These were identified by lymphoscintigraphy using a gamma probe and methylene blue.

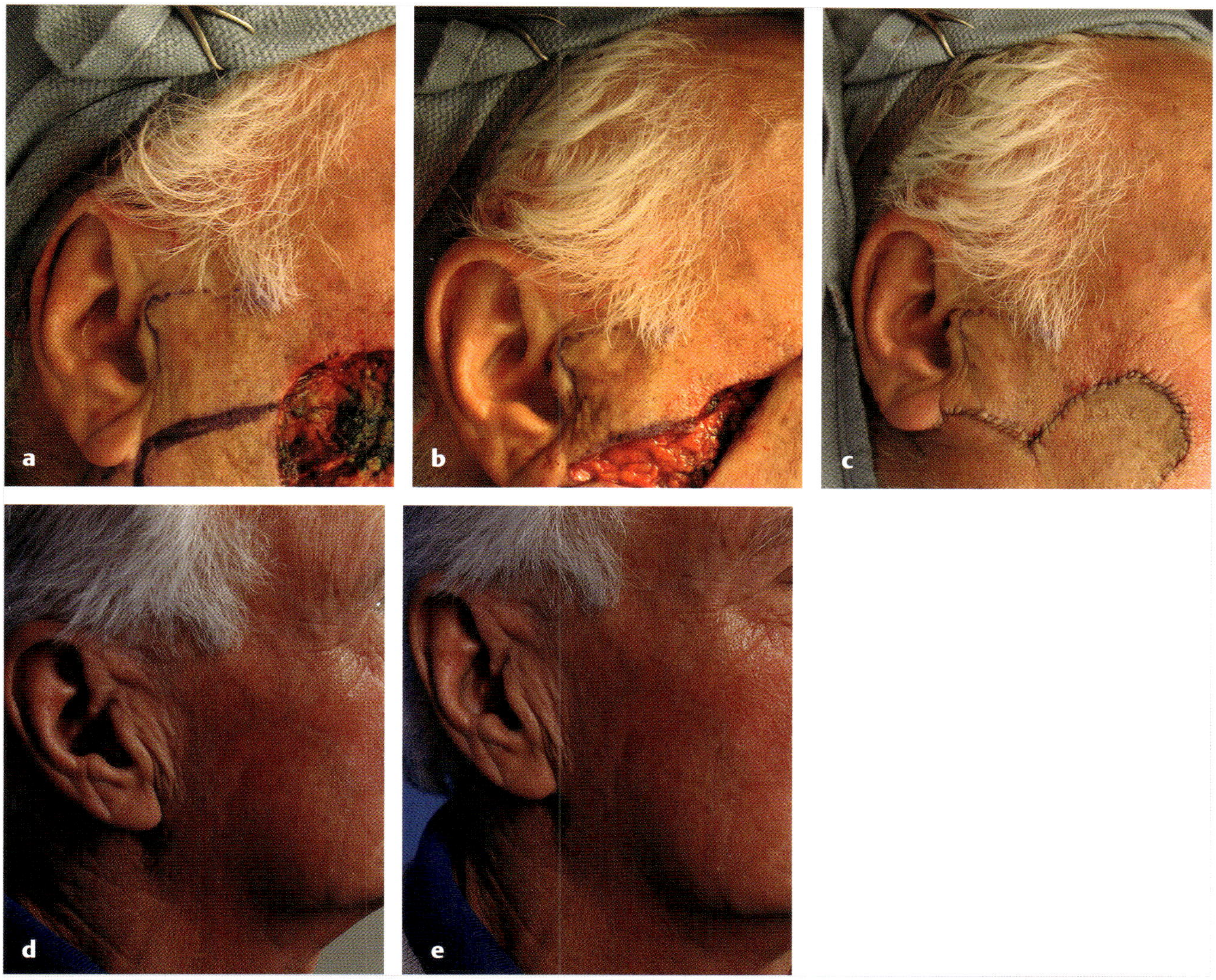

Fig. 5.5 Wide excision of Merkel cell carcinoma in the right cheek of a 68-year-old male. The skin around the lesion was injected interdermally with technician-labeled sulfur colloid and methylene blue for sentinel lymph node localization. The planned reconstruction with **(a)** rhomboid flap is marked. **(b)** The sentinel lymph node (x) in zone 3 of the neck was harvested through the reconstruction incision. **(c)** The rhomboid flap rotated and sutured into place. **(d)** Lateral view 4 months postoperatively after completion of radiation therapy. The sentinel lymph node biopsy showed no metastasis. **(e)** Oblique view 4 months postoperatively.

For patients with a positive sentinel lymph node or positive clinical nodes on exam, therapeutic regional lymph node dissection is recommended. Improved survival is seen in some studies.[19]

Type I interferons have been found to inhibit the proliferation of MCV positive Merkel cell carcinoma, inducing apoptosis in vitro and in vivo.[20] More research is needed before treatment recommendations can be made.

5.2.8 Radiation Therapy

Radiation to the primary site and/or the regional nodes may decrease local recurrence and improve disease-free survival.[6,21,22] This is controversial since other studies show no change in recurrence or overall survival.[12,23] The NCCN recommends radiation to the primary site (and the nodal basin in head and neck tumors) for patients with negative SLNB. If SLNB is not obtained or is positive, the primary site and nodal basin should be radiated.[9] Radiation should be given as soon as the surgical wounds have healed.

5.2.9 Chemotherapy

Traditional chemotherapy regimens including carboplatin and etoposide are poorly tolerated and have not been shown to decrease mortality; they have therefore not been recommended for routine use by the NCCN9. Immunotherapy has recently shown promising results in both MCV positive and MCV negative patients. These new medications include pembrolizumab and nivolumab, which inhibit programmed death-1 (PD-1), and avelumab, which inhibits programmed death ligand-1 (PD-L1). Immunotherapy should be initiated early in patients with metastatic disease.[24]

5.2.10 Prognosis

The overall 5-year survival rate is poor, at only about 50%. Immunosuppressed patients have an even worse prognosis, with only 43% alive 3 years after their diagnosis.[7] Worse survival rates are seen in men and the elderly.[19] Tumors on the limb are often diagnosed at an earlier stage than those on the trunk, and patients with tumors of the upper extremity have improved survival.[25] Most patients present with stage I or stage II disease. Staging is indeed predictive of survival, with patients diagnosed with stage I disease having an 86% 2-year survival rate, compared to 32% in patients with stage II disease.[2] Although patients with an unknown primary are stage III due to nodal involvement, these patients have a better survival rate than patients with a known primary who are stage III.[10] Node status and the corresponding pathologic stage are the most important predictors for prognosis.

SLNB itself may be therapeutic in addition to being prognostic, with SLNB patients having improved overall survival rate compared to patients with positive nodes and also those who did not have a lymph node evaluation. This is particularly true for tumors that were not on the head and neck,[22,26] whereas head and neck tumors have less predictable drainage patterns, possibly leading to a high false-negative SLNB rate.[18]

Up to half of patients have local or regional recurrence, usually in the nodal basin.[7,12] This occurs in an average of 9 months, with over 90% of recurrences occurring within 2 years. In patients with distant metastases, average survival is less than 1 year.[12]

Patients should be evaluated every 3 to 6 months for the first 2 years after treatment, and then at least yearly.[9]

5.2.11 Summary

Merkel cell carcinoma is a rare, but locally and regionally aggressive skin cancer that most commonly affects elderly white males. It is difficult to diagnose clinically, and histological diagnosis is assisted by special stains. Merkel cell carcinoma should be treated with wide local excision using at least 1-cm margins. SLNB should be mandatory, given it determines staging, which predicts prognosis. Radiation therapy is often indicated, while chemotherapy has not proven to be effective. MCV is often present in the tumor, but has yet to be effectively targeted therapeutically.

5.3 Dermatofibrosarcoma Protuberans

5.3.1 Background

Dermatofibrosarcoma protuberans (DFSP) is a malignant cutaneous tumor characterized by a low risk of distant metastasis but a high local recurrence rate if not treated appropriately. It is a mesenchymal tumor, stimulated by mutations in stem cells in skin appendages.[27]

DFSP was first described by Taylor in 1890 as a sarcoma "resembling in some aspects keloids." It was later given its name by Hoffman in 1925.[28]

5.3.2 Epidemiology

DFSP has an incidence of 1 to 4 cases per million people per year in the United States, accounting for 0.1% of all cancers.[29] It affects males and females nearly equally, with a slight predominance in women. Among American Caucasians, the highest incidence is in Hawaii[29]; however, a quarter of cases occur in non-Caucasian patients, with African Americans being disproportionately affected. DFSP is most commonly diagnosed in patients 30 to 50 years old,[29] but up to 20% of cases occur in pediatric patients. Congenital lesions are also reported.[30]

5.3.3 Diagnosis

DFSP lacks defining features, and is often present for many years before it is biopsied and diagnosed. It usually presents as an asymptomatic, firm plaque or nodule that has been slowly enlarging for a long time, sometimes with a recent rapid growth period.[29] Some patients describe a history of trauma preceding the lesion, but this has not been correlated with development of DFSP.[30] DFSP may be skin-toned, red-blue, brown-yellow, erythematous, sclerodermiform, telangiectatic, or atrophic. It is adherent to the skin but usually freely mobile over deeper structures.[31] Long-standing lesions may become painful or develop ulcerations.[28]

DFSP can present anywhere, but most commonly is found on the trunk. Thirty percent of tumors appear in the extremities (upper more often than lower), and 15% in the head and neck. The distribution in children is similar.[32]

Incisional or excisional biopsy should be performed. H&E stain shows a uniform proliferation of spindle cells with low mitotic activity. These form a characteristic "storiform" or "cartwheel" pattern (▶ Fig. 5.6), with projections invading underlying fat, fascia, muscle, and even bone, like tentacles. This creates a honeycomb appearance within subcutaneous fat. It may be difficult to distinguish DFSP from dermatofibroma, fibrosarcoma, atypical fibroxanthoma (AFX), and nodular fasciitis.[28] Immunohistochemistry can be helpful. CD34 is often strongly expressed in DFSP (▶ Fig. 5.7) and is used to differentiate it from dermatofibromas, which do not express CD34. Conversely, dermatofibromas

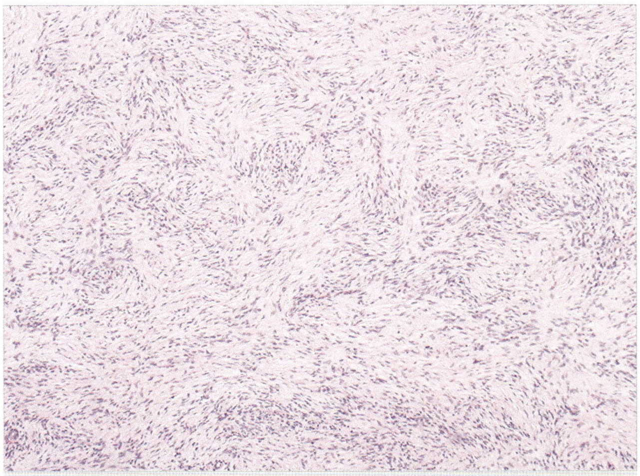

Fig. 5.6 Storiform pattern of dermatofibrosarcoma protuberans.

express coagulation factor XIIIa, while DFSP does not.[28] Other stains including stromolysin-3, S100, CD68, and apolipoprotein D may also be used to rule out other diagnoses.

The differential diagnosis may also include neurofibroma, leiomyoma, epidermal cyst, malignant melanoma, basal cell carcinoma, keloid, desmoids, Kaposi's sarcoma, and sarcoidosis.[28] In children, DFSP may be confused with vascular malformations and hamartomas, as well as congenital aplasia cutis, dermoid cyst or teratoma, and infantile fibromatosis.[32]

5.3.4 Workup

A thorough history and physical exam is usually sufficient prior to treatment of DFSP, given it is generally a local disease. DFSP metastasizes in only 1% of patients, mostly to the lungs. It does not commonly spread to the lymph nodes, and therefore SLNB is not recommended. MRI accurately depicts the depth of lesions, but underestimates the lateral extent.[33] The NCCN does not recommend any diagnostic imaging.[34]

5.3.5 Subtypes

Several variants exist, including the Bednar's tumor, a pigmented variant making up 1% of DFSP cases, as well as myxoid, myoid, granular cell, neuorfibromatous, sclerotic, giant cell fibroblastoma, and atrophic. A more aggressive subtype, fibrosarcomatous DFSP (DFSP-FS), has more frequent mitoses and areas of cellular atypia, with a herringbone pattern. This variant accounts for 10 to 15% of cases and is aggressive, with higher local recurrence rates, more frequent metastasis, and greater mortality.[35]

5.3.6 Chromosomal Abnormalities

Over 90% of cases have supernumerary ring chromosomes or translocations (t[17;22] [q22;q13]), combining parts of chromosomes 17 and 22. This results in an oncogenic fusion of collagen type I alpha 1 gene (COL1A1) with platelet-derived growth factor B-chain gene (PDGFB), resulting in lack of regulation of production of the PDGFB protein.[36] In turn, the PDGFB receptor, a tyrosine kinase, is overstimulated. The chromosomal changes are confirmed with karyotype analysis and fluorescence in situ hybridization (FISH), and the gene fusion is discovered with polymerase chain reaction (PCR).[27]

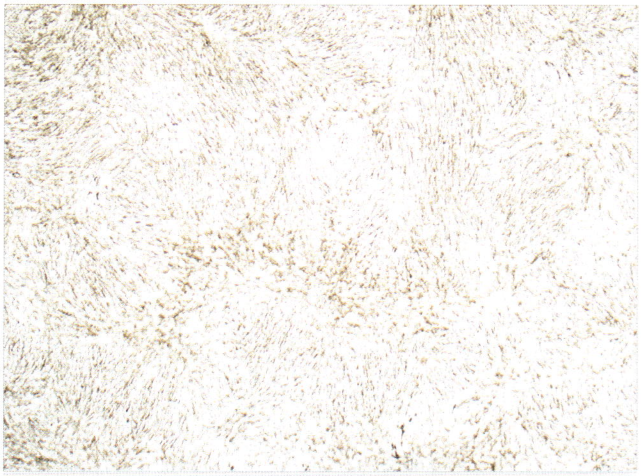

Fig. 5.7 Positive CD34 stain, typically found in dermatofibrosarcoma protuberans.

5.3.7 Staging

Several staging systems have been devised for DFSP, but none accurately predict outcomes.[27] The American Musculoskeletal Tumor Society system uses histologic grade, local extension, and metastases. The American Joint Committee on Cancer includes tumor size and depth, lymph node involvement, and distant metastasis. The Short German Guidelines are also available.[28] Ninety-nine percent of cases present with local or regional involvement only.[29]

5.3.8 Surgical Treatment

Treatment consists of complete excision of tumor. This can be difficult due to projections coursing microscopically much further than are visible clinically, sometimes over 10 cm.[37] Recurrence rates after wide local excision are reported to be as high as 60%.[28] With careful analysis of margins, recurrence rates after wide local excision can be as low as 1%, but may require multiple excisions and delayed wound closure.[38] The NCCN recommends margins of 2 to 4 cm when performing wide local excision, taking specimens down to investing fascia.[34]

Due to the difficulty in obtaining clear margins, Mohs micrographic surgery (MMS) has become the standard of care for DFSP, particularly in the head and neck. Recurrence rates after Mohs controlled excision are reported at about 0 to 1%.[39,40] Mohs defects are on average four times larger than the clinical lesion.[40] Treating all patients with conventional wide excision results in excessive resection in 80% of patients and inadequate resection in 5%, supporting MMS as the treatment of choice.[31]

While MMS is effective, it takes longer, requires a dermatologic surgeon who is familiar with DFSP frozen sections, and is expensive. Frozen sections can be difficult to interpret for an inexperienced dermatopathologist, with about 90% accuracy when compared to permanent pathology.[38] Many surgeons send the final stage as a permanent specimen for confirmation of negative margins (modified Mohs), especially in recurrent cases.

Reconstruction with tissue rearrangement should be delayed until negative margins are confirmed[34] (▶ Fig. 5.8a-h).

5.3.9 Radiation Therapy

DFSP is radiosensitive; however, due to the reasonably low recurrence rates with adequate resection, radiation therapy should be reserved for unresectable, recurrent, or metastatic cases.[34] Patients with microscopically positive margins have a 33% recurrence rate.[41] Treating all of these patients can potentially confer more risk than benefit, as the majority do not go on to develop local or distant metastases.

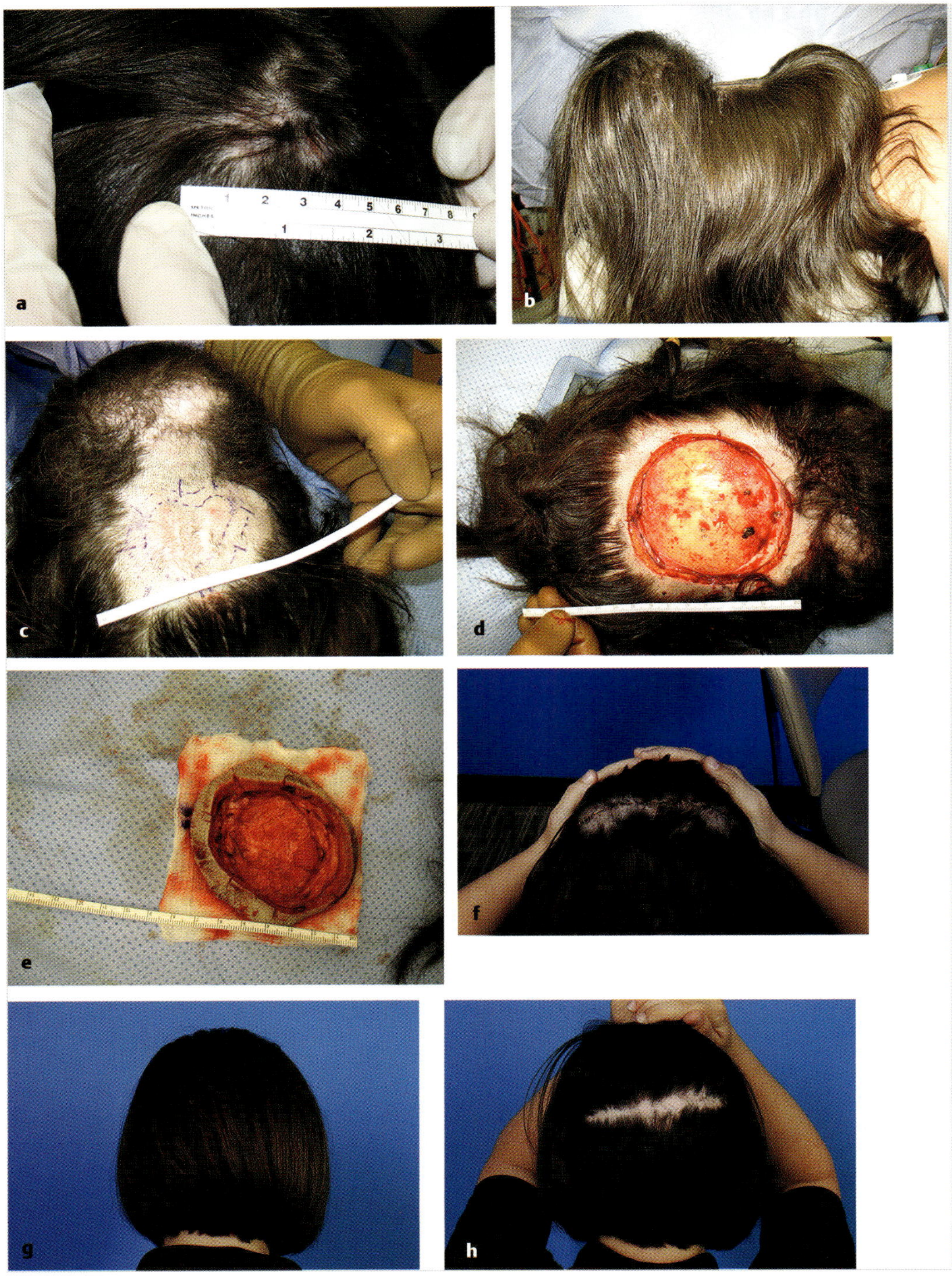

Fig. 5.8 (a) A 38-year-old female with a 2-year history of a painless enlarging nodule on her scalp. She sought the attention of several physicians who treated her for eczema. A biopsy revealed a dermatofibrosarcoma protuberans. **(b)** Because of the slow-growing nature of the lesions, two tissue expanders were placed prior to definitive excision and expanded over 3 months. Shown is the patient positioned prone on the operating table with the expanders fully inflated. **(c)** Marking of the palpable lesion and first stage of the excision with Mohs controlled margins. **(d)** Final excision after two stages of Mohs processing. The patient remained asleep in the operating room during the Mohs processing. **(e)** Additional rim of tissue with deep main is removed after completion of the Mohs processing and sent for permanent section evaluation. **(f)** Tissue expanders are removed and the flaps are rotated to close the defect. Results 1 week after surgery. **(g)** One year after surgery, the scar is well hidden. **(h)** Minimal incisional alopecia is present.

5.3.10 Chemotherapy

Patients with the COL1A1-PDGFB fusion gene may benefit from imatinib mesylate, a tyrosine kinase inhibitor. Up to two-thirds of patients will have tumor regression. Neoadjuvant therapy may make reconstruction simpler, but can change the appearance on histology by decreasing cellularity.[27] While this drug is well tolerated by most, patients should be screened for the fusion gene prior to treatment to prevent side effects in patients who will not have a response.[42] The NCCN recommends imatinib in unresectable, recurrent, or metastatic cases.[34]

Traditional chemotherapy is only recommended in patients with metastatic disease.[34]

5.3.11 Prognosis

Although DFSP is known for high recurrence rates, distant spread is rare, with only about 1% of patients developing distant metastasis. Metastases usually follow local recurrences, often in

DFSP-FS.[35] Patients have an overall 5-year survival of 99%, and a disease-specific 5-year survival of over 99%.[29] Recurrent disease is associated with decreased disease-free survival.[41]

Patients with DFSP are at increased risk for a second DFSP lesion, as well as for subsequent primary malignancies of other types. These are most often skin cancers, but also include breast cancer.[43]

Patients should be seen for follow-up every 6 to 12 months. Twenty percent of recurrences occur over 3 years after resection of the primary lesion.[27] Because of the possibility for late recurrence, as well as the increased risk of other cancers, follow-up should continue indefinitely.

5.3.12 Summary

DFSP is a locally aggressive skin cancer that affects men and women in their 30s to 50s, with an increased prevalence in African Americans. It often presents in a delayed fashion due to its slow growth and indistinct form, and is diagnosed with a biopsy using H&E and immunohistochemistry. Treatment consists of complete excision, either by wide local excision or with MMS. Imatinib may be useful in some patients with a specific gene fusion. Overall survival is excellent, and distant metastasis is rare.

5.4 Cutaneous Angiosarcoma

5.4.1 Background

Cutaneous angiosarcoma is a rare mesenchymal malignancy of vascular origin. It is one of the most aggressive skin cancers, with high rates of local recurrence and distant metastases, as well as high mortality rate.

5.4.2 Epidemiology

Cutaneous sarcomas account for 5% of skin malignancies, and angiosarcomas account for less than 2% of all soft tissue sarcomas.[44,45] More than half of angiosarcomas occur in the skin and superficial subcutaneous tissues,[46] with an overall incidence of 0.01/100,000 per year.[47] Cutaneous angiosarcoma occurs in three settings: spontaneously, following radiation therapy, and in the setting of chronic lymphedema (known as Stewart–Treves syndrome). The spontaneous category includes malignant degeneration of a vascular malformation.[48] Other possible contributing factors are excessive UV light,[49] immunosuppression,[45] and polyvinyl chloride, arsenic, or thorium dioxide exposure.[50] Spontaneous cases affect men more often; however, many of the cases related to radiation and lymphedema occur in women after breast cancer treatment. Cutaneous angiosarcoma usually occurs in Caucasian patients over 50 years old, peaking in the seventh or eighth decade of life. It has also been reported in children as young as 6 weeks, accounting for 0.3% of pediatric sarcomas.[51]

5.4.3 Diagnosis

Cutaneous angiosarcoma often looks like a bruise initially, which seems to enlarge over time. It may become nodular, painful, edematous, friable, or ulcerate.[46] Patients often have symptoms for several months prior to diagnosis.[46] At the time of diagnosis, the size of the lesion can range from less than 1 cm to over 10 cm.[45,48] The differential diagnosis includes pyogenic granuloma, Kaposi's sarcoma, lymphoma, malignant melanoma, recurrent breast cancer, or radiation-related morphea.[48,52] Lesions occur most commonly on the scalp and face, followed by the trunk, lower extremity, and upper extremity.[45] The high propensity for the scalp is thought to be influenced by increased UV exposure to this area combined with a relatively increased vascularity.[48] Lesions on the breast are most commonly associated with prior radiation for treatment of breast cancer, and lesions on the arm are often in the setting of Stewart–Treves syndrome.

Diagnosis is made by excisional or incisional biopsy. Histology shows vascular channels lined by endothelial cells, often dissecting collagen in the dermis and extending into the subcutaneous tissue[46,52] (▶ Fig. 5.9). Blood-filled channels or clefts are sometimes present with hemorrhage and necrosis.[52] Lesions range from well to poorly differentiated. On histology, the lesion may be difficult to distinguish from other vascular and epithelial tumors including spindle cell carcinoma, malignant melanoma, and AFX; therefore, immunohistochemistry, and in particular vascular markers, should be used.[53] Cutaneous angiosarcoma often stains positive for CD31 and Ets family transcription factor (ERG).[54] Less sensitive stains include vascular endothelial growth factor receptor 3 (VEGFR-3), factor VIII, and D2–D40 monoclonal antibody.[47,54] Angiosarcomas are usually negative for cytokeratin, S100, and desmin. Cutaneous angiosarcoma subtypes including the epithelioid subtype are diagnosed by histology and immunohistochemistry.

5.4.4 Workup

A careful history and physical exam should be performed, searching for multifocal or satellite disease, which is present in over one-third of patients, as well as locoregional and distant metastases. Metastasis eventually occurs in over 50% of patients, with metastasis most commonly to the lungs, as well as bone, liver, spleen, and less commonly to lymph nodes.[48] MRI may be used as an adjunct, but it shows greater local

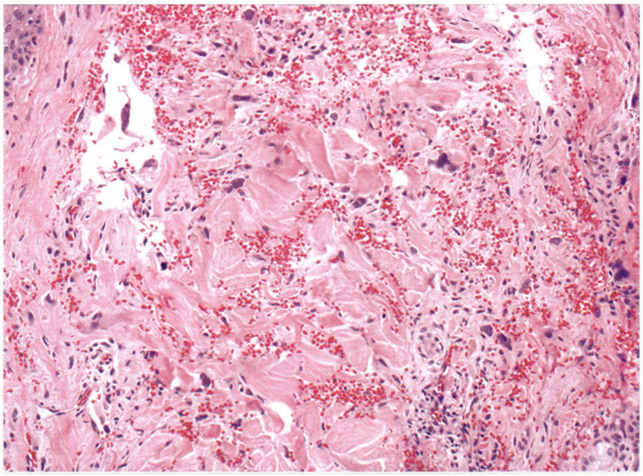

Fig. 5.9 Vascular channels are prominent in cutaneous angiosarcoma.

involvement than seen grossly.[46] MRI, CT, or PET-CT can detect local or distant metastases.

5.4.5 Radiation-Associated Cutaneous Angiosarcoma and Stewart–Treves Syndrome

Twenty-six percent of patients with cutaneous angiosarcoma have a prior primary cancer, with about 50% of these patients having a history of breast cancer.[45] In most of these instances, the lesion is ipsilateral to the previous breast cancer.[45] Stewart and Treves reported cutaneous angiosarcoma in six women with lymphedema after breast cancer treatment in 1948. The first report of cutaneous angiosarcoma attributed to radiation therapy was in the 1980s.[55] The lag between initial breast cancer treatment and development of angiosarcoma in these patients is often 5 to 15 years.[44]

Radiation-associated angiosarcoma presents as late edema or thickening of the radiated mastectomy skin flap with violaceous or erythematous macules or nodules.[52] In contrast, patients with Stewart–Treves syndrome have a history of lymphedema, most commonly from mastectomy with axillary lymph node dissection, and these angiosarcomas occur in the ipsilateral shoulder or upper extremity, not in the previously irradiated tissue. They present with variable changes in the lymphedematous skin, with a nodule or nonhealing eschar.[56] Stewart–Treves syndrome has also been described in patients with lower extremity lymphedema and congenital lymphedema. It is speculated to occur due to a relative immunodeficiency locally from lymphatic disruption.[44,56] Stewart–Treves syndrome occurs in less than 0.5% of patients who have a radical mastectomy, and its incidence is decreasing due to the relatively conservative surgical treatments for breast cancer favored today.[56]

5.4.6 Staging

There is no accepted staging system for cutaneous angiosarcoma. Histologic grade is not very predictive of prognosis.

5.4.7 Treatment

Surgical treatment is associated with improved survival and consists of wide local excision, with at least 1-cm margins (► Fig. 5.10). Patients with radiation-associated angiosarcoma of the breast should have a mastectomy.[52] MMS is an option; however, current data do not show improved outcomes compared to conventional surgery.[50]

Adjuvant radiation is also recommended. It should be delivered to the primary site and regional nodal basins. When the primary lesion is located on the scalp, it should target the entire scalp.[46]

Chemotherapy has not been shown to improve outcomes, and should be reserved for palliative or unresectable cases.

5.4.8 Prognosis

After proper treatment, patients have about 40% 3-year and 30% 5-year recurrence-free survival.[44] The overall survival is 51% at 5 years and 43% at 10 years.[45] Recurrence occurs after a median of 1 year.[44] Patients with distant metastases have less than a 10% chance of surviving 5 years.[45] Those who die of the disease have a median survival of less than 2 years.[44] Pediatric patients have similarly dismal survival rates.[51]

Tumor size less than 5 cm, single focus disease, age less than 50, and negative surgical margins are associated with improved survival.[44,45,46,47] Tumors on the scalp and neck have a worse prognosis.[45]

5.4.9 Summary

Cutaneous angiosarcoma is a very rare skin cancer, affecting elderly males, most often on the scalp. It also occurs in previously radiated sites, as well as in the setting of chronic lymphedema. It is one of the most aggressive skin cancers, with very poor recurrence-free and overall survival rates. Recommended treatment includes wide local excision and radiotherapy.

5.5 Cutaneous Leiomyosarcoma

5.5.1 Background

Leiomyosarcoma is a rare malignant mesenchymal tumor that arises from the arrector pili in the superficial subtype, and from the smooth muscle of blood vessels in the deep subtype.[57]

5.5.2 Epidemiology

Patients present at an average age of 50 to 70 years.[58] The disease has a male predilection.[58] Some patients have a history of prior radiation therapy in the same location.[59]

5.5.3 Diagnosis

The lesion is typically an erythematous, brown, or skin-toned nodule. Pain, ulceration, and bleeding are present in some.[58] The superficial subtype has a predilection for the head and neck, while the deep subtype is more commonly found on the lower extremities.[59]

The differential diagnosis is broad, and the lesion is commonly clinically misdiagnosed as a dermatofibroma.[57] On histology, fascicles of spindle-shaped cells within an eosinophilic cytoplasm are seen. Cigar-shaped nuclei are present, as are mitotic figures.[60] Immunohistochemistry shows near 100% expression of smooth muscle actin, and high expression of desmin and caldesmon.[59]

Three-quarters of these neoplasms are confined to the dermis (superficial subtype), and one-quarter extend into the superficial subcutaneous fat (deep subtype).[57]

5.5.4 Treatment

Most surgeons perform wide local excision with lateral margins of at least 2 cm[61] with the fascia as the deep margin. Success has been reported with MMS.[62] Radiation therapy is used as an adjunct in high-risk tumors, but with little evidence to support its efficacy.

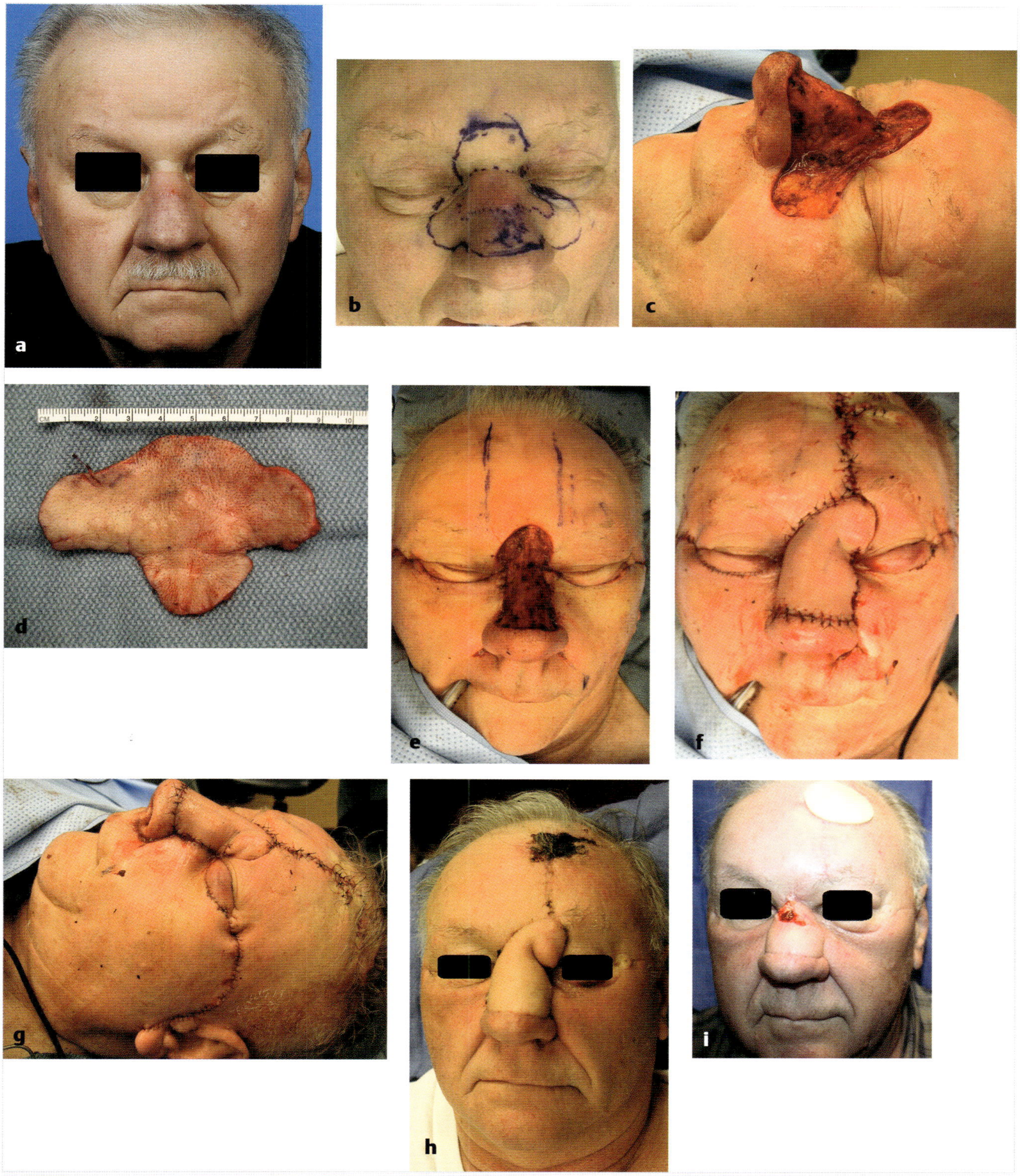

Fig. 5.10 **(a)** An 80-year-old male with a 1-year history of lesion on his nasal dorsum. Biopsy showed a cutaneous angiosarcoma. **(b)** Inner dotted line delineates palpable margins of the lesion, outer line shows planned 2-cm margin of excision. **(c)** Defect after resection. **(d)** Surgical specimen. **(e)** Bilateral facial flaps are used to cover the cheek defects. **(f)** Left paramedical forehead flap reconstruction of nasal defect. **(g)** Lateral view at completion of surgery. **(h)** Two weeks postoperative. Final pathology report showed a positive deep margin in the center of the specimen. The forehead flap donor site is allowed to heal by secondary intension. **(i)** The forehead flap was divided at 3 weeks and radical thinned with skeletonization of the nasal dorsum. Permanent sections showed no residual tumor. Photo is 2 weeks postdivision.

5.5.5 Prognosis

Reported recurrence rates after wide local excision range from 6 to 70%. Recurrence is much more common in the deep subtype, and inadequate margins are correlated with recurrence.[57] Most recurrences are found within 1 year of initial treatment. Distant metastases are exceedingly rare, and survival rates are above 90%.[63]

5.5.6 Summary

Primary cutaneous leiomyosarcoma is a rare cutaneous malignancy with variable presentation. Diagnosis is made by histology, and treatment consists of wide local excision. Local recurrence rates are low in purely dermal tumors, but moderate in those that extend into the subcutis. Distant metastases are rare and overall prognosis is favorable.

5.6 Cutaneous Adenoid Cystic Carcinoma

5.6.1 Background

Adenoid cystic carcinoma is most often a tumor of the salivary glands, but can also present primarily in other locations including the skin. Primary cutaneous adenoid cystic carcinoma is a rare, indolent adnexal neoplasm, first described by Boggio in 1975.[64]

5.6.2 Epidemiology

Patients are diagnosed at a median age of 63 years. Most cases occur in Caucasians, affecting men and women equally.[65]

5.6.3 Diagnosis

Cutaneous adenoid cystic carcinoma lacks characteristic features. It typically presents as a slow-growing, flesh-colored nodule, and most often occurs on the scalp. Other common locations include the ear, face, and eyelid.[65] Lesions may be asymptomatic, but can cause local alopecia or pain.[64]

Diagnosis is made by histology, which shows basaloid cells with an "adenoid or cribiform [sic] pattern occupying the mid to reticular dermis."[64] Glandlike spaces or pseudocysts have secretions that frequently stain positive for Alcian blue, a marker for sialomucin.[66] Perineural invasion is common and is associated with higher recurrence rates.[64] Immunohistochemistry is positive for epithelial membrane antigen (EMA), and often S100 and cytokeratin as well.[64] The histological differential diagnosis includes adenoid cystic carcinoma that is metastatic to the skin, cylindroma, adenoid basal cell carcinoma, and mucinous apocrine carcinoma.[64]

5.6.4 Treatment

Treatment is surgical and consists of wide local excision with negative margins. There are reports of successful treatment with MMS.[67]

5.6.5 Prognosis

Seventy percent of patients have localized disease at the time of presentation, and only 5% have distant metastases.[65] The 5-year overall survival is 96%, and is better in patients with lesions on the head and neck than those with lesions on the trunk.[65]

Local recurrence is common, with rates from 20 to 40%.[64] As recurrence can occur many years after excision, long-term follow-up is necessary.[64]

5.6.6 Summary

Cutaneous adenoid cystic carcinoma is a slow-growing adnexal tumor. Diagnosis is made by histology, and treatment consists of wide local excision. Recurrence rates are relatively high; however, distant metastases are rare and overall survival is excellent.

5.7 Sebaceous Carcinoma

5.7.1 Background

Sebaceous carcinoma is a rare adnexal tumor with occasionally aggressive behavior, also known as sebaceous gland carcinoma, sebaceous cell carcinoma, and meibomian gland carcinoma.[68]

5.7.2 Epidemiology

Sebaceous carcinoma accounts for less than 1% of skin cancers in the United States.[68] In the United States, it predominantly affects Caucasians with a slight predilection for men. Patients are diagnosed at an average age of 72 years.[69] There may be a higher incidence in Asian patients worldwide.[68]

Sebaceous carcinoma is associated with Muir–Torre syndrome, which is a hereditary disorder that leads to the development of cutaneous tumors and visceral tumors. Other risk factors include a history of radiation, immunosuppression, and familial retinoblastoma.[68]

5.7.3 Diagnosis

Sebaceous carcinoma usually presents as a painless nodule.[68] It occurs most often on the eyelid where there is a high density of sebaceous glands. Other common locations include the face, scalp or neck, ear, and lip.[69]

The clinical differential diagnosis includes chalazion, keratoconjunctivitis, blepharoconjunctivitis, basal cell carcinoma, and squamous cell carcinoma.[68] A biopsy should be obtained, particularly if the lesion becomes symptomatic.

Histology shows unencapsulated, lobular neoplasms composed of sebaceous and undifferentiated cells. Vacuolated cells are present in the epidermis and dermis with lipid granules in the cytoplasm, giving a frothy appearance[68] (► Fig. 5.11). Pagetoid spread is common.[68] Adipophilin expression is common on immunohistochemistry.

Histologic differential diagnosis includes sebaceous adenoma, sebaceoma, and basal cell carcinoma with sebaceous differentiation.[68]

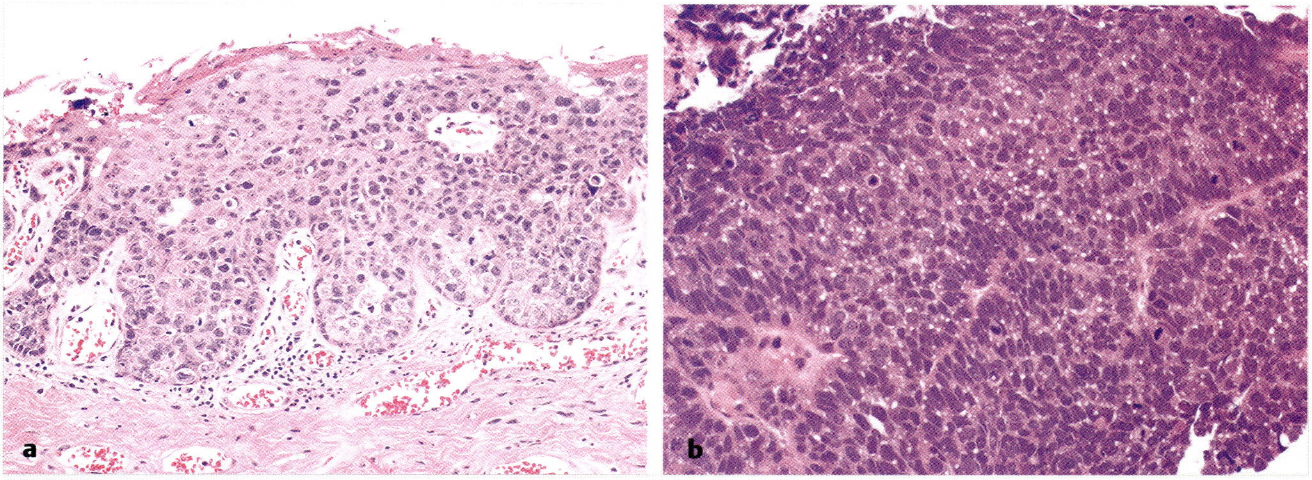

Fig. 5.11 (a) Sebaceous carcinoma, with vacuolated cells in the epidermis and dermis. (b) Sebaceous cell differentiation.

Patients with sebaceous carcinoma should be screened for Muir–Torre syndrome for increased suspicion and early detection of visceral malignancies.

Imaging may be considered in patients with palpable lymphadenopathy or lesions with aggressive histological features.[68]

5.7.4 Staging

The American Joint Committee on Cancer TNM Staging System is used for sebaceous carcinoma.

5.7.5 Treatment

Treatment consists of wide local excision with at least 5-mm margins[70]; however, local recurrence occurs in up to a quarter of patients. MMS is also an option,[70] with similar disease-specific survival rates.[69] At this time, SLNB is not required, but should be considered in periorbital cases, given that these have a greater tendency to metastasize.[68] Patients with positive nodes often undergo completion lymphadenectomy.[68]

Radiation therapy is reserved for patients unable to undergo surgical excision and for patients with recurrence or metastasis.

5.7.6 Prognosis

Lymph node metastasis occurs in up to a quarter of patients with sebaceous carcinoma.[68] Distant metastases are diagnosed in about 1%.[69] On histology, pagetoid spread, multicentric tumors, tumors over 10 mm, and tumors with perivascular, perineural, or perilymphatic invasion have worse prognosis.[68] Overall disease-specific mortality is about 5%.[68]

5.7.7 Summary

Sebaceous carcinoma is a rare adnexal tumor associated with Muir–Torre syndrome. It occurs most commonly in elderly Caucasians, with a predilection for the head and neck, particularly the eyelid. Diagnosis is made by histology, and treatment is excision. Local recurrence rates are relatively high, and regional metastases are not uncommon; however, overall survival is very good.

5.8 Microcystic Adnexal Carcinoma

5.8.1 Background

Microcystic adnexal carcinoma is a rare adnexal tumor with both follicular and sweat gland differentiation, first described by Goldstein et al in 1982.[71] Other names used to describe this tumor include sclerosing sweat duct carcinoma, malignant syringoma, and syringomatous carcinoma. It is believed to begin as a pluripotent adnexal keratinocyte.[72] It is slow growing but locally aggressive, and typically does not metastasize.

5.8.2 Epidemiology

Microcystic adnexal carcinoma has an incidence of 1.6 to 6.5 per 10,000,000. It disproportionately affects Caucasians.[72] The tumor has a slight predilection for females. The diagnosis is typically made in older patients, with an average age of 62 years[72]; however, the disease has been described in all ages; a congenital case has even been reported.[73] Significant sun exposure may be a risk factor, given that Americans tend to be affected on the left side of the face more often than the right.[72,74] This is believed to be due to increased sun exposure on the left side of the face when driving. A history of radiation also seems to be a risk factor for developing microcystic adnexal carcinoma.[75]

5.8.3 Diagnosis

Microcystic adnexal carcinoma presents as a slow-growing subcutaneous, yellow to flesh-colored nodule or plaque. Tumors can occur anywhere on the body, but most often on the face, specifically the central region of the face including the lips and nose.[72,75] Patients may experience pain or paresthesias.[71] The clinical differential diagnosis includes squamous cell carcinoma, cyst, and morpheaform basal cell carcinoma.[71]

Diagnosis is made by incisional or excisional biopsy. Adequate biopsy depth is critical; superficial biopsies result in a misdiagnosis rate of up to 27%.[74] Because of its lack of characteristic features both clinically and by histology when an inadequate superficial biopsy is obtained, the diagnosis of microcystic adnexal carcinoma is often delayed for years.[71] On biopsy, the tumor involves the skin and may invade the subcutaneous fat, muscle, and bone.[72] It involves tissue beyond what is clinically apparent, especially on lateral margins.[76] Perineural invasion is present in about half of cases.[77] Histology shows keratinous cysts superficially with strands of cells penetrating deeper, surrounded by dense fibrous stroma[78] (▶ Fig. 5.12). Cellular atypia and mitoses are rare.[79] The histological differential diagnosis includes morpheaform basal cell carcinoma, trichoadenoma, eccrine carcinoma, metastatic breast carcinoma, syringoma, and desmoplastic trichepithelioma.[71,80]

Immunohistochemical stains can be used to differentiate microcystic adnexal carcinoma from other cutaneous neoplasms. Microcystic adnexal carcinoma usually stains positive for carcinoembryonic antigen, EMA, and cytokeratin.[80]

5.8.4 Treatment

Treatment consists of complete excision with negative margins. Because of its indistinct borders and unpredictable lateral spread, MMS is often utilized, particularly in areas of cosmetic concern.[81] Slow Mohs (using paraffin sections) or modified Mohs (frozen sections until negative margins, followed by one layer sent as a permanent specimen) may increase sensitivity, especially when operating on a persistent tumor.[82]

Microcystic adnexal carcinoma is thought to be relatively radioresistant, but radiation therapy may be considered when negative margins cannot be obtained.[83]

Chemotherapy has no role in treatment for microcystic adnexal carcinoma.

5.8.5 Prognosis

Local recurrence is common, with up to a 60% recurrence rate with local excision; this is improved to 12% with MMS.[77] Perineural invasion is associated with higher recurrence rates.[80]

Metastases to regional lymph nodes and distant sites are extremely rare. Morbidity is usually due to local effects of the tumor, and mortality is almost always from other causes, with no difference in relative survival when comparing affected patients to those without microcystic adnexal carcinoma.[72]

Lifelong follow-up is a must, as tumors may recur up to 30 years after treatment.[79]

5.8.6 Summary

Microcystic adnexal carcinoma is an adnexal tumor with follicular and sweat gland components. It typically affects older Caucasian patients with a history of sun exposure. It is often misdiagnosed, and an adequate biopsy is required for accurate diagnosis. This tumor is locally aggressive, but usually does not metastasize.

5.9 Atypical Fibroxanthoma

5.9.1 Background

AFX is a rare spindle cell cutaneous malignancy, first described in 1961 by Helwig. It has previously been called many names, including the following: pseudocarcinoma, paradoxical fibrosarcoma, pseudosarcomatous dermatofibroma, and superficial malignant fibrous histiocytoma.[84] It has an intermediate malignancy potential, with a low local recurrence rate and very rare metastases.[84]

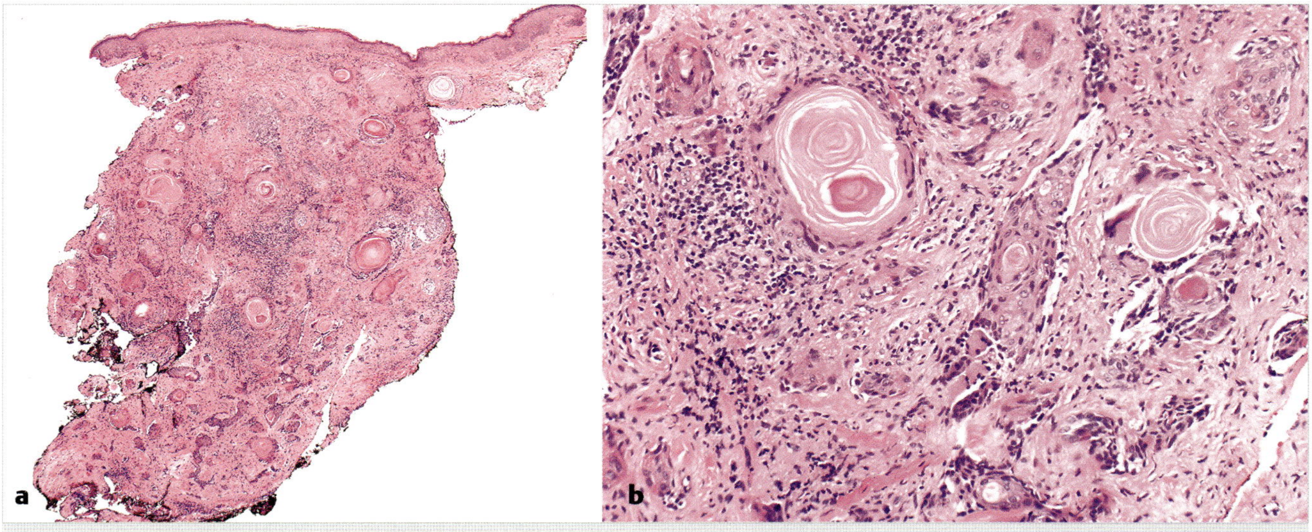

Fig. 5.12 **(a)** Low-power view of microcystic adnexal carcinoma with keratinous cysts present in the superficial dermis. **(b)** Higher-power view of keratinous cysts.

5.9.2 Epidemiology

Atypical fibroxanthoma most commonly affects elderly men, often around the seventh decade of life.[85,86] Caucasians are disproportionately affected, particularly those with excessive UV light exposure and solar elastosis.[85] Prior radiation, trauma, and immunosuppression also seem to infer increased risk[84] (▶ Fig. 5.13).

5.9.3 Diagnosis

The lesion does not have a characteristic appearance. It often appears as a yellow, tan, or erythematous nodule on the scalp, ears, face, or neck.[86,87,88] Less commonly, it may occur on the trunk or extremity. It grows rapidly, and 50% ulcerate as they outgrow their blood supply.[89,90] At the time of diagnosis, it is typically less than 2 cm in diameter[87] (▶ Fig. 5.14).

An incisional or excisional biopsy should be obtained. The diagnosis is one of exclusion. The differential diagnosis includes squamous cell carcinoma, basal cell carcinoma, keratoacanthoma, melanoma, leiomyosarcoma, DFSP, and pyogenic granuloma.

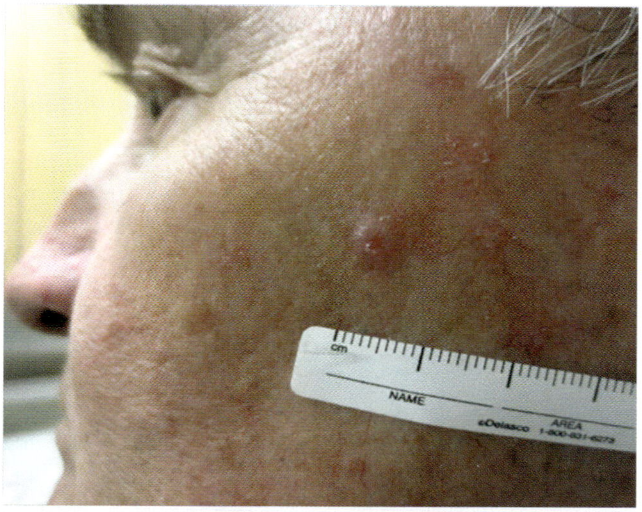

Fig. 5.14 A 79-year-old male with a 6-month history of asymptomatic, growing, pink papule on the L zygomatic cheek. Biopsy showed an atypical fibroxanthoma.

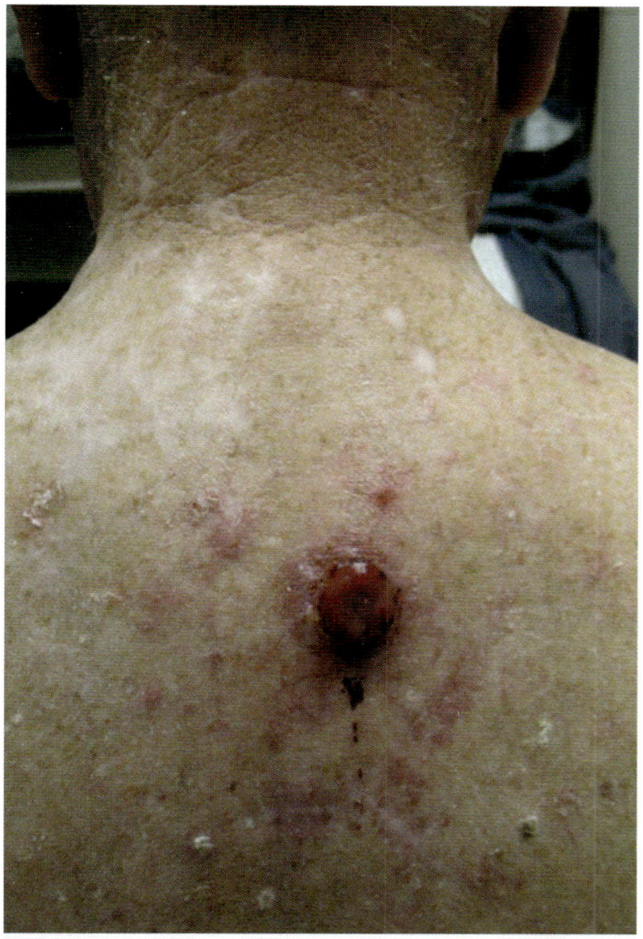

Fig. 5.13 A 68-year-old male with a history of renal transplantation presented with a 4-week history of a rapidly enlarging mass on his back. Biopsy confirmed the diagnosis of atypical fibroxanthoma.

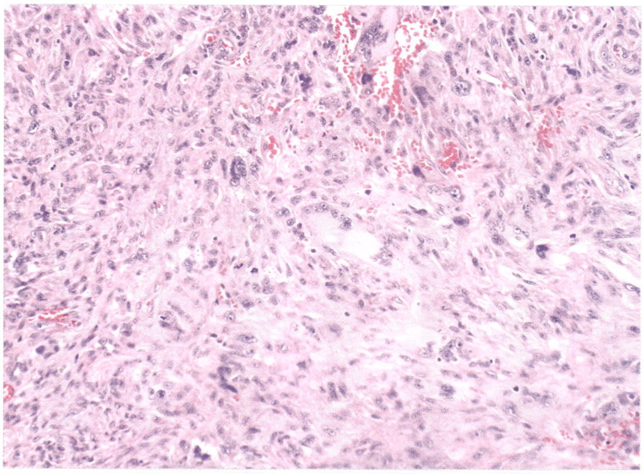

Fig. 5.15 Atypical fibroxanthoma with pleomorphic spindle cells. Bizarre nuclei and mitotic figures are present.

Histology shows a well-circumscribed dermal nodule with limited subcutaneous infiltration. Atypical spindle cells are present with multinucleated giant cells, pleomorphism, and mitoses[85] (▶ Fig. 5.15). Immunohistochemical stains are useful for ruling out other diagnoses. Atypical fibroxanthoma is often positive for vimentin and CD68, and it is negative for S100 and CD34.[90]

5.9.4 Treatment

Treatment consists of complete excision of the tumor, either by wide local excision with 1- to 2-cm margins, including some of the subcutaneous tissue, or by MMS.[88] Excision is typically curative when negative margins are achieved. Radiation therapy may be considered for patients who are not candidates for surgery or for patients with recurrence or metastasis.[84,91]

5.9.5 Prognosis

Prognosis is favorable, with recurrence rates around 8% and metastasis in less than 2%. Local recurrences usually occur less than a year after initial presentation, and more often in patients with positive margins.[86]

5.9.6 Malignant Fibrous Histiocytoma

Malignant fibrous histiocytoma, or undifferentiated pleomorphic sarcoma, is considered to be a deeper and more aggressive variant of atypical fibroxanthoma.[91] It also occurs more commonly in older men, but is found more often on the extremities, and usually within the subfascial or subcutaneous tissue layers.[92] These tumors are similar to atypical fibroxanthoma histologically, with the exception that malignant fibrous histiocytoma extends into the subcutaneous tissue and may have vascular and perineural invasion.[87] Malignant fibrous histiocytoma has high rates of recurrence (30–40%) and distant metastasis (40%).[92] Some authors argue that any case of atypical fibroxanthoma that metastasizes should be reclassified as malignant fibrous histiocytoma.[84,87]

5.9.7 Summary

Atypical fibroxanthoma is a cutaneous malignancy that typically occurs in older men with a history of excessive sun exposure. It is usually cured by a conservative excision with negative margins, with low local recurrence and rare metastasis. Histologically, it is similar to and may be confused with malignant fibrous histiocytoma.

5.10 Spitz Nevus, Atypical Spitzoid Neoplasm, and Spitzoid Melanoma

5.10.1 Background

Sophie Spitz first described the Spitz nevus in 1948, noting it to be benign and naming it "juvenile melanoma."[93] It was later found to exist on a continuum with atypical spitzoid neoplasm (also known as atypical Spitz nevus or atypical Spitz tumor) and spitzoid melanoma, which are proliferations of spindled or epithelioid melanocytes.[94] While these lesions have similar histopathologic characteristics, they clinically range from benign to malignant and therefore must be distinguished. The terminology can be confusing, and proper histological review must be performed to distinguish benign from malignant disease.

5.10.2 Epidemiology

Spitz nevi can present at any age, but they occur most commonly in children and adolescents. They are most often described in Caucasians; however, they can occur in any ethnicity. Lesions occur anywhere, but are most often found on the face and thighs.[94]

In contrast, spitzoid melanomas are more likely to appear in adulthood and do not appear to have a predilection for a specific location.[94]

5.10.3 Diagnosis

Spitz nevus presents as a solitary erythematous, tan, brown, or black macule, nodule, papule, or plaque.[93] The pigmented lesions form a subtype known as pigmented spindle cell Spitz nevi or Reed's nevi, which is the most common variant.[93] Spitz nevus grows rapidly and then remains stable in size, most often less than 6 mm in diameter.[94] Bleeding or pruritus may occur[95] (▶ Fig. 5.16).

Spitzoid melanoma is usually greater than 6 mm at the time of presentation. It also presents as a papule, nodule, or plaque, and may have variable pigmentation or be amelanotic.[94] Unlike Spitz nevus, it may change in appearance after a stable phase.[95]

Atypical spitzoid neoplasms are indistinct neoplasms and may be mistaken clinically for Spitz nevus or spitzoid melanoma.

Clinical features are correlated with histopathology. Even experienced dermatopathologists can have difficulty determining the accurate diagnosis.[95] On histology, Spitz nevus is

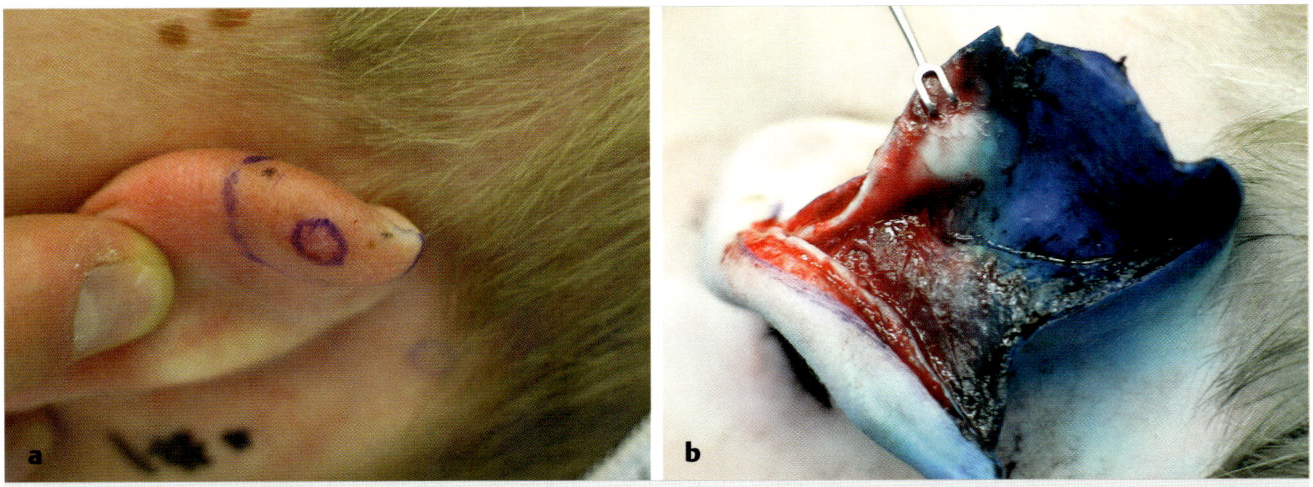

Fig. 5.16 (a) A 14-year-old male with nonhealing tan nodule on his left ear. Biopsy showed an atypical spitz neoplasm with moderate atypia. Fluorescence in situ hybridization (FISH) suggested a malignant tumor and Sentinel lymph node biopsy (SLNB) was recommended. **(b)** The tumor was excised with a 1-cm margin and SLNB was performed. The ear was reconstructed with a helical advancement (Antia) flap.

symmetric, well circumscribed, and has uniform nests and cells that are smaller and deeper in the dermis.[94] It is associated with Kamino bodies, pericellular clefts, and epidermal hyperplasia.[94] It may have mitotic figures; however, usually these are few and superficial.[93]

The histology of spitzoid melanoma is very similar to Spitz nevus, but is more asymmetric and has interruption in circumscription. It usually lacks Kamino bodies and has more frequent and deeper atypical mitotic figures.[94] Ulceration or necrosis may be present.[95]

Atypical spitzoid neoplasm has dense cellularity, cellular atypia, and mitotic figures.[94]

Immunohistochemistry shows expression of S100 protein and Melan-A (MART-1) in Spitz nevi and spitzoid melanomas, and is therefore of limited help.[94] Comparative genomic hybridization and fluorescence in situ hybridization (FISH) may be increasingly helpful in the future; although expensive, they can detect genome alterations present in melanoma[94] (▶ Fig. 5.16).

5.10.4 Treatment and Prognosis

Conservative management for children with lesions that are small and stable and consistent with Spitz nevus is appropriate.[93] For all other cases, excisional biopsy is recommended, taking 5-mm margins if possible.[95] This allows for adequate histological examination.

Sentinel lymph node biopsy (SLNB) is controversial in atypical spitzoid neoplasm and spitzoid melanoma. It is positive in a quarter of patients with atypical spitzoid neoplasm and in one-third with spitzoid melanoma. In children and adolescents with spitzoid melanoma, distant metastases are exceedingly rare. A positive biopsy, then, does not appear to change prognosis. In adults, spitzoid melanoma has a similar prognosis as other malignant melanomas of similar Breslow's depth,[94] and therefore SLNB should be performed.[95] Completion lymph node dissection has not been shown to alter disease-free or overall survival, but may be offered to patients with significant disease burden or atypia found within their sentinel lymph nodes.[95]

Radiation therapy and chemotherapy do not currently have a role in the treatment of spitzoid lesions.

5.10.5 Summary

Spitz nevus is a benign cutaneous proliferation of melanocytes that most often occurs in children and adolescents. It is part of a spectrum that includes atypical spitzoid neoplasm and spitzoid melanoma, which do have malignant potential. These lesions are difficult to distinguish clinically and histologically, and should be excised.

5.11 Websites

5.11.1 Patient Resources

- http://www.skincancer.org
- http://www.mayoclinic.org
- https://www.aad.org/dermatology-a-to-z
- http://www.merkelcell.org

5.11.2 Physician Resources

- http://www.cancer.org/index
- http://www.cancer.gov
- http://www.guideline.gov/index.aspx
- http://www.nccn.org

5.11.3 Acknowledgments

Special thanks to Dr. Jose Plaza for providing histology images.

References

[1] Erovic I, Erovic BM. Merkel cell carcinoma: the past, the present, and the future. J Skin Cancer. 2013; 2013:929364

[2] Agelli M, Clegg LX. Epidemiology of primary Merkel cell carcinoma in the United States. J Am Acad Dermatol. 2003; 49(5):832–841

[3] Senchenkov A, Moran SL. Merkel cell carcinoma: diagnosis, management, and outcomes. Plast Reconstr Surg. 2013; 131(5):771e–778e

[4] Penn I, First MR. Merkel's cell carcinoma in organ recipients: report of 41 cases. Transplantation. 1999; 68(11):1717–1721

[5] Heath M, Jaimes N, Lemos B, et al. Clinical characteristics of Merkel cell carcinoma at diagnosis in 195 patients: the AEIOU features. J Am Acad Dermatol. 2008; 58(3):375–381

[6] Asgari MM, Sokil MM, Warton EM, Iyer J, Paulson KG, Nghiem P. Effect of host, tumor, diagnostic, and treatment variables on outcomes in a large cohort with Merkel cell carcinoma. JAMA Dermatol. 2014; 150(7):716–723

[7] Tarantola TI, Vallow LA, Halyard MY, et al. Prognostic factors in Merkel cell carcinoma: analysis of 240 cases. J Am Acad Dermatol. 2013; 68(3):425–432

[8] Bobos M, Hytiroglou P, Kostopoulos I, Karkavelas G, Papadimitriou CS. Immunohistochemical distinction between merkel cell carcinoma and small cell carcinoma of the lung. Am J Dermatopathol. 2006; 28(2):99–104

[9] National Comprehensive Cancer Network. NCCN Clinical Practice Guidelines in Oncology (Version 1.2014): Merkel Cell Carcinoma. Fort Washington, PA: National Comprehensive Cancer Network; 2013

[10] Chen KT, Papavasiliou P, Edwards K, et al. A better prognosis for Merkel cell carcinoma of unknown primary origin. Am J Surg. 2013; 206(5):752–757

[11] Lemos BD, Storer BE, Iyer JG, et al. Pathologic nodal evaluation improves prognostic accuracy in Merkel cell carcinoma: analysis of 5823 cases as the basis of the first consensus staging system. J Am Acad Dermatol. 2010; 63(5):751–761

[12] Allen PJ, Bowne WB, Jaques DP, Brennan MF, Busam K, Coit DG. Merkel cell carcinoma: prognosis and treatment of patients from a single institution. J Clin Oncol. 2005; 23(10):2300–2309

[13] Siva S, Byrne K, Seel M, et al. 18F-FDG PET provides high-impact and powerful prognostic stratification in the staging of Merkel cell carcinoma: a 15-year institutional experience. J Nucl Med. 2013; 54(8):1223–1229

[14] Feng H, Shuda M, Chang Y, Moore PS. Clonal integration of a polyomavirus in human Merkel cell carcinoma. Science. 2008; 319(5866):1096–1100

[15] Amber K, McLeod MP, Nouri K. The Merkel cell polyomavirus and its involvement in Merkel cell carcinoma. Dermatol Surg. 2013; 39(2):232–238

[16] Faust H, Andersson K, Ekström J, Hortlund M, Robsahm TE, Dillner J. Prospective study of Merkel cell polyomavirus and risk of Merkel cell carcinoma. Int J Cancer. 2014; 134(4):844–848

[17] American Joint Committee on Cancer. Merkel cell carcinoma. In: Edge SB, Carducci M, Byrd DR, eds. AJCC Cancer Staging Manual, 7th ed. New York: Springer-Verlag; 2009

[18] Fritsch VA, Camp ER, Lentsch EJ. Sentinel lymph node status in Merkel cell carcinoma of the head and neck: not a predictor of survival. Head Neck. 2014; 36(4):571–579

[19] Tseng J, Dhungel B, Mills JK, et al. Merkel cell carcinoma: what makes a difference? Am J Surg. 2015; 209(2):342–346

[20] Willmes C, Adam C, Alb M, et al. Type I and II IFNs inhibit Merkel cell carcinoma via modulation of the Merkel cell polyomavirus T antigens. Cancer Res. 2012; 72(8):2120–2128

[21] Kang SH, Haydu LE, Goh RYH, Fogarty GB. Radiotherapy is associated with significant improvement in local and regional control in Merkel cell carcinoma. Radiat Oncol. 2012; 7:171

[22] Lewis KG, Weinstock MA, Weaver AL, Otley CC. Adjuvant local irradiation for Merkel cell carcinoma. Arch Dermatol. 2006; 142(6):693–700
[23] Kim JA, Choi AH. Effect of radiation therapy on survival in patients with resected Merkel cell carcinoma: a propensity score surveillance, epidemiology, and end results database analysis. JAMA Dermatol. 2013; 149 (7):831–838
[24] Terheyden P, Becker JC. New developments in the biology and the treatment of metastatic Merkel cell carcinoma. Curr Opin Oncol. 2017; 29:221-226
[25] Soltani AM, Allan BJ, Best MJ, Panthaki ZJ, Thaller SR. Merkel cell carcinoma of the hand and upper extremity: current trends and outcomes. J Plast Reconstr Aesthet Surg. 2014; 67(3):e71–e77
[26] Sattler E, Geimer T, Sick I, et al. Sentinel lymph node in Merkel cell carcinoma: to biopsy or not to biopsy? J Dermatol. 2013; 40(5):374–379
[27] Johnson-Jahangir H, Ratner D. Advances in management of dermatofibrosarcoma protuberans. Dermatol Clin. 2011; 29(2):191–200, viii
[28] Bogucki B, Neuhaus I, Hurst EA. Dermatofibrosarcoma protuberans: a review of the literature. Dermatol Surg. 2012; 38(4):537–551
[29] Criscione VD, Weinstock MA. Descriptive epidemiology of dermatofibrosarcoma protuberans in the United States, 1973 to 2002. J Am Acad Dermatol. 2007; 56(6):968–973
[30] Tsai YJ, Lin PY, Chew KY, Chiang YC. Dermatofibrosarcoma protuberans in children and adolescents: clinical presentation, histology, treatment, and review of the literature. J Plast Reconstr Aesthet Surg. 2014; 67(9):1222–1229
[31] Loghdey MS, Varma S, Rajpara SM, Al-Rawi H, Perks G, Perkins W. Mohs micrographic surgery for dermatofibrosarcoma protuberans (DFSP): a single-centre series of 76 patients treated by frozen-section Mohs micrographic surgery with a review of the literature. J Plast Reconstr Aesthet Surg. 2014; 67 (10):1315–1321
[32] Kornik RI, Muchard LK, Teng JM. Dermatofibrosarcoma protuberans in children: an update on the diagnosis and treatment. Pediatr Dermatol. 2012; 29 (6):707–713
[33] Serra-Guillén C, Sanmartín O, Llombart B, et al. Correlation between preoperative magnetic resonance imaging and surgical margins with modified Mohs for dermatofibrosarcoma protuberans. Dermatol Surg. 2011; 37(11):1638–1645
[34] Miller SJ, Alam M, Andersen JS, et al. National Comprehensive Cancer Network. Dermatofibrosarcoma protuberans. J Natl Compr Canc Netw. 2012; 10 (3):312–318
[35] Liang CA, Jambusaria-Pahlajani A, Karia PS, Elenitsas R, Zhang PD, Schmults CD. A systematic review of outcome data for dermatofibrosarcoma protuberans with and without fibrosarcomatous change. J Am Acad Dermatol. 2014; 71(4):781–786
[36] Simon MP, Pedeutour F, Sirvent N, et al. Deregulation of the platelet-derived growth factor B-chain gene via fusion with collagen gene COL1A1 in dermatofibrosarcoma protuberans and giant-cell fibroblastoma. Nat Genet. 1997; 15(1):95–98
[37] Ratner D, Thomas CO, Johnson TM, et al. Mohs micrographic surgery for the treatment of dermatofibrosarcoma protuberans. Results of a multiinstitutional series with an analysis of the extent of microscopic spread. J Am Acad Dermatol. 1997; 37(4):600–613
[38] Farma JM, Ammori JB, Zager JS, et al. Dermatofibrosarcoma protuberans: how wide should we resect? Ann Surg Oncol. 2010; 17(8):2112–2118
[39] Goldberg C, Hoang D, McRae M, Chung C, Leffell DJ, Narayan D. A strategy for the successful management of dermatofibrosarcoma protuberans. Ann Plast Surg. 2015; 74(1):80–84
[40] Foroozan M, Sei JF, Amini M, Beauchet A, Saiag P. Efficacy of Mohs micrographic surgery for the treatment of dermatofibrosarcoma protuberans: systematic review. Arch Dermatol. 2012; 148(9):1055–1063
[41] Fields RC, Hameed M, Qin LX, et al. Dermatofibrosarcoma protuberans (DFSP): predictors of recurrence and the use of systemic therapy. Ann Surg Oncol. 2011; 18(2):328–336
[42] Ugurel S, Mentzel T, Utikal J, et al. Neoadjuvant imatinib in advanced primary or locally recurrent dermatofibrosarcoma protuberans: a multicenter phase II DeCOG trial with long-term follow-up. Clin Cancer Res. 2014; 20(2):499–510
[43] Kurlander DE, Martires KJ, Chen Y, Barnholtz-Sloan JS, Bordeaux JS. Risk of subsequent primary malignancies after dermatofibrosarcoma protuberans diagnosis: a national study. J Am Acad Dermatol. 2013; 68(5):790–796
[44] Perez MC, Padhya TA, Messina JL, et al. Cutaneous angiosarcoma: a single-institution experience. Ann Surg Oncol. 2013; 20(11):3391–3397
[45] Albores-Saavedra J, Schwartz AM, Henson DE, et al. Cutaneous angiosarcoma. Analysis of 434 cases from the Surveillance, Epidemiology, and End Results Program, 1973–2007. Ann Diagn Pathol. 2011; 15(2):93–97
[46] Mendenhall WM, Mendenhall CM, Werning JW, Reith JD, Mendenhall NP. Cutaneous angiosarcoma. Am J Clin Oncol. 2006; 29(5):524–528
[47] Donghi D, Kerl K, Dummer R, Schoenewolf N, Cozzio A. Cutaneous angiosarcoma: own experience over 13 years. Clinical features, disease course and immunohistochemical profile. J Eur Acad Dermatol Venereol. 2010; 24 (10):1230–1234
[48] Morgan MB, Swann M, Somach S, Eng W, Smoller B. Cutaneous angiosarcoma: a case series with prognostic correlation. J Am Acad Dermatol. 2004; 50(6):867–874
[49] Köhler HF, Neves RI, Brechtbühl ER, Mattos Granja NV, Ikeda MK, Kowalski LP. Cutaneous angiosarcoma of the head and neck: report of 23 cases from a single institution. Otolaryngol Head Neck Surg. 2008; 139(4):519–524
[50] Buehler D, Rice SR, Moody JS, et al. Angiosarcoma outcomes and prognostic factors: a 25-year single institution experience. Am J Clin Oncol. 2014; 37 (5):473–479
[51] Deyrup AT, Miettinen M, North PE, et al. Pediatric cutaneous angiosarcomas: a clinicopathologic study of 10 cases. Am J Surg Pathol. 2011; 35(1):70–75
[52] Rao J, Dekoven JG, Beatty JD, Jones G. Cutaneous angiosarcoma as a delayed complication of radiation therapy for carcinoma of the breast. J Am Acad Dermatol. 2003; 49(3):532–538
[53] Mobini N. Cutaneous epithelioid angiosarcoma: a neoplasm with potential pitfalls in diagnosis. J Cutan Pathol. 2009; 36(3):362–369
[54] Wood A, Mentzel T, van Gorp J, et al. The spectrum of rare morphological variants of cutaneous epithelioid angiosarcoma. Histopathology. 2015; 66 (6):856–863
[55] Rubin E, Maddox WA, Mazur MT. Cutaneous angiosarcoma of the breast 7 years after lumpectomy and radiation therapy. Radiology. 1990; 174 (1):258–260
[56] Sharma A, Schwartz RA. Stewart-Treves syndrome: pathogenesis and management. J Am Acad Dermatol. 2012; 67(6):1342–1348
[57] Kraft S, Fletcher CDM. Atypical intradermal smooth muscle neoplasms: clinicopathologic analysis of 84 cases and a reappraisal of cutaneous "leiomyosarcoma". Am J Surg Pathol. 2011; 35(4):599–607
[58] Fields JP, Helwig EB. Leiomyosarcoma of the skin and subcutaneous tissue. Cancer. 1981; 47(1):156–169
[59] Massi D, Franchi A, Alos L, et al. Primary cutaneous leiomyosarcoma: clinicopathological analysis of 36 cases. Histopathology. 2010; 56(2):251–262
[60] Bellezza G, Sidoni A, Cavaliere A, Scheibel M, Bucciarelli E. Primary cutaneous leiomyosarcoma: a clinicopathological and immunohistochemical study of 7 cases. Int J Surg Pathol. 2004; 12(1):39–44
[61] Tsutsumida A, Yoshida T, Yamamoto Y, Itoh T, Minakawa H, Sugihara T. Management of superficial leiomyosarcoma: a retrospective study of 10 cases. Plast Reconstr Surg. 2005; 116(1):8–12
[62] Starling J, III, Coldiron BM. Mohs micrographic surgery for the treatment of cutaneous leiomyosarcoma. J Am Acad Dermatol. 2011; 64(6):1119–1122
[63] Rouhani P, Fletcher CDM, Devesa SS, Toro JR. Cutaneous soft tissue sarcoma incidence patterns in the U.S.: an analysis of 12,114 cases. Cancer. 2008; 113 (3):616–627
[64] Naylor E, Sarkar P, Perlis CS, Giri D, Gnepp DR, Robinson-Bostom L. Primary cutaneous adenoid cystic carcinoma. J Am Acad Dermatol. 2008; 58 (4):636–641
[65] Dores GM, Huycke MM, Devesa SS, Garcia CA. Primary cutaneous adenoid cystic carcinoma in the United States: incidence, survival, and associated cancers, 1976 to 2005. J Am Acad Dermatol. 2010; 63(1):71–78
[66] Ramakrishnan R, Chaudhry IH, Ramdial P, et al. Primary cutaneous adenoid cystic carcinoma: a clinicopathologic and immunohistochemical study of 27 cases. Am J Surg Pathol. 2013; 37(10):1603–1611
[67] Xu YG, Hinshaw M, Longley BJ, Ilyas H, Snow SN. Cutaneous adenoid cystic carcinoma with perineural invasion treated by Mohs micrographic surgery-a case report with literature review. J Oncol. 2010; 2010:469049
[68] Kyllo RL, Brady KL, Hurst EA. Sebaceous carcinoma: review of the literature. Dermatol Surg. 2015; 41(1):1–15
[69] Thomas WW, Fritsch VA, Lentsch EJ. Population-based analysis of prognostic indicators in sebaceous carcinoma of the head and neck. Laryngoscope. 2013; 123(9):2165–2169
[70] Hou JL, Killian JM, Baum CL, et al. Characteristics of sebaceous carcinoma and early outcomes of treatment using Mohs micrographic surgery versus wide local excision: an update of the Mayo Clinic experience over the past 2 decades. Dermatol Surg. 2014; 40(3):241–246
[71] Ongenae KC, Verhaegh MEJM, Vermeulen AHM, Naeyaert JM. Microcystic adnexal carcinoma: an uncommon tumor with debatable origin. Dermatol Surg. 2001; 27(11):979–984

[72] Yu JB, Blitzblau RC, Patel SC, Decker RH, Wilson LD. Surveillance, Epidemiology, and End Results (SEER) database analysis of microcystic adnexal carcinoma (sclerosing sweat duct carcinoma) of the skin. Am J Clin Oncol. 2010; 33(2):125–127

[73] Smart DR, Taintor AR, Kelly ME, et al. Microcystic adnexal carcinoma: the first reported congenital case. Pediatr Dermatol. 2011; 28(1):35–38

[74] Chiller K, Passaro D, Scheuller M, Singer M, McCalmont T, Grekin RC. Microcystic adnexal carcinoma: forty-eight cases, their treatment, and their outcome. Arch Dermatol. 2000; 136(11):1355–1359

[75] Snow S, Madjar DD, Hardy S, et al. Microcystic adnexal carcinoma: report of 13 cases and review of the literature. Dermatol Surg. 2001; 27(4):401–408

[76] LeBoit PE, Sexton M. Microcystic adnexal carcinoma of the skin. A reappraisal of the differentiation and differential diagnosis of an underrecognized neoplasm. J Am Acad Dermatol. 1993; 29(4):609–618

[77] Yu Y, Finn DT, Rogers GS. Microcystic adnexal carcinoma: a rare, locally aggressive cutaneous tumor. Am J Clin Oncol. 2010; 33(2):196–197

[78] Hoang MP, Dresser KA, Kapur P, High WA, Mahalingam M. Microcystic adnexal carcinoma: an immunohistochemical reappraisal. Mod Pathol. 2008; 21(2):178–185

[79] Diamantis SA, Marks VJ. Mohs micrographic surgery in the treatment of microcystic adnexal carcinoma. Dermatol Clin. 2011; 29(2):185–190, viii

[80] Leibovitch I, Huilgol SC, Selva D, Lun K, Richards S, Paver R. Microcystic adnexal carcinoma: treatment with Mohs micrographic surgery. J Am Acad Dermatol. 2005; 52(2):295–300

[81] Wetter R, Goldstein GD. Microcystic adnexal carcinoma: a diagnostic and therapeutic challenge. Dermatol Ther (Heidelb). 2008; 21(6):452–458

[82] Palamaras I, McKenna JD, Robson A, Barlow RJ. Microcystic adnexal carcinoma: a case series treated with Mohs micrographic surgery and identification of patients in whom paraffin sections may be preferable. Dermatol Surg. 2010; 36(4):446–452

[83] Pugh TJ, Lee NY, Pacheco T, Raben D. Microcystic adnexal carcinoma of the face treated with radiation therapy: a case report and review of the literature. Head Neck. 2012; 34(7):1045–1050

[84] Iorizzo LJ, III, Brown MD. Atypical fibroxanthoma: a review of the literature. Dermatol Surg. 2011; 37(2):146–157

[85] Beer TW, Drury P, Heenan PJ. Atypical fibroxanthoma: a histological and immunohistochemical review of 171 cases. Am J Dermatopathol. 2010; 32 (6):533–540

[86] Davidson JS, Demsey D. Atypical fibroxanthoma: clinicopathologic determinants for recurrence and implications for surgical management. J Surg Oncol. 2012; 105(6):559–562

[87] Gru AA, Santa Cruz DJ. Atypical fibroxanthoma: a selective review. Semin Diagn Pathol. 2013; 30(1):4–12

[88] Sakamoto A. Atypical fibroxanthoma. Clin Med Oncol. 2008; 2:117–127

[89] Mirza B, Weedon D. Atypical fibroxanthoma: a clinicopathological study of 89 cases. Australas J Dermatol. 2005; 46(4):235–238

[90] Singh M, Mann R, Ilankovan V, Hussein K, D'arrigo C. Atypical fibroxanthoma–a retrospective immunohistochemical study of 42 cases. J Oral Maxillofac Surg. 2012; 70(11):2713–2718

[91] Withers AHJ, Brougham NDL, Barber RM, Tan ST. Atypical fibroxanthoma and malignant fibrous histiocytoma. J Plast Reconstr Aesthet Surg. 2011; 64(11): e273–e278

[92] Marcet S. Atypical fibroxanthoma/malignant fibrous histiocytoma. Dermatol Ther (Heidelb). 2008; 21(6):424–427

[93] Ferrara G, Gianotti R, Cavicchini S, Salviato T, Zalaudek I, Argenziano G. Spitz nevus, Spitz tumor, and spitzoid melanoma: a comprehensive clinicopathologic overview. Dermatol Clin. 2013; 31(4):589–598, viii

[94] Zedek DC, McCalmont TH. Spitz nevi, atypical spitzoid neoplasms, and spitzoid melanoma. Clin Lab Med. 2011; 31(2):311–320

[95] Joyce DP, Prichard RS, Gulmann C, Hill ADK. The surgical management of Spitz naevi and atypical spitzoid neoplasms: a review of the literature. Surgeon. 2013; 11(4):205–209

6 Mohs Micrographic Surgery's Role in the Treatment of Skin Cancer

Charlene Lam, Christine Poblete-Lopez, and Elizabeth M. Billingsley

6.1 Introduction

Mohs micrographic surgery (MMS) is a specialized skin cancer excision technique that combines surgery with pathology. It is most commonly performed under local anesthesia in an outpatient setting and offers the advantages of higher cure rates for cutaneous tumors (▶ Table 6.1) along with maximal tissue preservation. Conceptualized by general surgeon, Dr. Frederic E. Mohs, the method is based on the theory that a tumor arises from a single focus and has contiguous spread. By utilizing fresh frozen tissue processing and horizontal sectioning techniques, the Mohs surgeon excises the tumor and examines 100% of the microscopic tissue margin. The complete surgical margin examination in MMS provides the highest, evidence-based cure rate for cutaneous malignancies, while conserving the maximum amount of normal tissue (tissue-sparing). From a functional, aesthetic, and reconstructive perspective, tissue-sparing is especially important for skin cancers near the orbit, nose, lips, ears, anogenital region, and digits (▶ Fig. 6.1a, b). The proven higher cure rate provided by MMS is especially valuable for recurrent tumors and those with more aggressive histologic features and subclinical extension (see list below).

Advantages of Mohs micrographic surgery:

- Tissue sparing.
- Superior cure rates.
- 100% margin examination.
- Continuity of care: surgeon and pathologist.
- Outpatient.
- Local anesthesia.
- Closure after histologic confirmation of clear margins.
- Cost-effective.

Table 6.1 Cure rates for skin cancers depending on treatment modalities

Method	Tumor type		
	BCC[1]	SCC[1]	MIS[2]
	5 y (%)		3–5 y (%)
Mohs surgery	99	96.9	92.7–100
Surgical excision	91–95	91.9	80–94
Cryotherapy	92.5	NA	66–93
Electrodessication and curettage	74–92	96.3	NA
Radiotherapy	89–96.1	90	81–100
Imiquimod[3]	69[4]	71[5,a]	56–100[6,7]
5-Fluoruracil[3]	NA	85[8,b]	NA

Abbreviations: BCC, basal cell carcinoma; MIS, melanoma in situ; SCC, squamous cell carcinoma.

[a]Invasive SCC and follow-up period was 28 months.

[b]Squamous cell carcinoma in situ (SCCIS) with mean follow-up of 4.6 years.

Skin cancer is the most common cancer. Of the nonmelanoma skin cancers (NMSCs), 95% are basal cell carcinomas (BCCs) and squamous cell carcinomas (SCCs). MMS has an evidence-based, 5-year cure rate of 99% for BCC[9,10] and 94% for cutaneous SCC (▶ Table 6.1).[1,11] MMS is also the preferred treatment method for skin cancers that are clinically poorly defined, recurrent, and/or have a higher risk of recurrence because of higher-risk histologic features, or specific anatomic location (▶ Fig. 6.2a,b).

The mounting evidence of the benefits of MMS provides patients with quality, evidence-based care (see list above). However, MMS is one treatment modality in the large armamentarium of a cutaneous surgical oncologist. It is important to understand the advantages and disadvantages of multiple techniques including standard excision, MMS, radiotherapy, chemotherapy, and oral hedgehog pathway inhibitors. The objective of this chapter is to familiarize one with the MMS technique, illustrate histologic examination of the surgical margins in MMS, and discuss variations as well as tactics to allow integration in a multidisciplinary setting.

6.2 Training

Mohs surgery training can be obtained through an Accreditation Council for Graduate Medical Education (ACGME) approved fellowship,[12] which has been renamed "micrographic surgery and dermatologic oncology" in September 2014. These fellowship-trained Mohs surgeons undergo 1 to 2 years of additional training after a 4-year dermatology residency. The fellowship involves gaining proficiency in cutaneous oncology, tumor resection with orientation on maps, tissue preparation, dermatopathology and histologic interpretation on frozen sections, and wound reconstruction. Dermatology residency, as a prerequisite, establishes a substantial clinical, surgical, and pathologic foundation for fellows to achieve expertise in clinicopathologic correlation. The dermatologic surgeon must also develop a mastery of frozen section histology interpretation, cutaneous and soft tissue anatomy, and advanced facial reconstruction.

6.3 Surgical Margins: Tissue Processing Techniques

Central to surgical treatment of cutaneous neoplasms is the concept of surgical margins. It is crucial for the surgeon to be familiar with histologic grossing techniques and their

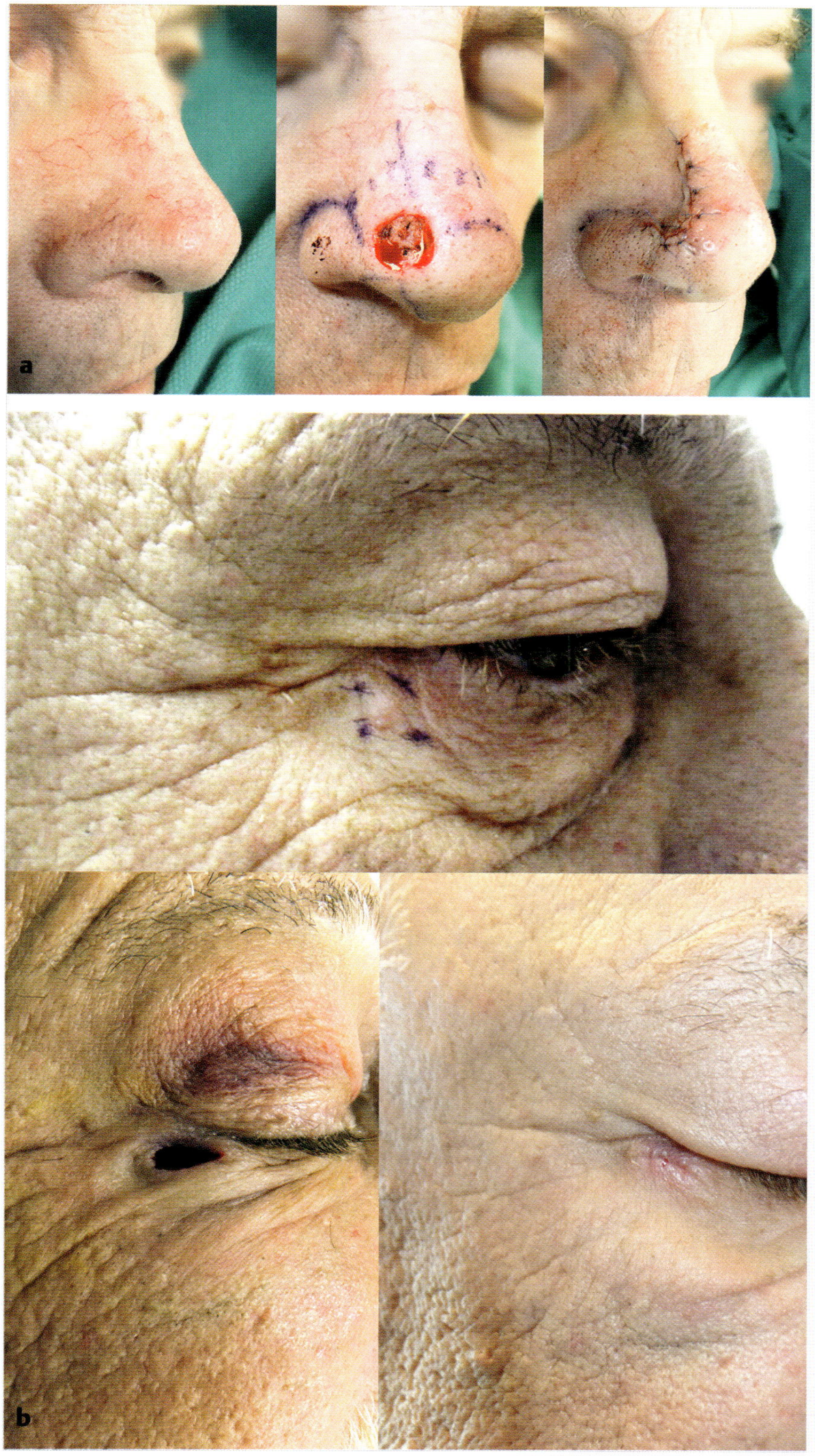

Fig. 6.1 (a, b) Examples of tissue sparing potential of Mohs micrographic surgery while achieving clear margins.

implications. The final histologic reading of a surgical margin is only as informative as the method in which tumor tissue is processed and what is actually examined. Developing a false sense of security regarding negative margins may result in unexpected tumor recurrence. Strong communication between the surgeon and the pathologist is critical given there may be subjectivity and inconsistencies in the histologic interpretation of surgical margins. A clinical margin is defined as the clinically apparent edge of the tumor, while a surgical margin refers to the specific measurement of the tissue surrounding the

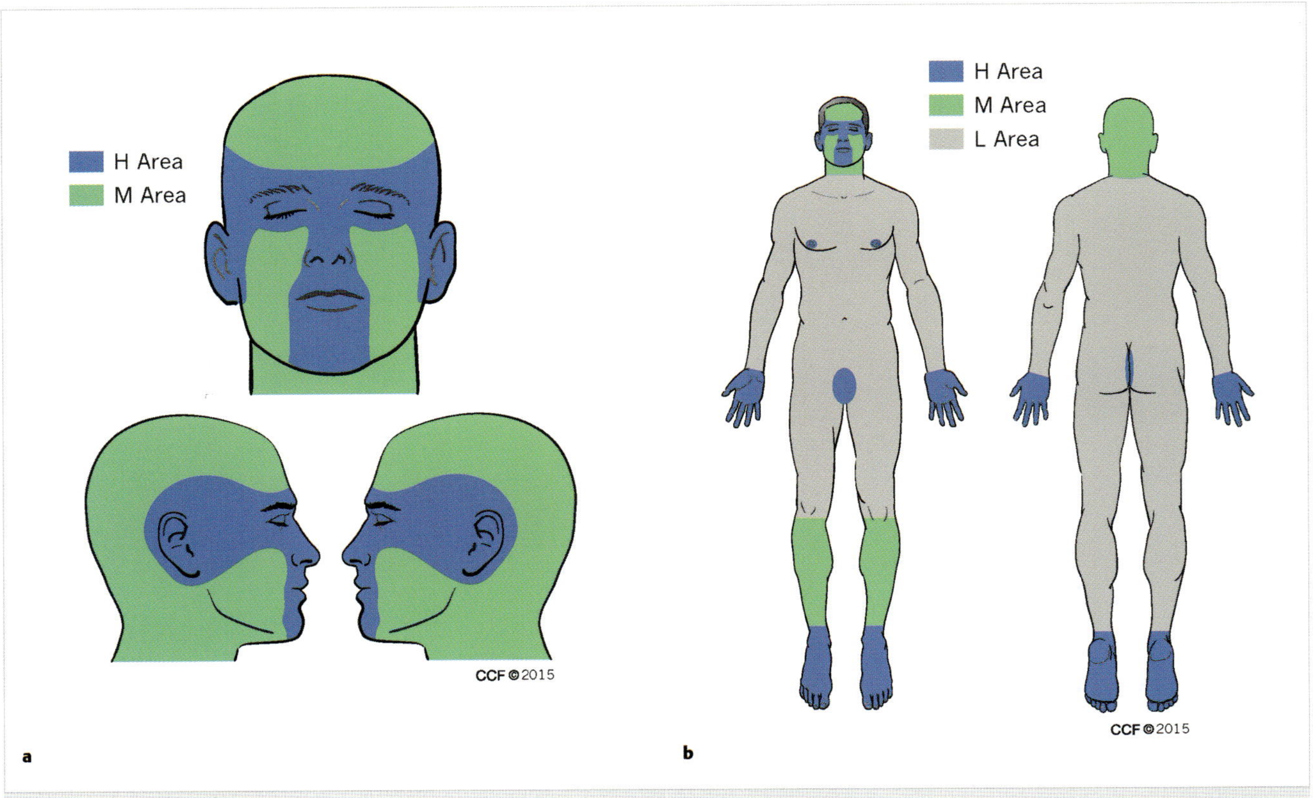

Fig. 6.2 Areas of the body divided according to risk. **(a)** Head and neck divided into H Area (central face, eyelids, eyebrows, nose, chin, ear, periauricular skin/sulci, and temple) and M Area (cheeks, forehead, scalp, and jawline). **(b)** Full body divided into H Area (genitalia, hands, feet, nail units, ankles, and areola), M Area (pretibial surface), and L Area (trunk and extremities). Reprinted with permission from CCF.

clinically evident tumor.[13] The term "close to the margin" illustrates the existing ambiguity. In a survey of pathologists, the definition of "close" surgical margins varied from tumor involvement of within a few cells to 0.1 to 5 mm adjacent to the tumor edge. In these cases of "close" surgical margins, SCCs were re-excised, while BCCs were not.[14] Surgeons need to be aware of pathologists' interpretation of margins because it will affect the need for subsequent surgical therapy or adjunctive therapy. Furthermore, regardless of the surgical technique, without clear understanding of how the tissue is processed, the final reading of clear margins is limited by the processing technique.

A thorough discussion regarding laboratory techniques is discussed in Chapter 11. The focus here will be on the comparison between the most commonly used histological grossing method, vertical (perpendicular/bread loafing), and horizontal (Mohs) sectioning.

6.3.1 Vertical (Bread Loafing) Sectioning

The routinely utilized technique to process excision specimens involves transverse, vertical sections often compared to slices in a loaf of bread ("bread loafing"). This technique allows great visualization of both the tumor and the margins of each examined section. Its limitation is only a small percentage of the true surgical margin is viewed with this sectioning technique (► Fig. 6.3). The specimen is typically placed in formalin, divided into 2 to 3 mm in width sections, placed in numbered cassettes and embedded in paraffin (formalin-fixed, paraffin-embedded [FFPE]). Within each section, a sample of tissue is sliced with the knife perpendicular to the epidermis and cut down to the base. Step sectioning cuts tissue at specified intervals, which can allow a faster view of different levels but can result in skip areas, while serial sectioning completely processes the specimen with unbroken sequence. With vertical sections, it is estimated that approximately 1% of the true surgical margin is evaluated. In theory, serial vertical sectioning could be done in a fashion that 100% of the margin is evaluated. This would be highly impractical, requiring sectioning and examination of hundreds of slices, and is not normally done in practice.[15] For example, 1 cm of tumor would produce 2,000 5-µm sections. One study demonstrated that vertical sectioning is about 44% sensitive for distinguishing residual facial BCC at the surgical margin excised with a 2-mm margins.[16]

It is important to note that many laboratories are willing to cut more sections at narrower intervals to gain more precise important diagnostic information on specimens when indicated. Good communication is key and may require discussion with the dermatopathologist prior to grossing of the specimen. Of note, the actual grossing of the specimen may not actually be done by the dermatopathologist but may be done by a technician or resident.[15]

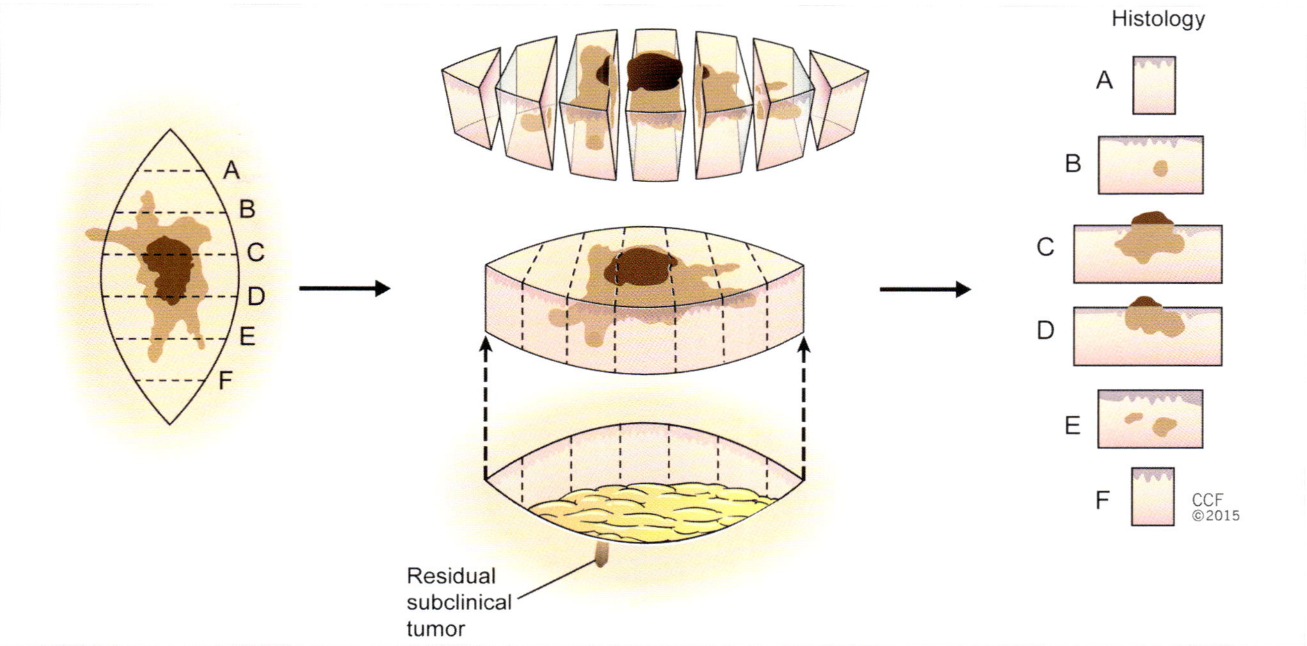

Fig. 6.3 Surgical elliptical excision of tumor and pathologic examination of tissue margins with vertical sectioning ("bread loafing"). Serial transverse cross-sectioning is utilized to section the specimen at specified intervals and embedded in paraffin. The cross-sections are cut and stained. This method can miss tumor at the surgical margin. The horizontal parallel lines indicate where transverse sections would be cut. There is tumor at the incision line that is not transected by the cross-section cuts; therefore, the tumor would be histologically missed. Reprinted with permission from CCF.

6.3.2 Horizontal (Mohs) Sectioning

With the Mohs processing technique, 100% of the deep and peripheral margins are evaluated (▶ Fig. 6.4). Tissue is excised with a surgical bevel of approximately 45 degrees. After the layer is removed and inked, the epidermal edge is pressed down to be in the same plane as the deep margin. The tissue is embedded in mounting medium (optimum cutting temperature [OCT] compound) and frozen. This frozen tissue block is sectioned in a horizontal fashion so that the knife is parallel to the deep margin of the subcutaneous tissue and the newly pressed epidermis. This bottom-up approach represents the true deep and peripheral surgical margin. Therefore, the specimen represents the entire deep and peripheral margin in one plane. Some critics argue that no tissue processing technique including Mohs consistently examines 100% of the margin due to incomplete sections, fragmented tissue, or orientation problems.[15] However, with Mohs sectioning, at least 95 to 99% of the margin can be evaluated, which is far more precise than the 1% margin examined in the vertical sectioning.[17,18] This complete margin examination is the basis for the maximal normal tissue preservation and higher cure rate for challenging tumors.

Tumors may have contiguous but asymmetric growth patterns and margins may be difficult to predict. The surgical margin is determined by the clinical margin, and with asymmetrical and infiltrative growth patterns, some tumors may extend histologically beyond the clinically evident margins. With standard vertical sectioning technique, areas of asymmetric infiltrative tumor growth may be missed (▶ Fig. 6.3).

Another advantage of MMS is the same physician serves as the pathologist and surgeon. The physician is in control of the specimen and is directly involved in sectioning and inking, and may assist in the grossing of the specimen. The Mohs surgeon is able to appreciate the histology during the procedure, which can be overlooked with the sampling errors in biopsies. For example, a biopsy of a tumor may reveal nodular BCC, but with the Mohs processing, it is common to discover that the tumor is actually an infiltrative BCC with further histologic extension than originally predicted. Mohs surgeons can correlate the clinical appearance of the tumor and note any discordance between the diagnosis of the biopsy sample and the tumor seen under frozen sections. Certain staging criteria like perineural invasion can also be appreciated during MMS, and adjunctive treatment can be recommended.

6.4 Indications and Contraindications for Mohs Micrographic Surgery

Currently, approximately 25% of skin cancers are treated with MMS.[19] MMS is ideally suited for skin cancers at high risk of recurrence, those located in regions requiring tissue conservation, and/or when complete margin control is necessary. Many NMSCs have aggressive local growth patterns and can invade vital structures such as the eye, nose, lips, and ears, leading to significant destruction and impairment. With time and neglect, metastasis may develop in more aggressive tumors. Fortunately,

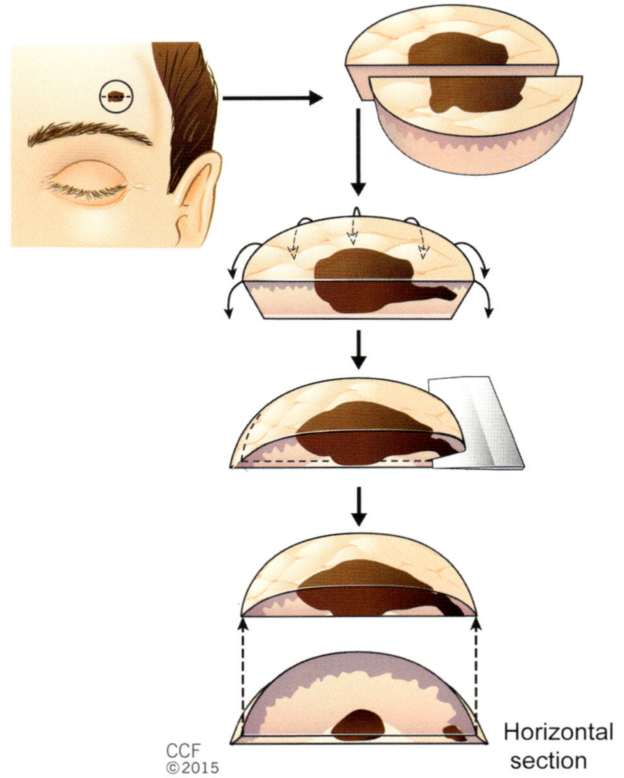

Fig. 6.4 Mohs layer excision with narrow margin and subsequent flattening of skin edges. The tissue is horizontally sectioned so the skin edge (epidermis) is in the same plane as the deep margin, thus ensuring complete lateral and deep margin assessment. As 100% of the margin is examined, there is no concern that tumor may be missed with serial sectioning. Reprinted with permission from CCF.

many of the NMSC are low risk and can be treated with superficial ablative techniques (e.g., electrodesiccation and curettage) with comparable cure rates and cost-effectiveness (see Section 6.4.3 Cost-Effective Care). Cutaneous tumors that can be treated with MMS are listed in ▶ Table 6.2. The indications for MMS are not absolute, and any treatment decision needs to be made in collaboration with the patient's preferences, performance status, and understanding of other available treatment options and cure rates (▶ Table 6.1).

The definition of "high-risk" skin cancer is dependent on multiple factors: clinical and histologic characteristics of the tumor, the anatomic site, and history of prior treatments (see text box). MMS has the ability to track unpredictable superficial or deep projections of tumor with the meticulous and complete histologic examination of the surgical margins. Additionally, tumors that involve embryonic fusion planes, periorbital, nerves, and bone can be followed with MMS. In these situations, the adeptness of this technique is most evident as deep and irregular tumor extensions are responsible for the higher recurrence rates with other techniques. With recurrent tumors, it is especially difficult to achieve clear margins with recommended margins, given that the subclinical extension is often prominent and clinically it is difficult to delineate the tumor from scar. MMS has a superior cute rate for recurrent tumors (▶ Table 6.2). The dilemma to clear the tumor with larger surgical margin resulting in a larger surgical defect and possible less aesthetic outcome and reduced functionality versus a more conservative margin with the possibility of positive margins and another surgery is a constant challenge for those treating facial tumors.[37]

Table 6.2 Cutaneous tumors treated with Mohs surgery and reported cure rates

Cutaneous tumors treated with Mohs surgery and reported cure rates		
Cutaneous tumors	Cure rates	
	5 y	10 y
Basal cell carcinoma • Primary • Recurrent	 • 99%[9] • 93%[10]	 • 95.6%[20] • 96.1%[20]
Squamous cell carcinoma • Primary • Recurrent • Erythroplasia of Queyrat • Keratoacanthoma	 • 92–99%[11] • 90%[1] • 90%[21] • 97.5%[22] (2 y)	
Melanoma in situ, including lentigo maligna	92.7–100%[23,24,25]	
Atypical fibroxanthoma	93–100%[26]	
Dermatofibrosarcoma protuberans	98–100%[27,28,29]	
Merkel cell carcinoma	84%[30]	
Microcystic adnexal carcinoma	90%[31,32,33]	
Sebaceous carcinoma	89%[34]	
Extramammary Paget's disease (EMPD)	92%[35]	
Leiomyosarcoma (superficial)	87%[36]	
Malignant fibrous histiocytoma	–	
Angiosarcoma	–	
Melanoma	–	
Apocrine carcinoma	–	
Lymphoepithelioma-like carcinoma	–	
Eccrine porocarcinoma	–	

Indications for Mohs Surgery for Basal Cell Carcinoma and Squamous Cell Carcinoma[38]

Tumor Characteristics

- High-risk* anatomic location (Area H): "Mask areas" of face (central face, eyelids, eyebrows, nose, lips, chin, ear, and periauricular skin/sulci, temple), genitalia (perineal and perianal), hands, feet, nail units, ankles, and nipples/areola (▶ Fig. 6.2a, b).
- Large size: Area L ≥ 20 mm, Area M ≥ 10 mm, Area H ≥ 6 mm (▶ Fig. 6.2a, b).
- Aggressive histologic subtype:
  - BCC: morpheaform (sclerosing), micronodular, or infiltrating.
  - SCC: poorly or undifferentiated, spindle cell, acantholytic, sclerosing, metatypical, small cell, clear cell, desmoplastic, KA type (central face), lymphoepithelioma-like, and sarcomatoid.
- Recurrent.
- Positive margin on excision.
- Poorly defined clinical border.
- Perineural/vascular* invasion.
- Breslow depth ≥ 2 mm.*
- Rapid growth.*
- Neurologic symptoms.*

Patient Characteristics

- Prior exposure to ionizing radiation.*
- Chronic inflammatory process (scar).*
- Immunocompromised: human immunodeficiency virus (HIV), organ transplant, hematologic malignancy, or pharmacologic immunosuppression.
- Predisposing genetic syndromes: xeroderma pigmentosa, basal cell nevus syndrome.
- Patient known to have high-risk tumors without other health risk factors.

*Squamous cell carcinoma (SCC) specific.

According to the National Comprehensive Cancer Network (NCCN), a multidisciplinary expert panel, MMS is the preferred surgical technique for high-risk BCCs and SCCs as it provides superior intraoperative surgical margin analysis.[39] This signifies the importance of complete tissue margin analysis for high-risk tumors. If MMS is not available, a viable alternative would be excision with recommended margins and complete circumferential peripheral and deep-margin (CPDM) assessment using intraoperative frozen sections. A meta-analysis of MMS demonstrated a 5-year disease-free survival rate of 99% for BCC and 97% for SCC.[1,9] A prospective, randomized controlled trial with 10-year follow-up revealed significantly lower recurrence rates for recurrent and primary facial BCC treated with MMS compared to standard excision.[20]

In addition to BCCs and SCCs, MMS has been utilized effectively for recurrent benign tumors that tend to recur, such as desmoplastic trichoepithelioma, infantile digital fibroma, and granular cell tumor, as well as other rare cutaneous malignancies[26,27,28,29,30,31,32,33,34,35,36] (▶ Table 6.2). In these cases, the complete margin examination MMS provides enhanced tumor clearance.

6.4.1 Melanoma Including Lentigo Maligna

The role of MMS with only frozen sections for the treatment of cutaneous melanoma is controversial because the margin taken is often narrower than published guidelines as well as the challenge in detecting atypical melanocytes in frozen sections (freeze artifact).[40] The use of special immunohistochemical (IHC) stains, such as human melanoma black 45 (HMB-45), Mel-5, Melan-A (MART-1), and S100, can increase histologic sensitivity during MMS for melanocytic lesions (▶ Table 6.3).[41] Many dermatologic surgeons still advocate for the examination of FFPE tissue margins to confirm that the final MMS margin is negative.[42] Some Mohs surgeons with extensive experience with management of melanoma with MMS suggest that outcomes are equivalent to standard margins.[43,44] MMS for melanoma may be advantageous in certain clinical scenarios such as locally recurrent melanoma, large diameter tumors, ill-defined or amelanotic melanoma, and melanoma near critical anatomic structures such as the genitals, digits, eyelids, nose, and ears.

The lentigo maligna subtype of melanoma in situ is considered an exception and MMS as a treatment is becoming increasingly accepted. Lentigo maligna (melanoma in situ) is often a clinically ill-defined tumor typically found on the head and neck with a high local recurrence rate with standard wide local excision, due to the unpredictable histologic tumor extension beyond the clinically predicted margins. Several studies have found the recommended 5-mm margin for melanoma in situ inadequate for complete removal of lentigo maligna.[40,45] Given these challenges, conventional MMS is one possibility for treatment of lentigo maligna because it offers the possibility of complete margin examination and higher cure rate along with tissue sparing in critical areas. A challenge is that frozen tissue processing may result in morphologic artifacts where keratinocytes can resemble melanocytes and the true margin can be difficult to interpret. Rapid IHC stains[41] are helpful, but it still may be challenging to reliably detect single cell change and nests without significant training and experience. One review demonstrated that nearly 25% of lesions initially diagnosed as melanoma in situ were found to have a dermal component upon re-excision.[23] Therefore it is recommended that the debulked clinical tumor be sent for permanent sections to evaluate for dermal invasion.

Due to these challenges, there are several modifications to MMS for treatment of lentigo maligna and melanoma. Some techniques include wide excision Mohs surgery, "slow" Mohs staged excision using FFPE sections, and geometric staged excision (GSE; see the "Modifications of Mohs Micrographic

Table 6.3 Commonly used rapid immunohistochemical stains for Mohs micrographic surgery

Tumor	Immunohistochemical stains
Melanoma	HMB-45, Melan-A (MART-1), S100
Squamous cell carcinoma	Cytokeratin (AE1/AE3)
Extramammary Paget's disease	Cytokeratin 7
Dermatofibrosarcoma protuberans	CD34

Abbreviation: HMB-45, human melanoma black 45.

Surgery" section),[41,42,45] which aim to achieve complete margin control with FFPE pathology.[46,47]

6.4.2 Appropriate Use Criteria

In 2012, evidence-based appropriate use criteria for Mohs micrographic surgery (Mohs AUC) was developed using the RAND Corp protocol with direction of the NCCN guidelines.[38,48] Two hundred and seventy clinical scenarios based on tumor location (▶ Fig. 6.2a, b), size, recurrence history, histology, and patient health status were presented to an expert panel to be graded as appropriate, inappropriate, or uncertain based on available evidence. The goal of the Mohs AUC was to provide guidance in the rational use of MMS.[38,49] The Mohs AUC tables can be downloaded at the American Academy of Dermatology World Wide Web site (http://www.aad.org/education/appropriate-use-criteria/mohs-surgery-auc). There is also a smartphone app (Mohs AUC) that can be downloaded and referenced for point-of-care decisions (http://www.aad.org/education/appropriate-use-criteria/mohs-auc-app).

6.4.3 Cost-Effective Care

With the escalating cost of health care, it is important to be mindful of meaningful use of therapies while providing evidence-based quality care to patients. The studies on the cost-effectiveness of MMS compared to standard excision with local anesthesia are variable depending on the study location and methods.[50,51] With the use of the Mohs AUC in addition to the aforementioned advantages of the procedure, MMS is a cost-effective treatment for skin cancer.[9,10] When standard excision with FFPE sections and immediate repair is compared with MMS, the cost differential is comparable or slightly less expensive with the former (standard excision with immediate repair). However, when factoring the physical location of where the surgery is performed (office-based vs. ambulatory center vs. operating room), type of anesthesia used (local vs. general), processing method for the specimen (frozen vs. permanent), type of reconstruction (immediate vs. delayed), the size of the defect (tissue-sparing vs. wide local excision), the need for additional surgery for recurrence, and the intangible aspects (stress associated with waiting for the results of permanent sections, returning for a second surgery), MMS is an economical skin cancer treatment.[19,50,51,52,53]

6.4.4 Contraindications

There are no absolute contraindications to MMS. There are limitations and challenges to the technique such as discontiguous tumors, certain histologic features, and patient characteristics. As the basis of MMS is grounded on a contiguous tumor, discontiguous tumors can result in false-negative margins and inadequate margin control. However, this is also a concern with other methods of evaluating surgical margins. If a tumor cannot reliably be identified histologically, especially on frozen sections, this can also be a relative contraindication. Patients who are unwilling or unable to undergo a time-intensive surgery may do better with a nonsurgical approach such as radiotherapy or standard excision. Nevertheless, for some patients with complex medical conditions and comorbidities, MMS done under local anesthesia may be preferable over surgery performed under general anesthesia.[54,55,56] MMS may not offer a decreased morbidity or mortality in cases of metastases or tumors deeply invading structures such as the orbit, parotid, or bone. MMS can assist in peripheral margin clearance in conjunction with surgical colleagues performing the more extensive deep tumor resection possibly under general anesthesia. These cases are rare and MMS can be utilized to decrease tumor burden and prevent possible invasion of vital structures[57] or assess peripheral margins (see below, Case 2).

6.5 Mohs Micrographic Surgery Technique

During MMS, the Mohs surgeon has complete control of the excised tissue, including laboratory processing and interpretation of the tissue sections, as well as precise mapping. MMS involves four major components: tumor extirpation, histopathologic examination, precise mapping, and wound management (▶ Fig. 6.5 and ▶ Fig. 6.6). The *tumor extirpation* component consists of removing a disc of tissue, often referred to as "layer" or "stage," with a beveled surgical margin (▶ Fig. 6.6c). This ensures that the entire 360 degrees of tumor margin is circumferentially removed and examined. A beveled plane of excision allows the tissue specimen sides to be flattened completely into a single plane, allowing complete examination of the peripheral and deep margin of the excised tissue (▶ Fig. 6.4 and ▶ Fig. 6.6d). The *histopathologic* component involves cutting horizontal sections and mounting them onto glass slides, followed by staining and microscopic examination for residual tumor (▶ Fig. 6.6f). Precise *mapping* involves marking any residual tumor on the "map" of the excision (▶ Fig. 6.6g). This three-step process is then repeated until there is no residual tumor identified microscopically (▶ Fig. 6.5). In the fourth step, *wound management*, the tumor-free defect is surgically closed (▶ Fig. 6.6k) or allowed to heal by second intention. The specific way each step is achieved may vary between individual surgeons.

6.5.1 Preoperative Assessment

After a given tumor is deemed appropriate for MMS, a consultation including a history and focused skin examination should be performed, which may be done the same day as the surgery. Indications for preoperative and postoperative antibiotic prophylaxis should be evaluated.[58] The management of any implanted devices including pacemakers, defibrillators, and deep brain stimulators should be considered and affect choice of hemostatic device. Medication and supplement history is noted. The use of anticoagulants should be managed accordingly. Typically, patients are asked to continue anticoagulants especially if used to prevent a life-threatening event as the risk/benefit ratio favors anticoagulation.[59,60] However, in collaborative cases, it is important to discuss with other physicians involved. Patient should be thoroughly questioned regarding

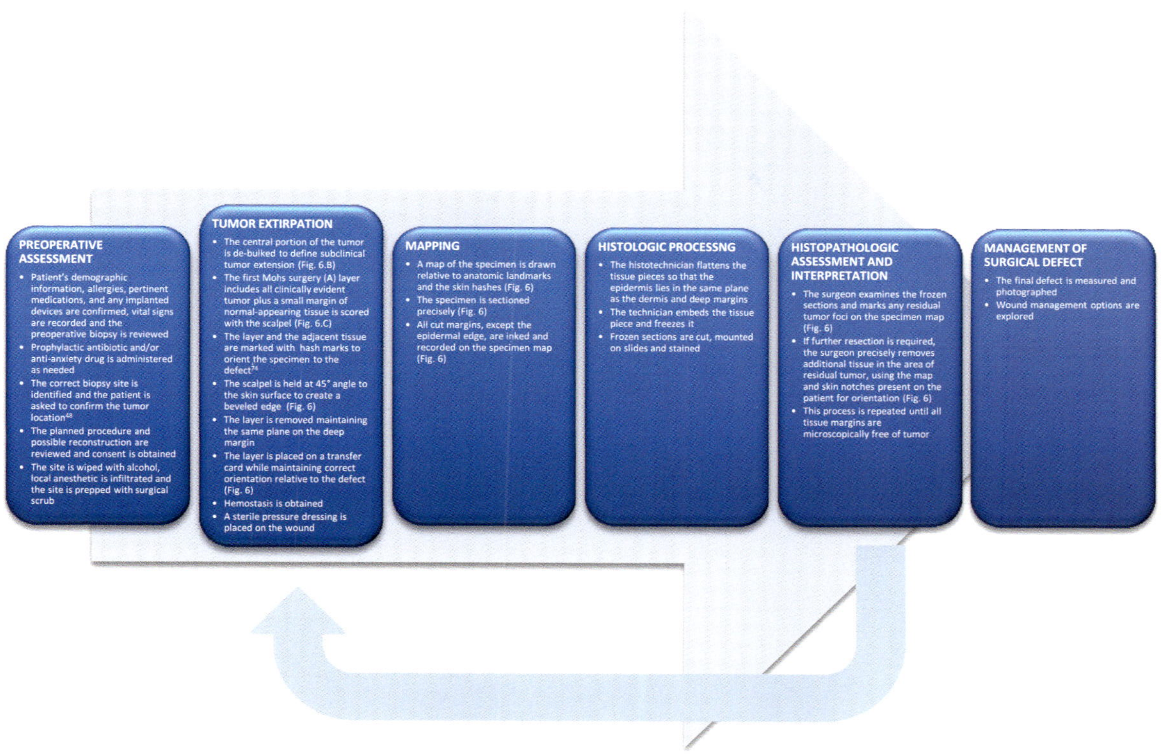

Fig. 6.5 Mohs micrographic surgery flow sheet.

allergies including local anesthetics, antibiotics, iodine, latex, and tape products. A social history regarding smoking, alcohol use, and home assistance with wound care is necessary. Chronic alcohol dependence or abuse can result in increased intraoperative bleeding, and smoking can result in poor wound healing due to decreased tissue oxygenation. Gaining an appreciation of the patient's understanding of the procedure will be important to prevent patient dissatisfaction.

Based on the tumor's characteristics (extremely large, recurrent, fixed, deeply invasive tumors) or clinical symptoms (pain, numbness, facial muscle asymmetry), preoperative radiologic imaging may be warranted.[61] Preoperative consultations with other subspecialties (e.g., oculoplastics, otolaryngology, neurosurgery, plastic surgery) may be considered for complicated cases.

Photographs of biopsy sites and patient identification of precise biopsy location are extremely important to prevent wrong-site surgery.[62] All treatment options are discussed including wide local excision performed by a non-MMS physician. Most patients prefer to know that their tumor is completely removed prior to reconstruction.[63] Wound management and options for defect repair should be explained. Typically, patients are asked to continue regular medications and eat a light meal on the morning of surgery, unless conscious sedation is planned. Most patients spend approximately 3 to 4 hours from same-day consultation to discharge, dependent on size of the tumor, number of layers required for clearance, and type of closure.

Intraoperative considerations include anxiety, pain (with local anesthesia injection), bleeding, nerve damage, and allergic reactions need to be managed appropriately. If warranted, oral midazolam can be given in the range of 5 to 15 mg for healthy adults. Knowledge of vascular, muscular, and neural anatomy, especially in "danger zones" of the face, will help surgeons avoid complications and improve outcomes. Hemorrhage can be minimized with the addition of epinephrine (adrenaline) in local anesthetic, meticulous hemostasis, and pressure bandaging. Injury to cutaneous sensory nerves occurs during all cutaneous surgery. Transection of significant motor nerves may be occasionally necessary for invasive tumors, especially in the temporal region. During consultation, patients should be informed of the possibility of loss of function if the tumor lies over or in proximity to a motor nerve. There may also be temporary sensation loss or paresthesias.

6.5.2 Tumor Extirpation

MMS is considered a "clean" rather than "sterile" procedure. After the patient verifies the site of the biopsied tumor, the clinically apparent tumor margins are marked with a surgical pen along with skin tension lines or cosmetic subunits (▶ Fig. 6.1a).

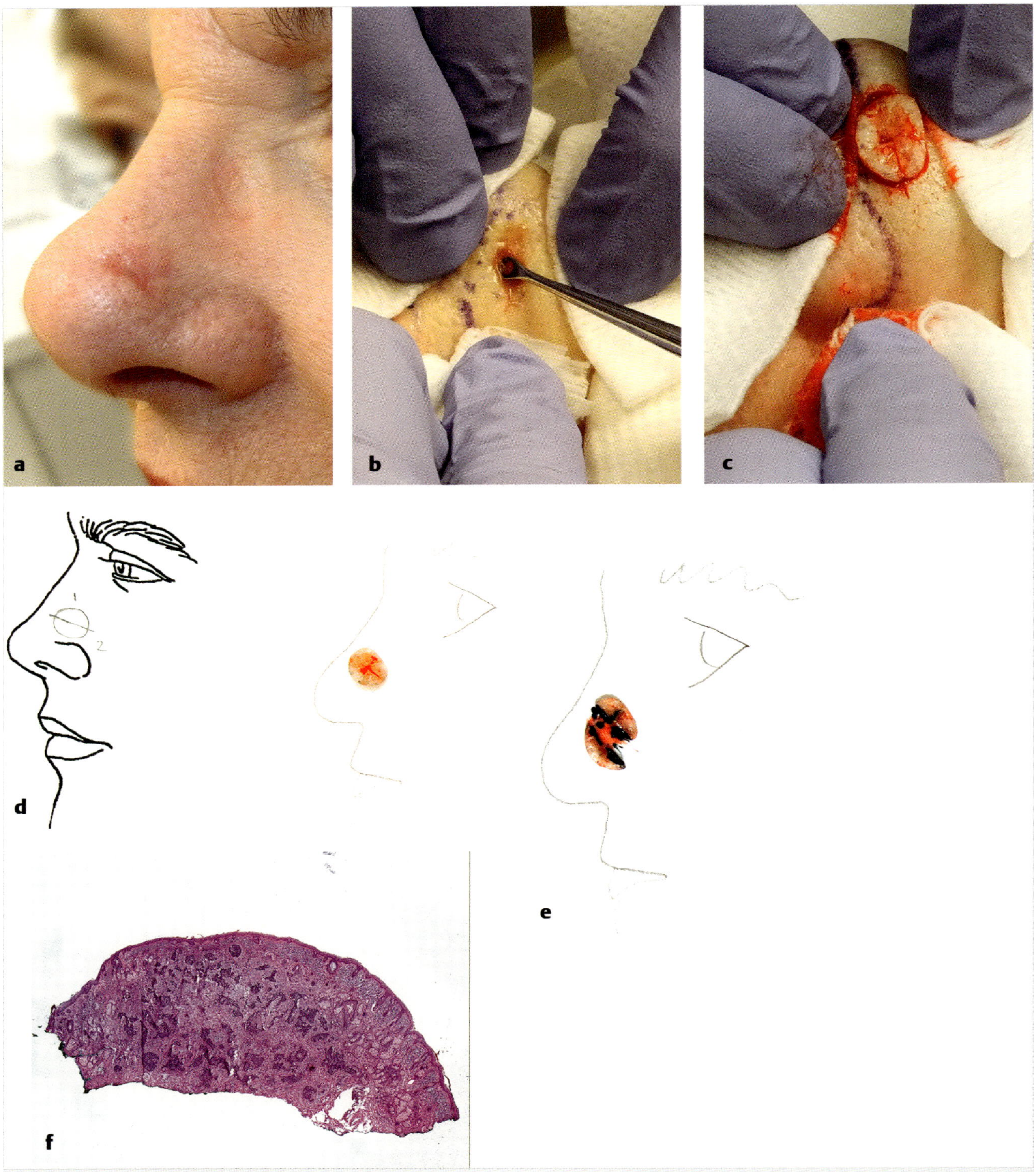

Fig. 6.6 Mohs micrographic surgery technique. **(a)** Preoperative appearance of a basal cell carcinoma on the nose. **(b)** Debulking of the tumor via curettage. **(c)** Beveled excision (with scalpel at a 45-degree angle) of all clinically evident tumor plus a small margin of normal-appearing skin. Placement of skin notches at 10 and 4 o'clock positions in adjacent surrounding tissue. **(d)** Orientation of the excised specimen on an anatomic card. **(e)** Specimen sectioned into two pieces and flattened. The superior portions of the specimens are marked as blue and the inferior aspects are marked as green. Matching Mohs map and tissue specimen ready for histologic preparation. **(f)** Histopathologic section with positive tumor.

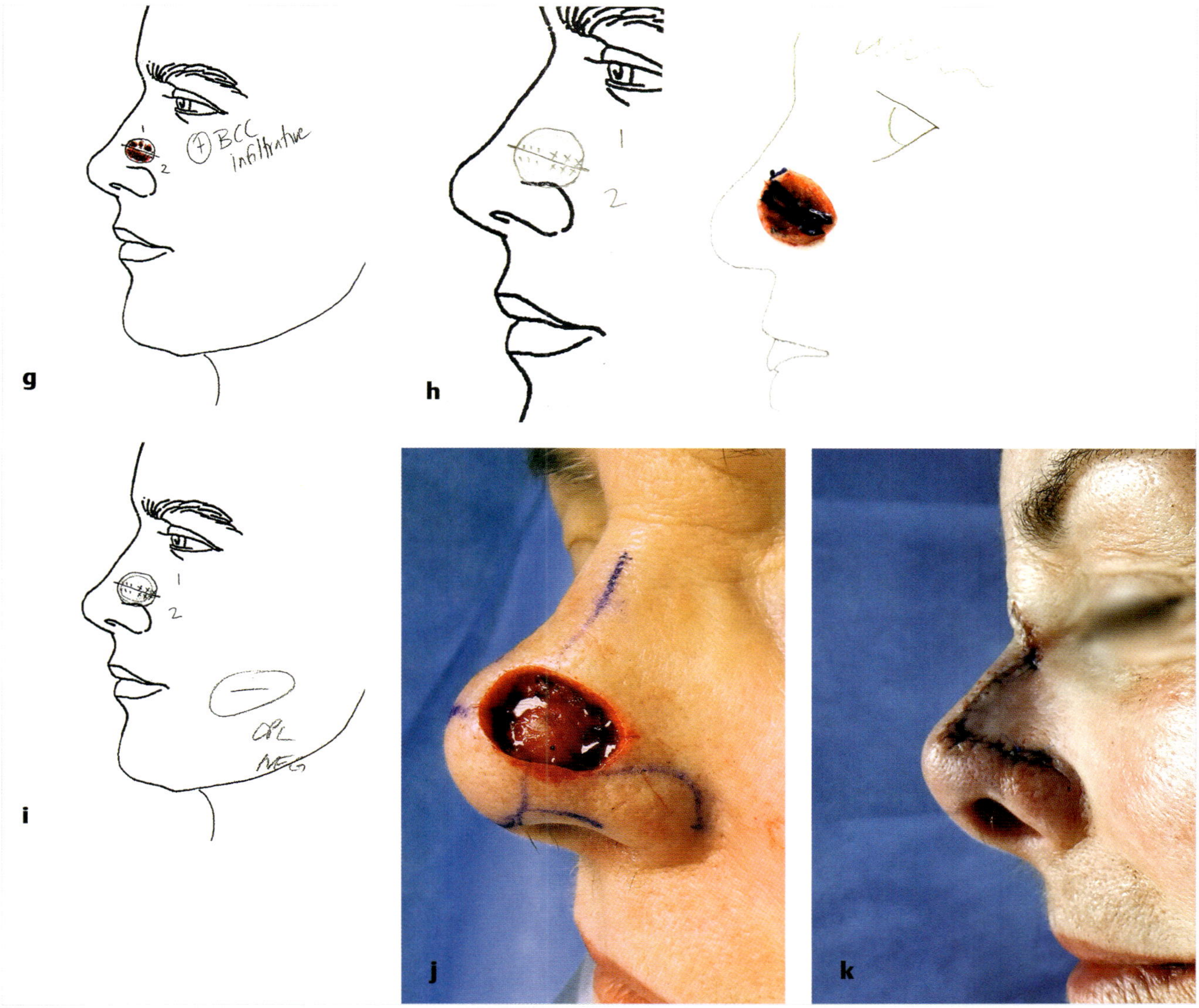

(g) Mohs map marked with red at the site of cancer. (h) Re-excision of the area of residual basal cell carcinoma (second "B" layer) and accompanying Mohs map from the second layer with corresponding tissue. (i) Mohs map for second layer denoting the tumor is clear. (j,k) Postoperative tumor-free defect and repair.

Local anesthetic typically 1 or 0.5% lidocaine with 1:100,000 epinephrine is infiltrated in the area. The lidocaine can also be buffered with sodium bicarbonate (10 lidocaine:1 sodium bicarbonate) to alkalinize the pH and minimize the discomfort of the injection. The anesthetic is usually allowed to penetrate for 10 to 15 minutes, enabling anesthesia for the larger nerves and vasoconstrictive effects of epinephrine. The identified surgical site is cleansed with surgical scrub (povidone-iodine or chlorhexidine).

Debulking of the tumor is the initial step. Typically, a curette is utilized to remove the friable tissue of the tumor and delineate it from the normal tissue (▶ Fig. 6.6b). This helps the surgeon estimate the tumor width and depth prior to removing the initial Mohs specimen (layer/stage). Not all surgeons curette the tumor as they argue that curettage does not reliably delineate the tumor.[64] Large tumors may be removed with a scalpel or scissors.

Initial (A) Layer

A scalpel is used to score around the tumor with a 1- to 2-mm margin of clinically normal skin (▶ Fig. 6.6c). Margins may vary depending on the tumor type, tumor location, patient characteristics, and other factors. Small skin incisions (hash marks) are made on the skin and the tumor for orientation purposes. The scalpel is then beveled at 45 degrees to cut through the dermis and subcutaneous tissue, and the base is transected, maintaining the same plane in the deep margin. Hemostasis is achieved if necessary. A temporary pressure bandage is placed on the wound while the tissue is processed in the Mohs lab. At this point, the bandaged patient can comfortably rest and join his/her family members or friends in the waiting room.

6.5.3 Mapping

The layer is carefully placed on a blotter that may have a drawing of the patient's tumor site to maintain orientation (▶ Fig. 6.6d). The *Mohs map* is a schematic representation of tumor and its relation to the patient. This map will detail the site, size, specimen orientation, number of pieces, and ink markings on the specimen. The accuracy and precision of the Mohs map is critical to the Mohs procedure. Specimens are typically bisected and ink applied to the medial (cut) edges of the specimens (▶ Fig. 6.6e). Often one color is applied to the superior or medial aspect and another color used for the inferior or lateral aspect of the specimen. The specimens are then numbered. The Mohs map is marked to reflect the specimen numbers and ink placement. The number of specimens depends on the size of the resected tissue. Tissue shrinkage is about 20% in frozen sections.[16] Smaller specimens can be processed in toto.

6.5.4 Histologic Examination/ Interpretation

The inked tissue sections are given to the histotechnician who begins to process the tissue by grossing it or flattening it so that the epidermis is laid down in the same plane as the dermis and subcutaneous tissue. With the orientation preserved, the specimen is embedded with embedding medium, and attached to a specimen holder button or chuck.[65] Once the embedded specimen is frozen, it is mounted on the stage of the cryostat. It is sectioned in the microtome and placed on the slide. The histotechnician obtains sections that contain a complete layer extending from the epidermis to the deepest section of the resected tissue. Multiple complete sections are normally harvested and placed on each slide. The slides are then stained with hematoxylin and eosin (H&E). Some surgeons utilize toluidine blue[66] or other immunostains depending on the tumor type. The number of slices and slides per specimen vary with the preference of the surgeon. Cartee and Monheit reported that on average, Mohs surgeons prefer three to six slices per specimen with the average thickness of the slices of 5 to 6 µm.[67] With the usual 5- to 6-µm thickness of slices, most prefer to view at least four full successive slices to establish that the sections are clear from the tumor.[68] If residual tumor is present, then an additional Mohs layer is required.

Understanding tissue orientation and embedding is crucial to interpretation and localization of any residual tumor in the layer. When viewing the slide, it is important to remember as one looks from the top to bottom of the slice (epidermis to dermis to subcutaneous tissue), it also moves centripetally from the margins (epidermis) to the tumor center (subcutaneous tissue). Therefore, if residual tumor appreciated at the epidermis and dermis, it means that in the subsequent layer, the surgical margin needs to be laterally extended (▶ Fig. 6.6h). However, if the tumor is only appreciated in the deep subcutaneous tissue, then in the subsequent layer, only the base needs to be excised. A small rim of epidermis may be taken to help orient the subsequent layer.

6.5.5 Wound Management

When complete tumor removal has been achieved, reconstruction or wound management can be planned (▶ Fig. 6.6jk). Closure techniques are discussed in Chapter 9. Large defects, certain anatomic locations, depth of the defect, and detection of perineural involvement are factors that may require collaboration with other specialties, such as plastic surgery, oculoplastic surgery, otolaryngology, neurosurgery, and radiation oncology. Mohs surgeons generally manage the majority of the surgical defects with second intention healing, primary closure, skin grafts, and flaps (▶ Fig. 6.7abc). Allowing wounds to heal by secondary intention or granulate with epithelialization especially those that are superficial or in concave areas can produce acceptable if not superior cosmetic results (▶ Fig. 6.8ab). Other advantages of secondary intention healing include lack of donor site involvement, less postoperative pain, lower costs, greater safety, and fewer complications.[69] Additionally, many patients prefer second intention healing and are pleased with the cosmetic result. Second intention healing can also be used in high-risk tumors where a complex flap or graft may hinder surveillance of recurrence. Possible disadvantages of secondary intention healing of large wounds are the following: delayed healing, longer wound care, and possible distortion of nearby structures due to contraction. Second intention healing with delayed closure is also an option for deep wounds. The wound contracts, shrinking the size of the defect and the base granulates, improving the survival of grafts and flaps.

Fellowship-trained Mohs surgeons are educated on advanced facial reconstructive techniques. The confirmed clear surgical margins prior to wound reconstruction and maximal preservation of normal skin are significant advantages of MMS. These advantages are particularly important for the head and neck region where recurrences and/or positive margins can be devastating and reconstructions especially challenging.

6.5.6 Postoperative Evaluation

Antibiotics may be given postoperatively for wound infection prophylaxis if indicated.[58] Substantial pain following MMS is uncommon and acetaminophen is often sufficient for postoperative discomfort, especially for smaller defects and simple repairs. Oral narcotic analgesics may be necessary for larger tumors, complex reconstruction, or wounds in anatomic locations of high tension or sensitivity (e.g., lip, nose, scalp, and ear).[70] A randomized controlled trial comparing acetaminophen, acetaminophen and ibuprofen, and acetaminophen with codeine demonstrated the combination of acetaminophen and ibuprofen was superior in controlling postoperative pain compared to the other two arms.[70]

Patients are also recommended to have ongoing surveillance at least annually for new primary and recurrent skin cancers, given that 50% of patients with NMSC will experience another skin cancer during the subsequent 5 years.

Complications

Serious complications and adverse events due to MMS are rare. MMS is a safe procedure with an undetected mortality rate.[71,72] A large, multicenter, prospective cohort study of

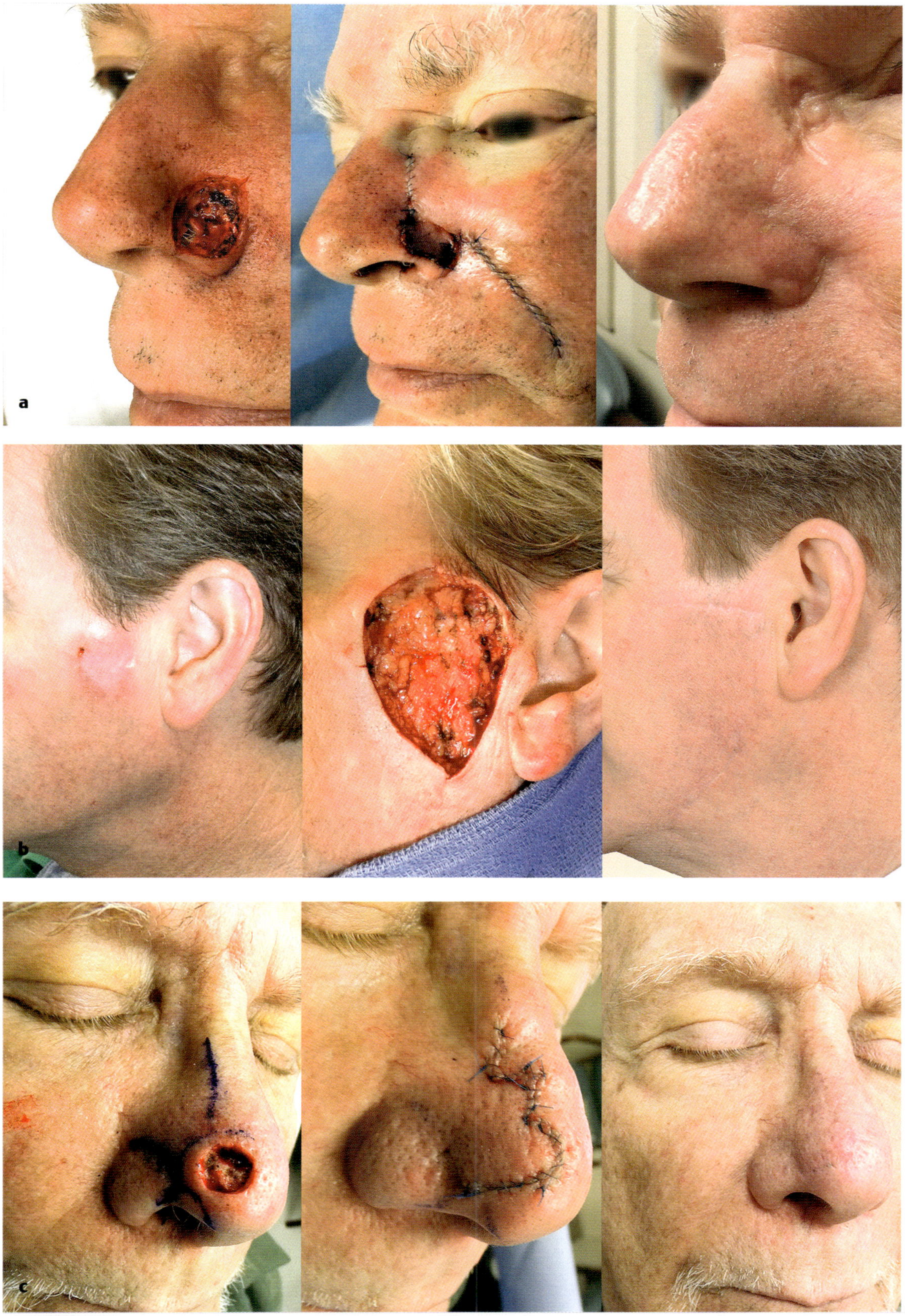

Fig. 6.7 (a–c) Examples of typical closures done by fellowship trained Mohs surgeons.

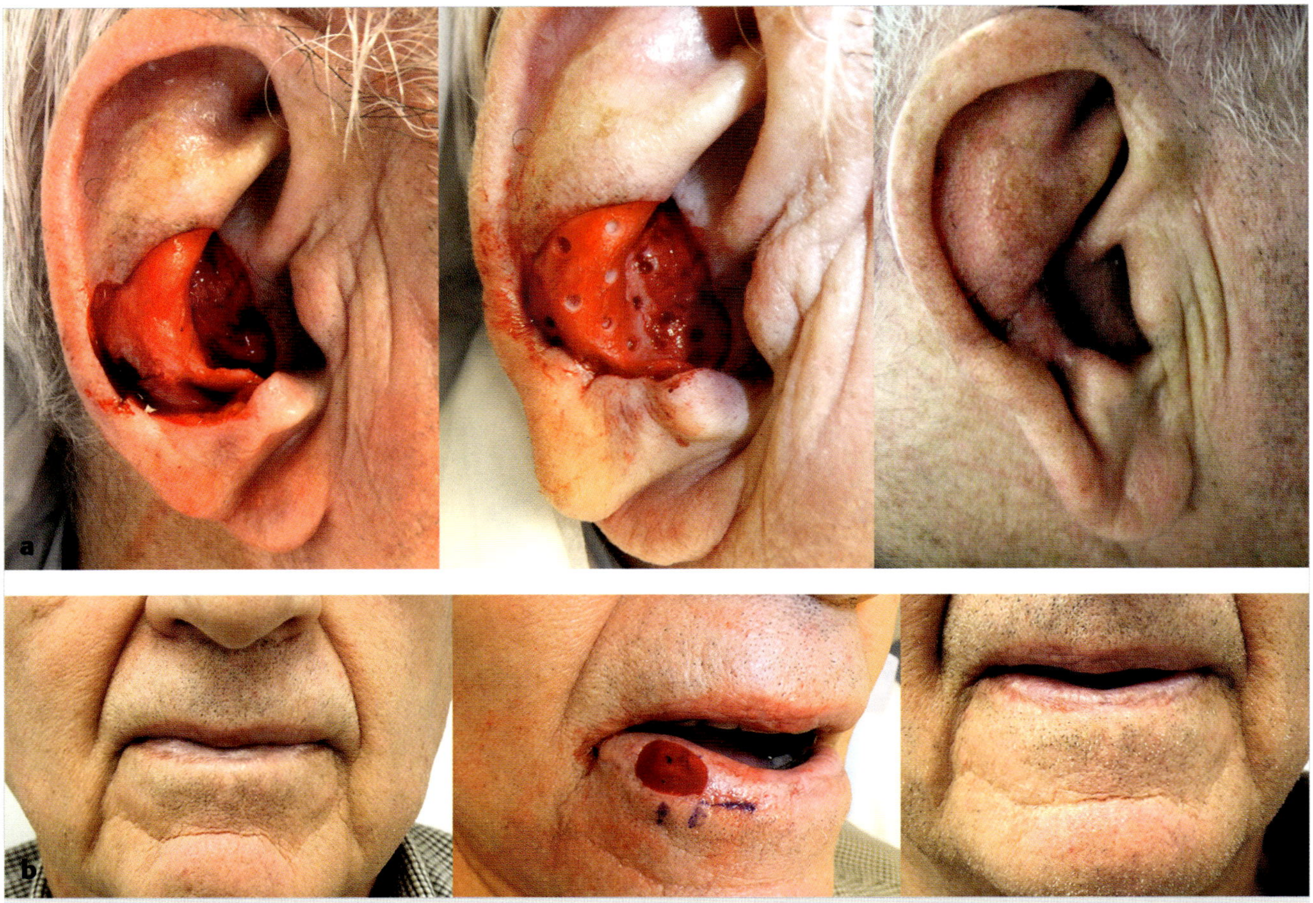

Fig. 6.8 Examples of defects left to heal by second intent. (a) Large defect on the ear that healed with second intent. There was some contraction, but the patient was very satisfied with the results. (b) Example of tissue sparing potential at lip with second intent healing.

adverse events in MMS found the rate of adverse events was less than 1%, with the majority of events being minor.[71] Postoperative complications include infection, dehiscence, partial or full necrosis, bleeding, and hematoma/seroma formation. The infection rate post-MMS is very low (0.7%) despite being a "clean" procedure and the duration of the procedure.[73]

6.6 Modifications of Mohs Micrographic Surgery

There are several modifications/variations in the MMS technique to improve the speed of tissue processing,[66] the efficiency of tumor removal, and the recognition of individual tumor cells in order to increase cure rates. Surgical modifications include (1) the single section method; (2) "slow" Mohs/GSE; (3) nonbeveled 90-degree incisions; and (4) wide excision. Variations to better recognize tumor cells include (1) IHC stains for frozen sections (▸ Table 6.3) and (2) submission of tissue specimens for routine histology ("rush" FFPE sections) and immunohistochemistry.

6.6.1 Single Section Method

The single section method can be used for smaller tumors.[74] The single section involves a highly beveled specimen with relaxing incisions on the superior, tumor-bearing portion that allow all peripheral edges to fold outward into a single plane. It can be particularly useful for small, superficial tumors where a shallow Mohs layer can be taken, with the goal of allowing the resulting wound to heal by second intention. Additionally, the unaltered examination of the complete deep margin reduces the possibility of areas missed by tissue subdivision.

6.6.2 "Slow" Mohs and Geometric Staged Excision for Melanoma

"Slow" Mohs staged excision is a technique where the tissue specimen is sent for "rush" FFPE sections that are read by a dermatopathologist the next day.[40] This variation of MMS is typically used for melanomas, but it can also be utilized for challenging tumors that can be difficult to read under frozen histology such as dermatofibrosarcoma protuberans (DFSP), extramammary Paget's disease (EMPD), and poorly differentiated SCC. FFPE sections require an average of 7 hours of processing time.[40] If there are residual tumor cells, another layer is removed until a negative (tumor-free) margin is achieved. A close working relationship with the dermatopathologist is essential.[40] This technique avoids the keratinocyte freeze artifact in frozen sections and the margin evaluation is performed by a dermatopathologist. The persistence rate for staged excision of melanoma ranges from 0 to 7%.[40]

GSE is a technique that involves excising the tumor with perpendicular skin margins.[45] Some surgeons use two closely spaced, parallel blades to create a square-shaped defect (thin and frame-like) with the tumor and presumed adequate margins left intact. If the excised peripheral tissue is found to contain no tumor cells, then the central square is excised. Others have found it easier to excise the entire specimen in a geometric pattern, ink the margins, and then cut off strips along the margins; the latter are then oriented, inked, processed, and cut en face, while the central portion is cut vertically to determine the thickness of the tumor. Some dermatopathologists prefer GSE method because it may be easier to process the tissue to examine the entire perpendicular epidermal margin.[40] A recent retrospective study and review of literature of this technique found GSE to be optimal for removal of lentigo maligna and lentigo maligna melanoma because of its low rate of recurrence (1.7%) and ability for complete examination of peripheral and deep margins.[45] In order to maintain the straight lengths of tissue, a few millimeters of skin may be sacrificed. In smaller tumors, this disadvantage is marginal. Cases requiring several layers may result in an irregularly shaped defect, leading to a more complex reconstruction.

6.6.3 Wide Excision Mohs Surgery

In wide excision MMS ("wide Mohs"), a larger, clinically tumor-free margin (5–20 mm) is taken during the first layer. It can be used for tumors that have a high propensity for recurrence or metastases (including satellite metastases), in particular melanoma, Merkel cell carcinoma, and cutaneous sarcomas,[21] and when tissue sparing is less of a concern.[15] In these challenging cases, tissue sparing is not the primary goal, but the advantage of precise margin evaluation offered by MMS is extremely valuable.

6.6.4 Rapid Immunohistochemical Stains

Rapid IHC stains can be utilized to assist in histologic evaluation of NMSC, melanocytic neoplasms, DFSP, EMPD, microcystic adnexal carcinoma (MAC), as well as other rare tumors.[76] They can be especially helpful in these challenging and high-risk tumors (▶ Table 6.2).[41,77,78] Conventional immunoperoxidase staining technique on FFPE sections requires several hours to process. In comparison, rapid IHC staining technique done on frozen tissue in MMS requires approximately 30 to 90 minutes depending on the protocol and can prevent the loss of antigens on the tissue.[77] However, rapid IHC stains are not without constraints. A recent survey of fellowship-trained Mohs surgeons found many barriers to routine use of IHC in Mohs labs including time consumption, lack of experience with IHC, and costs.[76] Nonetheless, the introduction of IHC stains has advanced the field of MMS in recent years and can be extremely helpful in locating tumor with subtle histologic features or those hidden in brisk inflammation. With continued use and research, the use of IHC may be routine for challenging tumors.

6.7 Integrating Mohs Micrographic Surgery into Your Practice

Collaboration between a Mohs micrographic surgeon and plastic surgeon can go beyond the traditional approach where the plastic surgeon repairs the defect after the cutaneous tumor is cleared.[79] By understanding the methods used by Mohs surgeons to process the tissue and read the histology, the technique can be tailored to provide optimal care for the patient. The following two cases are excellent examples of effective multidisciplinary collaboration.

6.7.1 Case 1

A 57-year-old Caucasian female presented as a plastic surgery consult for a tumor on her nose. It started as a pimple approximately 8 years ago and has progressively grown in size. She has been smoking for 45 years. On physical exam, a 4 × 4 cm pink, translucent, ulcerated tumor on the nasal dorsum extending through bilateral alar rims down onto columella and over bilateral nasal sidewalls and upper third of nasal dorsum was appreciated. There were no signs of intranasal involvement and the septum appeared intact (▶ Fig. 6.9abc). There was no lymphadenopathy. A computed tomography (CT) scan with and without contrast of the head and neck demonstrated soft tissue thickening and irregularity present along the nasal ala bilaterally, nasal septum, and dorsal aspect of the nose with no adjacent bony destruction. A screening chest radiograph was also obtained and found to be within normal limits. Dermatology was consulted and options were discussed including wide local excision, MMS, radiotherapy, and medical therapy with vismodegib. With the extensive soft tissue and cartilage damage, radiotherapy and oral vismodegib would not allow normal cutaneous tissue to recreate the nasal structure. Wide local excision would likely require complete rhinectomy with margins encroaching the orbits, leaving the possibility of incomplete resection and a challenging repair. The patient, therefore, agreed to MMS with reconstruction by plastic surgery.

The patient presented for MMS and was premedicated with diazepam. Infraorbital nerve blocks were placed with 1% lidocaine with 1:100,000 epinephrine. The area was also infiltrated with 1% lidocaine with 1:100,000 epinephrine and 0.5% bupivacaine. The "A" layer was removed, carefully mapped, and divided (▶ Fig. 6.9d–f). Eight specimens were found to be positive with infiltrative and nodular BCC (▶ Fig. 6.9g). The "B" layer was removed for a total of seven specimens and 1 specimen was found to be positive (▶ Fig. 6.9h, i). The "C" layer was excised and found to be clear of tumor (▶ Fig. 6.9j, k). Her final defect was extensive including bilateral medial cheeks and the entire surface of the nasal dorsum, a portion of the caudal septum, bilateral lower lateral cartilages, and columella (▶ Fig. 6.9l, m). The patient tolerated the whole 7-hour procedure without difficulty. She was alert and awake through the entire process and had a family member present for support.

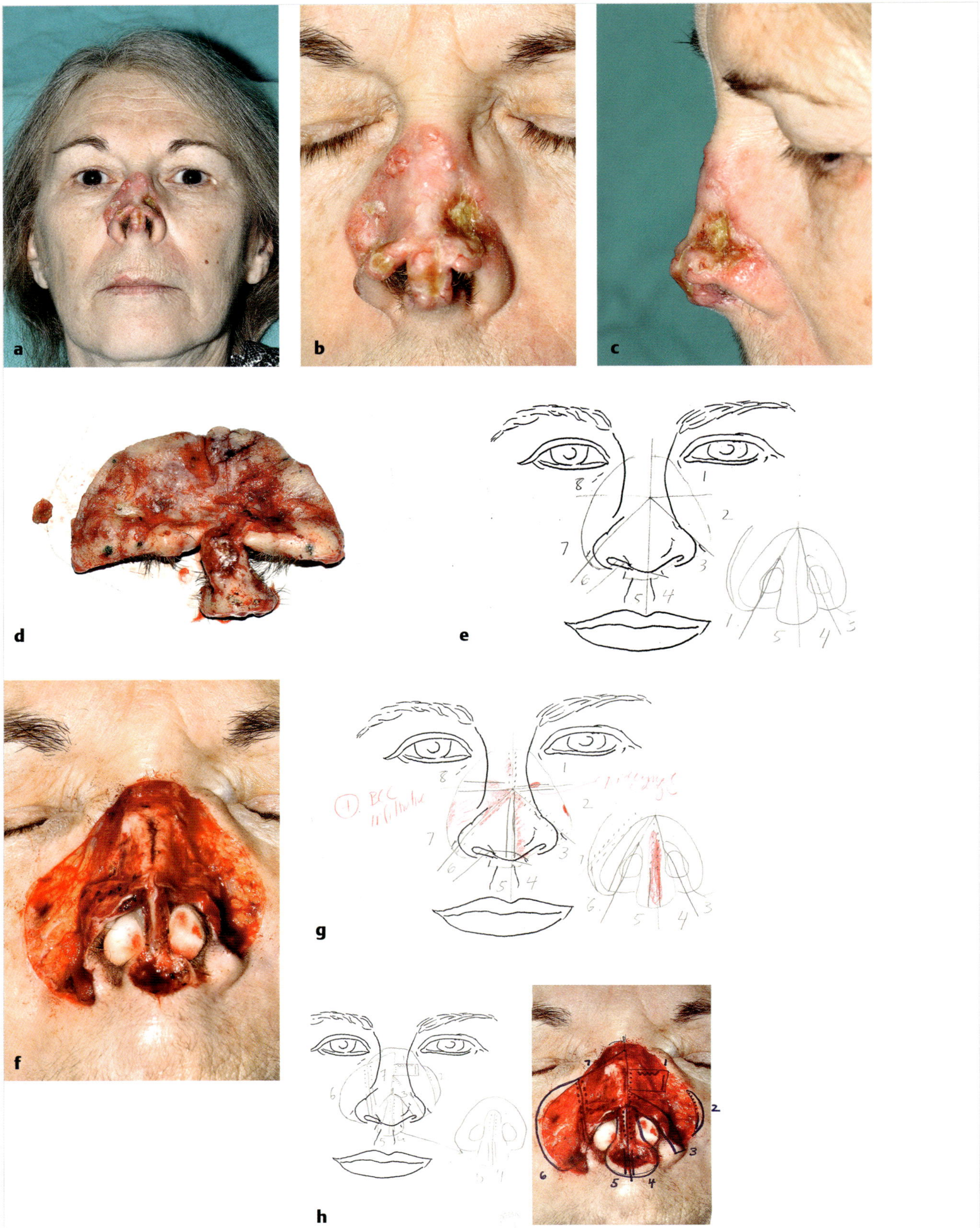

Fig. 6.9 Case 1. **(a–c)** Middle-aged female with large basal cell carcinoma (BCC) on nose. **(d)** Initial layer. **(e)** Map of "A" layer. **(f)** Defect after "A" layer. **(g)** Marked tumor positivity on "A" layer map. **(h)** Map of "B" layer.

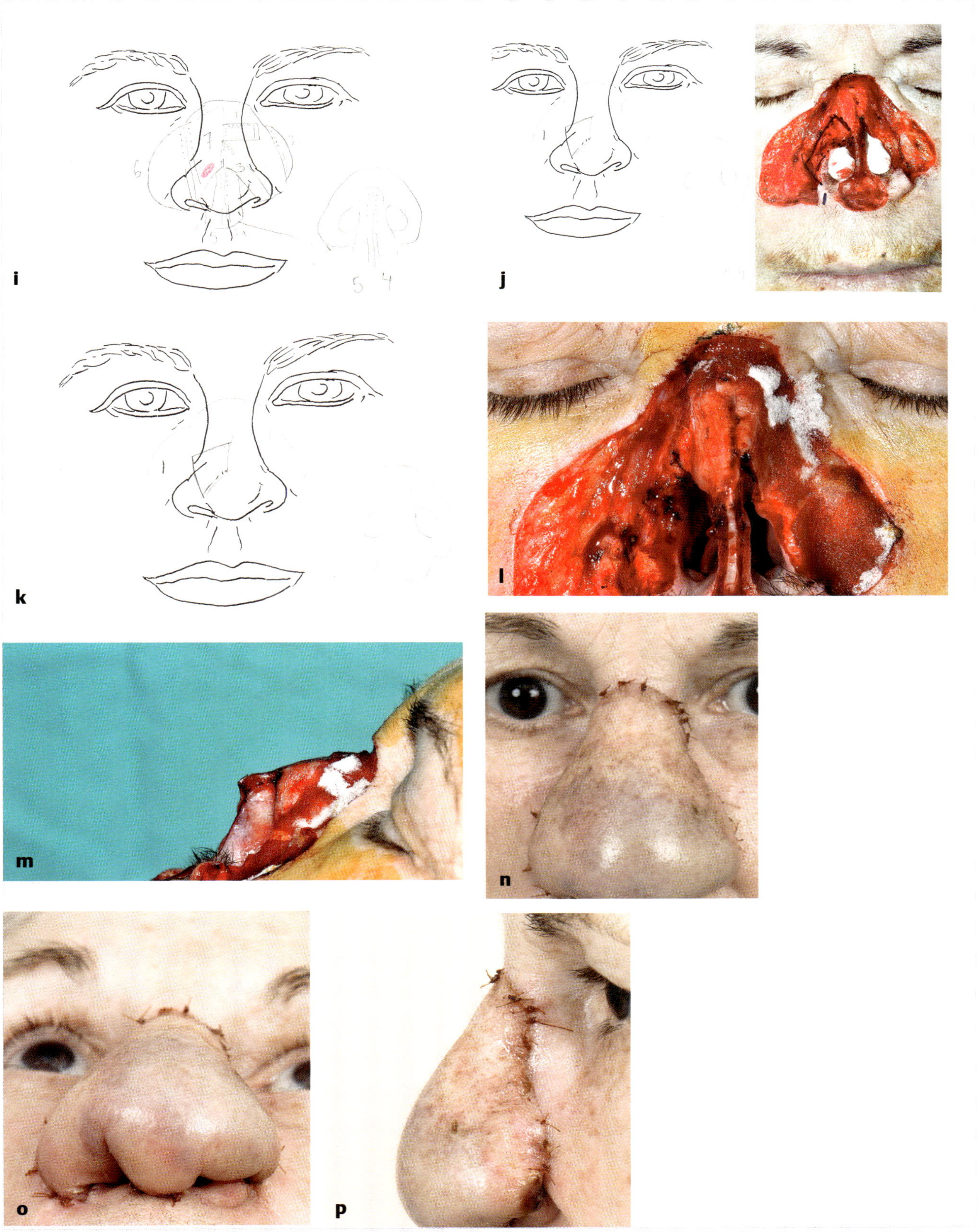

Fig. 6.9 (*continued*) **(i)** Marked tumor positivity on "B" layer map. **(j)** Map of "C" layer. **(k)** Tumor clearance as indicated by "C" map. **(l, m)** Final defect with tumor clearance. **(n–p)** Ongoing reconstruction with radial forearm free flap.

The patient was then placed under general anesthesia for staged reconstruction by the plastic surgeon. Initially, bilateral cheeks were advanced over the defect to the nasal sidewall and anchored to the nasal periosteum. A split thickness skin graft was placed over the nasal defect. Approximately, 3 weeks later, the patient returned for nasal reconstruction with a radial forearm free flap and is still in the process of reconstruction (▶ Fig. 6.9n–p). At two-year follow up, patient was doing well with no signs of clinical recurrence.

6.7.2 Case 2

An 86-year-old Caucasian male with a significant past medical history for hypertension, atrial fibrillation, and blindness in the left eye was admitted to the hospital for failure to thrive. The patient had a large tumor on his forehead, which was recently biopsied at an outside facility. The duration of time the patient had the tumor was unknown given the patient hid it under his hat. On examination, a 10 × 6 cm large ulcerative plaque with overlying hemorrhagic crust and rolled border extended from the left brow line inferiorly to the frontal hairline superiorly (▶ Fig. 6.10a). No lymphadenopathy was appreciated. The CT of the brain without contrast demonstrated a soft extracranial tissue mass on the left frontal region with underlying calvarial destruction. There was no hypermetabolic cervical lymphadenopathy or distant metastasis. The MRI of the brain showed extensive soft tissue prominence and ulceration overlying the left frontal region with underlying marrow infiltration in addition to a focal skull defect (▶ Fig. 6.10bc–e). There were no intracranial metastases. Subsequent biopsy demonstrated an invasive, moderate differentiated SCC, which was staged as pT3NxMx.

A multidisciplinary team involving a plastic surgeon, a neurosurgeon, a Mohs surgeon, and a radiation oncologist was assembled. The patient was placed under general anesthesia (▶ Fig. 6.10f) and the plastic surgeon resected the tumor and performed a left orbital exenteration (▶ Fig. 6.10g). The Mohs surgeon was present to assist in the mapping of the tumor and processed the excised tumor (▶ Fig. 6.10h). Since the underlying calvarium was involved, a craniectomy was performed by neurosurgery. The tissue was processed with the Mohs technique (frozen sections and horizontal sectioning), in which complete peripheral margins were examined. The deep margins were not assessed as the underlying bone was removed. After the peripheral margins were found to be clear, the plastic surgeon closed the defect with a vertical rectus abdominis myocutaneous and

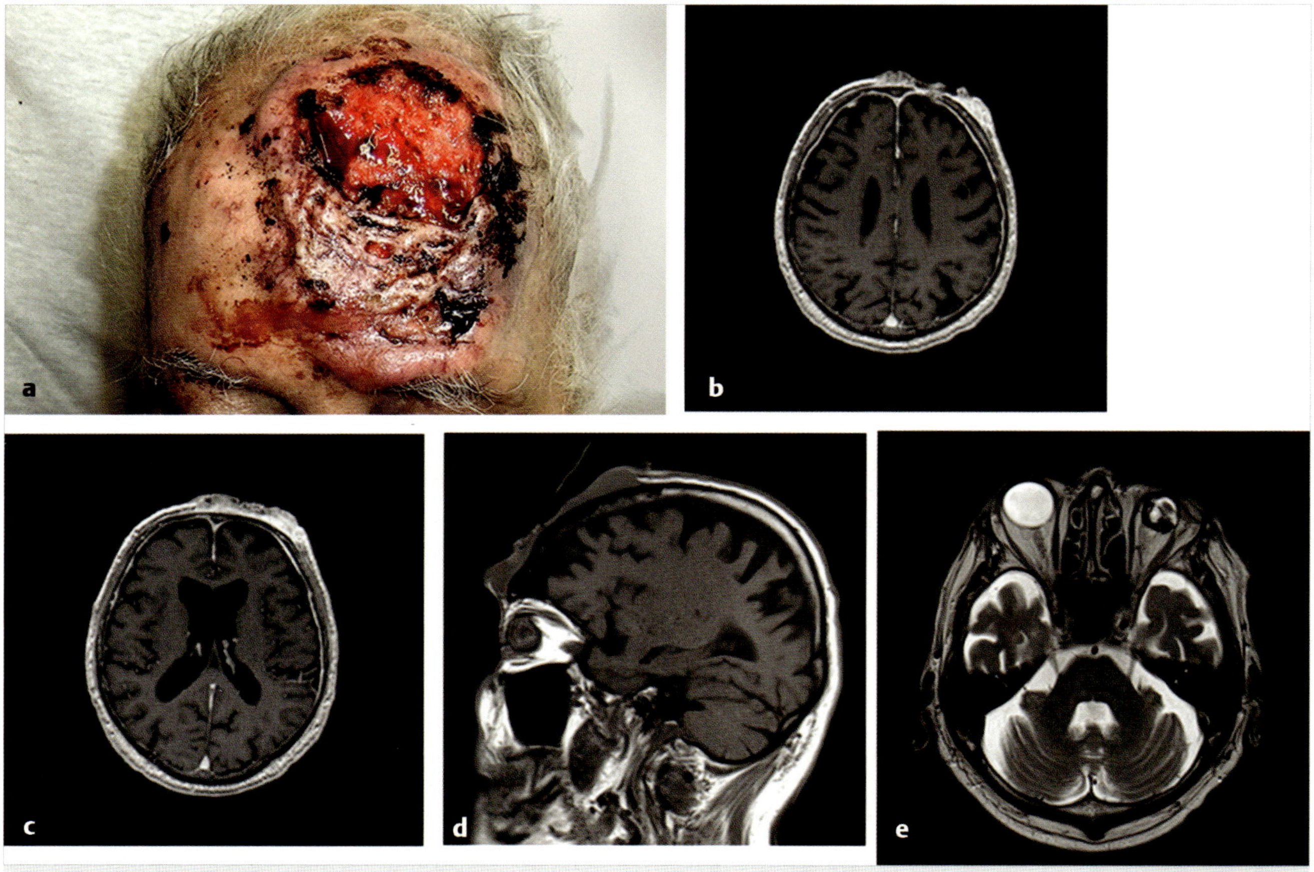

Fig. 6.10 Case 2: elderly male with neglected SCC (squamous cell carcinoma) on forehead. **(a)** Initial presentation. **(b)** T1-weighted scan with gadolinium. Scalp thickening in midline/left frontal region. Mild nonspecific dural thickening. **(c)** Axial postgadolinium T1 scan. Irregular scalp mass and focal penetration of skull by neoplasm in left frontal bone. Dural thickening is relatively uniform, and may be reactive or related to chronic low cerebrospinal fluid pressure. **(d)** Sagittal T1-weighted scan without gadolinium. Scalp mass is visible. Normal marrow hyperintense fat signal in the posterior calvarium is present, but is replaced adjacent to the scalp mass. **(e)** Axial T2 scan. Phthisis bulbi left globe.

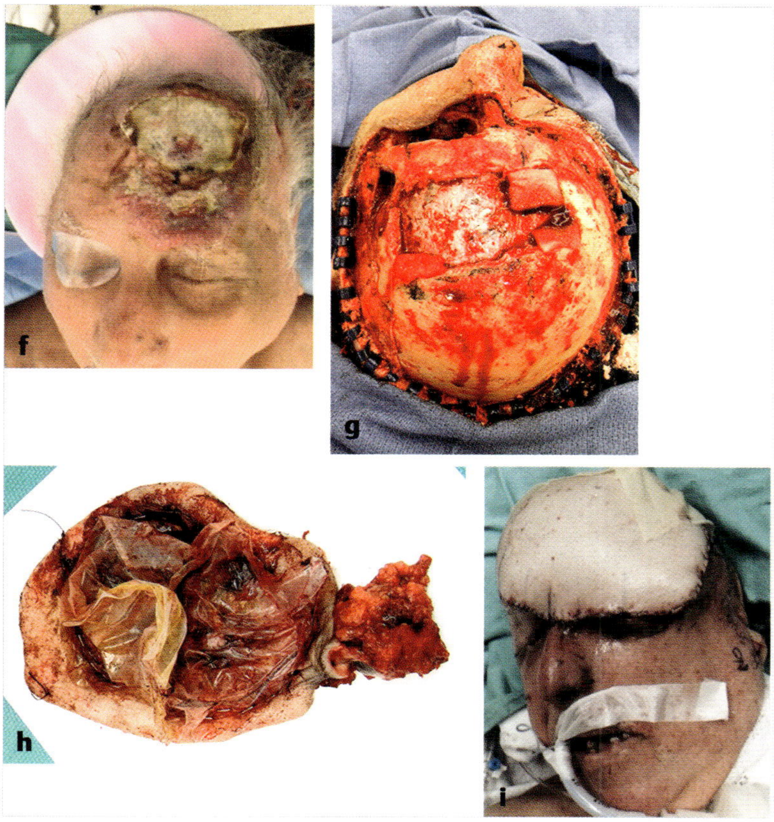

Fig. 6.10 (*continued*) **(f)** Crust and hemorrhage cleaned off and patient prepared for tumor extirpation. **(g)** Defect. **(h)** "A" layer for peripheral margin assessment by Mohs micrographic surgery. **(i)** Repair of defect.

latissimus myofascial free flaps (▶ Fig. 6.10i). The patient was discharged to a skill nursing facility and plans to follow up with radiation oncology. At nine-month follow up, patient's flap was healing well with no signs of recurrence.

6.8 Conclusion

The beauty of the MMS technique lays in the simplicity of each step that, when integrated, has transformed our view and consequent expectations of margin assessment in surgical cutaneous oncology. This is reflected in the highest cure rates of NMSC with MMS in both primary and recurrent tumors while simultaneously achieving maximal tissue conservation. For appropriate tumors, it is a cost-effective surgery that allows tumor clearance and reconstruction on the same day. Most commonly, this is done in the outpatient setting with local anesthesia. Patients also value these advantages and are very satisfied with the procedure.[63] In more complex cases, a multidisciplinary team involving Mohs surgery for the extirpation of the tumor and/or tissue processing is invaluable for complete margin control with conservation of tissue, followed by reconstruction expertise of colleagues in other surgical subspecialties.

References

[1] Rowe DE, Carroll RJ, Day CL, Jr. Prognostic factors for local recurrence, metastasis, and survival rates in squamous cell carcinoma of the skin, ear, and lip. Implications for treatment modality selection. J Am Acad Dermatol. 1992; 26 (6):976–990

[2] Kwon SY, Miller SJ. Mohs surgery for melanoma in situ. Dermatol Clin. 2011; 29(2):175–183, vii–viii

[3] Love WE, Bernhard JD, Bordeaux JS. Topical imiquimod or fluorouracil therapy for basal and squamous cell carcinoma: a systematic review. Arch Dermatol. 2009; 145(12):1431–1438

[4] Gollnick H, Barona CG, Frank RG, et al. Recurrence rate of superficial basal cell carcinoma following treatment with imiquimod 5% cream: conclusion of a 5-year long-term follow-up study in Europe. Eur J Dermatol. 2008; 18(6):677–682

[5] Peris K, Micantonio T, Fargnoli MC, Lozzi GP, Chimenti S. Imiquimod 5% cream in the treatment of Bowen's disease and invasive squamous cell carcinoma. J Am Acad Dermatol. 2006; 55(2):324–327

[6] Van Meurs T, Van Doorn R, Kirtschig G. Treatment of lentigo maligna with imiquimod cream: a long-term follow-up study of 10 patients. Dermatol Surg. 2010; 36(6):853–858

[7] Woodmansee CS, McCall MW. Recurrence of lentigo maligna and development of invasive melanoma after treatment of lentigo maligna with imiquimod. Dermatol Surg. 2009; 35(8):1286–1289

[8] Bargman H, Hochman J. Topical treatment of Bowen's disease with 5-Fluorouracil. J Cutan Med Surg. 2003; 7(2):101–105

[9] Rowe DE, Carroll RJ, Day CL, Jr. Long-term recurrence rates in previously untreated (primary) basal cell carcinoma: implications for patient follow-up. J Dermatol Surg Oncol. 1989; 15(3):315–328

[10] Rowe DE, Carroll RJ, Day CL, Jr. Mohs surgery is the treatment of choice for recurrent (previously treated) basal cell carcinoma. J Dermatol Surg Oncol. 1989; 15(4):424–431

[11] Roenigk RK, Roenigk HH, Jr. Current surgical management of skin cancer in dermatology. J Dermatol Surg Oncol. 1990; 16(2):136–151

[12] Hanke CW, Moy RL, Roenigk RK, et al. Current status of surgery in dermatology. J Am Acad Dermatol. 2013; 69(6):972–1001

[13] Bennett RG. The meaning and significance of tissue margins. Adv Dermatol. 1989; 4:343–355, discussion 356–357

[14] Abide JM, Nahai F, Bennett RG. The meaning of surgical margins. Plast Reconstr Surg. 1984; 73(3):492–497

[15] Rapini RP. Comparison of methods for checking surgical margins. J Am Acad Dermatol. 1990; 23(2, Pt 1):288–294

[16] Kimyai-Asadi A, Goldberg LH, Jih MH. Accuracy of serial transverse cross-sections in detecting residual basal cell carcinoma at the surgical margins of an elliptical excision specimen. J Am Acad Dermatol. 2005; 53(3):469–474

[17] Hanke CW, Menn H, O'Brian JJ. Chemosurgical reports: frozen-section processing with the Miami special. J Dermatol Surg Oncol. 1983; 9(4):260–262

[18] Hanke CW, Lee MW. Cryostat use and tissue processing in Mohs micrographic surgery. J Dermatol Surg Oncol. 1989; 15(1):29–32

[19] Rogers HW, Coldiron BM. Analysis of skin cancer treatment and costs in the United States Medicare population, 1996–2008. Dermatol Surg. 2013; 39(1, Pt 1):35–42

[20] van Loo E, Mosterd K, Krekels GA, et al. Surgical excision versus Mohs' micrographic surgery for basal cell carcinoma of the face: a randomised clinical trial with 10 year follow-up. Eur J Cancer. 2014; 50(17):3011–3020

[21] Mikhail GR. Cancers, precancers, and pseudocancers on the male genitalia. A review of clinical appearances, histopathology, and management. J Dermatol Surg Oncol. 1980; 6(12):1027–1035

[22] Larson PO. Keratoacanthomas treated with Mohs' micrographic surgery (chemosurgery). A review of forty-three cases. J Am Acad Dermatol. 1987; 16(5, Pt 1):1040–1044

[23] Dawn ME, Dawn AG, Miller SJ. Mohs surgery for the treatment of melanoma in situ: a review. Dermatol Surg. 2007; 33(4):395–402

[24] Bene NI, Healy C, Coldiron BM. Mohs micrographic surgery is accurate 95.1% of the time for melanoma in situ: a prospective study of 167 cases. Dermatol Surg. 2008; 34(5):660–664

[25] Hou JL, Reed KB, Knudson RM, et al. Five-year outcomes of wide excision and Mohs micrographic surgery for primary lentigo maligna in an academic practice cohort. Dermatol Surg. 2015; 41(2):211–218

[26] Davis JL, Randle HW, Zalla MJ, Roenigk RK, Brodland DG. A comparison of Mohs micrographic surgery and wide excision for the treatment of atypical fibroxanthoma. Dermatol Surg. 1997; 23(2):105–110

[27] Ratner D, Thomas CO, Johnson TM, et al. Mohs micrographic surgery for the treatment of dermatofibrosarcoma protuberans. Results of a multiinstitutional series with an analysis of the extent of microscopic spread. J Am Acad Dermatol. 1997; 37(4):600–613

[28] Gloster HM, Jr, Harris KR, Roenigk RK. A comparison between Mohs micrographic surgery and wide surgical excision for the treatment of dermatofibrosarcoma protuberans. J Am Acad Dermatol. 1996; 35(1):82–87

[29] Snow SN, Gordon EM, Larson PO, Bagheri MM, Bentz ML, Sable DB. Dermatofibrosarcoma protuberans: a report on 29 patients treated by Mohs micrographic surgery with long-term follow-up and review of the literature. Cancer. 2004; 101(1):28–38

[30] Boyer JD, Zitelli JA, Brodland DG, D'Angelo G. Local control of primary Merkel cell carcinoma: review of 45 cases treated with Mohs micrographic surgery with and without adjuvant radiation. J Am Acad Dermatol. 2002; 47(6):885–892

[31] Snow S, Madjar DD, Hardy S, et al. Microcystic adnexal carcinoma: report of 13 cases and review of the literature. Dermatol Surg. 2001; 27(4):401–408

[32] Leibovitch I, Huilgol SC, Selva D, Lun K, Richards S, Paver R. Microcystic adnexal carcinoma: treatment with Mohs micrographic surgery. J Am Acad Dermatol. 2005; 52(2):295–300

[33] Chiller K, Passaro D, Scheuller M, Singer M, McCalmont T, Grekin RC. Microcystic adnexal carcinoma: forty-eight cases, their treatment, and their outcome. Arch Dermatol. 2000; 136(11):1355–1359

[34] Spencer JM, Nossa R, Tse DT, Sequeira M. Sebaceous carcinoma of the eyelid treated with Mohs micrographic surgery. J Am Acad Dermatol. 2001; 44(6):1004–1009

[35] O'Connor WJ, Lim KK, Zalla MJ, et al. Comparison of mohs micrographic surgery and wide excision for extramammary Paget's disease. Dermatol Surg. 2003; 29(7):723–727

[36] Humphreys TR, Finkelstein DH, Lee JB. Superficial leiomyosarcoma treated with Mohs micrographic surgery. Dermatol Surg. 2004; 30(1):108–112

[37] Schell AE, Russell MA, Park SS. Suggested excisional margins for cutaneous malignant lesions based on Mohs micrographic surgery. JAMA Facial Plast Surg. 2013; 15(5):337–343

[38] Connolly SM, Baker DR, Coldiron BM, et al. Ad Hoc Task Force, Ratings Panel. AAD/ACMS/ASDSA/ASMS 2012 appropriate use criteria for Mohs micrographic surgery: a report of the American Academy of Dermatology, American College of Mohs Surgery, American Society for Dermatologic Surgery Association, and the American Society for Mohs Surgery. J Am Acad Dermatol. 2012; 67(4):531–550

[39] National Comprehensive Cancer Network. NCCN clinical guidelines in oncology: basal and squamous cell skin cancers (Version 2.2014). October 4, 2014. http://www.nccn.org/professionals/physician_gls/pdf/nmsc.pdf

[40] Whalen J, Leone D. Mohs micrographic surgery for the treatment of malignant melanoma. Clin Dermatol. 2009; 27(6):597–602

[41] Zalla MJ, Lim KK, Dicaudo DJ, Gagnot MM. Mohs micrographic excision of melanoma using immunostains. Dermatol Surg. 2000; 26(8):771–784

[42] Cohen LM, McCall MW, Zax RH. Mohs micrographic surgery for lentigo maligna and lentigo maligna melanoma. A follow-up study. Dermatol Surg. 1998; 24(6):673–677

[43] Zitelli JA, Brown C, Hanusa BH. Mohs micrographic surgery for the treatment of primary cutaneous melanoma. J Am Acad Dermatol. 1997; 37(2, Pt 1):236–245

[44] Bricca GM, Brodland DG, Ren D, Zitelli JA. Cutaneous head and neck melanoma treated with Mohs micrographic surgery. J Am Acad Dermatol. 2005; 52(1):92–100

[45] Abdelmalek M, Loosemore MP, Hurt MA, Hruza G. Geometric staged excision for the treatment of lentigo maligna and lentigo maligna melanoma: a long-term experience with literature review. Arch Dermatol. 2012; 148(5):599–604

[46] Huilgol SC, Selva D, Chen C, et al. Surgical margins for lentigo maligna and lentigo maligna melanoma: the technique of mapped serial excision. Arch Dermatol. 2004; 140(9):1087–1092

[47] Johnson TM, Headington JT, Baker SR, Lowe L. Usefulness of the staged excision for lentigo maligna and lentigo maligna melanoma: the "square" procedure. J Am Acad Dermatol. 1997; 37(5, Pt 1):758–764

[48] National Comprehensive Cancer Network. NCCN clinical guidelines in oncology. October 4, 2014. http://www.nccn.org/professionals/physician_gls/f_guidelines.asp

[49] Coldiron B. Commentary: implementation of the appropriate-use criteria will not increase Mohs micrographic surgery utilization. J Am Acad Dermatol. 2014; 71(1):36–37

[50] Tierney EP, Hanke CW. Cost effectiveness of Mohs micrographic surgery: review of the literature. J Drugs Dermatol. 2009; 8(10):914–922

[51] Seidler AM, Bramlette TB, Washington CV, Szeto H, Chen SC. Mohs versus traditional surgical excision for facial and auricular nonmelanoma skin cancer: an analysis of cost-effectiveness. Dermatol Surg. 2009; 35(11):1776–1787

[52] Cook J, Zitelli JA. Mohs micrographic surgery: a cost analysis. J Am Acad Dermatol. 1998; 39(5, Pt 1):698–703

[53] Ravitskiy L, Brodland DG, Zitelli JA. Cost analysis: Mohs micrographic surgery. Dermatol Surg. 2012; 38(4):585–594

[54] Alam M, Ricci D, Havey J, Rademaker A, Witherspoon J, West DP. Safety of peak serum lidocaine concentration after Mohs micrographic surgery: a prospective cohort study. J Am Acad Dermatol. 2010; 63(1):87–92

[55] Mason SE, Noel-Storr A, Ritchie CW. The impact of general and regional anesthesia on the incidence of post-operative cognitive dysfunction and post-operative delirium: a systematic review with meta-analysis. J Alzheimers Dis. 2010; 22 Suppl 3:67–79

[56] Pedersen T, Eliasen K, Henriksen E. A prospective study of mortality associated with anaesthesia and surgery: risk indicators of mortality in hospital. Acta Anaesthesiol Scand. 1990; 34(3):176–182

[57] Lam C, Wilkinson M, Billingsley E. Mohs micrographic surgery for cutaneous metastasis of breast cancer. Dermatol Surg. 2013; 39(10):1537–1539

[58] Maragh SL, Otley CC, Roenigk RK, Phillips PK, Division of Dermatologic Surgery, Mayo Clinic, Rochester, MN. Antibiotic prophylaxis in dermatologic surgery: updated guidelines. Dermatol Surg. 2005; 31(1):83–91

[59] Cook-Norris RH, Michaels JD, Weaver AL, et al. Complications of cutaneous surgery in patients taking clopidogrel-containing anticoagulation. J Am Acad Dermatol. 2011; 65(3):584–591

[60] Bordeaux JS, Martires KJ, Goldberg D, Pattee SF, Fu P, Maloney ME. Prospective evaluation of dermatologic surgery complications including patients on multiple antiplatelet and anticoagulant medications. J Am Acad Dermatol. 2011; 65(3):576–583

[61] Vidimos AT, Stultz TW. Imaging in cutaneous oncology: radiology for dermies. Dermatol Clin. 2011; 29(2):243–260, ix

[62] Alam M, Lee A, Ibrahimi OA, et al. Cutaneous Surgery Consensus Group. A multistep approach to improving biopsy site identification in dermatology: physician, staff, and patient roles based on a Delphi consensus. JAMA Dermatol. 2014; 150(5):550–558

[63] Chuang GS, Leach BC, Wheless L, Lang PG, Cook J. Preoperative expectations and values of patients undergoing Mohs micrographic surgery. Dermatol Surg. 2011; 37(3):311–319

[64] Jih MH, Friedman PM, Goldberg LH, Kimyai-Asadi A. Curettage prior to Mohs' micrographic surgery for previously biopsied nonmelanoma skin cancers: what are we curetting? Retrospective, prospective, and comparative study. Dermatol Surg. 2005; 31(1):10–15

[65] Thornton SL, Beck B. Setting up the Mohs surgery laboratory. Dermatol Clin. 2011; 29(2):331–340, xi

[66] Todd MM, Lee JW, Marks VJ. Rapid toluidine blue stain for Mohs' micrographic surgery. Dermatol Surg. 2005; 31(2):244–245

[67] Silapunt S, Peterson SR, Alcalay J, Goldberg LH. Mohs tissue mapping and processing: a survey study. Dermatol Surg. 2003; 29(11):1109–1112, discussion 1112

[68] Cartee TV, Monheit GD. How many sections are required to clear a tumor? Results from a web-based survey of margin thresholds in Mohs micrographic surgery. Dermatol Surg. 2013; 39(2):179–186

[69] Ellner KM, Goldberg LH, Sperber J. Comparison of cosmesis following healing by surgical closure and second intention. J Dermatol Surg Oncol. 1987; 13 (9):1016–1020

[70] Sniezek PJ, Brodland DG, Zitelli JA. A randomized controlled trial comparing acetaminophen, acetaminophen and ibuprofen, and acetaminophen and codeine for postoperative pain relief after Mohs surgery and cutaneous reconstruction. Dermatol Surg. 2011; 37(7):1007–1013

[71] Alam M, Ibrahim O, Nodzenski M, et al. Adverse events associated with mohs micrographic surgery: multicenter prospective cohort study of 20,821 cases at 23 centers. JAMA Dermatol. 2013; 149(12):1378–1385

[72] Merritt BG, Lee NY, Brodland DG, Zitelli JA, Cook J. The safety of Mohs surgery: a prospective multicenter cohort study. J Am Acad Dermatol. 2012; 67 (6):1302–1309

[73] Whitaker DC, Grande DJ, Johnson SS. Wound infection rate in dermatologic surgery. J Dermatol Surg Oncol. 1988; 14(5):525–528

[74] Randle HW, Zitelli J, Brodland DG, Roenigk RK. Histologic preparation for Mohs micrographic surgery. The single section method. J Dermatol Surg Oncol. 1993; 19(6):522–524

[75] Arnon O, Rapini RP, Mamelak AJ, Goldberg LH. Mohs micrographic surgery: current techniques. Isr Med Assoc J. 2010; 12(7):431–435

[76] Trimble JS, Cherpelis BS. Rapid immunostaining in Mohs: current applications and attitudes. Dermatol Surg. 2013; 39(1, Pt 1):56–63

[77] El Tal AK, Abrou AE, Stiff MA, Mehregan DA. Immunostaining in Mohs micrographic surgery: a review. Dermatol Surg. 2010; 36(3):275–290

[78] Miller CJ, Sobanko JF, Zhu X, Nunnciato T, Urban CR. Special stains in Mohs surgery. Dermatol Clin. 2011; 29(2):273–286, ix

[79] Dobke MK, Miller SH. Tissue repair after Mohs surgery. A plastic surgeon's view. Dermatol Surg. 1997; 23(11):1061–1066

7 Role of Radiotherapy in the Treatment of Skin Malignancies

Shlomo A. Koyfman, Bindu V. Manyam, Nikhil Purushottam Joshi, and Sue S. Yom

7.1 Introduction

Non-melanomatous skin cancers (NMSC), specifically basal cell carcinoma (BCC) and squamous cell carcinoma (SCC), are the most common malignancies in the United States. They are primarily managed surgically and carry an excellent prognosis, with a 1 to 5% rate of disease recurrence after complete excision and only exceedingly rare instances of distant metastasis. Historically, radiotherapy played a prominent role in the definitive management of these cancers as an alternative to surgical resection, especially in cosmetically sensitive areas. With the improvement in surgical techniques in recent decades, especially the widespread use of Mohs micrographic surgery (MMS), the use of curative radiation for skin cancers has declined. However, radiation is still commonly used in the definitive setting for patients with NMSC who are poor surgical candidates or have larger lesions in cosmetically sensitive regions of the face, and in the postoperative setting for more advanced tumors that have high-risk pathologic features that are associated with excessive risks of locoregional recurrence after surgery alone. Radiotherapy plays a similar role in the postoperative management of cutaneous melanoma. Radiation also offers excellent palliation for noncurable patients. This chapter reviews common indications, dose and fractionation schedules, techniques, and oncologic and cosmetic outcomes for radiotherapy for NMSC and melanoma (▶ Fig. 7.1).

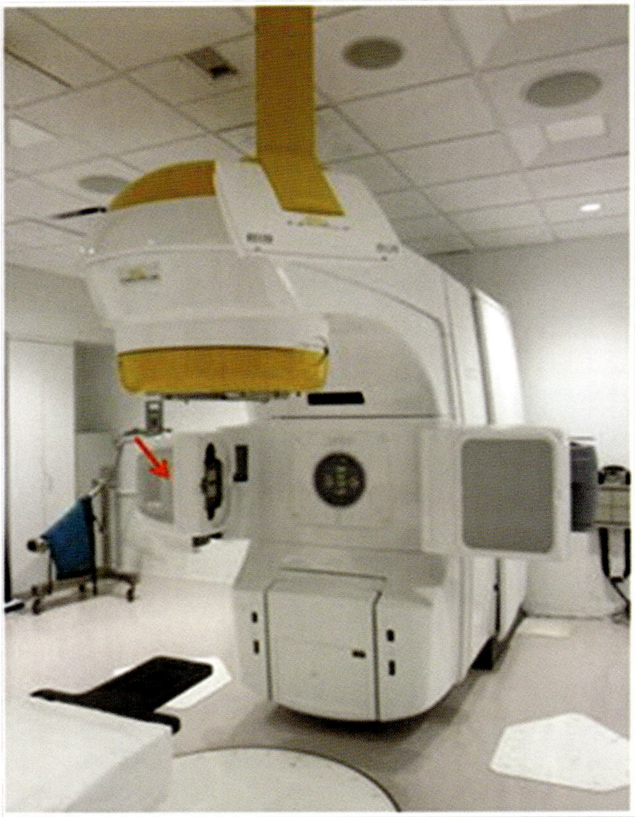

Fig. 7.1 A modern linear accelerator, capable of delivering photon and electron radiotherapy with image guidance provided by cone beam CT (red arrow).

7.2 Indications for Radiotherapy for NMSC

7.2.1 Indications for Definitive Radiotherapy

Both surgery and RT can offer excellent cure rates for the management of early-stage NMSC. Surgery is typically the preferred method of treatment, given it can be performed in a single session, and has been associated with superior oncologic and cosmetic outcomes. One prospective randomized study compared the outcomes of MMS and definitive RT in 347 patients with less than 4 cm BCC of the face. The local failure rate was 0.7% for patients treated with MMS and 7.5% for patients treated with RT. Additionally, the cosmetic outcome was rated "good" or better more often in those patients who underwent surgery (87 vs. 69%).[1] Though the technique of RT was not controlled (55% received interstitial brachytherapy and 45% received orthovoltage therapy), which could have affected the quality of the comparison, as the only randomized study, this trial remains pivotal in guiding medical decision making.

A variety of factors can influence the decision to favor RT rather than surgery for NMSC. Typical contraindications to definitive RT include very large tumors and those with bone and/or cartilage invasion, given that control rates are typically inferior, as well as recurrent tumors that have been previously radiated or arise in an area of previous radiotherapy. Radiation should also be avoided in patients with genetic radiosensitivity syndromes, such as xeroderma pigmentosum and basal cell nevus syndrome, and in those with active connective tissue diseases, such as scleroderma and systemic lupus erythematosus.[2] Patients who are candidates for definitive RT include those with unresectable disease, older patients with comorbidities limiting their surgical options, and patients with lesions involving the eyelid, canthi of the eye (especially those who carry surgical risk to the lacrimal duct), external ear (▶ Fig. 7.2 and ▶ Fig. 7.3), nose (▶ Fig. 7.4 and ▶ Fig. 7.5), brow (▶ Fig. 7.6), temple (▶ Fig. 7.7), or lip, which may incur significant cosmetic or functional defects from surgical resection.

A robust literature, much of it older when RT was more commonly used, supports the safety and efficacy of definitive RT for many of these aforementioned types of patients. A review of

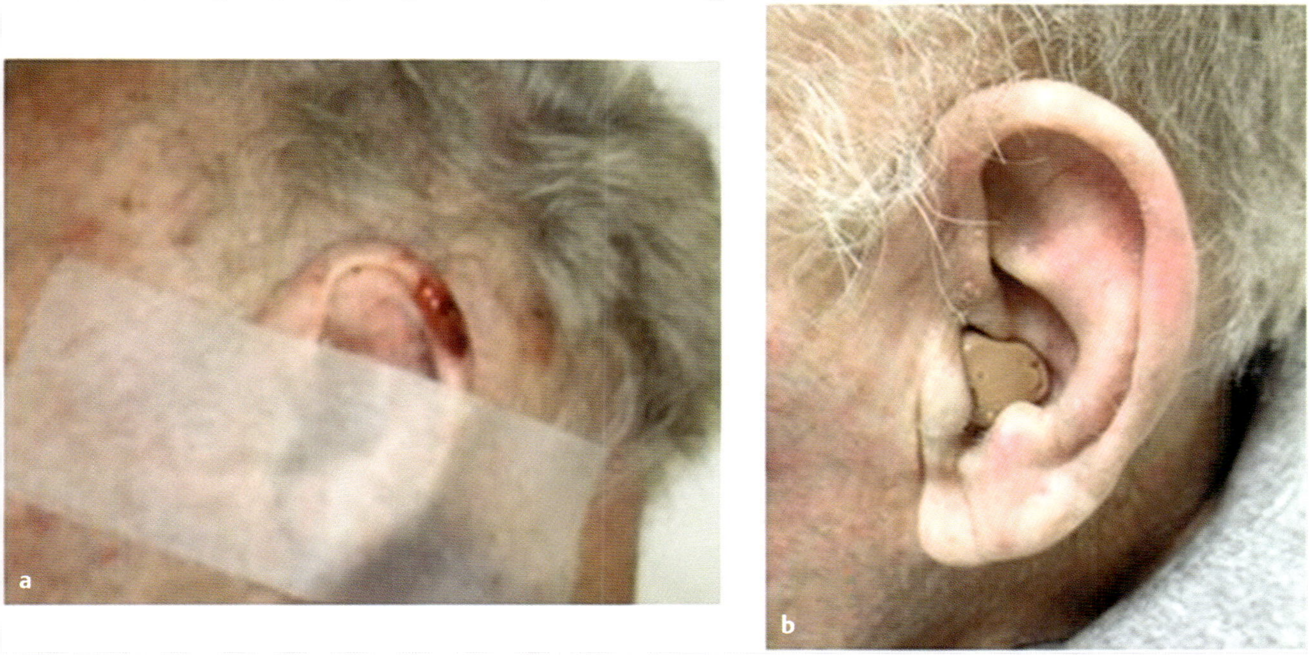

Fig. 7.2 **(a)** SCC of the helix of the left ear with bleeding (baseline). **(b)** After treatment with definitive radiation therapy (50 Gy in 20 fractions with electrons). There was complete remission with excellent cosmesis.

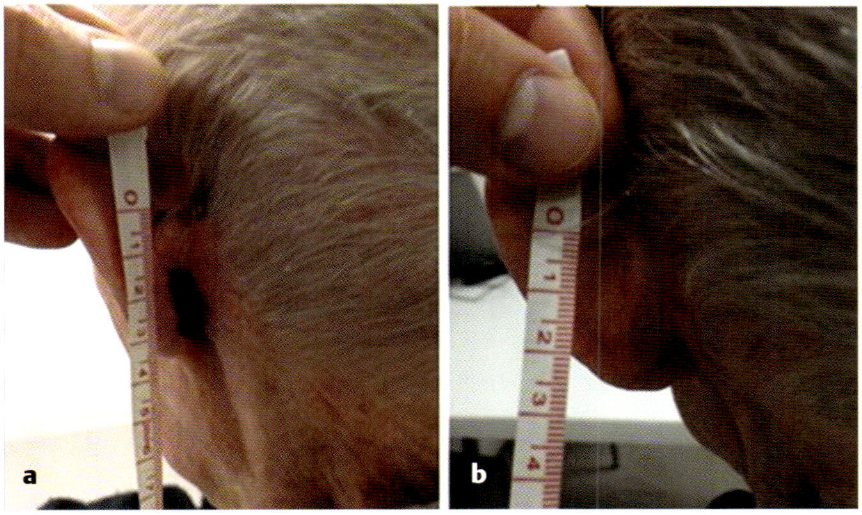

Fig. 7.3 **(a)** A 96-year-old patient with right retroauricular BCC, T2N0M0 (baseline). **(b)** One month after treatment with definitive radiation therapy (50 Gy in 20 fractions with electrons).

986 BCC and SCC of the skin overlying the eyelid treated with definitive RT demonstrated a 5-year cure rate of 96.4%.[3] A review of 334 BCC and SCC of the external ear at the Princess Margaret Hospital treated with definitive RT demonstrated a 2-year local control rate of 87%, with severe late toxicity noted in only 7% of patients.[4] A review of 100 patients with SCC of the nasal skin at the Princess Margaret Hospital treated with definitive RT demonstrated a 2-year local control rate of 90%, with no severe toxicities observed.[5]

While definitive RT monotherapy can provide effective tumor control for T1–3N0 NMSC, T4 tumors and those with nodal metastases demonstrate inferior outcomes. Initial surgical management is recommended in these patients, often followed by adjuvant radiotherapy. T4 disease is defined as tumor invasion into the axial or appendicular skeleton or perineural invasion (PNI) of the skull base. The University of Florida reported a local control rate of just 53% at 5 years in patients with T4 BCC and SCC.[6,7] In a review of 68 T4 BCC and SCC of the skin of the head and neck treated with definitive RT, local control rates were lower in patients with recurrent disease, compared to primary lesions (41 vs. 67%; $p = 0.07$) and the three most important prognostic indicators for inferior local control and cause-specific survival rates were bone involvement ($p < 0.01$), recurrent lesions ($p < 0.01$), and nerve involvement ($p < 0.02$).[6]

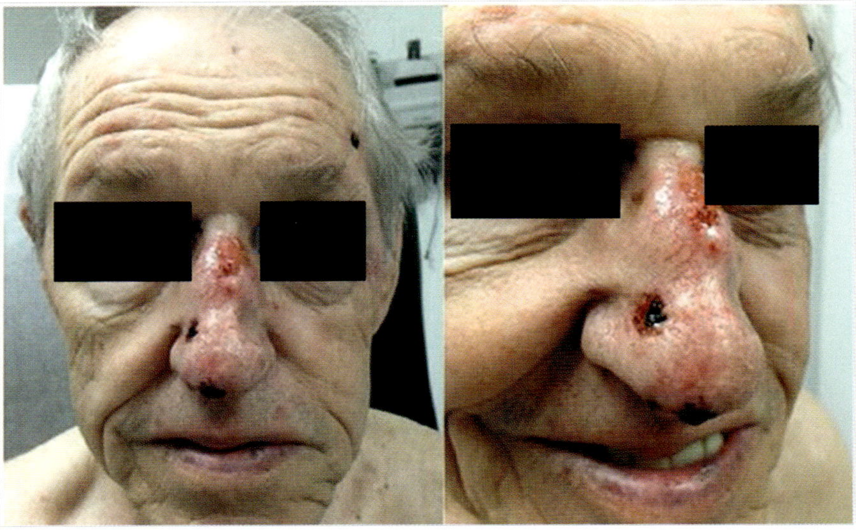

Fig. 7.4 A patient with multifocal BCC (baseline).

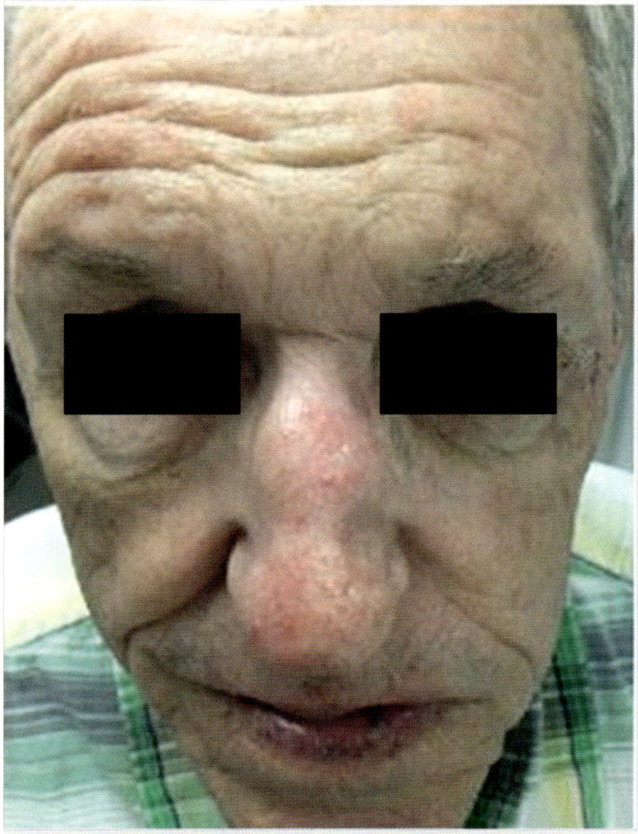

Fig. 7.5 A patient with multifocal BCC 3 months after treatment with definitive radiation therapy (40 Gy in 10 fractions with electrons).

Even the more favorable lesions had local control rates of less than 70%. Similarly, a large retrospective review which included 531 BCC and SCC treated with definitive RT demonstrated local control rates of 94 and 89% for primary BCC and SCC tumors, respectively, and 86 and 68% for BCC and SCC recurrent tumors, respectively.[8] In patients with nodal metastases, locoregional recurrence rates with definitive RT alone range from 30 to 50% and cancer-related mortality is as high as 30%.[9] Such suboptimal outcomes support the use of intensification of treatment and multimodal therapy for these patients with advanced disease. In patients who are not eligible for initial surgical resection, concurrent cisplatin-based chemotherapy can be considered to enhance the effectiveness of radiotherapy. While there is no high-quality evidence demonstrating clear benefit to such an approach in cutaneous malignancies, many head and neck oncologists extrapolate from the mucosal SCC of the head and neck, where concurrent chemotherapy significantly improves disease control and survival in the setting of locally advanced disease treated nonoperatively.[10]

Indications for Postoperative Radiotherapy

Postoperative RT is rarely used for BCC. Patients with BCC have an exceedingly low risk of recurrence after surgery alone, and even patients with a positive margin, focal cartilage invasion, or PNI are often still candidates for close observation and salvage re-resection if needed.[11,12] However, postoperative RT is often considered in cases where there are persistently positive margins after multiple resections, T4 disease that extensively invades bone or soft tissue, lymph node metastasis, or clinically apparent PNI (▶ Fig. 7.8).[13]

Postoperative RT is much more commonly used in resected SCC (▶ Fig. 7.9). Postoperative RT is indicated for patients with high-risk resected disease, such as T4 disease, in transit or satellite metastases, nodal metastases, persistently positive margins, and recurrent disease (▶ Fig. 7.10 and ▶ Fig. 7.11). In addition, patients with two or more intermediate-risk factors, including tumor size greater than 2 cm, poorly differentiated histology, ear and hair-bearing lip location, PNI, and immunosuppressed status, may also benefit from adjuvant RT.

Retrospective data have demonstrated high rates of local recurrence in patients with T4 tumors managed with surgery alone.[7] In addition, the rate of occult lymph node metastasis is high, ranging from 29 to 50%, in patients with advanced T-stage

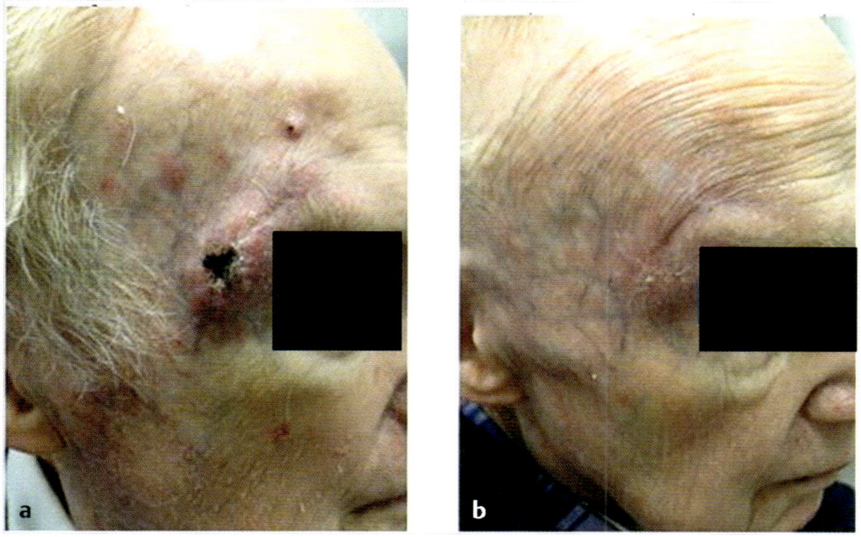

Fig. 7.6 **(a)** A patient with right brow/forehead SCC (baseline). **(b)** One month after definitive radiation therapy (45 Gy in 15 fractions with electrons).

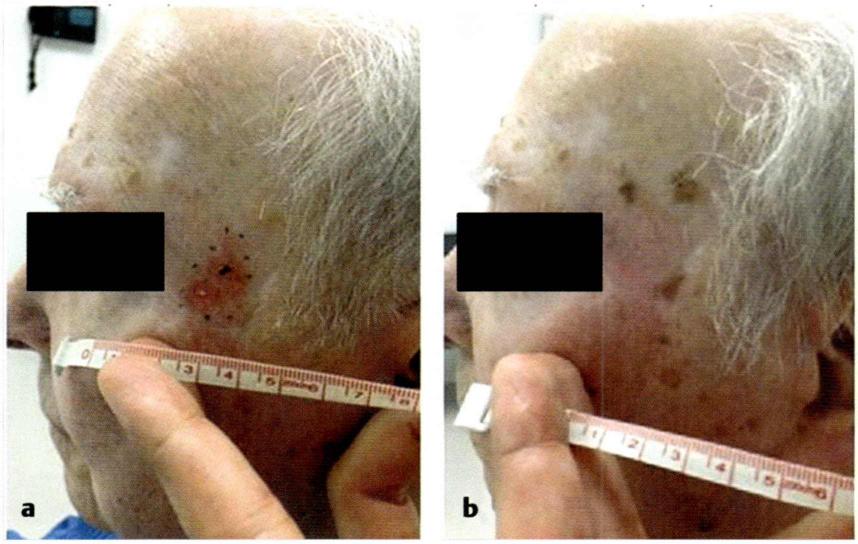

Fig. 7.7 **(a)** An 88-year-old man with left temporal SCC in situ (baseline). **(b)** One month after treatment with definitive radiation therapy (30 Gy in five fractions with electrons).

disease. In patients with deeply infiltrative (≥ 8 mm) tumors, or tumors that extensively invade deep subcutaneous fat, occult lymph node metastasis can be as high as 30%.[9] Patients with recurrent primary tumors, PNI, lymphovascular space invasion, and those that are immunosuppressed are at significantly higher risk for having lymph node metastases and should undergo careful evaluation for regional disease with a contrast-enhanced diagnostic neck computed tomography (CT) and/or a positron emission tomography scan.[14,15,16] In these patients, sentinel lymph node biopsy and/or neck dissection is recommended in conjunction with resection of the primary tumor. Postoperative RT can also be useful as an elective treatment to the undissected neck.

For patients with clinically involved lymph nodes, a therapeutic neck dissection followed by postoperative RT is the current standard of care. Although lymph node metastases are rare in SCC of the skin overall (~ 5%), they are clearly associated with a poor prognosis. After neck dissection alone, locoregional recurrence rates are 11 to 38% and even after multimodality therapy, the 5-year disease-free survival rates are 60 to 70%. Independent predictors of worse survival in this population include increased nodal size ≥ 3 cm, multiple lymph node involvement, extracapsular extension, incompletely excised nodes, and surgery monotherapy.[15,16,17] A review of 167 patients in Australia with SCC metastatic to the parotid or cervical nodes compared outcomes for surgery versus combination of surgery and postoperative RT at a median dose of 60 Gy in 30 fractions. The use of postoperative RT was associated with significantly lower rates of locoregional recurrence (20 vs. 43%), and higher 5-year disease free (73 vs. 54%; $p = 0.004$), and 5-year overall survival (66 vs. 27%; $p = 0.003$) compared to patients who received surgery alone.[16] Similar results supporting the benefit of postoperative RT for locoregional control and 5-year disease-free survival in patients with cutaneous SCC metastatic to lymph nodes and/or periparotid lymph nodes have been reproduced in a number of retrospective reviews.[18,19,20,21] For

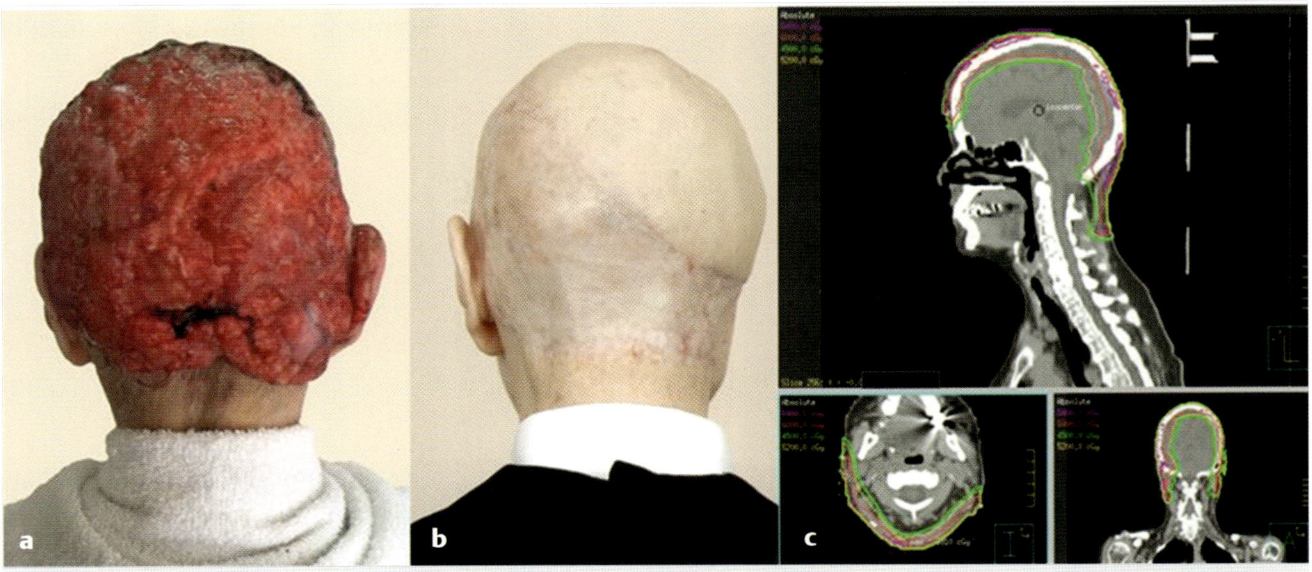

Fig. 7.8 A 75-year-old woman with a neglected T4 basal cell carcinoma of the scalp. **(a)** Preoperative disease. **(b)** Postoperative results after free flap reconstruction and postoperative radiation therapy. **(c)** Postoperative radiation plans (axial, sagittal, and coronal planning CT scans) demonstrating radiation dose distribution.

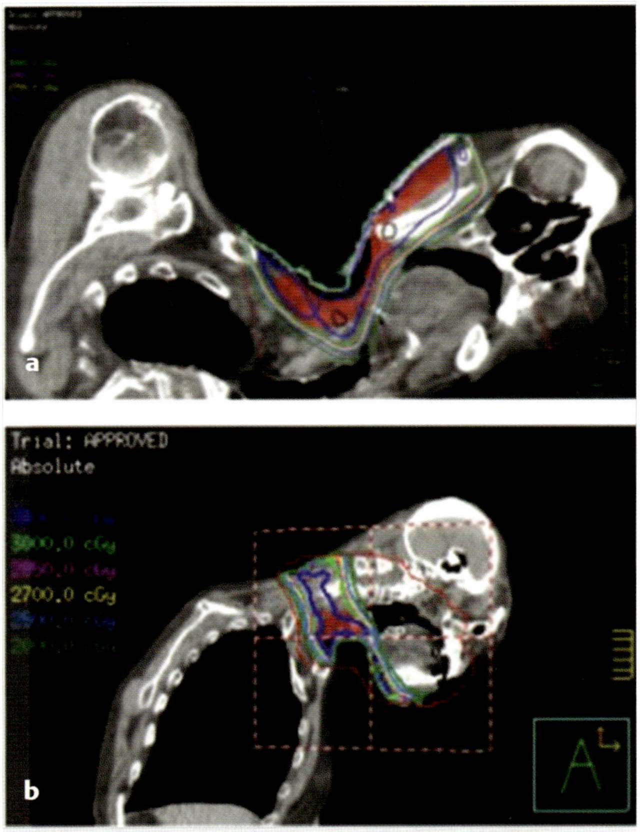

Fig. 7.9 A 91-year-old man with a history of extreme kyphosis and multiple facial SCC, who presented with a rapidly enlarging right neck mass, treated with surgical resection and free flap reconstruction. **(a)** Axial slice depicting isodose coverage of the neck bed with electron radiation therapy. **(b)** Extreme kyphosis dose coverage using 30 Gy in five fractions twice weekly.

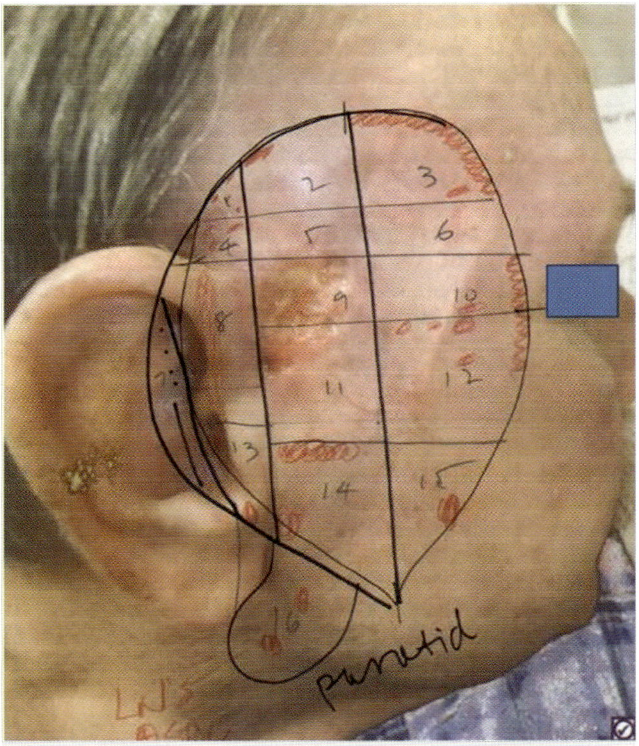

Fig. 7.10 A 63-year-old man with multiple recurrent SCC of the right temple with Mohs map overlying the site of the tumor.

patients who received lymph node dissection for primary SCC located on the trunk or extremities, postoperative RT is typically recommended when multiple nodes are involved or extracapsular extension is present. Similar to mucosal SCC of

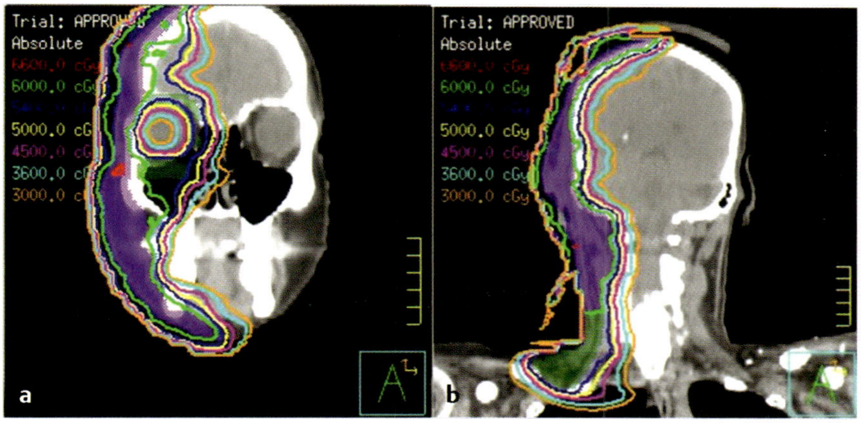

Fig. 7.11 **(a)** Coronal CT slice of dose distribution for postoperative radiation therapy after Mohs surgery for tumor depicted in ▶ Fig. 7.10. **(b)** Coronal slice of dose distribution for postoperative radiation therapy covering the ipsilateral cervical lymph nodes.

the head and neck, RT can be avoided in immunocompetent patients with a single involved lymph node, smaller than 3 cm, without extracapsular extension on parotidectomy or cervical lymph node dissection, as rate of regional recurrence is less than 5%.[22]

PNI, while not common (5–10% of SCC), is another important risk factor for recurrence that should be weighed in the decision to administer adjuvant RT. PNI is typically divided into clinical and microscopic PNI. Clinical PNI is defined by neurologic manifestations, most commonly involving the trigeminal or facial nerves, leading to pain, paresthesias, paralysis, formication (the sensation of bugs crawling on the skin), or radiographic evidence of nerve enhancement.[23,24] Microscopic PNI is appreciated only histologically and is identified after surgery in a patient who was asymptomatic preoperatively. PNI is important given it is associated with increased risks of local recurrence as well as regional and distant metastases. Factors associated with increased risk for SCC with PNI include male sex, tumor size greater than 2 cm, midfacial tumor location, recurrent tumor, and poorly differentiated subtypes.[25] The degree of PNI is predictive of risk of recurrence; therefore, a careful history as well as physical and imaging examination is critical. Magnetic resonance imaging (MRI) has the advantage of identifying the extent of macroscopic disease through nerve enlargement or enhancement or obliteration of the normal fat plane surrounding a nerve (▶ Fig. 7.12). CT offers the advantage of detecting whether bone erosion is present, particularly tumor invasion into foramina associated with cranial nerves.

The difference between clinical and microscopic PNI was highlighted in a series from the University of Florida which compared the outcomes of patients with PNI treated aggressively with surgery and postoperative RT. Those with clinical PNI had significantly lower 5-year rates of local control (57 vs. 90%; $p = < 0.001$) and overall survival (57 vs. 69%; $p = 0.03$) compared to those found to have microscopic PNI.[13,23] RT is therefore always recommended in cases of clinical PNI. The role of postoperative RT in patients with pathologic PNI is less clear. Lin et al found that focal versus extensive microscopic PNI carries different prognoses, with relapse-free survival better in the former group (86 vs. 74%; $p = 0.1$).[24] Unfortunately, the distinction between focal and extensive was not well defined. As such, adjuvant RT is not recommended in immunocompetent patients with nonrecurrent disease, in whom one or two isolated areas of PNI are found in small unnamed nerves, with a diameter of less than 0.1 mm, given the outcome is expected to be fairly good with surgery alone. However, patients with microscopic PNI, that is multifocal, involves larger nerves (> 0.1 mm in diameter) and named nerves, or occurs in immunosuppressed patients, are at higher risk and thus adjuvant RT is recommended.[2,25]

For irradiation of clinical PNI, the clinical target volume should include areas at high risk of failure, specifically the involved nerve, the portion of the nerve proximally at the skull base, the distal skin innervated by the nerve, major communicating branches, and the compartment in which the nerve is embedded.[26] For example, for patients with CN VII involvement, the area of treatment should be tracked back to the nerve's exit through the stylomastoid foramen, with care taken to administer adequate coverage of the geniculate ganglion by avoiding excessive restriction of the radiation dose delivered to the ipsilateral cochlea. Similarly, with V1/V2 nerve involvement, the gasserian ganglion in Meckel cave and the cavernous sinus should be targeted (▶ Fig. 7.13). Targeting the nerve root as it exits the brainstem should be considered for nerves that are radiographically involved at the skull base. For patients with unresectable disease invading the skull base, high-dose radiation (70 Gy), with or without concurrent chemotherapy, is required (▶ Fig. 7.14).

Another consideration highly relevant to radiation field design is the observation that PNI may also be associated with increased nodal failure in addition to recurrence in the tumor bed and along the nerve pathway. Lin et al demonstrated that patients who developed recurrent disease with pathologic PNI had a significantly higher risk of local recurrence (40 vs. 19%; $p < 0.01$) as well as regional recurrence (29 vs. 5%; $p = 0.02$).[24] It is important to consider the location of the lesion in such scenarios, given that tumors on the scalp, for example, may be less likely to metastasize to lymph nodes, compared to cheek, ear, or nasal skin lesions. Understanding the drainage patterns of these tumors is crucial (e.g., parotid nodes for head and neck sites, axilla for trunk and extremity lesions) and should be incorporated into radiation targeting.

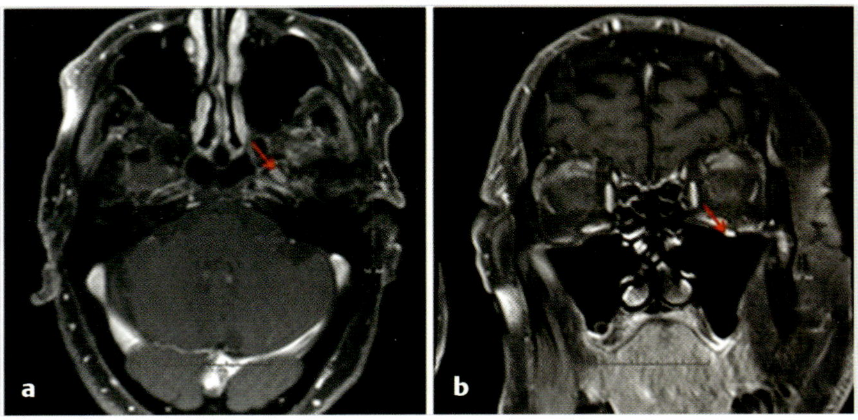

Fig. 7.12 A 64-year-old man with a history of chronic immunosuppression and pT2N0 SCC of left temple treated with surgery, with recurrence involving the trigeminal nerve. **(a)** Left V3 nerve enhancement is demonstrated at the foramen ovale (red arrow). **(b)** Left V2 enhancement is demonstrated at the infraorbital nerve (red arrow), with tracking back into Meckel's cave. He received post-salvage surgery IMRT with concurrent cetuximab with no evidence of disease at 8-month follow-up.

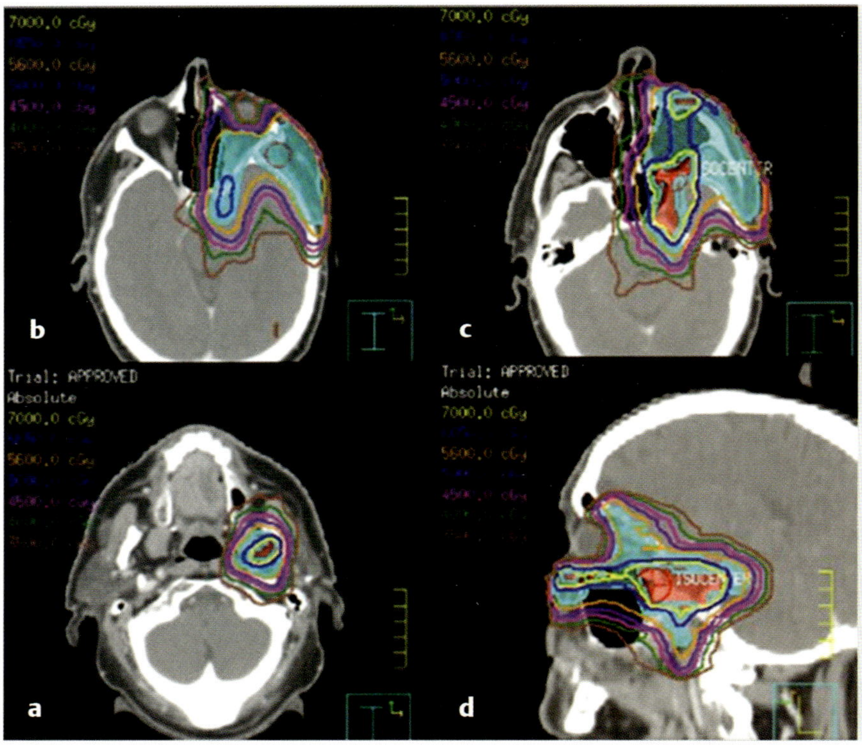

Fig. 7.13 **(a)** Axial radiation planning CT slice depicting inferior alveolar nerve (solid red) covered by isodose lines. **(b)** Axial radiation planning CT slice depicting left cavernous sinus and temporal musculature (solid light blue) covered by isodose lines. **(c)** Axial radiation planning CT slice depicting course of V2 into cavernous sinus (solid red) covered by isodose lines. **(d)** Sagittal radiation planning CT slice depicting coverage of V1 and V2 back to the cavernous sinus (solid red) covered by isodose lines.

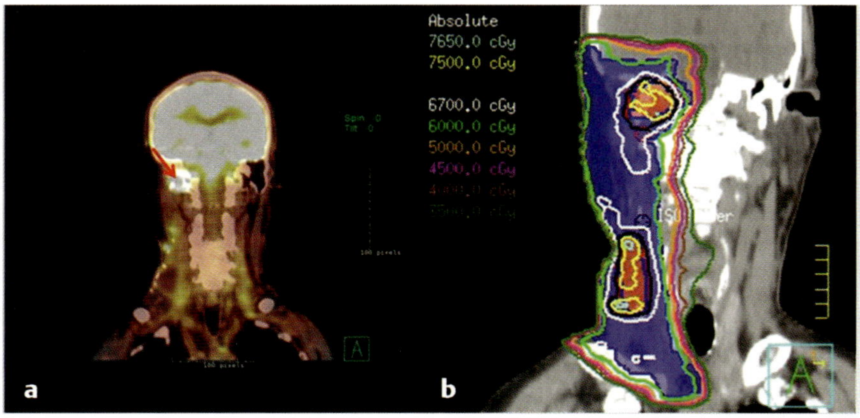

Fig. 7.14 **(a)** A 67-year-old man with history of recurrent right auricular SCC treated with multiple surgical resections and prior irradiation who presented with recurrent disease at the right skull base (red arrow). **(b)** Sagittal radiation planning CT slice depicting recurrent disease covered by 70 Gy isodose line (black line).

7.2.2 Indications for Radiotherapy for Cutaneous Melanoma

Indications for Definitive Radiotherapy

Melanoma is believed to be a relatively radioresistant malignancy. Therefore, maximal surgical resection is paramount in the management of these tumors. RT has limited benefit in achieving long-term control in the presence of gross disease. RT is delivered to gross melanoma in patients deemed to have unresectable disease, or those with rapid postoperative recurrence who have failed surgical management. In these cases, higher doses per fraction are generally preferable and the intent of treatment is largely palliative.

Indications for Postoperative Radiotherapy

Adjuvant radiotherapy to the primary tumor bed, nodal basin, or both, has been studied as a means of reducing locoregional recurrence. If adequate margins are obtained, local recurrence for primary melanoma is infrequent, with rates consistently reported to be less than 5%.[27,28] However, there is a smaller subset of patients with higher rates of failure in the tumor bed, including deeply invasive T4 disease, the presence of satellitosis, the presence of desmoplastic subtype, or persistently positive margins despite multiple attempts at excision. In these cases, adjuvant RT to the primary tumor bed should be considered (▶ Fig. 7.15 and ▶ Fig. 7.16).

O'Brien and colleagues analyzed 629 patients with head and neck melanoma and found that increased local recurrence rates were associated with increased tumor thickness: < 0.76 mm, 2%; 0.76 to 1.49 mm, 5%; 1.5 to 3.99 mm, 15%; and ≥ 4 mm, 20%.[29] Typically, adjuvant RT is considered for T4 tumors, although typically reserved for those with additional high-risk features. One of which is satellitosis, which represents discontiguous sites of disease within 2 cm of the primary tumor and is known to be a marker of increased recurrence risk.[30] Desmoplastic melanoma is a rare histologic subtype (1% of all melanomas) and is characterized by spindle-shaped cells with associated collagen production. This subtype is often associated with perineural spread and local recurrence rates have been reported as high as 20 to 50%.[31,32] In these cases, based on the relatively higher risk for local recurrence, adjuvant RT should be considered.

More extensive literature guides the use of adjuvant RT to nodal basins, both in the elective setting and following lymph node dissection.[33,34] Data supporting the benefit of RT in reducing regional recurrence come from the randomized phase III study by Burmeister et al in which higher risk patients were randomized to surgery and lymph node dissection with or without adjuvant radiation to the nodal basin.[35] Eligible patients had one of the following features associated with increased failure rates:

1. Serum lactate dehydrogenase < 1.5 times the upper limit of normal and the presence of extracapsular extension (ECE).
2. ≥ 1 involved parotid node of any size.
3. ≥ 2 involved cervical nodes and/or ≥ 3 cm of tumor within a node.
4. ≥ 2 involved axillary nodes and/or ≥ 4 cm of tumor within a node.
5. ≥ 3 involved inguinal nodes and/or ≥ 4 cm of tumor within a node, and/or recurrent disease.[27,30]

Importantly, no systemic therapy was delivered in this trial. In the 217 patients included on the study, those who received RT were significantly less likely to experience regional recurrence compared to those in the observation arm (18 vs. 33%; $p = 0.041$). As distant metastasis is the predominant mode of melanoma disease failure, it was not surprising that an improved rate of regional control did not translate into an overall survival average (54 vs. 44%; $p = 0.12$). The most common Grade 3 or 4 adverse events were seroma and wound infections, which were equivalent in both arms.[35] The lack of systemic therapy in this study as well as the lack of a survival difference

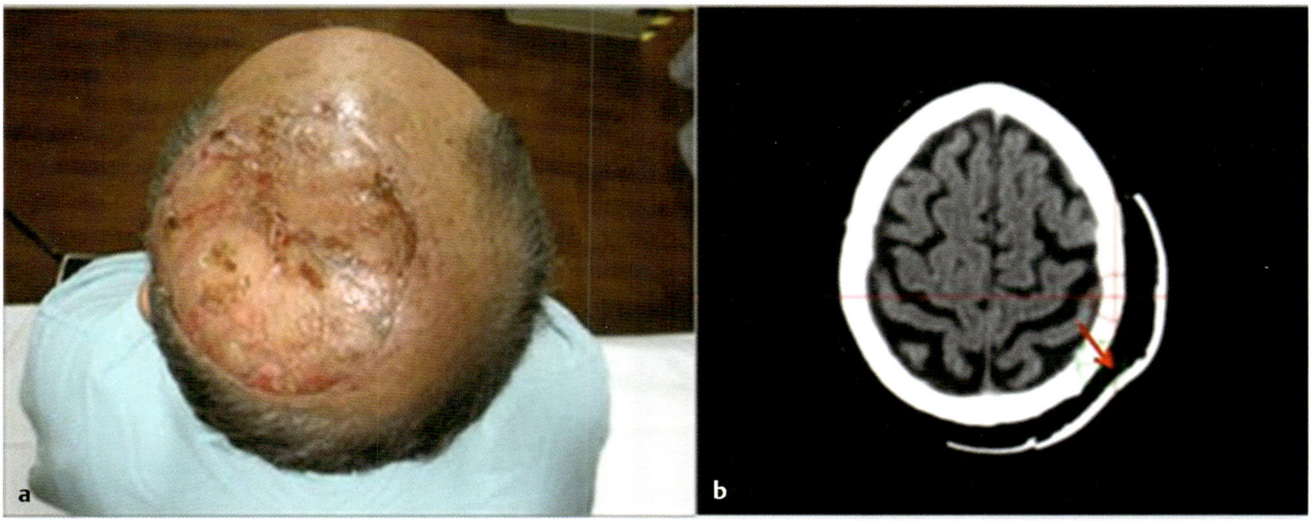

Fig. 7.15 A 72-year-old man with pT3N2cMx melanoma of the scalp with ulceration and satellitosis treated with wide local excision, free flap reconstruction, ipsilateral neck dissection, and adjuvant RT to the primary tumor bed. (a) Postoperative image. (b) Axial radiation planning CT slice demonstrating bolus material (red arrow) for achieving adequate surface dose.

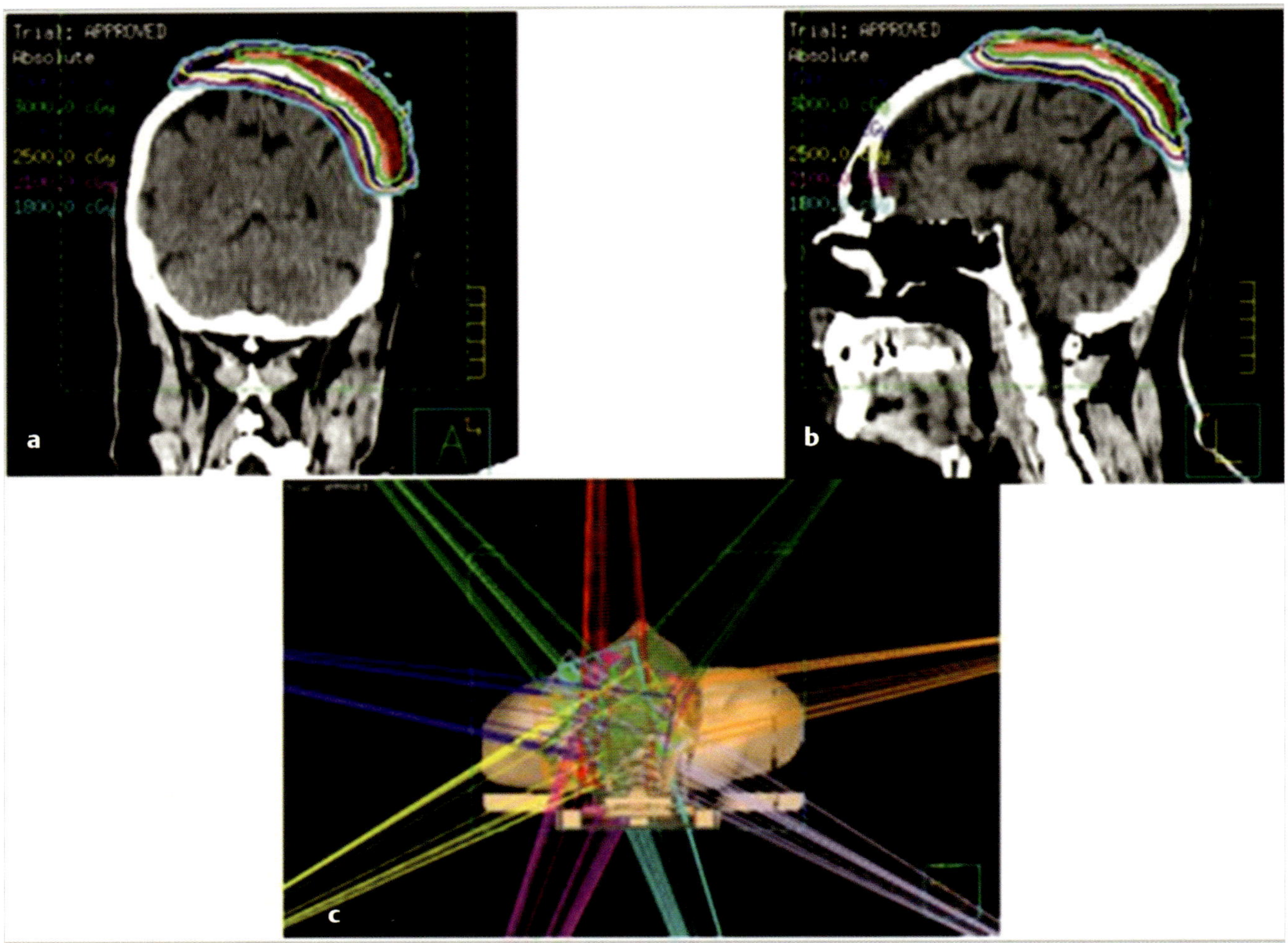

Fig. 7.16 **(a)** Coronal planning CT slice for postoperative radiation therapy to the primary tumor bed for scalp melanoma depicted in Fig. 16.15 with isodose lines covering the target (solid red). **(b)** Sagittal planning CT slice. **(c)** Nine-field intensity modulated radiation therapy arrangement (IMRT).

with the use of RT has raised the question of the true benefit of adjuvant RT for all patients eligible for this study. That said, it reinforces the guiding principle where locoregional control is a priority, and in a case with extensive nodal disease, especially with extranodal extension and significant soft-tissue involvement, adjuvant RT should be considered as a proven way to reduce rates of locoregional recurrence (▶ Fig. 7.17, ▶ Fig. 7.18, and ▶ Fig. 7.19).

7.2.3 Dose and Fractionation Paradigms

A crucial radiobiologic principle underlies the choice of dose and fractionation (the number of treatments chosen to deliver a given dose) for RT for skin cancers. While higher total doses typically yield better tumor control, nominal dose is less important than the radiobiologic effective dose. This refers to the fact that the dose per fraction (fx) also has a highly significant impact on control rates, as a lower total dose delivered using a higher daily dose per fraction can yield equivalent oncologic control rates as higher nominal doses in smaller doses per fraction. For example, while 66 Gy yields higher control rates than 40 to 45 Gy if the daily dose (e.g., 2 Gy) is kept constant, 40 to 45 Gy using 4 to 4.5 Gy per fraction over 10 fractions for 2 weeks has a fairly similar radiobiologic effect as does a total dose of 66 Gy using 2 Gy/fx over 33 treatments over 6.5 weeks.

However, the potential drawback of shorter courses of radiation using higher daily doses is that this schedule also delivers higher doses to normal tissue that overwhelm their repair capacity, leading to a higher risk of long-term side effects. As such, for skin cancer RT, there is a wide array of radiation schedules that are likely equally effective. However, shorter regimens using higher daily doses, while offering superior convenience, may be associated with increased risks of late effects.[36,37] A review of 1,149 irradiated fields for primary NMSC (85.7%) treated with definitive RT doses ranging from 45 to 80 Gy determined that hypopigmentation and telangiectases were the most common cosmetic changes after RT. Ninety days after RT, hypopigmentation was found in 64.7% of patients, telangiectases in 43.1% of patients, erythema in 24.8% of patients, and hyperpigmentation in 16.8% of patients. The frequency of certain cosmetic changes increased with time from RT, with hypopigmentation reported in 91.8% and telangiectases reported in

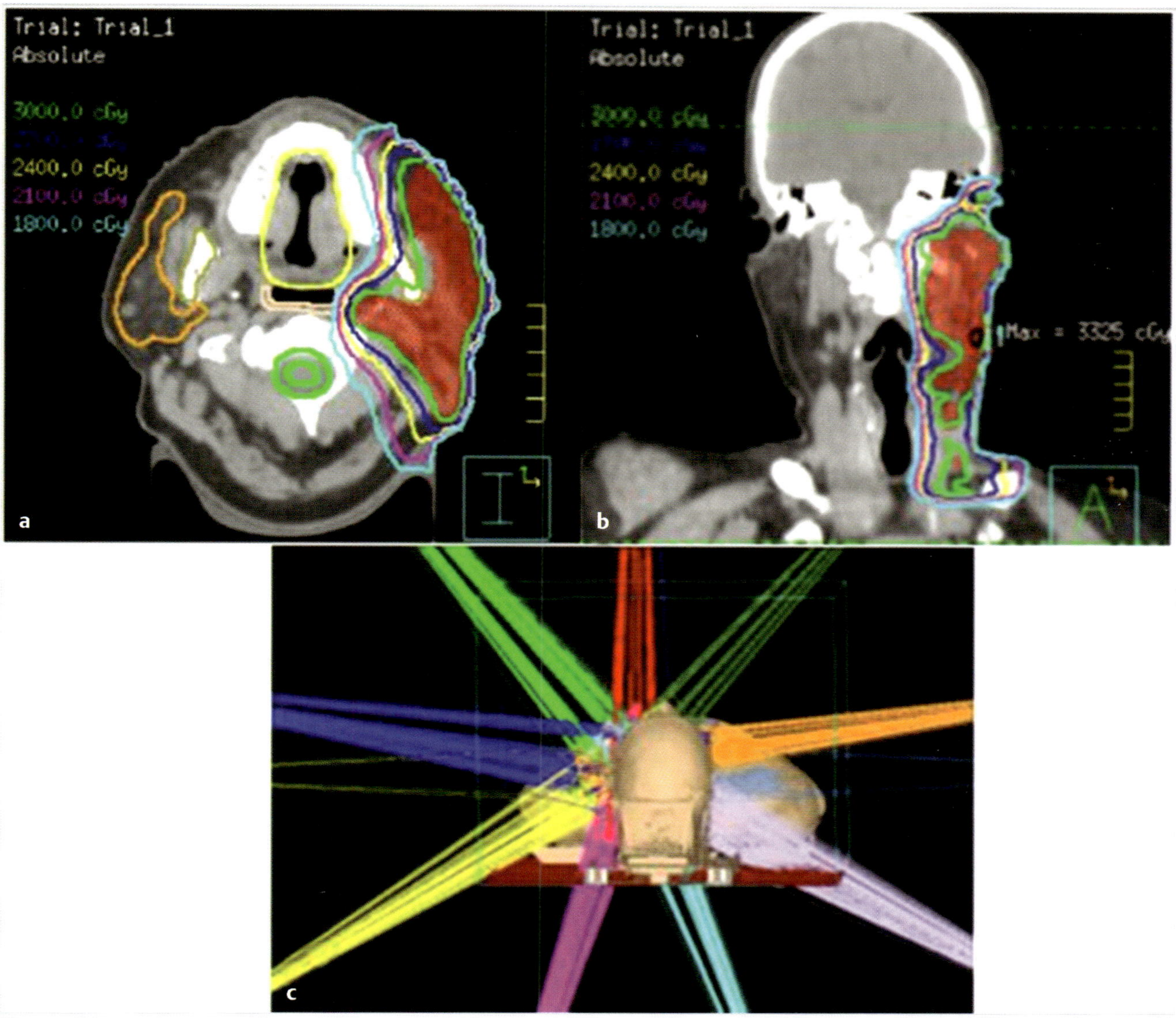

Fig. 7.17 A 40-year-old man with melanoma of the left cheek status treated with wide local excision, superficial parotidectomy, selective lymph node dissection (levels II–V), and postoperative radiation therapy to the primary tumor bed and ipsilateral cervical lymph nodes. **(a)** Axial radiation planning CT slice depicting isodose lines covering target (solid red). The right parotid (orange), oral cavity (yellow), and spinal cord (green) with a safety margin (green) are spared with the use of IMRT. **(b)** Coronal radiation planning CT slice depicting ipsilateral nodal coverage by the isodose lines. **(c)** Nine-field IMRT beam arrangement.

82.2% of patients 4 years after RT. This relationship was not observed for keratosis, erythema, and induration.[38] Modern series using either electron beam RT or electronic brachytherapy techniques report good to excellent cosmesis in 95 to 100% of patients, with low rates of long-term dermatitis, alopecia, or telangiectasias.[37] Other patient-related factors, such as the presence of skin folds within the radiation field, poor nutritional status, tobacco use, and diabetes can all contribute to increased risk for radiation-related morbidity.

While cosmetic outcomes may be significantly better with modern CT-based planning, the fundamental principle of fractionation is still a crucial one when considering the risk of late effects. Therefore, for cosmetically sensitive areas, in regions with adjacent radiosensitive tissue such as cartilaginous, orbital, and neural structures, and in younger patients with extended life spans, longer courses of RT using standard daily doses are preferable. However, for older patients with tumors that are not associated with cartilaginous, orbital, or neural tissues, or those with transportation or socioeconomic limitations, and for lesions in cosmetically noncritical locations, lower total dose RT using higher daily doses over 1 to 3 weeks can be an extremely attractive option.

As such, there are a wide variety of appropriate radiation schedules that can be used in the definitive and postoperative

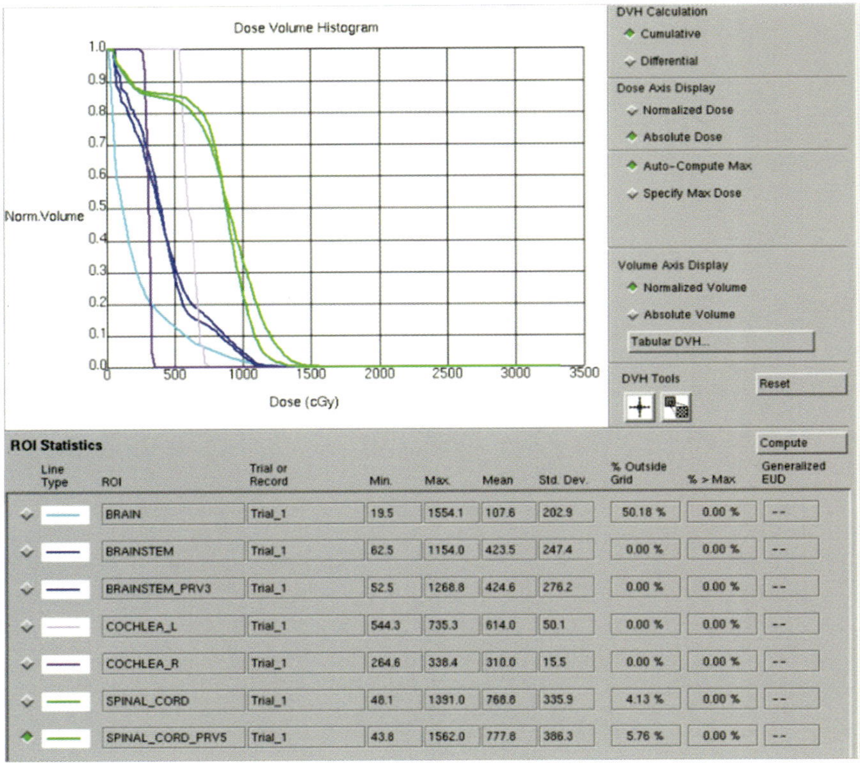

Fig. 7.18 A dose volume histogram illustrating representative normal organs at risk being spared using IMRT for the radiation treatment plan depicted in Fig. 17.17. The doses received by each of these structures are well below their tolerance.

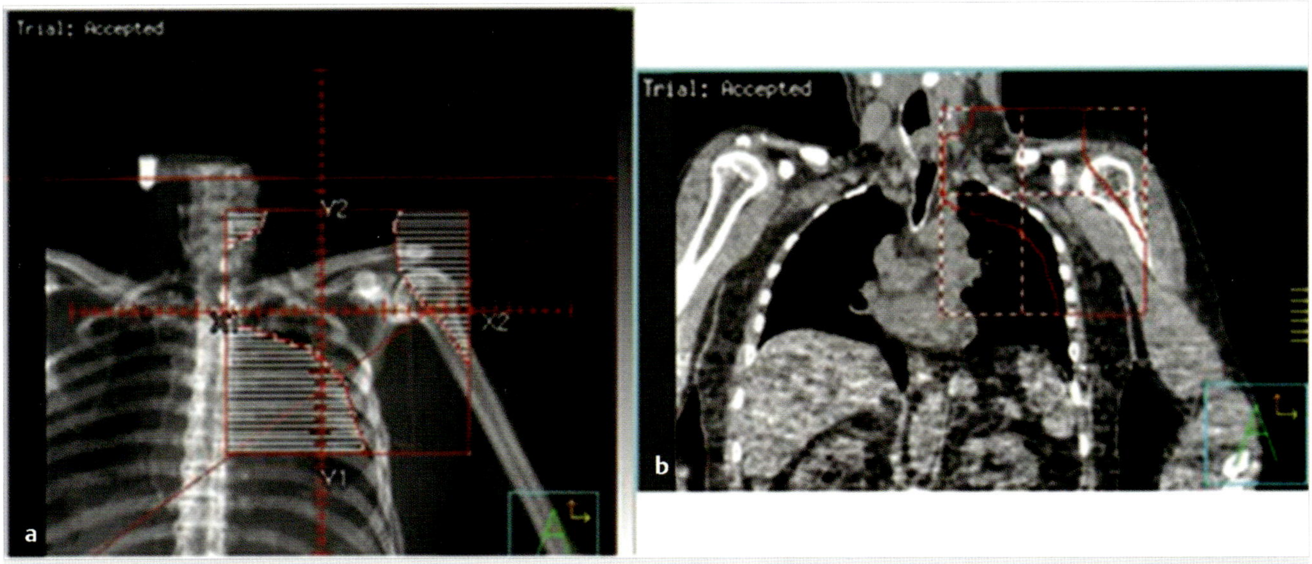

Fig. 7.19 **(a)** Digitally reconstructed radiograph depicting a left axillary radiation field for adjuvant radiation to the axilla for a patient with dermal melanoma. **(b)** Coronal CT image depicting the left axillary radiation treatment field.

settings. However, careful consideration should be given to the tumor size, location, proximity to critical structures, and importance of cosmesis before choosing appropriate dose and fractionation schemes. ▶ Table 7.1 and ▶ Table 7.2 provide representative schedules for the definitive and postoperative settings, respectively. When elective nodes are being targeted, typically 45 to 50 Gy in 1.8 to 2.0 Gy per fraction is appropriate, especially for the groin and axilla, while 54 to 60 Gy in 1.8 to 2.0 Gy per fraction is typically recommended for the head and neck region. Areas with positive margins and/or extracapsular extension typically demand a focal boost of an additional 6 to 10 Gy, for a total dose of 66 to 70 Gy, to try and achieve durable locoregional control.[2]

Table 7.1 Dose and fractionation paradigms for definitive radiation therapy of nonmelanomatous skin cancer

Gross primary tumor	Dose and fractionation regimen
	70 Gy in 35 fractions over 7 wk
	66 Gy in 30 fractions over 6 wk
	55 Gy in 20 fractions over 4 wk
	50 Gy in 15 fractions over 3 wk
	40 Gy in 5 fractions twice weekly
	30 Gy in 3 fractions once weekly
	20 Gy in single fraction
Regional nodes	**Dose and fractionation regimen**
• LN clinically (-), at risk for subclinical disease	50–54 Gy over 5–6 wk
	50 Gy over 4 wk
• LN clinically (+); Head and Neck	Surgical resection preferred
	70 Gy in 35 fractions over 7 wk
	66 Gy in 30 fractions over 6 wk
	55 Gy in 20 fractions over 4 wk
• LN clinically (+); axilla, groin	Surgical resection preferred
	60–66 Gy in 6 wk

Table 7.2 Dose and fractionation paradigms for postoperative radiation therapy of nonmelanomatous skin cancer

Primary tumor bed	Dose and fractionation regimen
• Margin negative	60 Gy in 30 fractions over 6 wk
	50 Gy in 25 fractions over 5 wk
	50 Gy in 20 fractions over 4 wk
• Margin positive	66 Gy in 33 fractions over 6.5 wk
	55 Gy in 20 fractions over 4 wk
Regional nodal bed	**Dose and fractionation regimen**
• Head and neck	
◦ Without ECE	60 Gy in 30 fractions over 6 wk
	50 Gy in 20 fractions over 4 wk
◦ With ECE	66 Gy in 33 fractions over 6.5 wk
• Axilla or groin	55 Gy in 20 fractions over 4 wk
◦ Without ECE	45–50 Gy in 25 fractions over 5 wk
◦ With ECE	60–66 Gy in 30–33 fractions over 6 wk

In addition to producing differential late effects, there is some data that hypofractionated (higher daily dose in less treatment) regimens are associated with superior tumor control rates in definitive RT for BCC and SCC. In a retrospective review of 531 BCC and SCC treated with definitive RT, patients with BCC who received ≤ 2 Gy per fraction had significantly lower local control compared with patients who received > 2 Gy per fraction (75 vs. 95.9%; $p = 0.01$). This was not the case in the SCC cohort.[39] However, other studies have shown conflicting data. In a retrospective review of 434 BCC and SCC, patients treated with 54 Gy in 18 fractions and 44 Gy in 10 fractions had similar 3-year local recurrence-free rate for BCC (97.6 vs. 96.9%) and SCC (97 vs. 93.6%).[8] In our experience, there is little rationale for a daily dose of < 2 Gy, as this unduly extends the treatment course for the patient. Excellent control can be achieved using shorter or longer courses with varying total dose prescriptions. The choice of dose and fractionation is primarily driven by proximity to normal tissues, long-term cosmetic impact, and patient tolerance and convenience factors.

The choice of total dose and dose per fraction in radiation for cutaneous melanoma is of particular relevance, given that this disease demonstrates radio-resistant properties in vitro. Numerous cell culture studies have demonstrated a broader shoulder on the dose–response curve, requiring and theoretically suggesting that higher doses per fraction would be required to achieve efficient tumor cell kill, especially in the presence of gross disease. A phase III Radiotherapy Therapy Oncology Group (RTOG) study investigated this question in the palliative setting by randomizing 137 patients with metastatic melanoma at any site other than the brain or abdomen to receive either 32 Gy in 4 fractions (8 Gy/fx) compared to 45 Gy in 20 fractions (4.5 Gy/fx). Despite the preclinical data suggesting that there would be a difference, the study failed to detect any difference in clinical response rate between the two arms.[40] However, this study failed to control for tumors of widely varying sizes, which may have reduced the ability to differentiate between the arms.

In the definitive setting, a common radiation schedule is to deliver 30 to 40 Gy in five to eight fractions. However, if the intended treatment area is adjacent to critical neural structures, standard fractionation over several weeks is advised[41] (▶ Table 7.3). Control rates for gross unresected melanoma are suboptimal.

In the postoperative setting, locoregional control rates are quite good, ranging from 80 to 90%. A few alternative regimens appear equally effective. In the study by Burmeister et al, 48 Gy in 20 fractions was used safely and effectively.[35] Ballo et al published the longstanding MD Anderson's approach which utilized 30 Gy in five fractions given twice weekly, for all sites not adjacent to critical neural organs at risk. In these cases, traditional doses of 60 to 66 Gy in 30 to 33 fx (2 Gy/fx) are typically used.[42]

7.2.4 Radiation Techniques and Targeting

The primary goal of radiotherapy is to precisely deliver a maximum dose of radiation, to a defined tumor volume, that eradicates disease and results in minimal damage to surrounding, normal tissue. This can be accomplished in a variety of ways, generally broken up into two categories: (1) external beam radiation using electrons or photons and (2) internal radiation known as brachytherapy, using radioactive sources. A lack of understanding of these differences has caused an under-appreciation of the distinct modes of treatment available to patients, and may very well have contributed to excessive treatment failures and/or poor cosmetic results in some older published series in which suboptimal techniques were used.

Table 7.3 Dose and fractionation paradigms for postoperative radiation therapy of melanoma

Primary tumor/Nodal bed	Dose and fractionation regimen
• Adjacent to critical neural structures	60–66 Gy in 30–33 fractions over 6.5 wk
• Not adjacent to critical neural structures	48 Gy in 20 fractions over 4 wk
	30 Gy in 5 fractions twice weekly

External Beam Radiotherapy

Technologic advances over the second half of the 20th century have produced an evolution in the types of machines that deliver external radiation used to treat skin cancers. Contact radiation therapy can be accomplished using a Grenz ray machine which produces low energy X-rays that operate with beam energies of 10 to 50 kilovolt Peak (kVp). Grenz rays have very low penetration and are absorbed within the first 2 mm of skin. Given its superficial penetration, Grenz ray therapy is largely reserved for in situ malignancies, such as Bowen's disease, actinic keratosis, and lentigo maligna, and was also historically used for inflammatory processes, such as psoriasis and chronic eczema. While Grenz ray therapy can be used for the management of very superficial BCC and SCC, a high index of suspicion to rule out deeper infiltration is critical. Published treatment regimens with satisfactory outcomes include 6 Gy twice weekly for 12 fractions, 30 Gy in 1 fraction, 15 Gy every other day for 3 fractions, or 20 Gy every other day for 3 fractions. A cumulative dose of 100 Gy should not be exceeded. The advantage of Grenz ray therapy is fewer long-term side effects such as hypo- or hyperpigmentation, no alopecia after treatment, and a negligible risk of secondary RT-induced malignancy.[37]

Superficial X-rays have been used to treat slightly larger/deeper lesions with beam energies of 50 to 100 kVp). The larger or deeper the lesion, the higher the energy that is needed to dose the target. A customized lead shield is often placed over the skin surface with a central cutout to collimate, or accurately shape, the beam (▶ Fig. 7.20). With superficial X-rays, the maximum dose is deposited onto the skin surface, the scatter to surrounding normal tissue is fairly minimal, and the dose distribution is unlikely to be impacted by irregular or curved surfaces such as found on the nose, canthus, lip, and external ear. Therefore, superficial is an ideal treatment for some of the cosmetically sensitive areas where surgery may not be desirable to the patient. However, X-rays in this energy range are differentially absorbed in denser material like bone or cartilage, and therefore could carry an increased risk of osteo- or chondronecrosis if the fractionation schedule is overly aggressive. It should also be noted that orthovoltage is truly restricted to superficial lesions. At this range of photon energies, the coverage of the target tissue is very poor beyond several millimeters into tissue. In the past, the radiation exposure would be increased to drive more dose to the desired depth, which created significant hot spots, resulting in a surface dose 20 to 50% higher than the planned prescription dose, which may well have led to poorer cosmetic outcomes. This also may partially account for inferior outcomes in larger/deeper lesions treated with this technique, given the coverage at depth may have been suboptimal.[37] These issues are avoided with a proper understanding of the technology and its unique qualities which can make it ideal for superficial skin cancer treatment.

Orthovoltage units and Cobalt units produce higher energy X-rays and were also commonly used in the past. However, all of these modalities have largely fallen into disuse and been replaced by electron and photon therapy produced by linear accelerators. Electron beam therapy has the advantage of having rapid dose fall off at depth, akin to some of the lower energy X-rays, but can also achieve deeper penetration in tissue (▶ Fig. 7.21). Electron energy ranges are quite broad, ranging

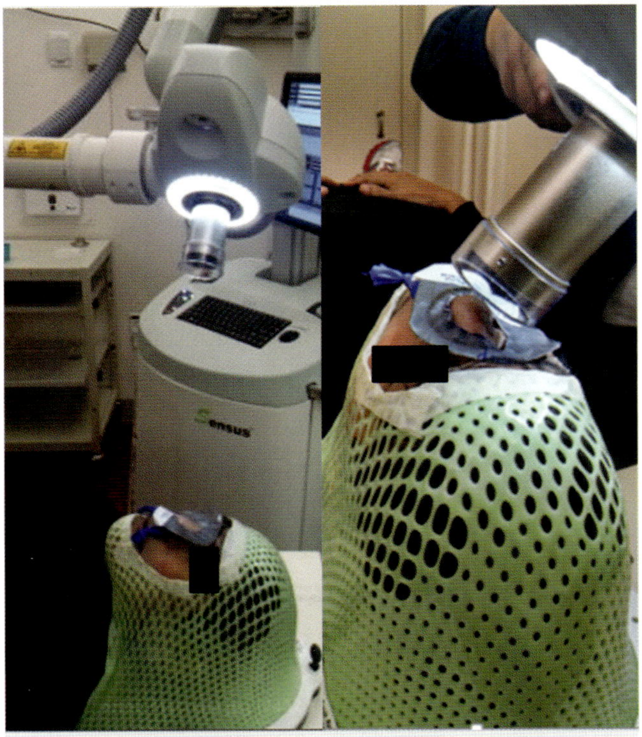

Fig. 7.20 Superficial radiation machine with customized lead shield for treatment of nasal skin SCC.

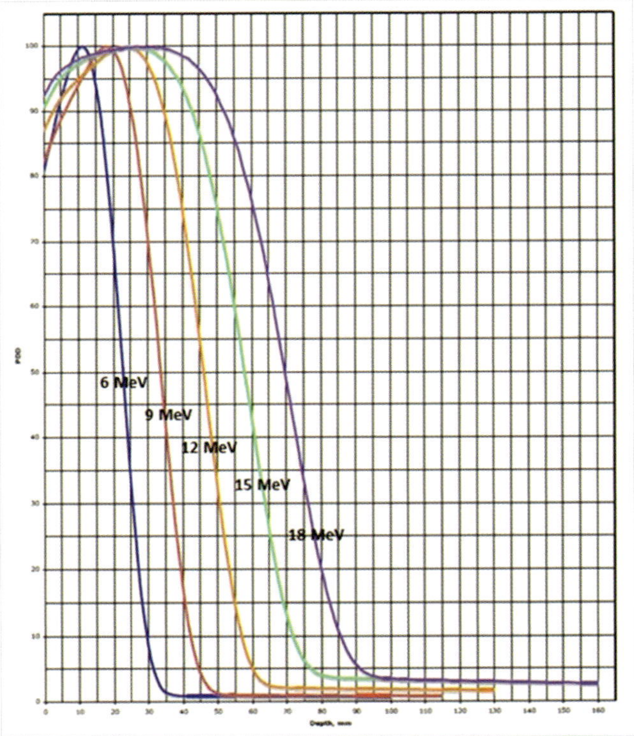

Fig. 7.21 Electron energies. The depth dose profiles for different electron energies (dose on *x*-axis and depth on *y*-axis) is depicted. As electron energy increases, the maximum dose is deposited deeper in tissue with higher exit doses. Lower energy electrons are ideal to spare underlying normal tissue.

from 6 Megaelectron volts (MeV) up to 21 MeV in clinical practice, and the higher energy beams can cover targets at depths up to 4 to 5 cm. Electrons are especially useful for skin cancer, given the surface dose is quite high and can be augmented to achieve 100% of the prescription dose with the use of customized bolus material. En face electrons work best on flat surfaces that provide homogeneous and predictable dose distributions. Surfaces with significant concavity can be treated, but often multiple matching fields are required which introduce additional planning complexity and the possibility of hot spots at the match line.

Photons have energy ranges that are nominally similar to electrons (6–18 Megavolts), but they are typically skin sparing, with entrance doses at the skin of only 15 to 35% of prescription dose at depth in tissue (▶ Fig. 7.22). However, photons are useful when treating targets with complex sloping or concave shapes, and they are the most appropriate modality for treating deeper tissues such as lymphatic beds, or nerve pathways. Skin dose can be augmented by using multiple tangential fields, and with the addition of customized bolus material. For more complex plans for deep-seated tumors, the advent of intensity modulated radiotherapy (IMRT) has been a huge advance in treatment planning capability. By using multiple beam angles and allowing for beam modulation and consequent differential radiation deposition in complex shapes in tissues, high doses are able to be delivered to very complex targets with rapid dose falloff and superior sparing of normal tissue. This has particular importance when treating the neck and skull base, given avoidance of salivary glands, swallowing organs, bone, orbits, optic nerves, and brainstem is routinely achievable. This technologic advance, coupled with daily image guidance using cone beam CT to reduce daily setup error, has been associated with significant decreases in radiation-induced morbidity and has provided greater opportunities to treat large infiltrative tumors adjacent to critical organs, or those tracking into the skull base, with greater success.[37]

Brachytherapy

Brachytherapy involves the placement of a radioactive source on a body surface (surface-mold technique) or the placement of a radioactive source into a body tissue (interstitial technique). It has particular application to lesions of the lip, eyelid, or pre/post-auricular skin given their irregular contour and proximity to critical structures. Brachytherapy can achieve very steep dose falloff to avoid organs at risk that are only several millimeters away. Brachytherapy is predominantly used in the definitive setting, but can also be used postoperatively, in the setting of a positive margin.

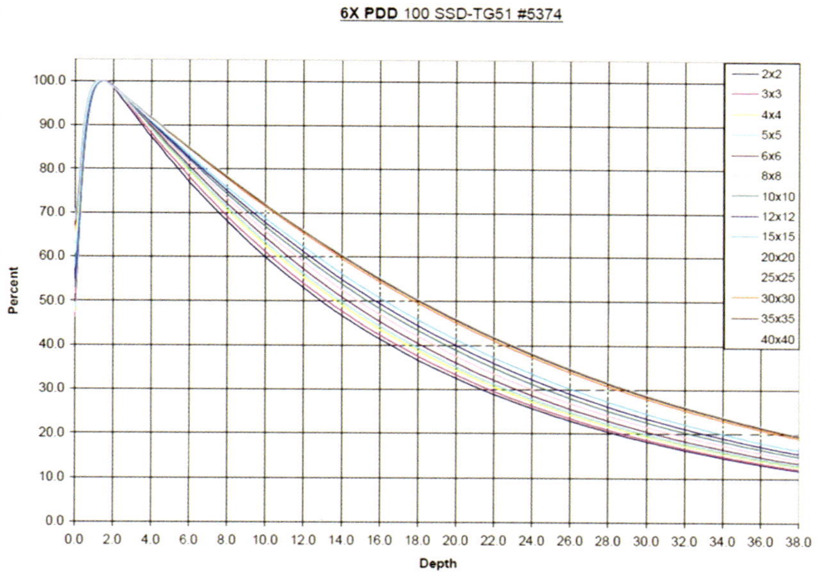

Fig. 7.22 Photon beam dose profile for 6-MV photons. Different field sizes are shown on the left. Note that the dose falloff is more gradual compared to electrons (shown in ▶ Fig. 7.20).

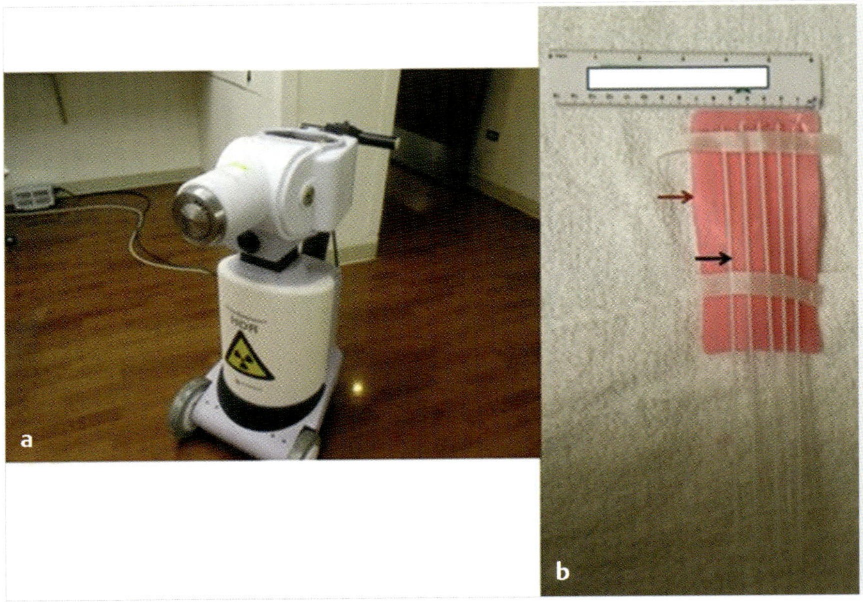

Fig. 7.23 (a) High dose rate brachytherapy machine. **(b)** Surface mold brachytherapy device using catheters fashioned on a wax bolus material to provide adequate surface dose and photon energy buildup (catheter—black arrow; gel bolus material—red arrow).

Brachytherapy can be accomplished using interstitial implants or surface mold techniques (▶ Fig. 7.23). Interstitial brachytherapy involves placing radioactive wires or seeds directly into the target tissue. Interstitial implants may be permanent or temporary. It can be accomplished using low-dose rate (LDR) over 48 to 72 hours, or high-dose rate (HDR) delivery using multiple fractions delivered over 5 to 15 minutes. The latter is far more commonly used currently due to the much wider availability of HDR delivery units in the radiation oncology community. In a review of 147 BCC and SCC of the eyelid, canthus, nose, or external ear, patients were treated with interstitial wire implant brachytherapy with ^{192}Ir for primary tumors or recurrent tumors after surgery. The locoregional recurrence rate at 5 years was 12.7% and was well tolerated. Mild to moderate hypopigmentation, skin atrophy, telangiectasias, and eyelid dysfunction were observed, without severe toxicities. No severe toxicities were observed. As expected, outcomes were worse for patients with recurrent disease.[43]

Surface mold brachytherapy is an alternative technique that is particularly useful in superficial lesions with limited tissue penetration at depth (1 cm). It involves the placement of a mold constructed from pliable materials which later harden into a customized cast-like material onto the target region. The mold is impregnated with catheters through which radioactive sources can be precisely directed for discreet time periods, allowing for precise dose deposition to tumors. The radiation is typically delivered using a HDR afterloader device, typically with ^{192}Ir. This technique is particularly advantageous for tumors of the nasal tip or ala, in which the sloping surface can interfere with homogeneous dose distributions with electrons or photons (▶ Fig. 7.24). Mold brachytherapy allows for the customized

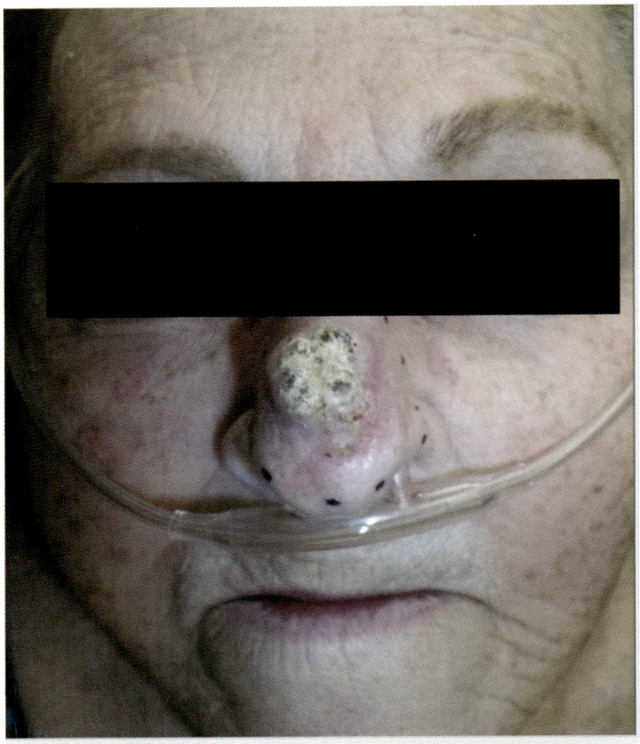

Fig. 7.24 A 94-year-old woman, medically inoperable, with SCC of the nasal tip treated with external beam radiation therapy with electrons. Pictured is a 2 × 1.8 cm recurrent SCC, T1N0M0, which was treated with surface-mold brachytherapy.

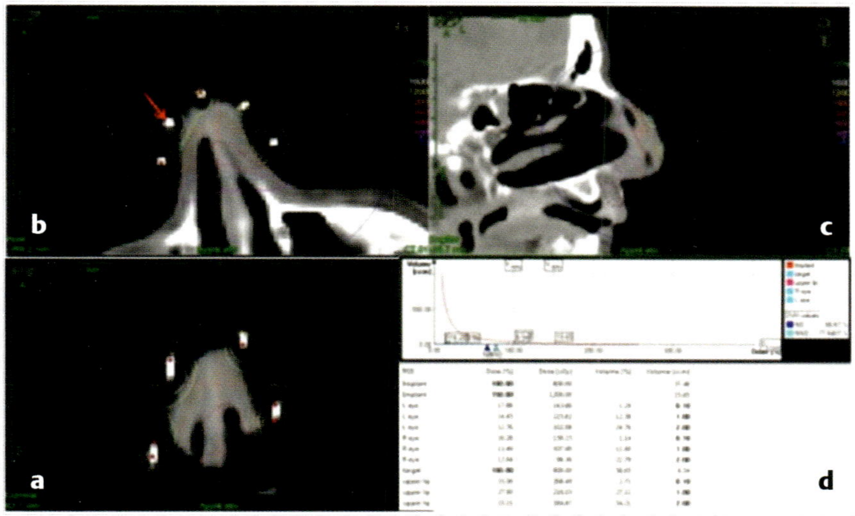

Fig. 7.25 Brachytherapy plan for SCC of the nasal tip depicted in ▶ Fig. 7.22. **(a)** Axial radiation planning CT scan slice of the mold implant. **(b)** Five catheters (red arrow) are incorporated in the plan. The catheters are resting on a layer of red bees wax bolus, not seen here. **(c)** Sagittal radiation planning CT scan slice with isodose lines covering the lesion. **(d)** Dose volume parameters for the target and normal organs at risk. The prescription dose was 8 Gy in five fractions.

bending of the wax to conform to the complex nasal contour of the patients and ensures homogeneous dose delivery to the target (▶ Fig. 7.25).[44] HDR surface-mold brachytherapy for treatment of NMSC has been studied in both prospective and retrospective studies and shown to be safe and effective. In a prospective series of 136 patients with BCC and SCC of the face treated with HDR brachytherapy via external surface mold, a 5-year local control rate of 99% for primary tumors and 87% for recurrent tumors was observed. Good or excellent cosmesis was reported in 98% of patients 6 months after treatment.[45]

7.2.5 Considerations in Immunosuppressed Patients with NMSC

Chronic immune suppression is associated with a higher incidence of cutaneous SCC and BCC. This increased risk has been observed in solid organ transplant recipients (OTRs) on chronic immunosuppressive therapy, patients with chronic lymphocytic leukemia (CLL), and exposure to chronic corticosteroid therapy. OTRs demonstrate up to a 65- to 100-fold increase in incidence of SCC compared to the immunocompetent population.[11] Once immunosuppressed patients develop a skin cancer, more than 75% will develop additional lesions within 5 years, often within months of each other.[46] In addition to being at increased risk for malignancy, the chronically immunosuppressed population more often develop SCC with high-risk features, including PNI, LVSI, tumors located on the head and neck, nodal metastasis, and deep tissue involvement. SCC in these patients may demonstrate more aggressive behavior with poorer outcomes. Skin cancer in these patients may even account for 5 to 10% of mortality.[47] As modern immunosuppressive therapy has become more potent and efficacious, posttransplant survival time and duration of immunosuppressive therapy has increased, which has led to an increase in the incidence of SCC in these patients. Therefore, aggressive management of these patients is of increasing importance.

Postoperative RT is recommended for high-risk SCC and plays an important role in the management of this patient population. Whether disease control rates and tolerance of RT differ according to immune status has not been well defined; however, available literature suggests that even with postoperative RT, immunosuppressed patients have worse outcomes than immunocompetent patients.[48] Manyam et al recently reported a retrospective comparison of 38 immunocompetent and 21 immunosuppressed patients treated for cutaneous SCC of the head and neck with resection and adjuvant RT. Most had nodal metastases (63%), 50% had PNI, and 15% were T3/4. Actuarial locoregional control (48 vs. 73%; $p = 0.01$) and disease-free survival (44 vs. 62%; $p = 0.03$) at 2 years were significantly inferior in the immunosuppressed population.[49] Immunosuppressed patients may be intrinsically more resistant to traditional adjuvant therapy. Whether these patients may benefit from intensification of therapy with earlier disposition to RT, dose-escalated RT, or concurrent systemic therapies requires future prospective study. SCC in immunosuppressed patients may also have a higher tendency toward discontinuous pattern of spread or satellitosis and recurrences can occur further away from the primary tumor. Therefore, the extent of surrounding tissue that must be involved in the RT field should be a consideration, especially in the setting of extensive PNI or LVSI.[50] Ultimately, evaluation of a chronically immunosuppressed patient with SCC should warrant a higher degree of caution, even in early-stage lesions.

Immunosuppressive regimens in this patient population are also an important consideration. OTRs are typically treated with calcineurin inhibitors, such as FK-506 and tacrolimus, for prevention of graft rejection; however, these agents have been shown to be promitotic and contribute to tumor development. On the other hand, mammalian target of rapamycin (mTOR) inhibitors, such as sirolimus, have been shown to have antineoplastic properties. A phase III randomized controlled trial involving renal transplant patients demonstrated that use of sirolimus resulted in significantly decreased incidence of new SCC (22 vs. 39%; $p = 0.02$) and introduced a significant delay in the development of new SCC (15 vs. 7 months; $p = 0.02$) compared to patients receiving calcineurin inhibitors. There were no significantly increased episodes of graft rejection with sirolimus, but there were significantly more side effects.[51] Therefore, the risks and benefits of transitioning to an mTOR inhibitor after a new diagnosis of SCC in this patient population should be discussed with the patient and their transplant physician.

7.2.6 Consideration of Concurrent Systemic Therapy with Radiotherapy

The risk of distant metastasis is extremely low for BCC; therefore, the role of systemic therapy has not been extensively studied. Vismodegib, a small molecule inhibitor of the hedgehog pathway, is the first approved systemic therapy for advanced BCC. The drug is indicated for recurrent or metastatic BCC that is not amenable to definitive surgery or RT. In a phase II study of vismodegib, patients with inoperable locally advanced BCC demonstrated a 43% response rate to the drug (95% CI: 31–56; $p < 0.0001$) and patients with metastatic BCC demonstrated a 30% response rate to the drug (95% CI: 16–48; $p = 0.001$), with serious adverse event rate of 25%. There are no data currently available regarding its efficacy as a concurrent therapy with postoperative or definitive RT, though clinical trials are underway to explore this application.[52]

The overall risk of distant metastasis with SCC is also extremely low, about 3.7%. Currently, there are no prospective phase III trials to evaluate the benefit of the addition of concurrent systemic therapy to definitive or postoperative RT for high-risk SCC. Much of the decision to include systemic therapy has been extrapolated from phase III randomized trials conducted in head and neck mucosal SCC treated with postoperative RT and concurrent platinum-based chemotherapy. These trials demonstrated significantly higher locoregional control and progression-free survival with concurrent postoperative RT and cisplatin compared to postoperative RT alone, though there were significantly higher rates of severe adverse effects.[53,54] Further analysis of these trials demonstrated that positive margins and lymph node extracapsular extension were the two risk factors for which concurrent chemotherapy was beneficial.[22] Patients with cutaneous SCC with these risk factors should consider multidisciplinary consultation to discuss supplementation of RT with cisplatinum-based chemotherapy.

Epidermal growth factor receptor (EGFR) inhibitors have been a source of interest as monotherapy or in combination with surgery and/or RT for cutaneous SCC. A phase II study investigated the use of neoadjuvant gefitinib followed by surgery, RT, or both in 22 patients with locally advanced cutaneous SCC. A complete response rate was observed in 18% of patients, a partial response rate was observed in 27% of patients, and a 2-year progression-free survival of 60% was observed.[55] Similarly, another EGFR inhibitor, cetuximab, used as a monotherapy demonstrated a 30% response rate and 70% disease stabilization rate in a phase II trial in patients with unresectable or metastatic cutaneous SCC.[56] However, there is an absence of data investigating the added utility of EGFR inhibition, given concurrent with radiation in either the definitive or adjuvant settings.[57,58]

In our practices, we consider the addition of concurrent cisplatin to adjuvant radiotherapy for patients with extranodal extension of disease and those with positive margins, and in conjunction with definitive RT for patients with unresectable disease (e.g., skull base invasion). For patients who are not candidates for cisplatin, either due to age and/or renal function concerns, we also consider concurrent cetuximab.

7.2.7 Palliative Radiotherapy for Metastatic Disease

Traditional principles of palliative radiotherapy apply to skin cancers of all varieties. Palliation is typically offered for focal symptomatic areas, such as pain, bleeding, and airway compression. Radiation therapy is also indicated in asymptomatic patients when metastases threaten to cause significant morbidity in the near future. This would include femoral lesions at risk of fracture, spinal lesions with epidural extension which can cause spinal cord compression, and brain metastases which can cause neurological morbidity and mortality when progressive. Typical palliative fractionation schemes include 30 Gy in 10 fractions, 24 Gy in 6 fractions, 20 Gy in 5 fractions, or 8 Gy in 1 fraction (▶ Fig. 7.26).[59]

Advanced radiation technologies using high-dose single-fraction stereotactic radiosurgery (SRS) or single or multifraction stereotactic body radiotherapy (SBRT) have an important role to play in several circumstances of metastatic disease. Brain metastases are a significant problem in malignant melanoma and account for 20 to 54% of deaths in these patients (▶ Fig. 7.27).[60] SRS, either through gamma knife radiosurgery, or linear accelerator-based radiosurgery, has been shown to be quite effective in the treatment of these lesions when the size of the metastasis remains small enough to be amenable to these approaches (▶ Fig. 7.28, ▶ Fig. 7.29, and ▶ Fig. 7.30).[61,62,63] Mori and colleagues analyzed 60 patients with metastatic melanoma to the brain treated with SRS (mean dose: 16.4 Gy) and found imaging-defined local control rate of 90%, with complete disappearance in 11% of patients.[61] Similarly, spine radiosurgery for spinal metastases has been reported to produce high rates of pain control and radiographic local control in melanoma patients, with minimal side effects (▶ Fig. 7.31). SBRT has also been shown to be highly effective and safe for patients with oligometastatic lung or liver metastases.

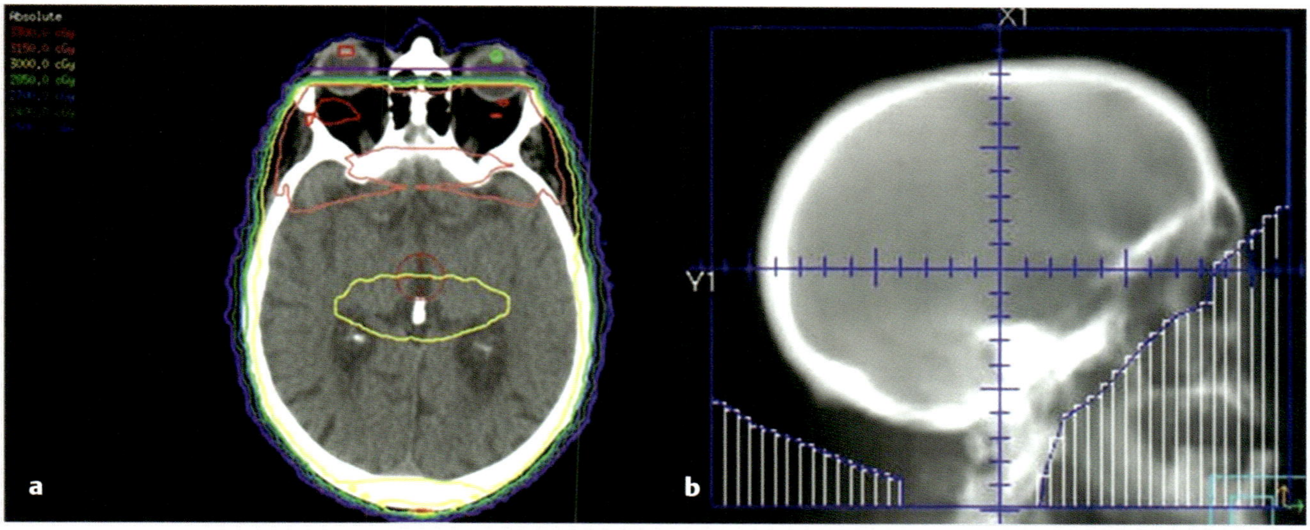

Fig. 7.26 (a) Axial radiation planning CT scan slice depicting whole-brain palliative radiation therapy for brain metastases from dermal melanoma with a prescription dose of 30 Gy in 10 fractions. **(b)** Whole brain radiation therapy lateral field.

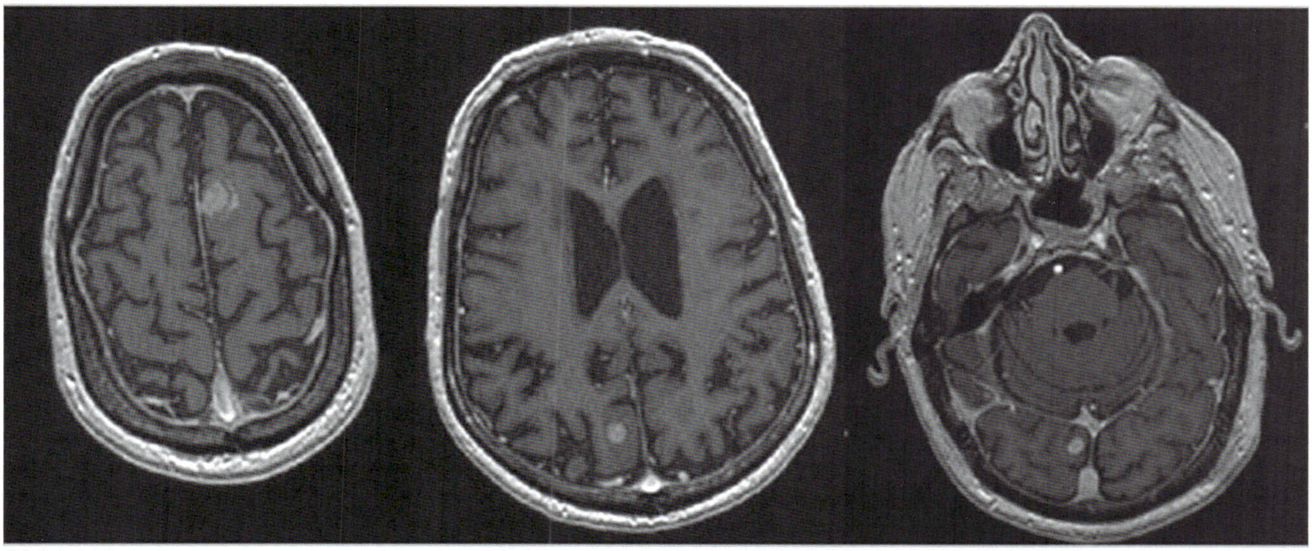

Fig. 7.27 Axial T1 contrast-enhanced MRI images showing multiple brain metastases from dermal melanoma.

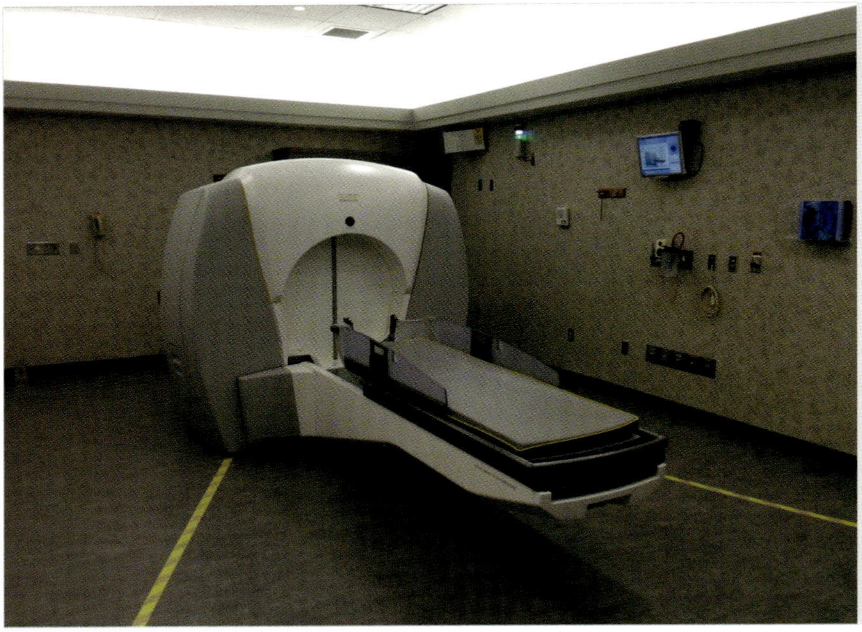

Fig. 7.28 Gamma knife radiosurgery delivery system (Perfexion model).

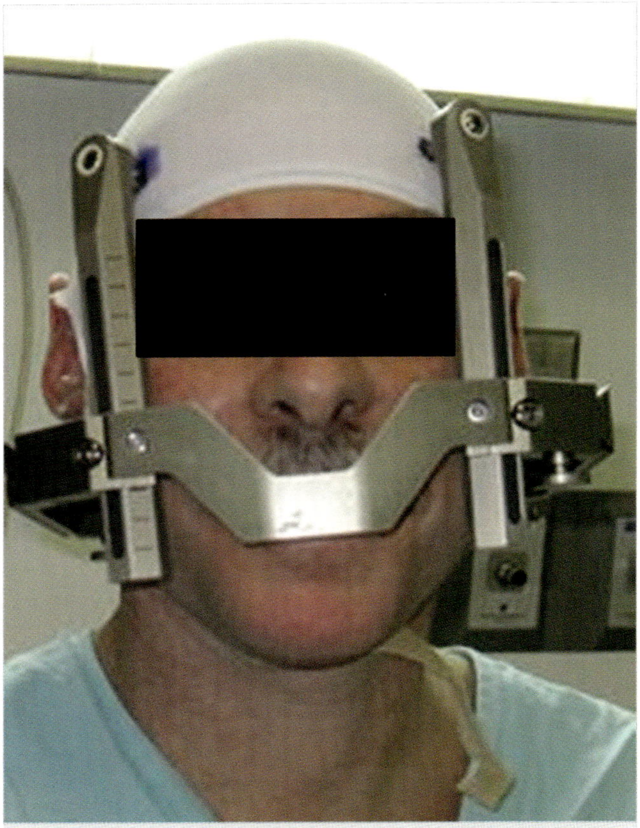

Fig. 7.29 Gamma knife head frame used for immobilization during gamma knife radiosurgery.

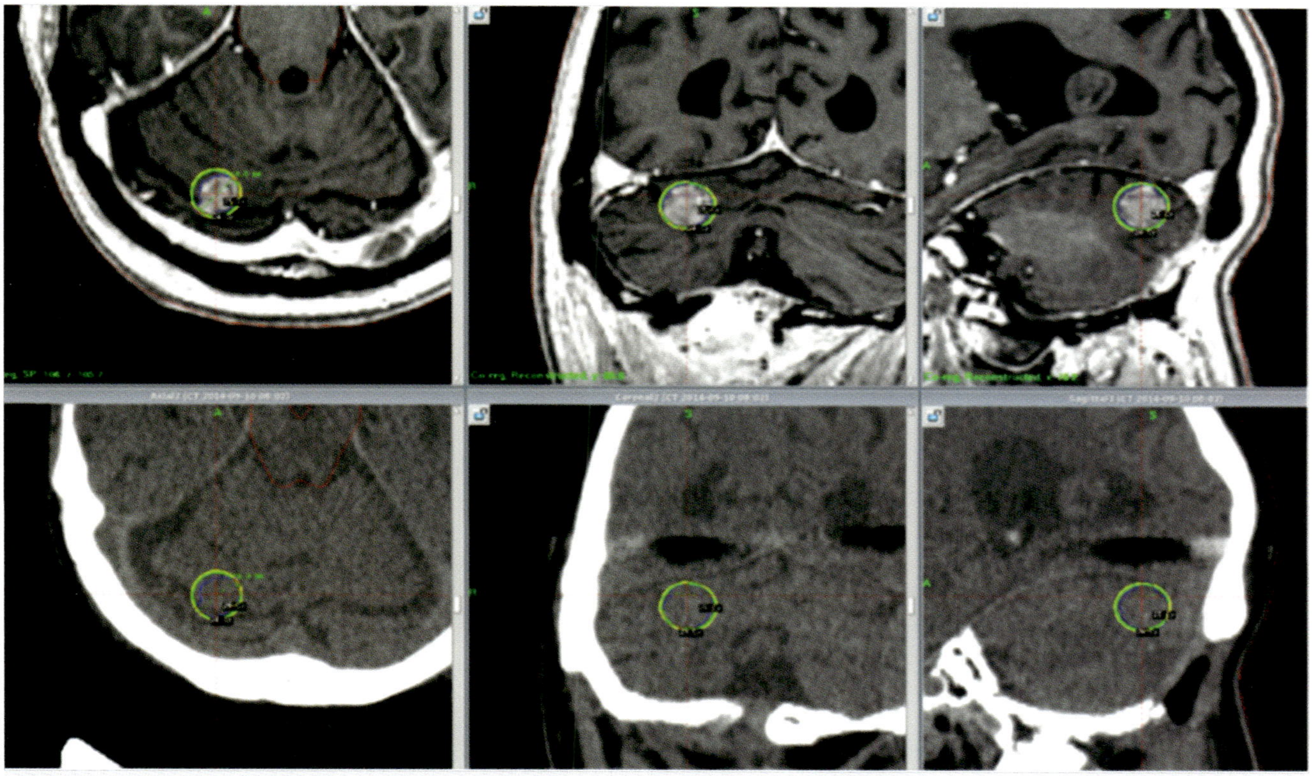

Fig. 7.30 A 58-year-old man with single brain metastasis from cutaneous melanoma treated with gamma knife radiosurgery to 24 Gy in one fraction. (Top panels—left to right: axial, coronal and sagittal MRI images depicting the lesion and 24 Gy isodose in light green; Bottom panel—corresponding CT images)

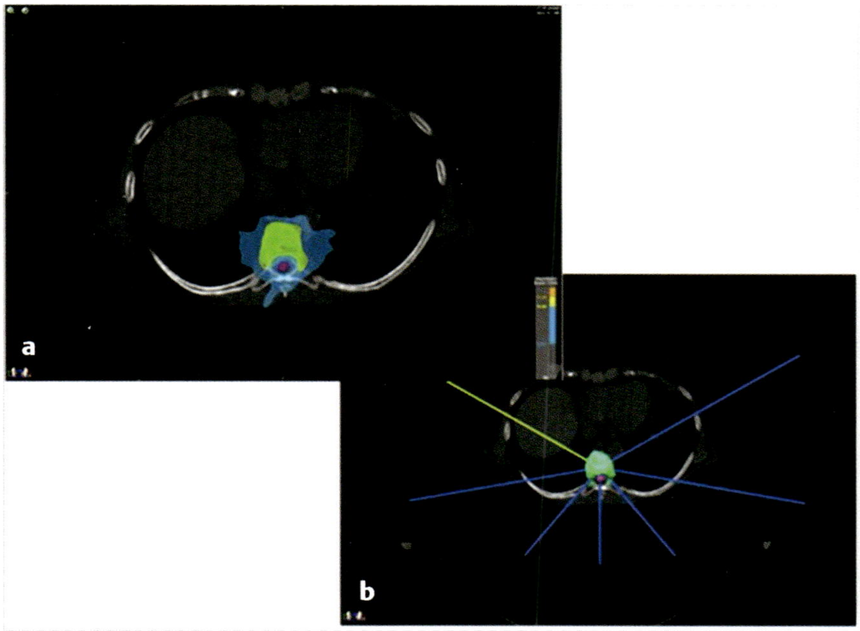

Fig. 7.31 **(a)** Axial slice of a radiation planning CT demonstrating delineation of a T8 vertebra metastasis from cutaneous melanoma treated with a single session of spine SBRT to 16 Gy in one fraction (target in green, spinal cord in pink, 16 Gy isodose line in yellow). **(b)** A seven-field IMRT beam arrangement for the lesion (target depicted in green and cord shown in pink).

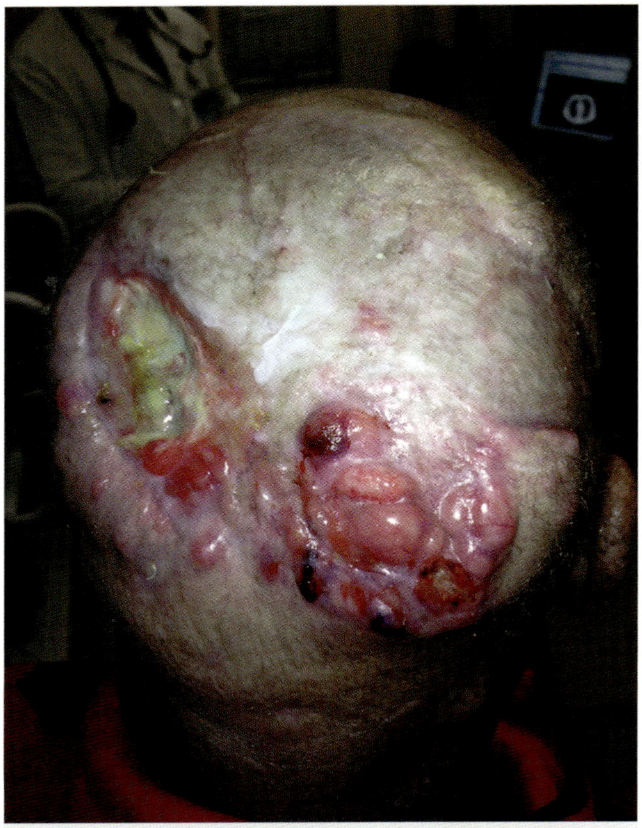

Fig. 7.32 A 58-year-old man with history of chronic immunosuppression, with recurrent, fungating scalp SCC treated with surgery and two courses of palliative stereotactic body radiotherapy.

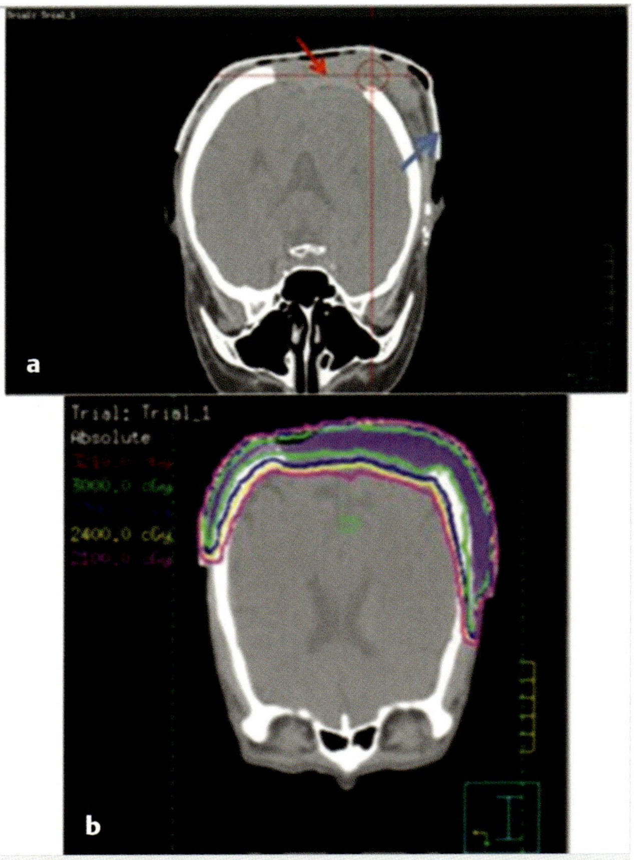

Fig. 7.33 Stereotactic body radiation therapy. (a) Axial radiation planning CT slice depicting the prone set up with soft-tissue extension through the skull (red arrow) and overlying bolus (blue arrow). (b) Isodose lines covering the target (solid purple) with a prescription of 30 Gy in five fractions.

For recurrent NMSC, often locoregional recurrence presents the greatest therapeutic challenge and is a primary cause of morbidity and mortality in the small number of patients who do not achieve cure. As this often occurs in the head and neck region, head and neck SBRT is an emerging therapeutic option to achieve durable locoregional salvage (▸ Fig. 7.32, ▸ Fig. 7.33, and ▸ Fig. 7.34).[64] After a phase I study demonstrated the safety of using up to 44 Gy in five fractions for recurrent, previously radiated head and neck SCCs, hundreds of patients were treated with this approach. Response rates were high at 50 to 75%, and morbidity was uniformly modest with grade 3/4 toxicity rates between 10 and 15% when delivered in an every-other-day regimen. Although the use of this regimen in skin cancer seems quite logical, one must extrapolate as the data apply only to mucosally based head and neck cancers at present.

7.2.8 Radiotherapy and Hyperthermia for Melanoma

For large, unresectable, often recurrent skin cancers being treated with radiotherapy, concurrent hyperthermia, using temperatures of 40 to 45°C, has been shown to offer a significant radiosensitization effect and direct cytotoxic effect, as it selectively damages cells in the S phase of mitosis, a time in the cell cycle that radiotherapy is particularly ineffective.[65,66] A study of metastatic or recurrent melanoma was conducted by the European Society of Hyperthermic Oncology in which 70 patients were randomized to RT with or without hyperthermia. Patients who received hyperthermia with RT (24–27 Gy in three fractions) had a significantly higher 2-year local control rate compared to patients who received RT alone (46 vs. 28%; $p = 0.008$). There was no significant difference in survival between the two groups.[67] This also is an important potential adjunct to radiotherapy for large unresectable skin cancers. In our experience, hyperthermia can be particularly useful as an adjunctive concurrent treatment to be used with RT in patients who have had prior radiation therapy to the area. With the use of hyperthermia, the efficacy of the radiation therapy increases, and thus the total doses of RT can be lower, which is advantageous for a scenario of reirradiation.

7.2.9 Conflict of Interest

Dr. Yom receives clinical trial support from Genentech, Inc.

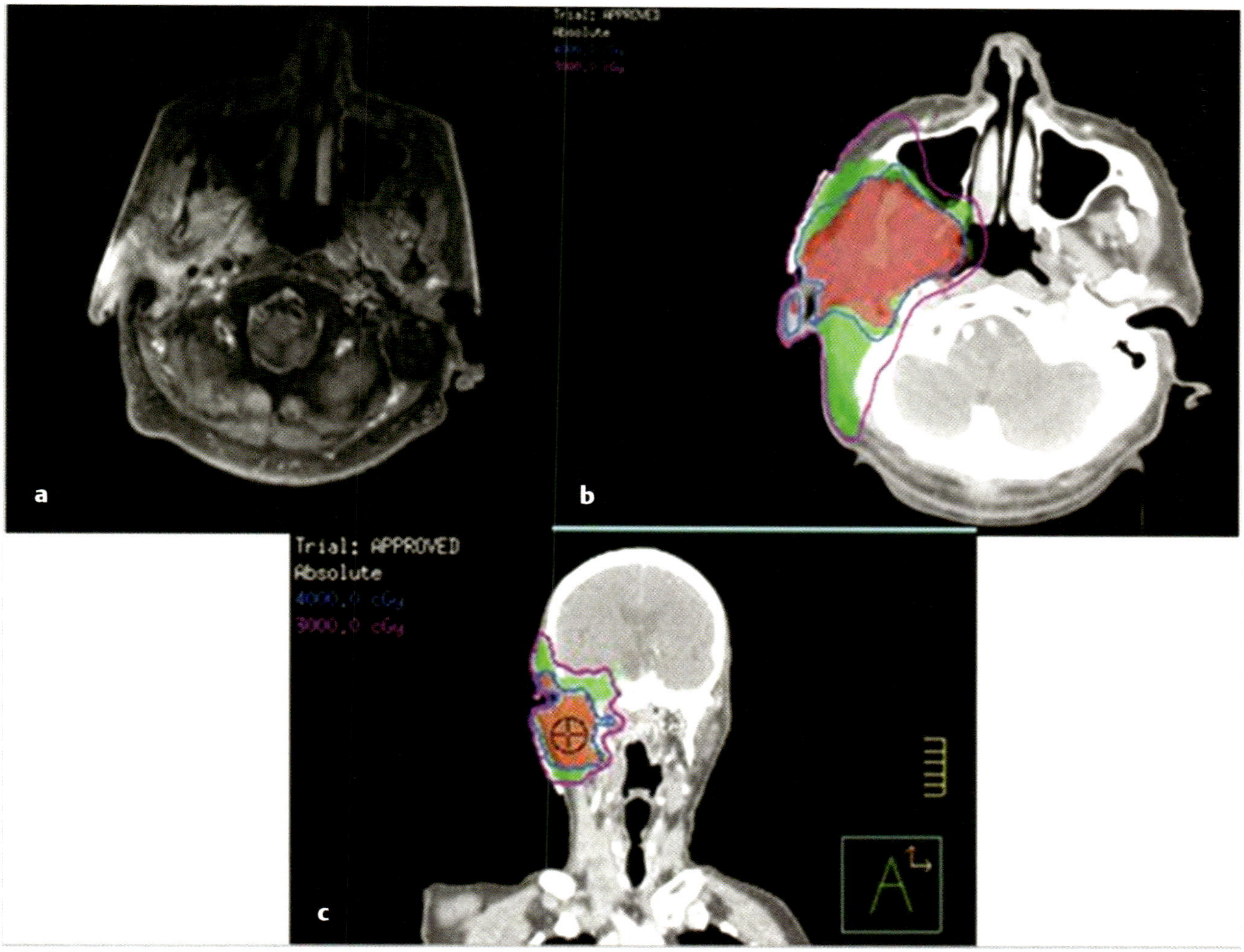

Fig. 7.34 A 70-year-old patient with a history of chronic immunosuppression presenting with a recurrent right parapharyngeal mass after definitive chemoradiation for an unresectable SCC of the skin with parotid nodal metastases, treated with SBRT for recurrence. **(a)** Axial T1 contrast-enhanced MRI. **(b)** Axial radiation planning CT scan slice depicting target (solid red) covered by 40-Gy isodose line. **(c)** Coronal radiation planning CT scan slice.

References

[1] Avril MF, Auperin A, Margulis A, et al. Basal cell carcinoma of the face: surgery or radiotherapy? Results of a randomized study. Br J Cancer. 1997; 76 (1):100–106

[2] Bichakjian CK, Olencki T, Aasi S, et al. NCCN Clinical Practice Guidelines in Oncology (NCCN Guidelines) Squamous Cell Skin Cancer; 2015

[3] Caccialanza M, Piccinno R, Gaiani F, Contini D. Relevance of dermatologic radiotherapy in the therapeutic strategy of skin epithelial neoplasms: excellent results in the treatment of lesions localized on eyelids and skin overlying the cartilage of the nose. G Ital Dermatol Venereol. 2013; 148(1):83–88

[4] Silva JJ, Tsang RW, Panzarella T, Levin W, Wells W. Results of radiotherapy for epithelial skin cancer of the pinna: the Princess Margaret Hospital experience, 1982–1993. Int J Radiat Oncol Biol Phys. 2000; 47(2):451–459

[5] Tsao MN, Tsang RW, Liu FF, Panzarella T, Rotstein L. Radiotherapy management for squamous cell carcinoma of the nasal skin: the Princess Margaret Hospital experience. Int J Radiat Oncol Biol Phys. 2002; 52(4):973–979

[6] Lee WR, Mendenhall WM, Parsons JT, Million RR. Radical radiotherapy for T4 carcinoma of the skin of the head and neck: a multivariate analysis. Head Neck. 1993; 15(4):320–324

[7] Al-Othman MO, Mendenhall WM, Amdur RJ. Radiotherapy alone for clinical T4 skin carcinoma of the head and neck with surgery reserved for salvage. Am J Otolaryngol. 2001; 22(6):387–390

[8] van Hezewijk M, Creutzberg CL, Putter H, et al. Efficacy of a hypofractionated schedule in electron beam radiotherapy for epithelial skin cancer: analysis of 434 cases. Radiother Oncol. 2010; 95(2):245–249

[9] Kwan W, Wilson D, Moravan V. Radiotherapy for locally advanced basal cell and squamous cell carcinomas of the skin. Int J Radiat Oncol Biol Phys. 2004; 60(2):406–411

[10] Blanchard P, Baujat B, Holostenco V, et al. MACH-CH Collaborative group. Meta-analysis of chemotherapy in head and neck cancer (MACH-NC): a comprehensive analysis by tumour site. Radiother Oncol. 2011; 100 (1):33–40

[11] Lott DG, Manz R, Koch C, Lorenz RR. Aggressive behavior of nonmelanotic skin cancers in solid organ transplant recipients. Transplantation. 2010; 90 (6):683–687

[12] Traywick C, O'Reilly FM. Management of skin cancer in solid organ transplant recipients. Dermatol Ther (Heidelb). 2005; 18(1):12–18

[13] Jackson JE, Dickie GJ, Wiltshire KL, et al. Radiotherapy for perineural invasion in cutaneous head and neck carcinomas: toward a risk-adapted treatment approach. Head Neck. 2009; 31(5):604–610

[14] Wang JT, Palme CE, Morgan GJ, Gebski V, Wang AY, Veness MJ. Predictors of outcome in patients with metastatic cutaneous head and neck squamous cell carcinoma involving cervical lymph nodes: improved survival with the addition of adjuvant radiotherapy. Head Neck. 2012; 34 (11):1524–1528

[15] Veness MJ, Palme CE, Smith M, Cakir B, Morgan GJ, Kalnins I. Cutaneous head and neck squamous cell carcinoma metastatic to cervical lymph nodes (nonparotid): a better outcome with surgery and adjuvant radiotherapy. Laryngoscope. 2003; 113(10):1827–1833
[16] Veness MJ, Morgan GJ, Palme CE, Gebski V. Surgery and adjuvant radiotherapy in patients with cutaneous head and neck squamous cell carcinoma metastatic to lymph nodes: combined treatment should be considered best practice. Laryngoscope. 2005; 115(5):870–875
[17] O'Brien CJ, McNeil EB, McMahon JD, Pathak I, Lauer CS, Jackson MA. Significance of clinical stage, extent of surgery, and pathologic findings in metastatic cutaneous squamous carcinoma of the parotid gland. Head Neck. 2002; 24(5):417–422
[18] Chua MS, Veness MJ, Morgan G, et al. Parotid lymph-node metastases from cutaneous squamous-cell carcinomas: treatment outcome and prognostic factors following surgery and adjuvant radiotherapy. Australas Radiol. 2002; 46(2):174–179
[19] Palme CE, O'Brien CJ, Veness MJ, McNeil EB, Bron LP, Morgan GJ. Extent of parotid disease influences outcome in patients with metastatic cutaneous squamous cell carcinoma. Arch Otolaryngol Head Neck Surg. 2003; 129 (7):750–753
[20] Jol JA, van Velthuysen ML, Hilgers FJ, Keus RB, Neering H, Balm AJ. Treatment results of regional metastasis from cutaneous head and neck squamous cell carcinoma. Eur J Surg Oncol. 2003; 29(1):81–86
[21] delCharco JO, Mendenhall WM, Parsons JT, Stringer SP, Cassisi NJ, Mendenhall NP. Carcinoma of the skin metastatic to the parotid area lymph nodes. Head Neck. 1998; 20(5):369–373
[22] Bernier J, Cooper JS, Pajak TF, et al. Defining risk levels in locally advanced head and neck cancers: a comparative analysis of concurrent postoperative radiation plus chemotherapy trials of the EORTC (#22931) and RTOG (# 9501). Head Neck. 2005; 27(10):843–850
[23] Mendenhall WM, Amdur RJ, Hinerman RW, Cognetta AB, Mendenhall NP. Radiotherapy for cutaneous squamous and basal cell carcinomas of the head and neck. Laryngoscope. 2009; 119(10):1994–1999
[24] Lin C, Tripcony L, Keller J, et al. Perineural infiltration of cutaneous squamous cell carcinoma and basal cell carcinoma without clinical features. Int J Radiat Oncol Biol Phys. 2012; 82(1):334–340
[25] Han A, Ratner D. What is the role of adjuvant radiotherapy in the treatment of cutaneous squamous cell carcinoma with perineural invasion? Cancer. 2007; 109(6):1053–1059
[26] Gluck I, Ibrahim M, Popovtzer A, et al. Skin cancer of the head and neck with perineural invasion: defining the clinical target volumes based on the pattern of failure. Int J Radiat Oncol Biol Phys. 2009; 74(1):38–46
[27] Guadagnolo BA, Zagars GK. Adjuvant radiation therapy for high-risk nodal metastases from cutaneous melanoma. Lancet Oncol. 2009; 10(4):409–416
[28] Burmeister BH, Smithers BM, Poulsen M, et al. Radiation therapy for nodal disease in malignant melanoma. World J Surg. 1995; 19(3):369–371
[29] O'Brien CJ, Coates AS, Petersen-Schaefer K, et al. Experience with 998 cutaneous melanomas of the head and neck over 30 years. Am J Surg. 1991; 162 (4):310–314
[30] Gonzalez RJ, Kudchadkar R, Rao NG, Sondak VK. Adjuvant immunotherapy and radiation in the management of high-risk resected melanoma. Ochsner J. 2010; 10(2):108–116
[31] Vongtama R, Safa A, Gallardo D, Calcaterra T, Juillard G. Efficacy of radiation therapy in the local control of desmoplastic malignant melanoma. Head Neck. 2003; 25(6):423–428
[32] Chen LL, Jaimes N, Barker CA, Busam KJ, Marghoob AA. Desmoplastic melanoma: a review. J Am Acad Dermatol. 2013; 68(5):825–833
[33] Corry J, Smith JG, Bishop M, Ainslie J. Nodal radiation therapy for metastatic melanoma. Int J Radiat Oncol Biol Phys. 1999; 44(5):1065–1069
[34] Agrawal S, Kane JM, III, Guadagnolo BA, Kraybill WG, Ballo MT. The benefits of adjuvant radiation therapy after therapeutic lymphadenectomy for clinically advanced, high-risk, lymph node-metastatic melanoma. Cancer. 2009; 115(24):5836–5844
[35] Burmeister BH, Henderson MA, Ainslie J, et al. Adjuvant radiotherapy versus observation alone for patients at risk of lymph-node field relapse after therapeutic lymphadenectomy for melanoma: a randomised trial. Lancet Oncol. 2012; 13(6):589–597
[36] Hymes SR, Strom EA, Fife C. Radiation dermatitis: clinical presentation, pathophysiology, and treatment 2006. J Am Acad Dermatol. 2006; 54(1):28–46
[37] Cognetta A, Mendenhall WM. Radiation Therapy for Skin Cancer. New York. Springer; 2013
[38] Rupprecht R, Lippold A, Auras C, et al. Late side-effects with cosmetic relevance following soft X-ray therapy of cutaneous neoplasias. J Eur Acad Dermatol Venereol. 2007; 21(2):178–185
[39] Locke J, Karimpour S, Young G, Lockett MA, Perez CA. Radiotherapy for epithelial skin cancer. Int J Radiat Oncol Biol Phys. 2001; 51(3):748–755
[40] Sause WT, Cooper JS, Rush S, et al. Fraction size in external beam radiation therapy in the treatment of melanoma. Int J Radiat Oncol Biol Phys. 1991; 20 (3):429–432
[41] Coit DG, Thompson JA, Andtbacka R, et al. NCCN Clinical Practice Guidelines in Oncology (NCCN Guidelines) Melanoma. 2015
[42] Ballo MT, Ross MI, Cormier JN, et al. Combined-modality therapy for patients with regional nodal metastases from melanoma. Int J Radiat Oncol Biol Phys. 2006; 64(1):106–113
[43] Ducassou A, David I, Filleron T, Rives M, Bonnet J, Delannes M. Retrospective analysis of local control and cosmetic outcome of 147 periorificial carcinomas of the face treated with low-dose rate interstitial brachytherapy. Int J Radiat Oncol Biol Phys. 2011; 81(3):726–731
[44] Wong JR, Wang CC. Radiation therapy in the management of cutaneous malignancies. Clin Dermatol. 2001; 19(3):348–353
[45] Guix B, Finestres F, Tello J, et al. Treatment of skin carcinomas of the face by high-dose-rate brachytherapy and custom-made surface molds. Int J Radiat Oncol Biol Phys. 2000; 47(1):95–102
[46] Wisgerhof HC, Edelbroek JR, de Fijter JW, et al. Subsequent squamous- and basal-cell carcinomas in kidney-transplant recipients after the first skin cancer: cumulative incidence and risk factors. Transplantation. 2010; 89 (10):1231–1238
[47] Buell JF, Hanaway MJ, Thomas M, Alloway RR, Woodle ES. Skin cancer following transplantation: the Israel Penn International Transplant Tumor Registry experience. Transplant Proc. 2005; 37(2):962–963
[48] Oddone N, Morgan GJ, Palme CE, et al. Metastatic cutaneous squamous cell carcinoma of the head and neck: the Immunosuppression, Treatment, Extranodal spread, and Margin status (ITEM) prognostic score to predict outcome and the need to improve survival. Cancer. 2009; 115 (9):1883–1891
[49] Manyam BV, Gastman B, Zhang AY, et al. Inferior outcomes in immunosuppressed patients with high-risk cutaneous squamous cell carcinoma of the head and neck treated with surgery and radiation therapy. J Am Acad Dermatol. 2015; 73(2):221–227
[50] Lang PG, Jr, Braun MA, Kwatra R. Aggressive squamous carcinomas of the scalp. Dermatol Surg. 2006; 32(9):1163–1170
[51] Euvrard S, Morelon E, Rostaing L, et al. TUMORAPA Study Group. Sirolimus and secondary skin-cancer prevention in kidney transplantation. N Engl J Med. 2012; 367(4):329–339
[52] Sekulic A, Migden MR, Oro AE, et al. Efficacy and safety of vismodegib in advanced basal-cell carcinoma. N Engl J Med. 2012; 366(23):2171–2179
[53] Bernier J, Domenge C, Ozsahin M, et al. European Organization for Research and Treatment of Cancer Trial 22931. Postoperative irradiation with or without concomitant chemotherapy for locally advanced head and neck cancer. N Engl J Med. 2004; 350(19):1945–1952
[54] Cooper JS, Pajak TF, Forastiere AA, et al. Radiation Therapy Oncology Group 9501/Intergroup. Postoperative concurrent radiotherapy and chemotherapy for high-risk squamous-cell carcinoma of the head and neck. N Engl J Med. 2004; 350(19):1937–1944
[55] Lewis CM, Glisson BS, Feng L, et al. A phase II study of gefitinib for aggressive cutaneous squamous cell carcinoma of the head and neck. Clin Cancer Res. 2012; 18(5):1435–1446
[56] Samstein RM, Ho AL, Lee NY, Barker CA. Locally advanced and unresectable cutaneous squamous cell carcinoma: outcomes of concurrent cetuximab and radiotherapy. J Skin Cancer. 2014; 2014:284582
[57] Kim S, Eleff M, Nicolaou N. Cetuximab as primary treatment for cutaneous squamous cell carcinoma to the neck. Head Neck. 2011; 33(2):286–288
[58] Maubec E, Petrow P, Scheer-Senyarich I, et al. Phase II study of cetuximab as first-line single-drug therapy in patients with unresectable squamous cell carcinoma of the skin. J Clin Oncol. 2011; 29(25):3419–3426
[59] Lutz ST, Lo SS, Chang EL, et al. Expert Panel On Radiation Oncology-Bone Metastases. ACR Appropriateness Criteria® non-spine bone metastases. J Palliat Med. 2012; 15(5):521–526
[60] Skibber JM, Soong SJ, Austin L, Balch CM, Sawaya RE. Cranial irradiation after surgical excision of brain metastases in melanoma patients. Ann Surg Oncol. 1996; 3(2):118–123

[61] Mori Y, Kobayashi T, Shibamoto Y. Stereotactic radiosurgery for metastatic tumors in the pituitary gland and the cavernous sinus. J Neurosurg. 2006; 105 Suppl:37–42
[62] Yu C, Chen JC, Apuzzo ML, et al. Metastatic melanoma to the brain: prognostic factors after gamma knife radiosurgery. Int J Radiat Oncol Biol Phys. 2002; 52 (5):1277–1287
[63] Selek U, Chang EL, Hassenbusch SJ, III, et al. Stereotactic radiosurgical treatment in 103 patients for 153 cerebral melanoma metastases. Int J Radiat Oncol Biol Phys. 2004; 59(4):1097–1106
[64] Lim CM, Clump DA, Heron DE, Ferris RL. Stereotactic Body Radiotherapy (SBRT) for primary and recurrent head and neck tumors. Oral Oncol. 2013; 49(5):401–406
[65] van der Zee J. Heating the patient: a promising approach? Ann Oncol. 2002; 13(8):1173–1184
[66] Kroon BB, Bergman W, Coebergh JW, Ruiter DJ, Dutch Melanoma Working Party. Consensus on the management of malignant melanoma of the skin in The Netherlands. Melanoma Res. 1999; 9(3):207–212
[67] Overgaard J, Gonzalez Gonzalez D, Hulshof MC, et al. Hyperthermia as an adjuvant to radiation therapy of recurrent or metastatic malignant melanoma. A multicentre randomized trial by the European Society for Hyperthermic Oncology. Int J Hyperthermia. 1996; 12(1):3–20

8 Surgical Implications of Systemic Therapy for Skin Cancer

Vadim P. Koshenkov, Oliver Eng, and Howard L. Kaufman

8.1 Introduction

Skin cancer is the most common form of cancer worldwide. Basal cell and squamous cell carcinomas represent the vast majority of these cancers and are associated with sun and ultraviolet radiation exposure. In the United States, it is estimated that 3.5 million nonmelanoma skin cancers are diagnosed annually, with 20% being squamous cell carcinoma.[1] While melanoma is far less frequent with 87,110 new cases expected in 2017, it accounts for at least 50% of mortality from all skin cancers. The incidence of melanoma has been steadily increasing by approximately 2.6% annually since the 1970s.[2] Skin cancer mortality has also been increasing, largely related to the recent increase in squamous cell carcinoma deaths. In 2017, it is expected there will be almost 9,730 deaths from melanoma and up to 8,800 deaths from squamous cell carcinoma.[2,3]

While the prognosis for most patients diagnosed with skin cancer is excellent, major challenges exist in treating advanced squamous cell carcinoma and metastatic melanoma. Approximately 5% of all patients with squamous cell carcinoma (nearly 30,000 patients annually) have high-risk tumors with significant rates of regional and distant metastases.[4] Most of the 8,791 deaths attributable to squamous cell carcinoma occur in these patients. Similarly, while 5-year survival rates for early-stage melanoma approach 98%, the overall survival for stage IV disease remains less than 20%.[5] In the past few years, however, major advances in the treatment of patients with metastatic melanoma have occurred. The developments in targeted therapeutics and tumor immunotherapy have revolutionized the management of metastatic melanoma. From 2011 to 2015, there have been seven new U.S. Food and Drug Administration (FDA)-approved agents. The roles of targeted therapy and immunotherapy are also being explored in nonmelanoma skin cancers.

During the 20th century and the first decade of the 21st century, only two agents were available for the treatment of metastatic melanoma. These were dacarbazine, an alkylating agent, and high-dose interleukin-2 (IL-2), an immunotherapy drug.[6] Since 2011, multiple agents have been shown to improve progression-free and/or overall survival for patients with advanced melanoma. These include ipilimumab (a first-generation T-cell checkpoint inhibitor), vemurafenib and dabarafenib (BRAF inhibitors), and trametinib (a selective MEK inhibitor).[7,8,9] Additionally, dramatic results with newer immunotherapy drugs, such as programmed death-1 (PD-1) and PD-1 ligand 1 (PD-L1) inhibitors, have been promising with two PD-1 inhibitors, pembrolizumab and nivolumab, being approved in 2014 for second-line treatment of metastatic melanoma. Several clinical trials are also under way to evaluate these new agents in the adjuvant treatment of melanoma and for the treatment of metastatic skin cancers, including squamous cell carcinoma and Merkel cell carcinoma. As the list of these agents grows and therapeutic efficacy improves, the number of people who are living longer with advanced melanoma is likely to rise. In these patients, the role of surgery in the treatment of metastatic disease will probably expand in order to augment the benefits of newer, more potent systemic therapies. Similarly, the surgeon must be familiar with the indications and toxicity profiles of these agents to maximize the benefit of surgical intervention in this new era of systemic cancer therapy. This chapter will briefly discuss the new systemic agents and highlight implications for surgical management, focusing on melanoma and squamous cell carcinoma.

8.2 Systemic Therapy of Melanoma

Treatment options for patients with metastatic melanoma include cytotoxic chemotherapy, targeted therapy, and immunotherapy. Surgical resection and radiotherapy are supplementary or palliative, and can be beneficial in carefully selected patients with minimal metastatic disease or isolated residual disease after systemic therapy. Consensus guidelines from the Society for Immunotherapy of Cancer (SITC) and the National Comprehensive Cancer Network (NCCN) are available to help choose the type and order of therapy for patients with advanced melanoma[10,11] (http://www.nccn.org/professionals/physician_gls/PDF/melanoma.pdf). A multidisciplinary team consisting of medical, surgical radiation oncology, and molecular pathology and radiology is pivotal in providing appropriate treatment of such patients. Patients with advanced melanoma should be evaluated with a serum lactate dehydrogenase level, for the purposes of staging and monitoring response to treatment as well as whole-body imaging, with particular attention to visceral organs, central nervous system (CNS), and bone. For patients with disease that can be completely resected with negative margins, metastasectomy is indicated and has been associated with 30 to 35% 5-year survival.[10,11] Radiation therapy has also been useful in patients with large, matted lymph node disease, especially in the neck and axillary nodal basins. It has also been beneficial in patients with painful bone lesions and CNS disease.

8.2.1 Chemotherapy

While cytotoxic chemotherapy is not as effective for melanoma as for other cancers, it may still play a role in the management of the disease. The only chemotherapy agent approved by the FDA for the treatment of metastatic melanoma is dacarbazine (DTIC). It has been available since 1974.[12] Less than 5% of patients experience a complete response, and 5-year survival rates range from 2 to 6%. However, objective response rates can be as high as 20%, and it is relatively well tolerated.[13] DTIC remains the single-agent chemotherapy drug of choice given that no high-quality trial has shown a survival benefit with another chemotherapy drug.

Temozolomide is an oral analog of dacarbazine with the added advantage of CNS penetrance. In a study that compared the two agents, there was no difference in objective response rate (21% with temozolomide vs. 18% with dacarbazine), overall survival (7.7 vs. 6.4 months; $p = 0.20$), or side effect profile.[14]

Temozolomide can be used in place of dacarbazine in the setting of brain metastases or if oral administration is desired.

Multiple combination chemotherapy regimens have been studied in attempts to improve on the minimal efficacy of the above-described monotherapy. A combination of cisplatinum, vinblastine, and dacarbazine (CVD) has been widely used, but it has yielded increased toxicity without a survival benefit.[15,16] A combination of carboplatin and paclitaxel in the setting of progression on dacarbazine or temozolomide has shown promising results in a phase II clinical trial.[17] An objective response rate of 26% and an overall survival of 7.8 months were reported. Biochemotherapy, in which interferon alfa-2b (IFNα2β) and low-dose IL-2 are added to CVD, has also been tested in attempts to improve outcomes. However, two large randomized clinical trials have demonstrated an increase in adverse events without improvement in overall survival when compared to standard chemotherapy.[18,19]

8.2.2 Targeted Therapy

BRAF and MEK Inhibitors

Multiple molecular pathways with gene mutations that drive tumor progression in melanoma cells have been identified, resulting in the development of molecular inhibitors. BRAF inhibitors, MEK inhibitors, vascular endothelial growth factor (VEGF) inhibitors, and CKIT inhibitors are all pertinent to the discussion of targeted therapy in melanoma. The BRAF pathway utilizes RAS-RAF-MEK-ERK signaling proteins (▶ Fig. 8.1). BRAF mutations lead to constitutive activation of the pathway and are critical to cell signaling, tumor growth. Activating mutations in BRAF occur in approximately 50% of cutaneous melanomas.[20] Mutations in RAS, BRAF, and MEK proteins lead to continuous activation of the pathway despite the absence of a growth ligand. The most common BRAF mutation is at amino acid position 600 resulting in an exchange of valine for glutamic acid (V600E). All patients with advanced melanoma should be tested for BRAF mutation because of its relatively high prevalence and potential pharmacologic treatment options.

The first BRAF inhibitor, vemurafenib, was approved by the FDA in 2011 for use in BRAF-mutated metastatic melanoma.[8] In a phase III clinical trial of 675 treatment-naive patients, vemurafenib was compared to dacarbazine, and was associated with an improvement in progression-free survival (5.3 vs. 1.6 months, $p < 0.001$) and 6-month survival (84 vs. 64%). Tumor regression was seen in up to 50 to 70% of patients across clinical trials.[8,21,22] Median time to response was short—approximately 4.5 weeks; however, resistance was common, typically within 7 to 8 months after the initiation of therapy. Several strategies, such as combination therapy and discontinuous dosing, are being attempted in order to lower the emergence of resistance. Dabrafenib is another BRAF inhibitor that has also demonstrated improved progression-free survival compared to dacarbazine (5.1 vs. 2.7 months, $p < 0.001$), with an objective response rate of 52%.[23] As a result of this trial, dabrafenib was approved by the FDA in 2013. Both vemurafenib and dabrafenib can be taken orally. Both have a slightly higher toxicity profile than dacarbazine, and dose reduction may be necessary in up to 38% of patients.[8] The adverse events of these agents include fatigue, arthralgias, myalgias, skin hypersensitivity, and development of skin lesions, such as acanthomas and cutaneous squamous cell carcinoma.

Trametinib, an oral MEK inhibitor that has been FDA-approved since 2013, was tested against dacarbazine or paclitaxel in a phase III clinical trial that included 322 patients with BRAF V600E or V600K mutation metastatic melanoma.[24] Progression-free survival (4.8 vs. 1.5 months, $p < 0.001$) and 6-month survival (81 vs. 67%, $p = 0.01$) were both superior with trametinib. Objective response rate was 22%, which was lower than with BRAF inhibitors, and reported side effects were fewer. Skin reactions were common, such as rash, dermatitis, acneiform, dry skin, pruritus, and paronychia. However, these were generally mild. Other side effects included diarrhea, stomatitis, abdominal pain, lymphedema, hypertension, and hemorrhage.

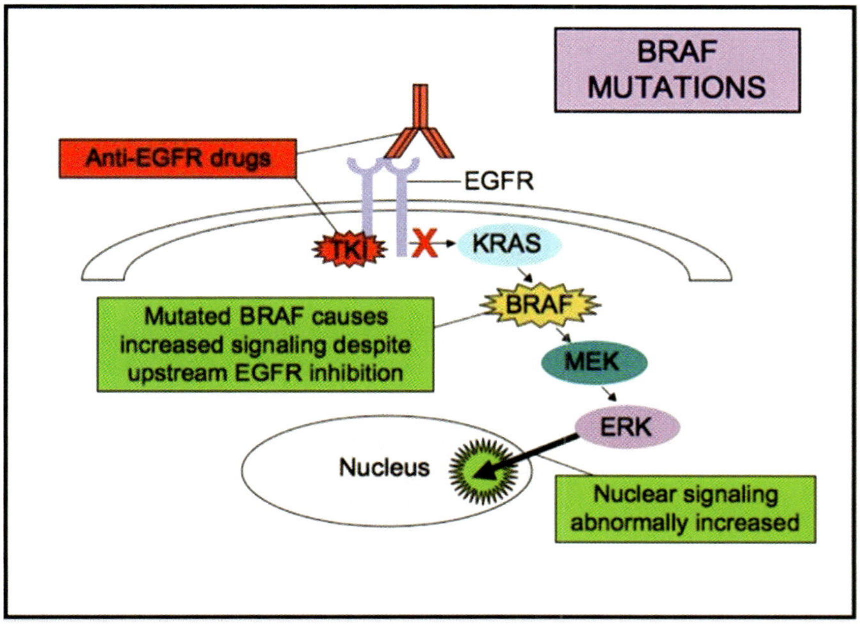

Fig. 8.1 BRAF pathway and cell signaling.

Mutations in MEK may be responsible for resistance to BRAF inhibitors. A phase II clinical trial was conducted in which 162 patients were treated with either dabrafenib alone or a combination of dabrafenib and trametinib.[9] Median progression-free survival was considerably improved with dual therapy from 5.6 to 9.4 months, while the objective response rate was 76 versus 54% ($p = 0.03$). Interestingly, the development of squamous cell carcinoma, which is seen in about 20% of patients with monotherapy BRAF inhibitors, was more than halved by the addition of the MEK inhibitor. Depending on the dose of trametinib, the incidence of squamous cell carcinoma ranged from 2 to 7% ($p = 0.004$ and 0.09). While other skin changes associated with BRAF inhibitors were less frequent in the combination therapy group, MEK inhibitor–associated toxicities were common. More recently, these findings were replicated in the setting of a phase III clinical trial that included 423 previously untreated patients.[25] In the dual therapy group, there was an improvement in progression-free survival (9.3 vs. 8.8 months, $p = 0.03$), objective response rate (67 vs. 51%, $p = 0.002$), and 6-month survival (93 vs. 85%, $p = 0.02$). Similarly, the incidence of squamous cell carcinoma was lower in the combination therapy group (2 vs. 9%).

Anti-VEGF and CKIT Inhibitors

VEGF and CKIT represent other possible therapeutic targets for drug development in melanoma. There has been lack of efficacy with anti-VEGF agents when used alone, and somewhat disappointing results when used in combination with cytotoxic chemotherapy.[26] In the setting of a phase II clinical trial, 214 patients were treated with carboplatin and paclitaxel with or without bevacizumab. The differences in progression-free survival (5.6 vs. 4.2 months), objective response rate (25.5 vs. 16.4%), and median overall survival (12.3 vs. 9.2 months) all failed to reach statistical significance.

Imatinib, a CKIT inhibitor, has significantly improved outcomes in patients with gastrointestinal stromal tumors and chronic myelogenous leukemia. CKIT mutations are present in approximately 6% of all melanomas, but higher rates have been reported in patients with mucosal and subungual lesions.[27] A phase II clinical trial was conducted in which 24 patients with CKIT-mutated melanoma were treated with imatinib, and an objective response rate of 29% was reported.[28] The disease control rate was 50%, but varied considerably between CKIT mutations and CKIT amplifications (77 vs. 18%).[28] These data suggest there may be a role for VEGF and CKIT inhibition, but to date, the results of clinical trials have not been sufficient to mandate clinical approval of these agents. Nonetheless, melanoma patients may be exposed to these drugs as part of clinical trials.

8.2.3 Immunotherapy

Immunotherapy can be defined as the augmentation of the host immune system to combat cancer cells. This is possible because B and T cells can recognize tumor-associated antigens, resulting in cytotoxicity of tumor cells. This process can initiate a cascade of immune responses against multiple antigens released by dying tumor cells leading to the eventual elimination of tumor. The important role of T cell–mediated immunity has been widely recognized, leading to the development of several immunotherapy agents designed to promote activation or prevent inhibition of T cell responses. These include cytokines, such as interferon and IL-2, and, more recently, inhibitors of T cell checkpoints, such as ipilimumab, pembrolizumab, and nivolumab. All five aforementioned agents, as well as a pegylated form of interferon, have been approved by the FDA for the treatment of metastatic melanoma. In contrast to chemotherapy and targeted therapy, which are associated with rapid onset of response with eventual resistance, immunotherapy may have a more delayed onset of activity without the association with resistance. It often can also induce durable responses, even in patients with advanced metastatic disease.

Interleukin-2

IL-2, which was approved by the FDA for metastatic melanoma treatment in 1998, had been extensively studied for three decades in mouse models as well as human clinical trials. The exact antitumor mechanism is unclear, but IL-2 appears to function by promoting large volume expansion of tumor-specific effector T cells. Two large trials were integral in testing the effectiveness of IL-2. A single-institution clinical trial, which included 409 patients with either metastatic melanoma ($n = 182$) or renal cell carcinoma ($n = 227$), demonstrated that high-dose IL-2 led to an objective response rate of 17.1%, with 8.1% of patients achieving a complete response.[29] A subsequent multi-institutional clinical trial in 270 patients with metastatic melanoma showed similar results, with an objective response rate of 16% and a complete response rate of 6%.[30] Perhaps, the most remarkable finding of the trial was the durability of the responses. In the responder group, the median duration of complete response was 59 months, and 40% of patients were disease-free for over 70 months.[31] Therapy with IL-2 is associated with considerable morbidity related to capillary leak syndrome. However, toxicities are usually reversible and guidelines exist to help clinicians manage these.[32]

Ipilimumab

Ipilimumab is a monoclonal antibody that targets the T cell checkpoint inhibitor, cytotoxic T-lymphocyte antigen-4 (CTLA-4), found on the surface of activated T cells (▶ Fig. 8.2). T cells are activated through a series of signals, with the first signal provided by the T cell receptor upon recognition of cognate antigen presented as processed peptides bound to major histocompatibility complexes. The second signal is provided by CD28, which is also found on the surface of T cells, activating proliferation and cytokine production upon binding to the costimulatory molecules, B7.1 and B7.2. After activation, CTLA-4 is mobilized to the T cell surface and modulates T cell activity by binding B7.1 and B7.2 with high affinity and inhibiting T cell proliferation and cytokine production. Ipilimumab prevents CTLA-4 from inhibiting T cell activity and hence prevents T cell inhibition, allowing a more prolonged, and thus potent, T cell response. In a phase III clinical trial of 676 patients with advanced melanoma, patients were randomized to ipilimumab alone, combination with a gp100 peptide vaccine, or both. There was an improvement in overall survival with ipilimumab (10 vs. 6 months, $p = 0.0026$) given alone or in combination compared to vaccine alone.[7] Interestingly, there was no

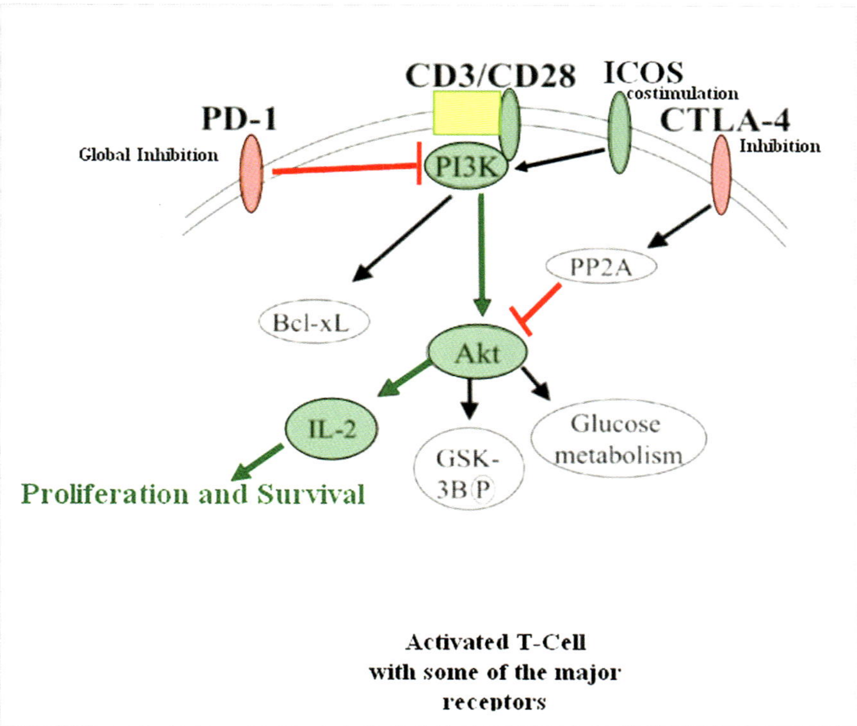

Fig. 8.2 Various T-cell pathways and sites of action of immunotherapy agents in melanoma.

significant difference in progression-free survival between treatment arms, suggesting a delayed therapeutic response with ipilimumab.

Ipilimumab has also been used in combination with dacarbazine or granulocyte-macrophage colony-stimulating factor (GM-CSF) in two large clinical trials.[33,34] When used in conjunction with dacarbazine, 1-year survival was significantly improved (47.3 vs. 36.3%).[33] However, grade 3 or higher adverse events were more than doubled in the combination group (56.3 vs. 27.5%, $p < 0.001$). When given together with GM-CSF, 1-year survival was significantly improved over ipilimumab alone (68.9 vs. 52.9%, $p = 0.01$), but the combination was paradoxically associated with fewer side effects.[34] Adverse events associated with ipilimumab include autoimmune dermatitis, colitis, hepatitis, hypophysitis, and rarely peripheral neuritis and pancreatitis. Early detection is paramount to treatment, as therapy discontinuation, administration of corticosteroids, and, in rare cases, infliximab have been shown to be successful in the management of the autoimmune-related toxicities.[35]

PD-1 and PD-L1 Inhibitors

The PD-1 receptor is another T cell checkpoint that is expressed on the surface of T cells after activation (▶ Fig. 8.2). Although PD-1 expression is observed shortly after T cell activation, it serves as a marker of T cell exhaustion and functions similarly to CTLA-4 in downregulating T cell responses. PD-1 signaling is triggered by binding to one of two ligands, called PD-L1 and PD-L2.[36] Inhibition of PD-1 binding to PD-L1 has been proposed as another strategy for preventing or reversing T cell exhaustion, and this has shown significant promise in the treatment of melanoma, non–small cell lung cancer, bladder cancer, Hodgkin's lymphoma, and other cancers. In 2014, two PD-1 inhibitors, pembrolizumab and nivolumab, were FDA-approved for the treatment of metastatic melanoma in the second-line setting.

In a phase I clinical trial, 135 melanoma patients were treated with an anti-PD-1 antibody in a dose escalation manner.[37] The objective response rate across all dose cohorts was 38%, with a rate of 52% at the highest dose. Importantly, prior therapy with ipilimumab did not appear to impact this effect. The median duration of response had not been reached at the time of the analysis, with a median follow-up time of 11 months, indicating a very durable response. The PD-1 inhibitor was well tolerated with few grade 3/4 toxicities. In another clinical phase I trial that included 52 patients with advanced cancer, an anti-PD-L1 antibody resulted in a 17.3% objective response rate.[38] Most of the responses lasted for longer than 1 year and only 9% of patients experienced grade 3/4 toxicity.[38] More recently, nivolumab, an anti-PD-1 antibody, was compared to dacarbazine in the setting of a clinical phase III trial of 418 previously untreated melanoma patients without a BRAF mutation.[39] One-year survival (72.9 vs. 42.1%, $p < 0.001$), progression-free survival (5.1 vs. 2.2 months, $p < 0.001$), and objective response rate (40.0 vs. 13.9%, $p < 0.001$) were all superior in nivolumab-treated patients. PD-L1 expression was present in 35.4% of pretreatment tumor samples in the 418 patients, and was associated with higher response rates in the nivolumab-treated group (52.7 vs. 33.1%), but not in the dacarbazine group (10.8 vs. 15.7%). Treatment-related grade 3 or higher toxicities were less frequent in the nivolumab cohort compared to the dacarbazine group (11.7 vs. 17.6%).

The clinical success of T cell checkpoint inhibitors has led to an interest in combination regimens. This was tested in a clinical phase I trial that included 53 melanoma patients who underwent concurrent therapy and 33 patients who received sequential therapy using ipilimumab and nivolumab.[40] The objective response rates were 40 and 20%, respectively. At maximal tolerable doses in the concurrent group, the response rate reached 53%, and 18% of patients underwent a rapid complete response. The toxicity profile in the concurrent group was no worse than what has been observed for monotherapy treatment with ipilimumab. A large randomized trial of this combination in melanoma is in progress.

Oncolytic Virus Immunotherapy

Another approach to immunotherapy involves directly infecting cancer cells with native or recombinant oncolytic viruses. These are viruses that preferentially replicate within tumor cells, induce lytic tumor cell death, release danger-associated molecular signals, and promote antitumor immunity by release of tumor-associated antigens in the context of a viral infection. Numerous vectors have shown promise in therapeutic murine models and early phase clinical trials, including adenovirus, adeno-associated virus, herpesvirus, reovirus, vaccinia virus, coxsackievirus, and Newcastle disease virus. Skin cancers, most notably melanoma, have been logical targets for oncolytic virus immunotherapy because patients often have accessible lesions for injection and these tumors are inherently immunogenic.

In terms of clinical development, there are considerable data supporting the use of a modified herpes simplex type I virus encoding human GM-CSF (termed talimogene laherparepvec or T-VEC). The T-VEC virus is attenuated by deletion of two pathogenic viral gene segments, which prevent neurotropism. T-VEC also encodes GM-CSF, which can help recruit and mature dendritic cells to engulf dying tumor cells and initiate a tumor-specific T cell response. A phase II clinical trial was conducted in 50 patients with advanced or metastatic melanoma with lesions accessible for direct intratumoral injection.[41] An objective response rate for both the injected and noninjected disease was 26%, and a mild toxicity profile was observed that included low-grade constitutional symptoms and injection site reactions.[41] One-year and 2-year survival rates were 58 and 52%, respectively, suggesting a durable response when present. Patients treated with T-VEC also demonstrated accumulation of melanoma-specific effector CD8 + T cells within injected tumors and a decrease number of suppressive regulatory CD4 + T cells and myeloid-derived suppressor cells.

T-VEC has also been tested in a phase III clinical trial enrolling 436 patients with advanced melanoma, who were randomized in a 2:1 fashion to receive T-VEC or recombinant GM-CSF.[42] The objective response rates were 26 and 6% in the two groups, while the durable response rate, the primary end point of the trial, was 16 versus 2% ($p < 0.0001$). Median overall survival was also higher in subjects treated with T-VEC (23.3 vs. 18.9 months, $p = 0.051$). Grade 3 or higher adverse events occurred in less than 3% of patients treated with T-VEC. Combination approaches using T-VEC and ipilimumab are now being studied in a clinical phase Ib/II trial with preliminary data demonstrating an earlier response onset than with ipilimumab alone and an improvement in the objective response rate.[43]

8.3 Adjuvant Therapy of Melanoma

8.3.1 Interferon Alfa-2b

Melanoma patients with metastasis to regional lymph nodes (stage III) are at high risk for recurrence. High-dose IFNα2β has been approved by the FDA for the adjuvant therapy of stage III melanoma since 1996. The exact mechanisms responsible for the antitumor activity of interferon are incompletely defined but likely include immunomodulation, direct antiproliferative, and proapoptotic effects, possibly through an antiangiogenesis mechanism. One of the first large clinical trials to investigate the efficacy of IFNα2β as an adjuvant agent for high-risk melanoma enrolled 287 patients who had undergone wide local excision and lymphadenectomy.[44] Both progression-free survival (20 vs. 12 months) and overall survival (45.6 vs. 33.6 months) were improved with high-dose IFNα2β when compared to placebo. Toxicities were significant in the majority of patients and dose modification was frequently required. The FDA approved interferon based on the results of this trial. A follow-up study that enrolled 642 patients compared high-dose IFNα2β with low-dose IFNα2β and placebo.[45] Progression-free survival, but not overall survival, was superior in the high-dose IFNα2β group. A subsequent phase III clinical trial that randomized patients to either induction therapy only with high-dose IFNα2β or placebo was conducted.[46] This trial was closed prior to completion because preliminary results showed no difference in progression-free survival and overall survival between the two groups.

Pegylated IFNα2β was evaluated as a strategy to optimize efficacy and limit toxicity because this type of drug formulation increases absorption and half-life. A phase III clinical trial that included 1,256 resected node-positive melanoma patients initially suggested a benefit in progression-free survival, which was most pronounced in patients with a single positive lymph node metastasis and in patients with ulcerated primary lesions. While this resulted in FDA approval, neither progression-free survival nor overall survival benefit was sustained after long-term follow-up of 90 months.[47] Additionally, the drug had to be discontinued in 37% of patients because of toxicity. Multiple meta-analyses have been performed in attempts to determine whether both progression-free survival and overall survival are improved with high-dose IFNα2β. Most have shown that while progression-free survival benefits from this therapy, this effect does not extend to overall survival when patients are followed up for a prolonged period.[48,49,50]

8.3.2 Ipilimumab

The limited improvement in outcomes seen with INFα2β in the adjuvant setting has prompted a search for a better agent. Ipilimumab, an immunotherapy drug that has been shown to improve overall survival in patients with metastatic melanoma with a durable response profile,[7] is being investigated in several clinical trials. In a setting of a phase III clinical trial of 951 resected stage III patients, ipilimumab is being compared to placebo in a 1:1 fashion. After a median follow-up of 2.7 years, 3-year progression-free survival rates were significantly higher in ipilimumab group (46.5 vs. 34.8%, $p = 0.0013$).[51] The higher dose of ipilimumab (10 mg/kg) used in this trial has resulted in a considerable grade 3/4 adverse event rate, particularly for endocrinopathies (8.5 vs. 0%). Of the patients started on ipilimumab, 52% discontinued treatment because of adverse events, most within 12 weeks of therapy initiation. Other phase II and phase III clinical trials investigating adjuvant ipilimumab are currently accruing patients.[52,53]

8.4 Systemic Therapy of Nonmelanoma Skin Cancer

8.4.1 Cetuximab

The vast majority of patients diagnosed with cutaneous squamous cell carcinoma have excellent prognosis, and surgical resection is usually sufficient therapy. However, in approximately 5% of the 700,000 annual cases, there are high-risk features that can result in regional and/or distant metastases. These high-risk features include size ≥ 2 cm, thickness ≥ 4 mm, head and neck location, poor differentiation, perineural invasion, tumor recurrence, and host immunosuppression.[4,54,55] Patients with these advanced squamous cell carcinomas have 5-year survival rates of 65 to 75% in the presence of regional metastases.[56,57]

Adjuvant therapies have been studied in attempts to improve upon the relatively poor survival outcomes with surgery alone for squamous cell carcinoma with regional metastatic disease.

Cetuximab has been explored with some success for such a purpose. In a setting of a phase II clinical trial of 36 chemotherapy (naive unresected patients), cetuximab demonstrated an objective response rate of 28%, with a disease control rate of 69% and a progression-free survival of 4.1 months.[58] The most common side effect was a rash, with no patient presenting with grade 3/4 toxicity. Other uncontrolled studies have shown a reduction in morbidity via tumor regression following cetuximab therapy, and associated improved clinical outcomes.[59,60] The limited data indicate potential for reducing morbidity of resection and improving survival, but larger well-designed controlled trials are needed to further confirm these outcomes.

8.4.2 Hedgehog Inhibitors

Basal cell cancer is the most common cutaneous malignancy.[1] These tumors rarely develop metastases but may grow locally, causing significant morbidity and disfigurement if not treated properly. Given these circumstances, an effective treatment had not been available until 2012, when vismodegib, a hedgehog inhibitor, was approved by the FDA. Most basal cell carcinomas have abnormalities in the hedgehog signaling pathway, and vismodegib inhibits signaling by blocking the activity of smoothened homologue. In a phase II clinical trial of 96 patients, vismodegib was shown to be effective for metastatic basal carcinoma (objective response rate of 30%, $p = 0.001$) and advanced basal carcinoma (objective response rate of 43%, $p < 0.001$).[61] The median progression-free survival was 9.5 months in both cohorts. The toxicity profile was significant, with serious adverse events occurring in 25% of patients. There were also seven deaths, although no definite pattern was identified, with the authors stating that the relationship between the study drug and the deaths was undetermined. This agent has also shown efficacy in preventing the development of new cancers in patients with basal cell nevus syndrome, although the adverse events were significant enough to warrant therapy discontinuation in approximately half of the patients.[62]

8.5 Implications of Systemic Therapy for the Surgeon

The surgeon may be called upon to help manage patients with metastatic melanoma with the goal of curative resection, palliative intervention, or management of complications from systemic therapy. Melanoma patients should be carefully evaluated for the ability to completely resect all tumor, the underlying metabolic and nutritional status of the patient, medical comorbidities, and the potential for durable responses with previous and subsequent systemic therapy. In general, patients should first be evaluated for curative operation, and if this is deemed not possible, then the goal may be palliative or designed to improve the patient's quality of life.

8.5.1 Surgery for Metastatic Disease

Over the past two decades, the role of surgery in the treatment of metastatic melanoma has continued to expand. Palliative resection of impending small bowel metastases and painful cutaneous lesions has become an accepted practice, with considerable retrospective reports suggesting clinical benefit and improvement in quality of life. Melanoma is the most common malignancy to metastasize to the small intestine, and reports of solitary and oligometastatic gastrointestinal metastasectomy have been associated with improved survival when compared to incomplete resection or observation.[63,64,65,66] Similarly, retrospective reports of curative resections for cutaneous, nodal, and pulmonary metastases have shown improved outcomes with surgery. The patients who benefitted most from an operative approach were those with a limited number of metastases that could be excised completely. These patients were associated with a long progression-free interval from the time of diagnosis.[67,68]

The role of metastasectomy was explored in a large cohort of patients who were enrolled in the Multicenter Selective Lymphadenectomy Trial-1 (MSLT-1). In this study, 291 patients developed metastatic disease. Metastasectomy was performed in 161 of these patients, and the 4-year survival rate was superior in this group than in a comparable nonoperated group (20.8 vs. 7%, $p < 0.0001$).[69] Operations were most beneficial in patients with stage M1a disease (cutaneous, subcutaneous, and nodal metastases). Curative resections have also been shown to be effective in improving survival of carefully selected patients with visceral oligometastatic disease, including brain, liver, and adrenal gland metastases.[70,71,72] A cohort of patients who underwent resection of brain metastases had a median survival of 8.5 months, which is an improvement over the expected 3- to 6-month survival in patients treated nonoperatively.[70]

More recently, the concept of considering metastasectomy in patients with an incomplete response to systemic therapy has been established. This has gained support due to the larger number of effective systemic agents and the durability associated with newer treatment regimens, most notable immunotherapy approaches. Data supporting the benefit of this strategy have been demonstrated in several small-cohort reports. Eleven patients with metastatic renal cell carcinoma treated with high-dose IL-2 had a partial response. These patients subsequently underwent an excision of residual disease in order to be rendered surgically no evidence of disease (SNED). Progression-free survival of these patients was comparable to complete responders and was found to be superior to partial responders who did not undergo operative intervention (100 vs. 76 vs. 35%).[73] Similar results were demonstrated for progression-free survival in 60 patients who were partial responders to IL-2 with metastatic melanoma and renal cell carcinoma.[74] With the recent introduction of more potent immunotherapy agents, such as ipilimumab and PD-1 and PD-L1 inhibitors, the approach of resecting residual disease with the intention of SNED in partial responders is likely to improve outcomes in a greater number of patients.

While metastasectomy for melanoma has been evaluated in retrospective series, there are even fewer reports on the role of metastasectomy for squamous cell carcinoma or other types of skin cancer. The use of cetuximab can result in objective, yet incomplete, clinical responses, and it is appropriate to consider resection of residual disease in those patients who exhibit a profound initial response to such therapy. Until further studies can be done, it is appropriate that patients with metastatic skin cancer who have incomplete responses to current systemic treatments be considered for resection of residual disease, especially if complete extirpation of all disease is possible.

8.5.2 Surgical Management of Toxicities of Systemic Therapies

The number of systemic agents available for the treatment of metastatic melanoma has increased with seven new agents approved by the U.S. FDA between 2011 and 2015. These drugs include molecularly targeted agents and immunotherapy drugs, which are both associated with unique side effects as discussed earlier. The surgeon may be placed in a position to manage various toxicities, although algorithms for standard management are not established. The most common surgical issues associated with systemic melanoma therapy are autoimmune gastrointestinal toxicities seen with immunotherapy and the management of squamous cell carcinomas in patients treated with BRAF inhibitors.

Ipilimumab has been associated with autoimmune enterocolitis, and occurs in about 21% of patients when the drug is used at the 3 mg/kg dose.[75] A higher rate of colitis has been reported with higher doses of ipilimumab, and lower rates of colitis have been seen with inhibitors of the PD-1/PD-L1 pathway. In general, colitis can be managed medically with antidiarrheals for limited symptoms. More serious or resistant cases can require high-dose corticosteroids and rarely infliximab. In all cases of significant diarrhea, management should include excluding other causes of colitis, such as *Clostridium difficile*–associated colitis, and efforts to rule out perforation should be done prior to initiating high-dose immunosuppressive medication.

Although medical management is usually effective for autoimmune colitis, about 2% of patients with ipilimumab-related colitis will develop bowel perforation. The surgeon should be aware of this difficult complication given its diagnostic challenges because many of the patients will already be on high doses of corticosteroids, potentially masking overt symptoms of an acute abdomen. Diarrhea and hematochezia are common, but not uniformly associated with autoimmune colitis related to tumor immunotherapy. Some patients can present with crampy abdominal pain without diarrhea. If there is doubt about the status of such patients, admission with serial abdominal examinations, fluid/electrolyte monitoring, repeat white blood cell counts, and consideration of intra-abdominal imaging should be performed. Patients may also require gentle endoscopy and a low threshold for surgical intervention.

The surgical approach to ipilimumab-related bowel perforation has not been uniformly established. A thorough exploratory laparotomy should be completed to ensure that there are no other causes for the colitis, and laparoscopy may be helpful as an initial approach. If the site of perforation can be identified either preoperatively or intraoperatively, primary repair may be possible if there is minimal contamination of the peritoneal cavity. Intraoperative endoscopy can also be a useful aid when the site of perforation is not known. In the event that the site cannot be found, a total colectomy may be necessary. Diversion may also be required depending on the degree of intraperitoneal contamination, status of the bowel, and security of the repair. Copious intraperitoneal irrigation should also be performed prior to closure. Patients may require stress doses of steroids if they have been on immunosuppressive agents for a prolonged time prior to operation. While the role of antibiotics has not been firmly established, early and perioperative antibiotics should also be considered in the management of severe autoimmune colitis once *C. difficile* colitis has been excluded.

Colonic perforation has also been reported with other forms of immunotherapy, although the incidence is much lower with PD-1 inhibitors and has been reported to occur in less than 0.45% of patients treated with high-dose IL-2 therapy.[76] Ipilimumab followed by high-dose IL-2 has even led to a bowel perforation rate of 13.6%.[77] Some clinicians recommend a colonoscopy after therapy with ipilimumab, but prior to the initiation of a second agent, such as IL-2, to rule out active colitis if patients have symptoms.[37] As different combination regimens continue to be evaluated, it is important for both the medical oncologist and the surgeon to remain vigilant and knowledgeable about possible complications of such therapy.

A unique side effect of BRAF inhibitor therapy is development of cutaneous acanthomas and, rarely, invasive squamous cell carcinoma. This has been observed with both vemurafenib and dabrafenib treatment.[78] While most of the cutaneous lesions that develop secondary to treatment with these agents are benign acanthomas, the potential for invasive squamous cell carcinoma mandates that all patients on BRAF inhibitor therapy have regular skin screening by a qualified dermatologist, who is comfortable differentiating between these two entities. Typically, the cutaneous lesions arise after 3 months of treatment, but can occur as early as 1 week into therapy. The incidence of squamous cell carcinoma has been reported to be as high as

26% in some series.[79] Large or painful benign acanthomas or documented invasive carcinomas should be treated by complete surgical excision. While metastases have not been reported, treatment should generally be discontinued or reduced and patients monitored more closely once a serious cutaneous manifestation has occurred. Interestingly, combination therapy with a BRAF and MEK inhibitor lowers the incidence of both benign and malignant cutaneous lesions, and the effect is dose-dependent.[9,25]

8.6 Conclusion

The impact of skin cancer continues to grow. Melanoma is now the fifth-most common malignancy in the United States, while the incidence of nonmelanoma skin cancers is higher than all the other cancers combined. The grim outlook for patients with advanced nonmelanoma skin cancer and metastatic melanoma is quickly changing because of the rapidly expanding armamentarium of agents available for systemic treatment. In addition to cytotoxic chemotherapy, there are an increasing number of new molecularly targeted therapy and immunotherapy agents available. The targeted therapy drugs have rapid onset and high response rates, although resistance is nearly universal. In contrast, tumor immunotherapy agents may take a longer time for a response to develop, but can induce very durable responses. The implications for the surgeon are two-fold. As the effectiveness of systemic therapy has improved the outcomes for patients with advanced and metastatic skin cancer, metastasectomy of all residual disease in patients with incomplete responses to systemic therapy may be advisable. Additionally, surgical complications of targeted therapy include benign and malignant skin neoplasms requiring surgical excision and careful skin surveillance. Immunotherapy, most notably with ipilimumab and combination approaches, has resulted in autoimmune colitis that may require careful clinical management and rarely surgical exploration and colectomy for bowel perforation. The surgeon will continue to be an important part of the team involved in caring for patients with metastatic melanoma and nonmelanoma skin cancer while on systemic therapy.

References

[1] Lomas A, Leonardi-Bee J, Bath-Hextall F. A systematic review of worldwide incidence of nonmelanoma skin cancer. Br J Dermatol. 2012; 166 (5):1069–1080

[2] Siegel R, Ma J, Zou Z, Jemal A. Cancer statistics, 2014. CA Cancer J Clin. 2014; 64(1):9–29

[3] Karia PS, Han J, Schmults CD. Cutaneous squamous cell carcinoma: estimated incidence of disease, nodal metastasis, and deaths from disease in the United States, 2012. J Am Acad Dermatol. 2013; 68(6):957–966

[4] Karia PS, Jambusaria-Pahlajani A, Harrington DP, Murphy GF, Qureshi AA, Schmults CD. Evaluation of American Joint Committee on Cancer, International Union Against Cancer, and Brigham and Women's Hospital tumor staging for cutaneous squamous cell carcinoma. J Clin Oncol. 2014; 32(4):327–334

[5] Edge SB, Byrd DR, Compton CC, Fritz AG, Green FL, Trotti A, eds. AJCC Cancer Staging Manual. 7th ed. New York, NY: Springer; 2010

[6] Ko JM, Fisher DE. A new era: melanoma genetics and therapeutics. J Pathol. 2011; 223(2):241–250

[7] Hodi FS, O'Day SJ, McDermott DF, et al. Improved survival with ipilimumab in patients with metastatic melanoma. N Engl J Med. 2010; 363(8):711–723

[8] Chapman PB, Hauschild A, Robert C, et al. BRIM-3 Study Group. Improved survival with vemurafenib in melanoma with BRAF V600E mutation. N Engl J Med. 2011; 364(26):2507–2516

[9] Flaherty KT, Infante JR, Daud A, et al. Combined BRAF and MEK inhibition in melanoma with BRAF V600 mutations. N Engl J Med. 2012; 367 (18):1694–1703

[10] Kaufman HL, Kirkwood JM, Hodi FS, et al. The Society for Immunotherapy of Cancer consensus statement on tumour immunotherapy for the treatment of cutaneous melanoma. Nat Rev Clin Oncol. 2013; 10(10):588–598

[11] Coit DG, Andtbacka R, Anker CJ, et al. National Comprehensive Cancer Network (NCCN). Melanoma, version 2.2013: featured updates to the NCCN guidelines. J Natl Compr Canc Netw. 2013; 11(4):395–407

[12] Bhatia S, Tykodi SS, Thompson JA. Treatment of metastatic melanoma: an overview. Oncology (Williston Park). 2009; 23(6):488–496

[13] Kim C, Lee CW, Kovacic L, Shah A, Klasa R, Savage KJ. Long-term survival in patients with metastatic melanoma treated with DTIC or temozolomide. Oncologist. 2010; 15(7):765–771

[14] Middleton MR, Grob JJ, Aaronson N, et al. Randomized phase III study of temozolomide versus dacarbazine in the treatment of patients with advanced metastatic malignant melanoma. J Clin Oncol. 2000; 18(1):158–166

[15] Legha SS, Ring S, Papadopoulos N, Plager C, Chawla S, Benjamin R. A prospective evaluation of a triple-drug regimen containing cisplatin, vinblastine, and dacarbazine (CVD) for metastatic melanoma. Cancer. 1989; 64 (10):2024–2029

[16] Buzaid A, Legha SS, Balch CM, et al. Pilot study of preoperative chemotherapy with cisplatin, vinblastine, and dacarbazine in patients with local-regional recurrence of melanoma. Cancer. 1994; 74(9):2476–2482

[17] Rao RD, Holtan SG, Ingle JN, et al. Combination of paclitaxel and carboplatin as second-line therapy for patients with metastatic melanoma. Cancer. 2006; 106(2):375–382

[18] Bajetta E, Del Vecchio M, Nova P, et al. Multicenter phase III randomized trial of polychemotherapy (CVD regimen) versus the same chemotherapy (CT) plus subcutaneous interleukin-2 and interferon-alpha2b in metastatic melanoma. Ann Oncol. 2006; 17(4):571–577

[19] Atkins MB, Hsu J, Lee S, et al. Eastern Cooperative Oncology Group. Phase III trial comparing concurrent biochemotherapy with cisplatin, vinblastine, dacarbazine, interleukin-2, and interferon alfa-2b with cisplatin, vinblastine, and dacarbazine alone in patients with metastatic malignant melanoma (E3695): a trial coordinated by the Eastern Cooperative Oncology Group. J Clin Oncol. 2008; 26(35):5748–5754

[20] Bauer J, Büttner P, Murali R, et al. BRAF mutations in cutaneous melanoma are independently associated with age, anatomic site of the primary tumor, and the degree of solar elastosis at the primary tumor site. Pigment Cell Melanoma Res. 2011; 24(2):345–351

[21] Bollag G, Hirth P, Tsai J, et al. Clinical efficacy of a RAF inhibitor needs broad target blockade in BRAF-mutant melanoma. Nature. 2010; 467 (7315):596–599

[22] Das Thakur M, Salangsang F, Landman AS, et al. Modelling vemurafenib resistance in melanoma reveals a strategy to forestall drug resistance. Nature. 2013; 494(7436):251–255

[23] Hauschild A, Grob JJ, Demidov LV, et al. Dabrafenib in BRAF-mutated metastatic melanoma: a multicentre, open-label, phase 3 randomised controlled trial. Lancet. 2012; 380(9839):358–365

[24] Flaherty KT, Robert C, Hersey P, et al. METRIC Study Group. Improved survival with MEK inhibition in BRAF-mutated melanoma. N Engl J Med. 2012; 367 (2):107–114

[25] Long GV, Stroyakovskiy D, Gogas H, et al. Combined BRAF and MEK inhibition versus BRAF inhibition alone in melanoma. N Engl J Med. 2014; 371 (20):1877–1888

[26] Kim KB, Sosman JA, Fruehauf JP, et al. BEAM: a randomized phase II study evaluating the activity of bevacizumab in combination with carboplatin plus paclitaxel in patients with previously untreated advanced melanoma. J Clin Oncol. 2012; 30(1):34–41

[27] Beadling C, Jacobson-Dunlop E, Hodi FS, et al. KIT gene mutations and copy number in melanoma subtypes. Clin Cancer Res. 2008; 14(21):6821–6828

[28] Hodi FS, Corless CL, Giobbie-Hurder A, et al. Imatinib for melanomas harboring mutationally activated or amplified KIT arising on mucosal, acral, and chronically sun-damaged skin. J Clin Oncol. 2013; 31(26):3182–3190

[29] Rosenberg SA, Yang JC, White DE, Steinberg SM. Durability of complete responses in patients with metastatic cancer treated with high-dose

interleukin-2: identification of the antigens mediating response. Ann Surg. 1998; 228(3):307–319
[30] Atkins MB, Lotze MT, Dutcher JP, et al. High-dose recombinant interleukin 2 therapy for patients with metastatic melanoma: analysis of 270 patients treated between 1985 and 1993. J Clin Oncol. 1999; 17(7):2105–2116
[31] Atkins MB, Kunkel L, Sznol M, Rosenberg SA. High-dose recombinant interleukin-2 therapy in patients with metastatic melanoma: long-term survival update. Cancer J Sci Am. 2000; 6 Suppl 1:S11–S14
[32] Schwartzentruber DJ. Guidelines for the safe administration of high-dose interleukin-2. J Immunother. 2001; 24(4):287–293
[33] Robert C, Thomas L, Bondarenko I, et al. Ipilimumab plus dacarbazine for previously untreated metastatic melanoma. N Engl J Med. 2011; 364(26):2517–2526
[34] Hodi FS, Lee S, McDermott DF, et al. Ipilimumab plus sargramostim vs ipilimumab alone for treatment of metastatic melanoma: a randomized clinical trial. JAMA. 2014; 312(17):1744–1753
[35] Fecher LA, Agarwala SS, Hodi FS, Weber JS. Ipilimumab and its toxicities: a multidisciplinary approach. Oncologist. 2013; 18(6):733–743
[36] Freeman GJ, Long AJ, Iwai Y, et al. Engagement of the PD-1 immunoinhibitory receptor by a novel B7 family member leads to negative regulation of lymphocyte activation. J Exp Med. 2000; 192(7):1027–1034
[37] Hamid O, Robert C, Daud A, et al. Safety and tumor responses with lambrolizumab (anti-PD-1) in melanoma. N Engl J Med. 2013; 369(2):134–144
[38] Brahmer JR, Tykodi SS, Chow LQ, et al. Safety and activity of anti-PD-L1 antibody in patients with advanced cancer. N Engl J Med. 2012; 366(26):2455–2465
[39] Robert C, Long GV, Brady B, et al. Nivolumab in previously untreated melanoma without BRAF mutation. N Engl J Med. 2015; 372(4):320–330
[40] Wolchok JD, Kluger H, Callahan MK, et al. Nivolumab plus ipilimumab in advanced melanoma. N Engl J Med. 2013; 369(2):122–133
[41] Senzer NN, Kaufman HL, Amatruda T, et al. Phase II clinical trial of a granulocyte-macrophage colony-stimulating factor-encoding, second-generation oncolytic herpesvirus in patients with unresectable metastatic melanoma. J Clin Oncol. 2009; 27(34):5763–5771
[42] Andtbacka RHI, Kaufman HL, Collichio F, et al. Talimogene laherparepvec induces durable responses in patients with advanced melanoma. J Clin Oncol 2015; 33(25):2780-2788
[43] Puzanov I, Milhem MM, Minor D, et al. Talimogene laherparepvec in combination with ipilimumab in previously untreated, unresectable stage IIIB-IV melanoma. J Clin Oncol 2016; 34(22):2619-2626
[44] Kirkwood JM, Strawderman MH, Ernstoff MS, Smith TJ, Borden EC, Blum RH. Interferon alfa-2b adjuvant therapy of high-risk resected cutaneous melanoma: the Eastern Cooperative Oncology Group Trial EST 1684. J Clin Oncol. 1996; 14(1):7–17
[45] Kirkwood JM, Ibrahim JG, Sondak VK, et al. High- and low-dose interferon alfa-2b in high-risk melanoma: first analysis of intergroup trial E1690/S9111/C9190. J Clin Oncol. 2000; 18(12):2444–2458
[46] Agarwala SS, Lee SJ, Yip W, et al. HYPERLINK "https://www.ncbi.nlm.nih.gov/pubmed/28135150" Phase III Randomized Study of 4 Weeks of High-Dose Interferon-α-2b in Stage T2bNO, T3a-bNO, T4a-bNO, and T1-4N1a-2a (microscopic) Melanoma: A Trial of the Eastern Cooperative Oncology Group-American College of Radiology Imaging Network Cancer Research Group (E1697). J Clin Oncol 2017; 35(8):885-892
[47] Eggermont AM, Suciu S, Testori A, et al. Long-term results of the randomized phase III trial EORTC 18991 of adjuvant therapy with pegylated interferon alfa-2b versus observation in resected stage III melanoma. J Clin Oncol. 2012; 30(31):3810–3818
[48] Lens MB, Dawes M. Interferon alfa therapy for malignant melanoma: a systematic review of randomized controlled trials. J Clin Oncol. 2002; 20 (7):1818–1825
[49] Verma S, Quirt I, McCready D, Bak K, Charette M, Iscoe N. Systematic review of systemic adjuvant therapy for patients at high risk for recurrent melanoma. Cancer. 2006; 106(7):1431–1442
[50] Mocellin S, Pasquali S, Rossi CR, Nitti D. Interferon alpha adjuvant therapy in patients with high-risk melanoma: a systematic review and meta-analysis. J Natl Cancer Inst. 2010; 102(7):493–501
[51] Eggermont AM, Chiarion-Seleni V, Grob JJ, et al. Ipilimumab versus placebo after complete resection of stage III melanoma: initial efficacy and safety results from the EORTC 18701 phase III trial. J Clin Oncol 2014;32(Suppl.). Abstract LBA9008
[52] National Cancer Institute, Ipilimumab or High-Dose Interferon Alfa-2b in Treating Patients With High-Risk Stage III-IV Melanoma That Has Been Removed by Surgery, Accessed June 16, 2017 http://clinicaltrials.gov/ct2/show/NCT01274338?term=ecog+1609&rank=1
[53] National Cancer Institute, Ipilimumab With or Without High-Dose Recombinant Interferon Alfa-2b in Treating Patients With Stage III-IV Melanoma That Cannot Be Removed by Surgery, Accessed June 16, 2017 http://clinicaltrials.gov/ct2/show/NCT01708941?term=ecog+3611&rank=1
[54] Jambusaria-Pahlajani A, Kanetsky PA, Karia PS, et al. Evaluation of AJCC tumor staging for cutaneous squamous cell carcinoma and a proposed alternative tumor staging system. JAMA Dermatol. 2013; 149(4):402–410
[55] Clayman GL, Lee JJ, Holsinger FC, et al. Mortality risk from squamous cell skin cancer. J Clin Oncol. 2005; 23(4):759–765
[56] Andruchow JL, Veness MJ, Morgan GJ, et al. Implications for clinical staging of metastatic cutaneous squamous carcinoma of the head and neck based on a multicenter study of treatment outcomes. Cancer. 2006; 106(5):1078–1083
[57] O'Brien CJ, McNeil EB, McMahon JD, Pathak I, Lauer CS, Jackson MA. Significance of clinical stage, extent of surgery, and pathologic findings in metastatic cutaneous squamous carcinoma of the parotid gland. Head Neck. 2002; 24(5):417–422
[58] Maubec E, Petrow P, Scheer-Senyarich I, et al. Phase II study of cetuximab as first-line single-drug therapy in patients with unresectable squamous cell carcinoma of the skin. J Clin Oncol. 2011; 29(25):3419–3426
[59] O'Bryan K, Sherman W, Niedt GW, et al. An evolving paradigm for the workup and management of high-risk cutaneous squamous cell carcinoma. J Am Acad Dermatol. 2013; 69(4):595–602.e1
[60] Kim S, Eleff M, Nicolaou N. Cetuximab as primary treatment for cutaneous squamous cell carcinoma to the neck. Head Neck. 2011; 33(2):286–288
[61] Sekulic A, Migden MR, Oro AE, et al. Efficacy and safety of vismodegib in advanced basal-cell carcinoma. N Engl J Med. 2012; 366(23):2171–2179
[62] Tang JY, Mackay-Wiggan JM, Aszterbaum M, et al. Inhibiting the hedgehog pathway in patients with the basal-cell nevus syndrome. N Engl J Med. 2012; 366(23):2180–2188
[63] Berger AC, Buell JF, Venzon D, Baker AR, Libutti SK. Management of symptomatic malignant melanoma of the gastrointestinal tract. Ann Surg Oncol. 1999; 6(2):155–160
[64] Gutman H, Hess KR, Kokotsakis JA, Ross MI, Guinee VF, Balch CM. Surgery for abdominal metastases of cutaneous melanoma. World J Surg. 2001; 25 (6):750–758
[65] Ollila DW, Essner R, Wanek LA, Morton DL. Surgical resection for melanoma metastatic to the gastrointestinal tract. Arch Surg. 1996; 131(9):975–979, 979–980
[66] Sanki A, Scolyer RA, Thompson JF. Surgery for melanoma metastases of the gastrointestinal tract: indications and results. Eur J Surg Oncol. 2009; 35 (3):313–319
[67] Neuman HB, Patel A, Hanlon C, Wolchok JD, Houghton AN, Coit DG. Stage-IV melanoma and pulmonary metastases: factors predictive of survival. Ann Surg Oncol. 2007; 14(10):2847–2853
[68] Wasif N, Bagaria SP, Ray P, Morton DL. Does metastasectomy improve survival in patients with Stage IV melanoma? A cancer registry analysis of outcomes. J Surg Oncol. 2011; 104(2):111–115
[69] Howard JH, Thompson JF, Mozzillo N, et al. Metastasectomy for distant metastatic melanoma: analysis of data from the first Multicenter Selective Lymphadenectomy Trial (MSLT-I). Ann Surg Oncol. 2012; 19(8):2547–2555
[70] Zacest AC, Besser M, Stevens G, Thompson JF, McCarthy WH, Culjak G. Surgical management of cerebral metastases from melanoma: outcome in 147 patients treated at a single institution over two decades. J Neurosurg. 2002; 96(3):552–558
[71] Mittendorf EA, Lim SJ, Schacherer CW, et al. Melanoma adrenal metastasis: natural history and surgical management. Am J Surg. 2008; 195(3):363–368, discussion 368–369
[72] Ryu SW, Saw R, Scolyer RA, Crawford M, Thompson JF, Sandroussi C. Liver resection for metastatic melanoma: equivalent survival for cutaneous and ocular primaries. J Surg Oncol. 2013; 108(2):129–135
[73] Kim B, Louie AC. Surgical resection following interleukin 2 therapy for metastatic renal cell carcinoma prolongs remission. Arch Surg. 1992; 127 (11):1343–1349
[74] Yang JC, Abad J, Sherry R. Treatment of oligometastases after successful immunotherapy. Semin Radiat Oncol. 2006; 16(2):131–135
[75] Beck KE, Blansfield JA, Tran KQ, et al. Enterocolitis in patients with cancer after antibody blockade of cytotoxic T-lymphocyte-associated antigen 4. J Clin Oncol. 2006; 24(15):2283–2289
[76] Heimann DM, Schwartzentruber DJ. Gastrointestinal perforations associated with interleukin-2 administration. J Immunother. 2004; 27(3):254–258

[77] Smith FO, Goff SL, Klapper JA, et al. Risk of bowel perforation in patients receiving interleukin-2 after therapy with anti-CTLA 4 monoclonal antibody. J Immunother. 2007; 30(1):130

[78] Chu EY, Wanat KA, Miller CJ, et al. Diverse cutaneous side effects associated with BRAF inhibitor therapy: a clinicopathologic study. J Am Acad Dermatol. 2012; 67(6):1265–1272

[79] Boussemart L, Routier E, Mateus C, et al. Prospective study of cutaneous side-effects associated with the BRAF inhibitor vemurafenib: a study of 42 patients. Ann Oncol. 2013; 24(6):1691–1697

9 Common Reconstructive Techniques after Facial Skin Cancer Excision

Neilendu Kundu and Brian R. Gastman

9.1 Introduction

Skin cancer represents a diverse collection of pathology. Skin cancer is the most common cancer in the United States, and it is estimated that 20% of Americans will develop at least one skin cancer in their lifetime.[1,2] According to published figures, the average annual treatment cost for skin cancer in the United States was approximately $8.1 billion from 2007 to 2011.[2] This figure continues to rise annually.

A large subsection of skin cancer affects the face, given it is one of the areas that is most exposed to the elements. Cutaneous defects of the face are unique for a variety of reasons. From a medical science standpoint, wounds tend to heal very well with a low rate of infection and often require minimal debridement compared to other areas of the body due to the exceptional vascularity of the face. As will be discussed later, cosmetically acceptable results can be achieved even with secondary intention. From a social science standpoint, the face is critical for communication, as well as negotiating complex social interactions that are part of daily activity. Thus, reconstruction of lesions of the face is crucial for patients to maintain normalcy. Tagliacozzi—one of the fathers of plastic surgery—described it best, "restore, repair, and make whole those parts which nature has given, but fortunate has taken away, not so much that it please the eye of the beholder, but that it buoys the spirit of the afflicted."[3]

Facial reconstruction allows for contributions from a range of specialties, including general and plastic surgery, dermatology, ophthalmology, and otolaryngology. In order to appropriately manage these defects, a multitude of options are necessary in the surgeon's armamentarium. This requires exposure to extensive modalities from primary closure to skin grafting to locoregional flaps and even free tissue transfer. While some reconstructive options extend beyond the scope of this chapter, common techniques are described, including pitfalls to avoid.

The face is one of the most anatomically complex aspects of the body. To aid surgeons in better elucidating areas of reconstruction, it has been divided into facial aesthetic regions based on landmarks and shadowing. The main aesthetic subunits of the face include the forehead, eyelids, cheeks, nose, lips, chin, and ears.[4] These subunits are then subsequently further subdivided. For example, the nose itself has nine subunits: the dorsum, paired lateral side walls, tip, paired soft tissue triangles, paired lobules, and the columella.[5] The ideal reconstruction for cutaneous defects provides coverage with like tissue, ideally from within the aesthetic unit itself. By manipulating the subunit principle, scars can be "hidden" within natural shadows to provide aesthetically pleasing outcomes for patients who present with initially intimidating facial defects.

9.2 Forehead

Experience in forehead reconstruction has revealed that large defects can be primarily closed with excellent results. Additionally, due to the rich vascularity, defects can also heal with secondary intention yielding cosmetically satisfying results (▶ Fig. 9.1). The forehead has been subdivided into paramedian, lateral, and lateral temporal subunits, with the eyebrows providing a mobile subunit of their own.[6]

Arterial and venous flow is provided by paired vessels. From the arterial standpoint, flow is distributed from both the external and internal carotid arteries by the paired frontal branches of the superficial temporal artery (external carotid artery system) and supratrochlear and supraorbital arteries (internal carotid artery system). Each supply is robust enough to allow for elevation of a flap utilizing this as the axial system. This allows for a variety of rotation and advancement flaps.

The forehead is innervated by the supraorbital nerve as well as by the frontal branch of the facial nerve. The supraorbital nerve provides sensory innervation to the forehead and has two divisions. There is a deep division that runs from the orbital rim (lateral) toward the superior temporal line of the skull, which then moves cranial (parallel) to the temporal line before taking a medial course to enter the scalp. The superficial division also courses over the orbital rim, but traverses anterior to the frontalis muscle to provide sensation to the scalp. Injury to these nerves can lead to paresthesias as well as itching. The frontal branch of the facial nerve is deep to the frontalis—which it innervates. It provides motor function and can be identified along a line—referred to as Pitanguy's line—that runs 0.5 cm below the tragus to a point 1.5 cm superior to the lateral position of the eyebrow.[7]

Small defects of the forehead—up to 1 to 2 cm—can be closed primarily or heal with secondary intention with satisfactory cosmetic results. This concept has been utilized in nasal reconstruction, where forehead flaps have been utilized for large nasal defects. The superior aspect of the forehead flap—which is based on an axial blood supply from the supratrochlear system—is left open to allow for granulation and healing. With standard wound care to ensure maintenance of a clean, moist environment, the forehead scarring is acceptable. The downside to leaving the wound open is that it may take up to 6 weeks to achieve complete healing.

Medium-sized defects of the forehead—up to 3 to 4 cm—can be approximated with primary closure. Primary closure of larger wounds is possible in this region due to the excellent vascularity. Wounds that may otherwise develop wound necrosis elsewhere on the body due to tension on the incision often heal without complication.

For relatively large defects of the forehead—up to 6 cm—advancement flaps provide excellent outcomes as they mobilize skin from relaxed skin tension lines (RSTL) of the forehead. While full-thickness, sheet skin grafts are also excellent options, "H-flaps" allow for reconstruction within the aesthetic principle without utilization of a separate donor site. H-flap also utilizes the benefit of increased laxity found within the lateral forehead skin, which helps to facilitate mobilization. In prospective case series studies, H-flap

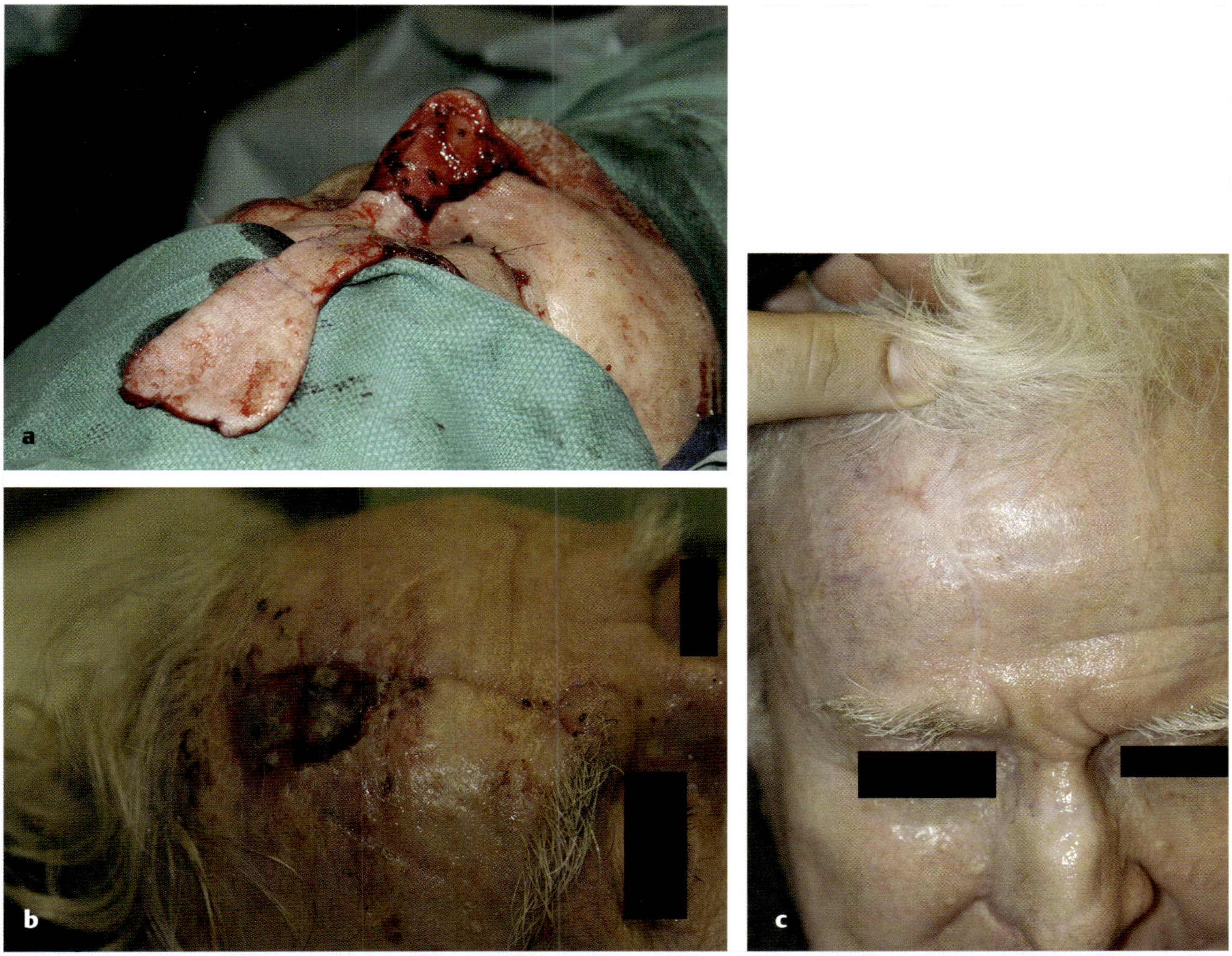

Fig. 9.1 (a,b) Secondary healing of a forehead after a paramedian forehead flap utilized for nasal reconstruction is common practice. Often, acceptable cosmetic results can be obtained using this method for the forehead. (c) The superior aspect was left to heal with secondary intention leaving a cosmetically acceptable result.

was found to have excellent cosmetic outcomes based on answers to a validated patient satisfaction questionnaire.[8] The flap is created by making incisions parallel to the RSTL and removing burrow triangles from each side. After removal of the triangles and undermining superficial to the temporal muscle to decrease the likelihood of injury to the supraorbital nerves, the wounds can be closed without undue tension, also allowing for aesthetic scars (▶ Fig. 9.2). The cosmesis can be improved further by designing the flap in such a way that the horizontal components are able to fit within the main transverse rhytids of the forehead that are created due to the natural movement of the frontalis muscle.

Temporal wounds of the forehead can also be reconstructed using local advancement flaps, as described earlier. A key aspect in this region is to maintain the position of the eyebrow as well as the temporal hairline. Regional flaps—including the cervicofacial flap, which will be discussed in detail later in this chapter—can provide one with the ability to solve both of these potential situations before they become an issue.

9.3 Cheeks

The cheek possesses the largest facial aesthetic region and is intimately related to social interaction as it allows for the ability to capture emotion on a large scale, in conjunction with the other aspects of the face. It marries the superior and inferior face to act as one unit.

Contour of the cheek is created by a synergy of fat distribution, underlying bony architecture, and the retaining ligaments of the face. Retaining ligaments of the cheek are critical for these subunits as they provide the structural framework that allows for youthful appearance. Thus, as one ages, these ligaments become increasingly lax, which can cause fat redistribution, leading to an older appearance. Several of these retaining ligaments have been described which has allowed for classification of the aforementioned creases. For example, the retaining ligaments of the zygoma have been referred to as McGregor's patch. These are osteocutaneous ligaments that provide support for the skin overlying the zygoma. Other examples include ligaments at the junction of the cheek and upper

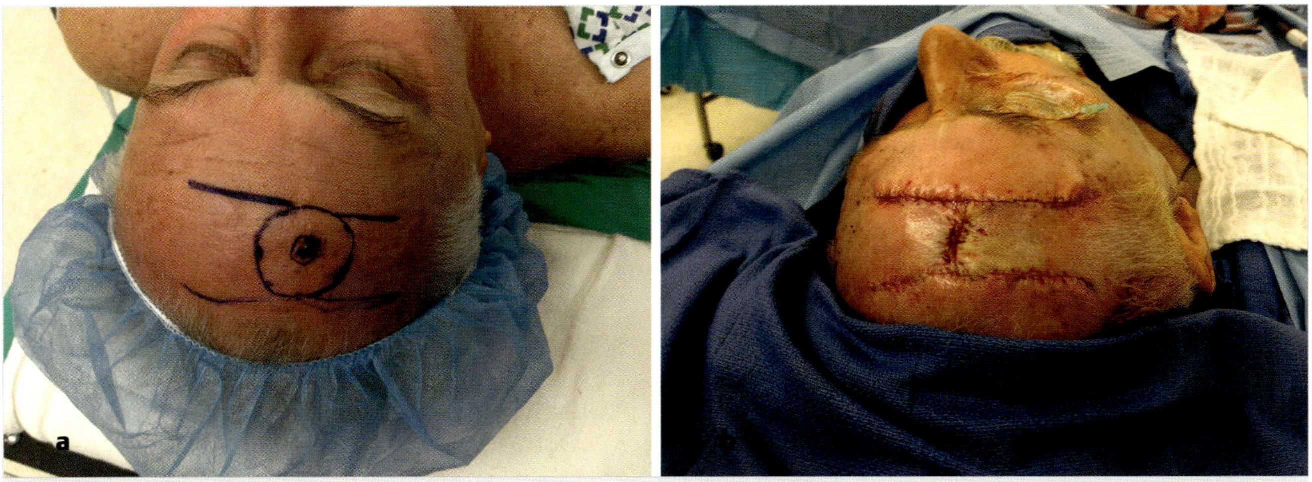

Fig. 9.2 A 2-cm squamous cell carcinoma excised leaving a 6-cm defect approximated with an H-flap under local anesthesia.

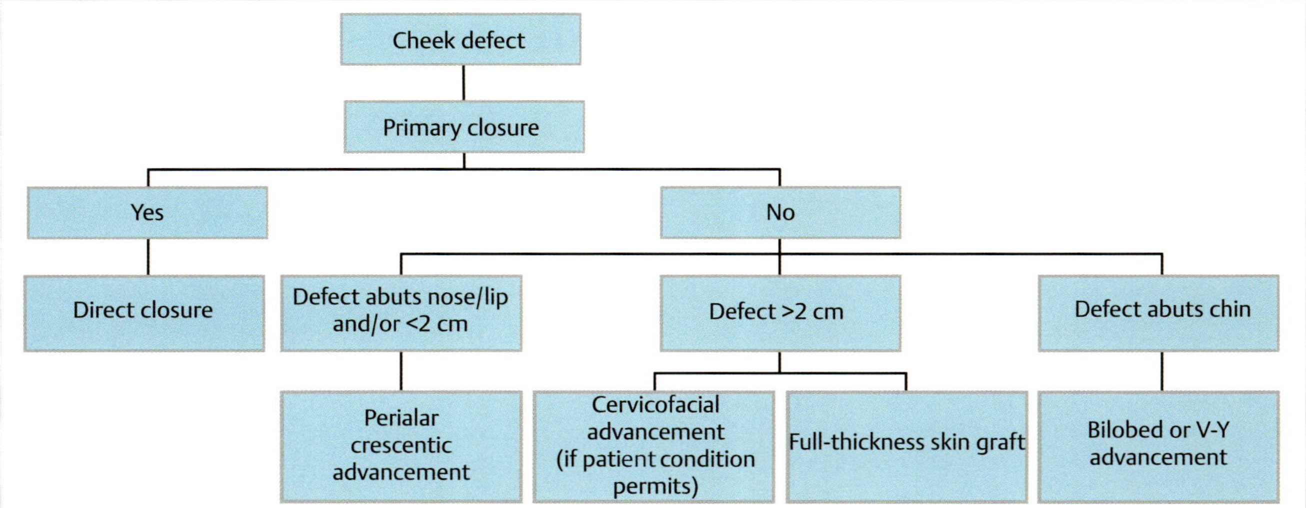

Fig. 9.3 An easy-to-follow cheek reconstruction algorithm. (Reproduced with permission from Rapstine et al.[11])

lip creating the melolabial (nasolabial) crease.[9] The anatomy of the cheek requires knowledge of the facial nerve as well because injury can be severely disfiguring for patients. As long as dissection proceeds anterior to the superficial musculo-aponeurotic system (SMAS), a safe plane—with respect to the nerves—is maintained.

The cheek receives its vascular supply from the external carotid system. Namely, it obtains the majority of its blood flow from branches of the facial artery. A minor supply is provided by the transverse facial artery, which is a branch of the superficial temporal artery. The venous drainage follows the arterial system, as it does in the forehead.

Innervation to the cheek is dependent on location. The medial aspect of the cheek from just lateral of the lateral limbus to the upper second premolar tooth is supplied by the infraorbital nerve (from the second division of the trigeminal cranial nerve). The nerve also provides sensation to the lower eyelid, upper lip, and nasal vestibule. The anterior branch of the great auricular nerve provides sensation for the lateral skin from the tragus to the lateral limbus.

Several classification systems of the cheek have been developed that divide the cheek into separate aesthetic subunits. One utilizes eight separate aesthetic subunits. They are the inferior bony orbital rim, nasofacial sulcus, melolabial crease, labiomandibular crease, inferior border of the mandible, preauricular crease, and a line extending from the lateral canthus to the root of the helix.[9] Roth et al divided the cheek into three overlapping aesthetic zones: zone 1 (suborbital), zone 2 (preauricular), and zone 3 (buccomandibular).[10] Based on these zones, reconstructive algorithms for the cheek have been described. ▸ Fig. 9.3 reveals an algorithm that is easy to follow in this author's opinion.[11] Many defects of the cheek—including a high percentage of Mohs defects—can be reconstructed using primary closure. An elliptical excision or simply creating

Burow's triangles at both ends of a Mohs defect, in the plane that is best fitting with the RSTL, allows for tension-free, primary closure with optimal cosmetic results. This is especially the situation in older patients because there is an increase in the amount of skin laxity, thus allowing for repair without concern for issues including ectropion or elevation of the modiolus.

Small defects that abut the nose/lip or chin can be closed using crescentic advancement, bilobed/VY advancement, or nasolabial fold flaps.

For patients who have large defects of the cheek—more than 3 to 4 cm—several options for reconstruction are feasible. While tissue expansion is an appropriate option and can lead to excellent results, it requires several weeks to months of painful expansion as well as substantial disfigurement in the time frame until the expansion process has reached its completion. Additionally, custom-made expanders are often required for the cheek, which can cause an increase in cost. Full-thickness skin grafting, harvested from the pre/postauricular or supraclavicular sites, provides a reasonable reconstructive option for older patients who possess multiple comorbidities. Skin grafting is not the preferred option given that it can be difficult to obtain a good color match with the native face. Furthermore, contracture of the skin graft can also lead to suboptimal results. Originally described by Mustarde for lower lid reconstruction, cervicofacial advancement flaps provide the ability to cover a large surface defect of the skin with tissue that possesses an ideal color, texture, and contour match.[12] Austen et al described 32 consecutive cervicofacial flaps that were performed without major complications and with satisfactory cosmetic results.[13] Additionally, dissection can be carried inferiorly beneath the neck to the level of the deltopectoral groove to assist in the recruitment of additional tissue for tension-free repair. This is of importance for wounds that are large and also are near the medial canthus, where excess tension of the wound can lead to ectropion (▶ Fig. 9.4). A significant aspect in the reconstructive decision tree is choosing between a cervicofacial and reverse

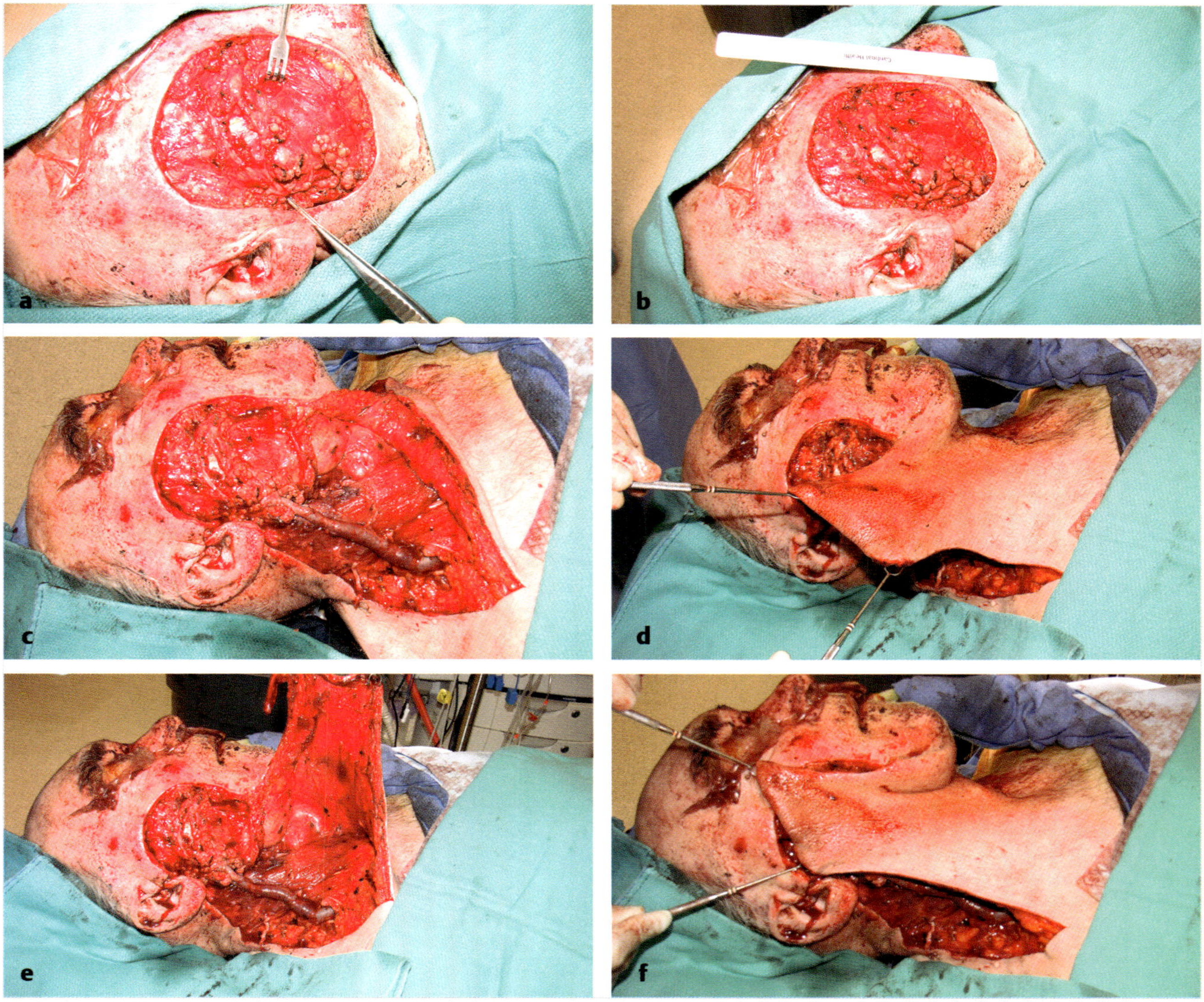

Fig. 9.4 An 8 × 8 cm cheek defect that was reconstructed using a cervicofacial flap.

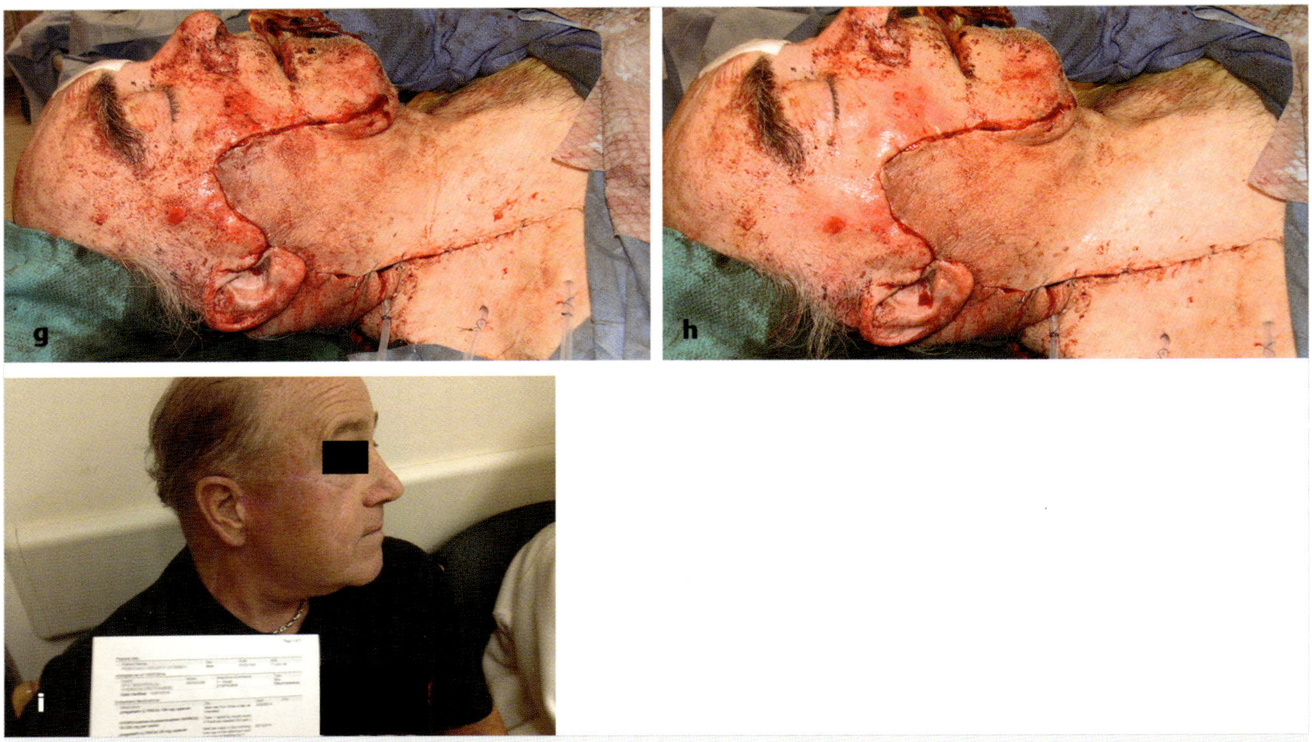

Fig. 9.4 *(continued)*

cervicofacial advancement flap.[14] The difference between the two types of flap stems from the directionality of the rotation. A cervicofacial flap rotates the lateral cheek and neck skin toward the nose. The reverse cervicofacial flap rotates the skin of the lower face in a cranial direction. The reverse flap is used in situations where the defect is medial to the midpupillary line (▶ Fig. 9.5).

Marking the cervicofacial flap requires a preauricular facelift incision that can be extended behind the ear and inferiorly toward the deltopectoral groove. The superior aspect of the marking should be above the level of the lateral canthus, as this is the point of maximal tension and can produce an ectropion if marked beneath the canthus. The incision can then be extended medially toward the defect. Elevation the flap is above the SMAS and can transition to a subplatysmal dissection in the neck for recruitment. A large standing cone ("dog ear") can then be excised in the medial aspect, which allows for appropriate insetting of the flap. However, one needs to be certain not to encroach into the base of the flap while excising the dog ear. If there is concern, then keep the standing cone and return in several weeks as division. As the flap can be large, a drain is usually placed and left until the output is less than 30 mL over a 24-hour period.

9.4 Eyelids

Eyelids are arguably the most complex facial subunits with respect to reconstruction due to the intricate interplay of musculature and thin skin. Besides being the thinnest skin in the body, the lids service as vital barriers that protect, lubricate, and clean the eyes.[15,16] The basic principles of reconstruction include maintenance of the aforementioned key functions for eye protection, as well as maintenance of eye mobility, using like tissue for replacement of deficiencies in soft tissue, all the while maintaining aesthetics. Local flaps and grafts serve as the workhorses

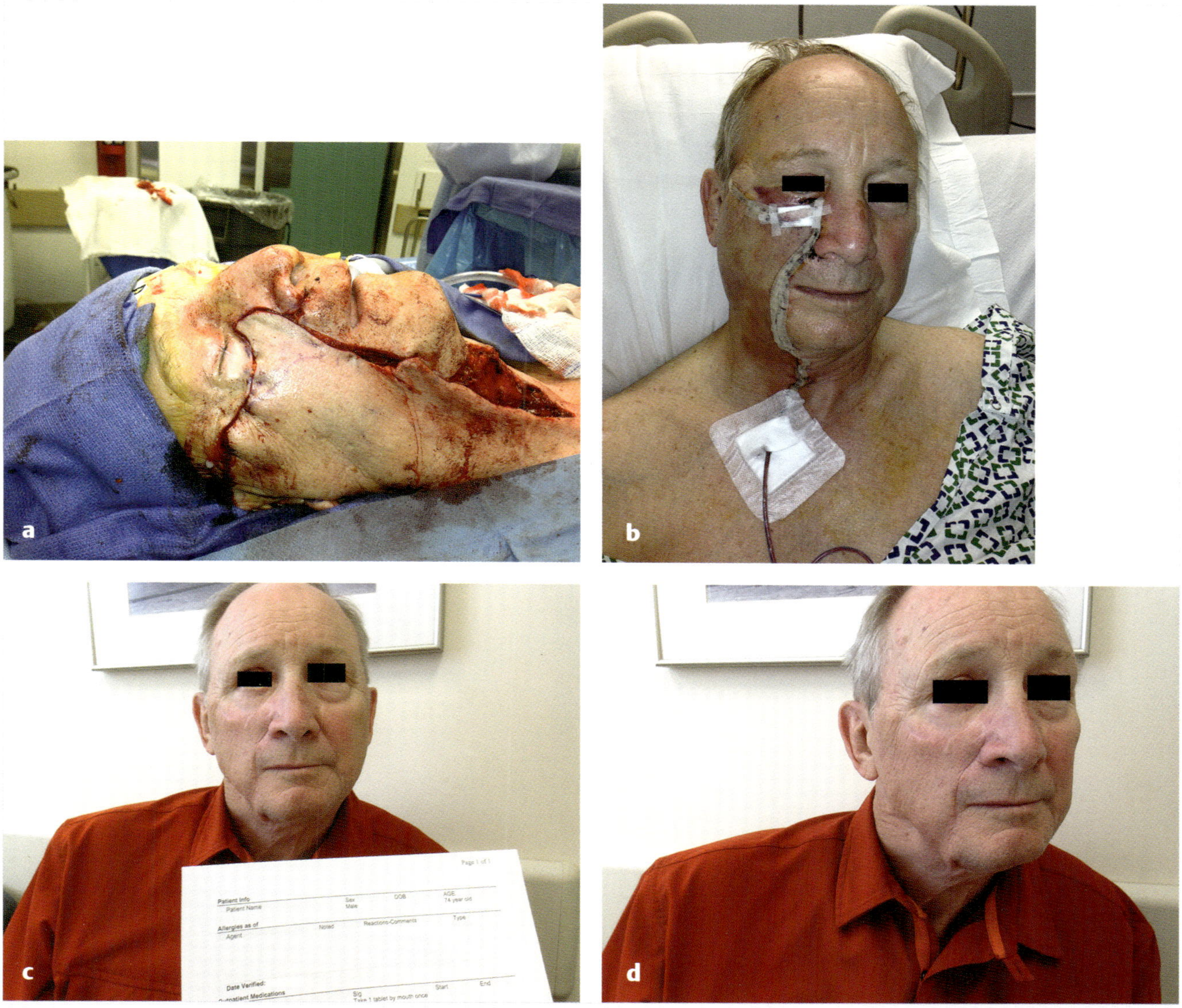

Fig. 9.5 A reverse cervicofacial flap can be used in situations where there exists large defects medial to the midpupillary line.

for the reconstructive surgeon (▸ Fig. 9.6). However, due to the complexity that is beyond the scope of this chapter, we will forego additional discussion regarding specific eyelid techniques.

9.5 Lips

The lips play a major functional role in sensation, facial expression, oral continence (including muscular integrity), and phonation, while serving as the focal point of the lower face. The lips interplay several aesthetic units, which are composed of skin, muscle, and mucosa. This can be particularly challenging from a reconstructive standpoint as it is difficult to produce tissue of the same quality, color, texture, etc., utilizing distant flaps.[17] Lip alignment needs to be precise as minute distortion of the vermilion—even at the level of 1 mm—can lead to obvious scarring that can be seen at conversation distance.[18]

The lip is divided into two aesthetic units: upper and lower lip. The upper lip has two units—the lateral and medial/philtral. The lower lip is one entire aesthetic unit itself. The external landmarks are the commissure, cupid's bow, philtral columns, tubercle, white roll, and red roll. Additionally, there are four key components. They are the skin and subcutaneous tissue, muscle (orbicularis oris), mucosa, and the vermilion border. From a cross-sectional standpoint, innervation—which consists of the mental and infraorbital nerves for sensation, as well as the inferior orbital nerve (upper) and the mental nerve (lower) for motor innervation—and vascular supply (labial artery branches of the facial artery) lie between the muscle and mucosa. The vermilion is the visible portion of the lip within the outer white roll and has a unique light reflection.[19] One of the key hallmarks to reconstruction of the lip is maintenance of this vermilion border.

Full-thickness lip reconstruction is carried out using the rule of thirds.[20] For the sake of this chapter, full-thickness complete

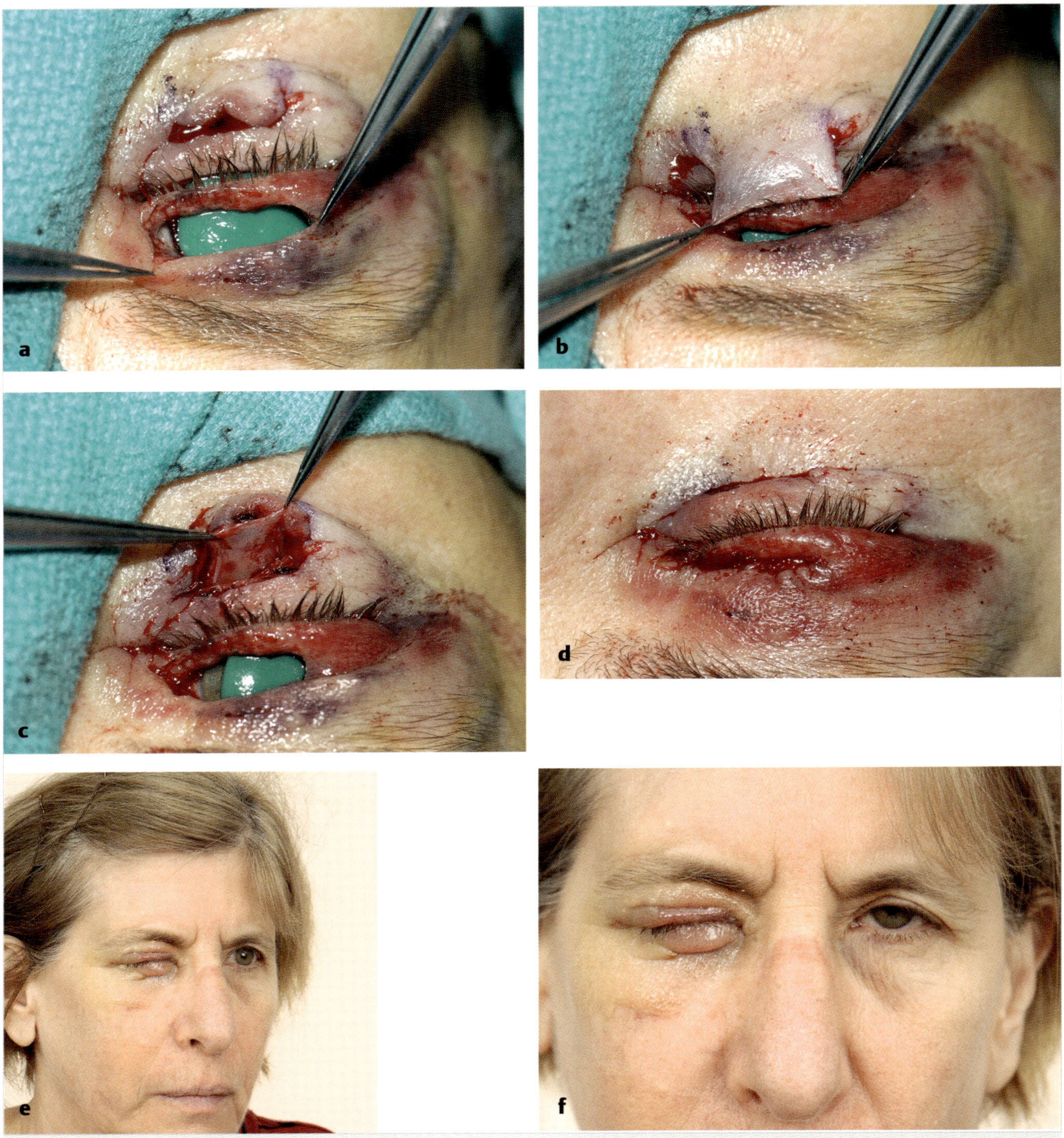

Fig. 9.6 A Cutler-Beard flap for upper eyelid reconstruction. (Subparts i and j reprinted with permission from CCF.)

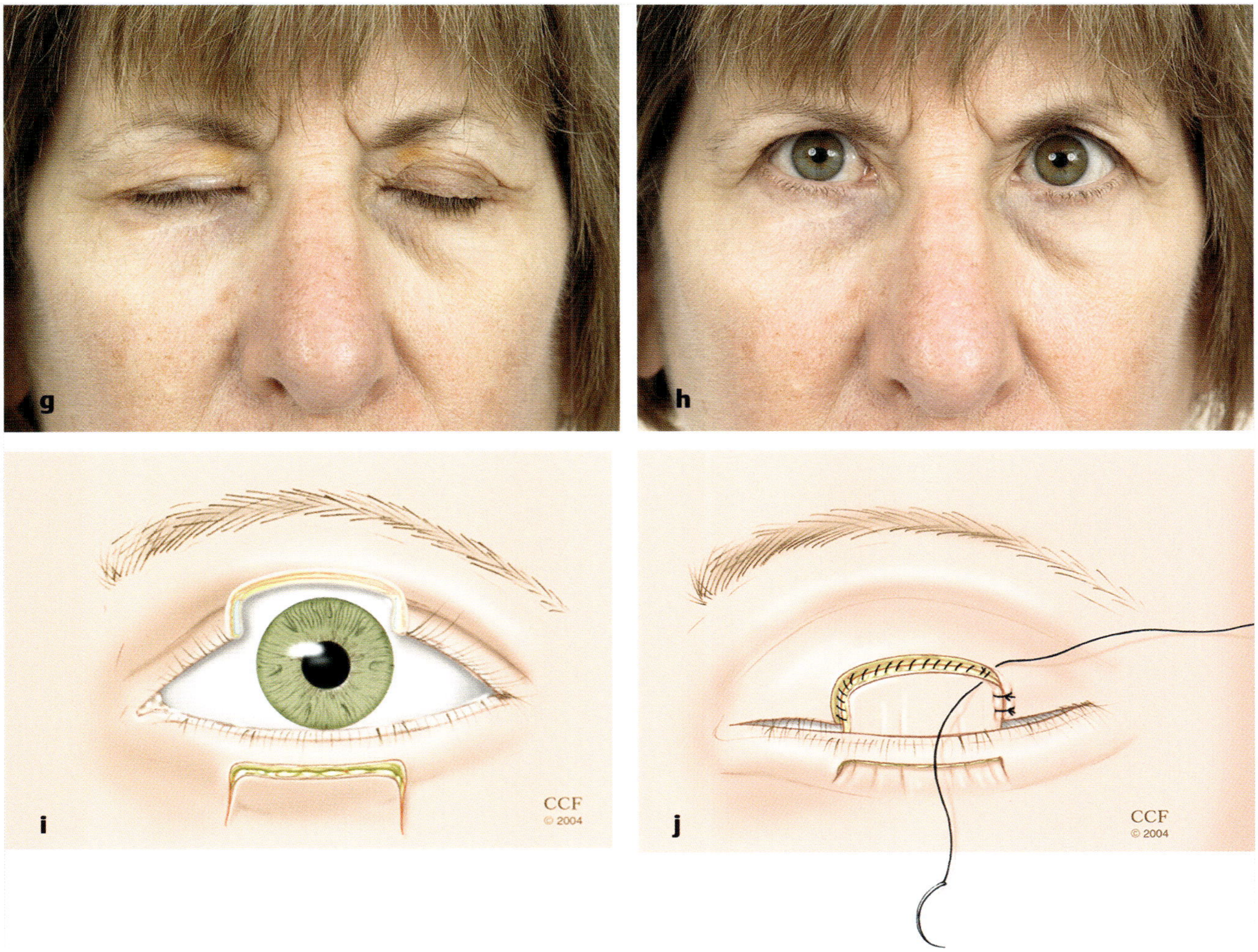

Fig. 9.6 *(continued)*

defects of the lips will be omitted. Free flap reconstruction with innervated, free radial forearm and palmaris longus has been the standard reconstruction modality for many years.[21,22] If the defect totals less than one-third of the lip, then primary closure can be performed with wedge excision. To obtain ideal results, one needs to ensure precise approximation of the tissues—including the vermilion border (▶ Fig. 9.7).

For defects that encompass between one-third and half of one lip with commissure preservation, one can utilize a staged, Abbe lip switch flap[23] (▶ Fig. 9.8). Prior to performing an Abbe flap, the patient needs to be alerted to the lack of postoperative sensation. When designing the flap, marking should be half the width of the defect to ensure the ability to close the donor site primarily. The flap is performed in a full-thickness manner through the mucosa and pivoted nearly 180 degrees on its pedicle. The patient is able to have parenteral nutrition limited to liquids until flap sectioning, which occurs usually in 3 weeks. Flap viability is evaluated prior to sectioning by compressing the flap to eliminate flow and evaluating the viability of the tissue that has been transplanted.

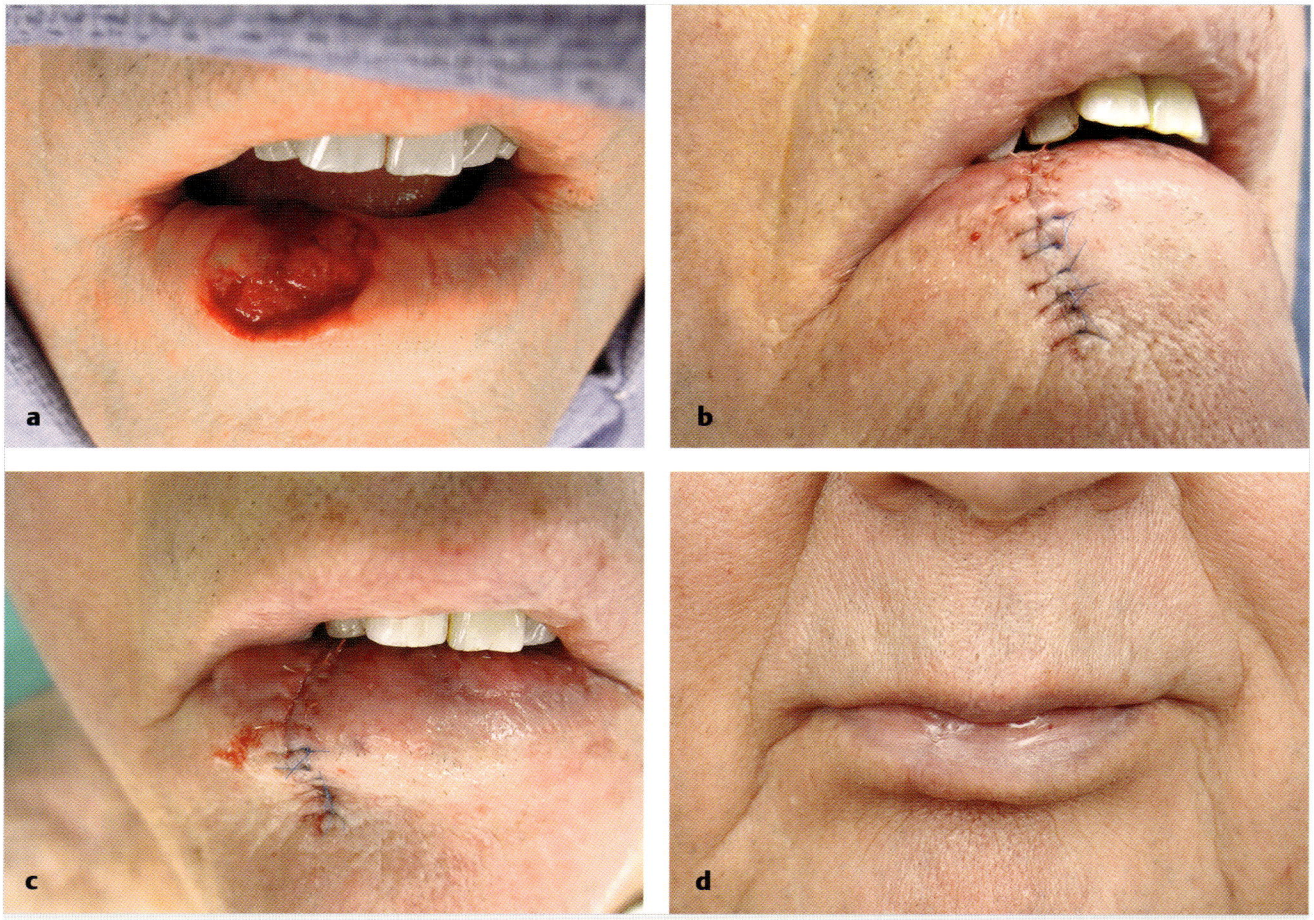

Fig. 9.7 Lip advancement flaps can be utilized to obtain excellent aesthetic results. Precise vermillion border approximation is the most critical aspect.

When defects involve the commissure and are less than half of the total width of either the upper or lower lip, then an Estlander flap can be performed.[24] While the flap is insensate—like the Abbe—it also suffers from distortion with oral animation as the modiolus is altered (▶ Fig. 9.9). This can often require secondary commissuroplasty. Similar to the Abbe, the donor site needs to be designed in a full-thickness manner and should be one-third to one-half the size of the defect.

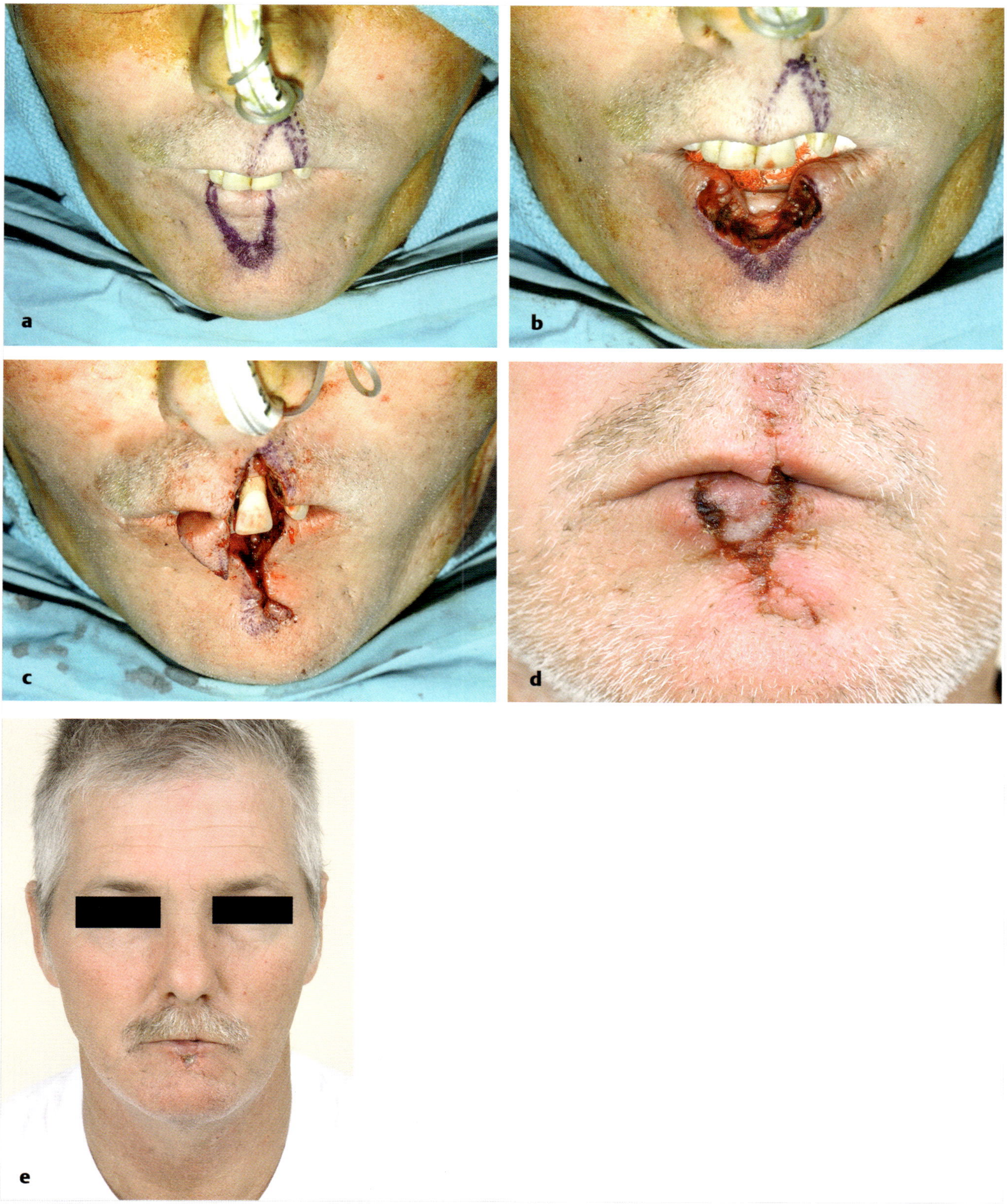

Fig. 9.8 An Abbe lip switch staged flap can be used for defects that encompass one-third to one-half of one lip.

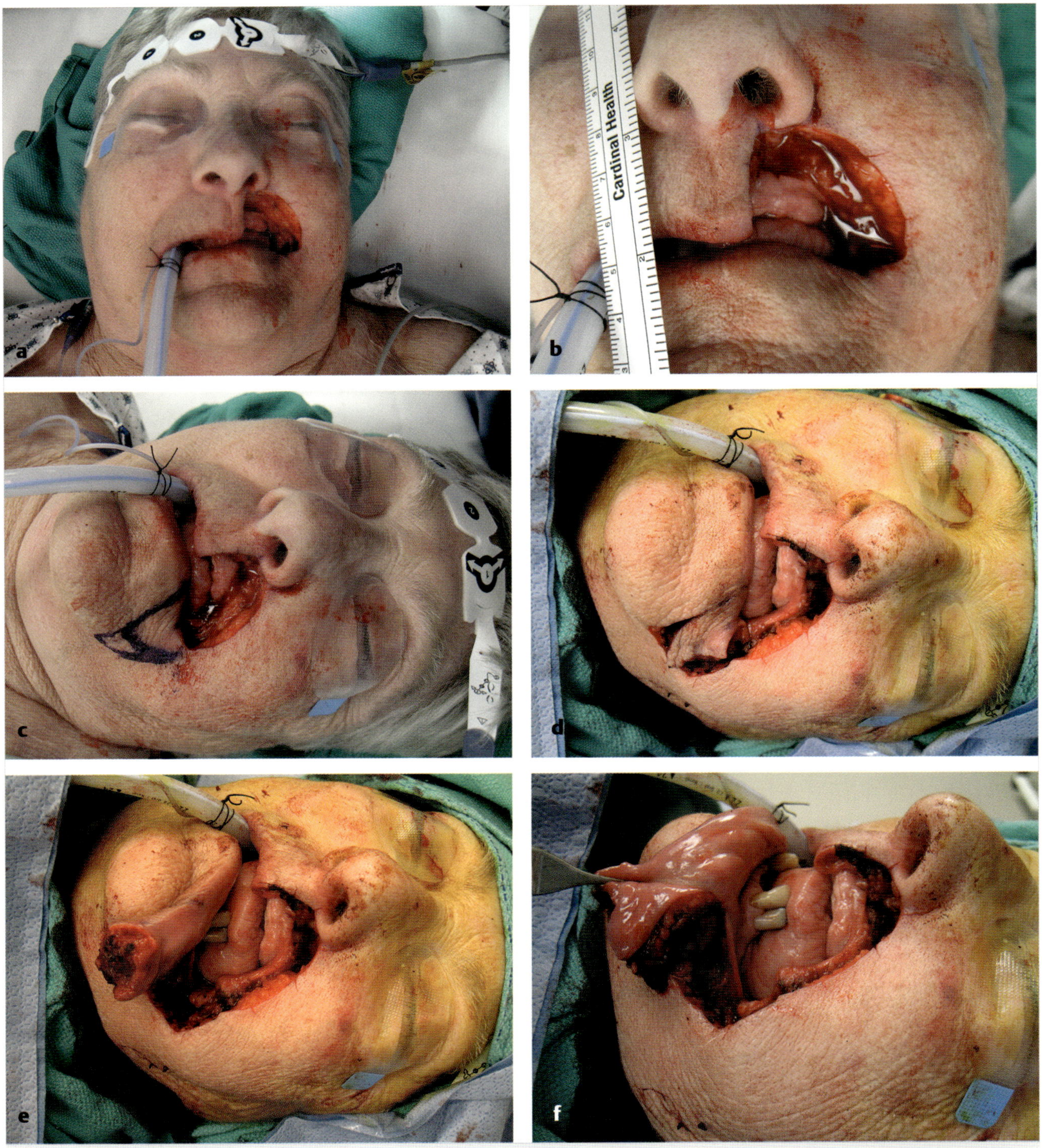

Fig. 9.9 When defects involve the commissure, an Estlander flap reconstruction can often be utilized to provide excellent reconstructive outcomes. These flaps can be used for defects that encompass half the total width of either one of the lips while simultaneously involving the commissure.

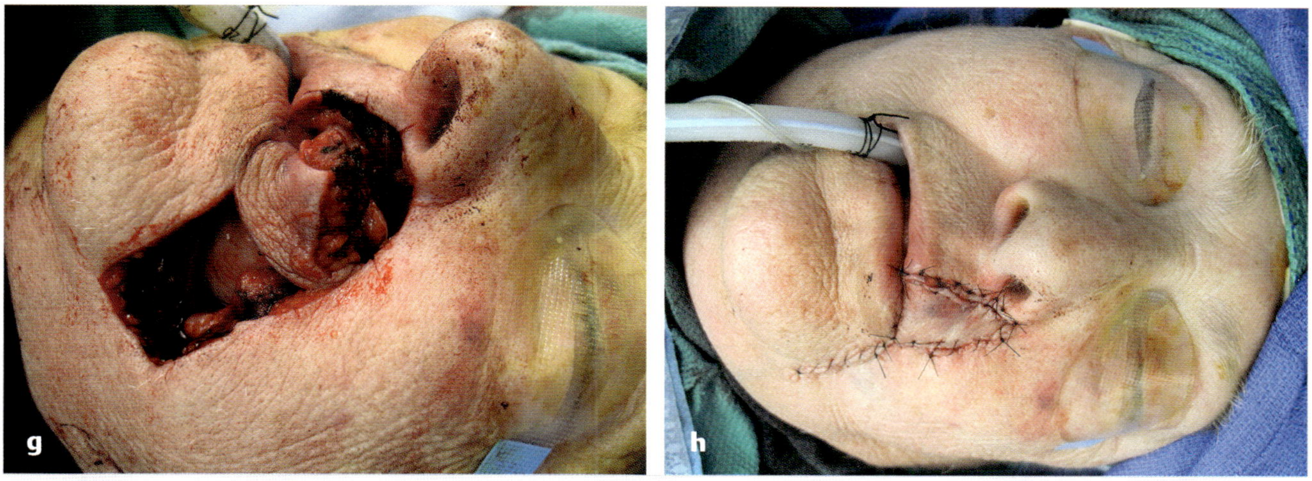

Fig. 9.9 (*continued*)

Central defects involving one-third to two-thirds of the lip can be reconstructed using a Karapandzic flap[25] (▶ Fig. 9.10). While larger defects that utilize a Karapandzic flap can lead to microstomia, the flap is ideal in that it is performed in a single stage that maintains competence of the oral sphincter as well as the modiolus and philtrum. Additionally, the flap is able to maintain sensation unlike the Estlander and Abbe flaps. Marking of this flap requires the width of the curvilinear incision to maintain—at a minimum—the height of the vertical component of the defect. This allows for appropriate rotation of the circumoral flaps to approximate the defect without substantial tension, all the while allowing for closure of the curvilinear incisions.

9.6 Nose

The nose occupies the most crucial place of the face as it occupies the (0,0) space from a Cartesian coordinate system standpoint. Alterations and changes to the nose can lead to poor cosmetic outcomes and, worse, compromised breathing if the deeper structures are involved. As discussed earlier in the chapter, the nose is subdivided into nine aesthetic subunits: the dorsum, the paired lateral side walls, tip, paired soft tissue triangles, paired lobules, and the columella.[5] One of the key concepts regarding nasal subunits for reconstruction is the emphasis on replacement of an entire subunit if the majority of one is missing. While it may seem counterintuitive, this may lead to making the wound larger. This concept has been stressed by Menick and relies on the principle of hiding incisions within the shadows created by the natural contours of the nose, thus increasing the camouflage to distract the eye.[26]

The nasal skin thickness and character vary in a cranial to caudal dimension with the skin becoming thicker with more sebaceous glands and less pliable when moving further caudally toward the tip. Additional differences are noted between the skin of men and women—with men having more glabrous and thicker skin. All of these factors dramatically affect the reconstructive options. Depth of defects affects the reconstructive modalities that would pertain to the best outcomes. For the majority of cutaneous malignancies, defects will be limited to the full thickness of the skin and subcutaneous tissues. Yet, there are situations in which deeper structures, such as

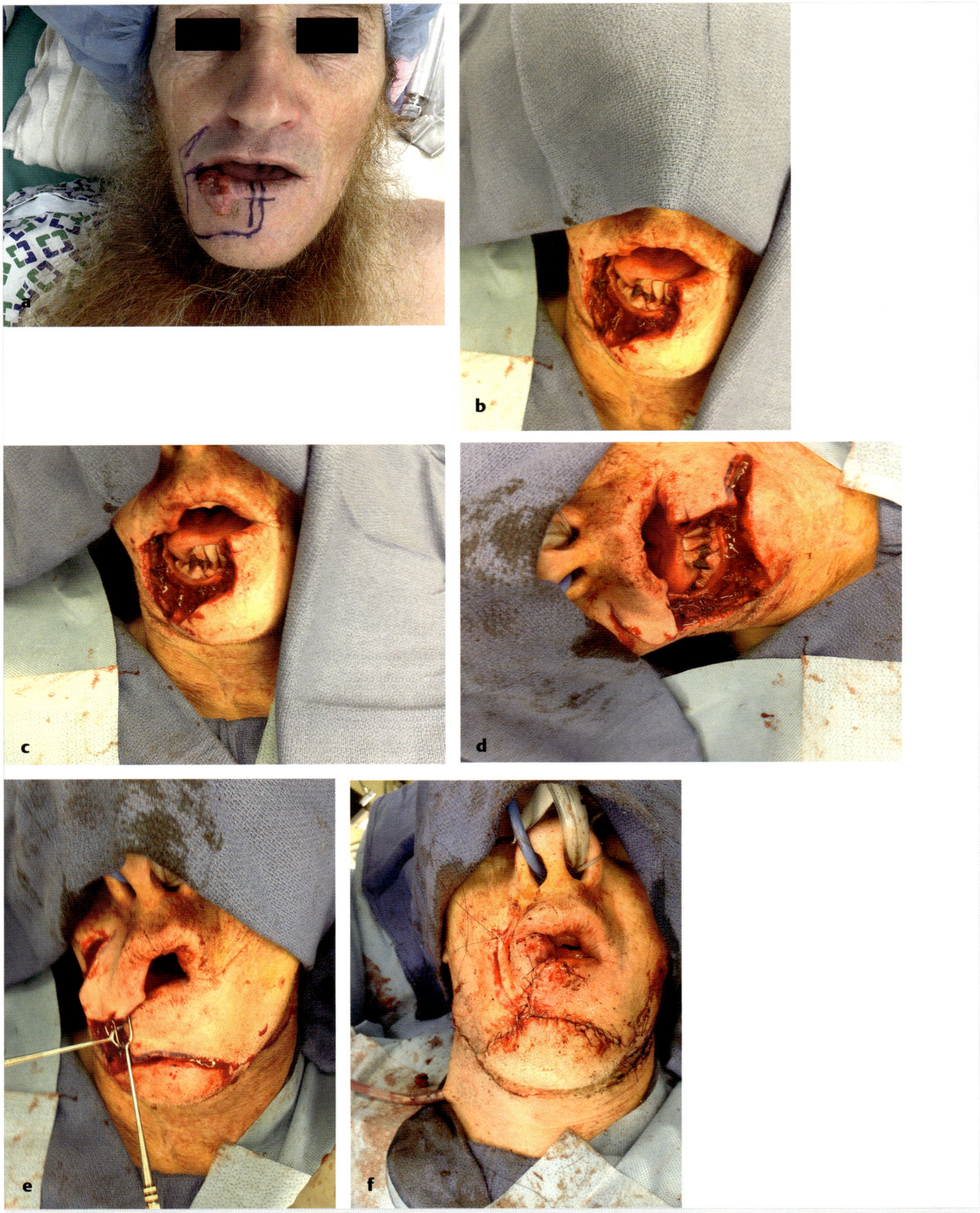

Fig. 9.10 Large central lip defects are reconstructed using Karapandzic flaps. However, care needs to be exercised as patients can develop microstomia.

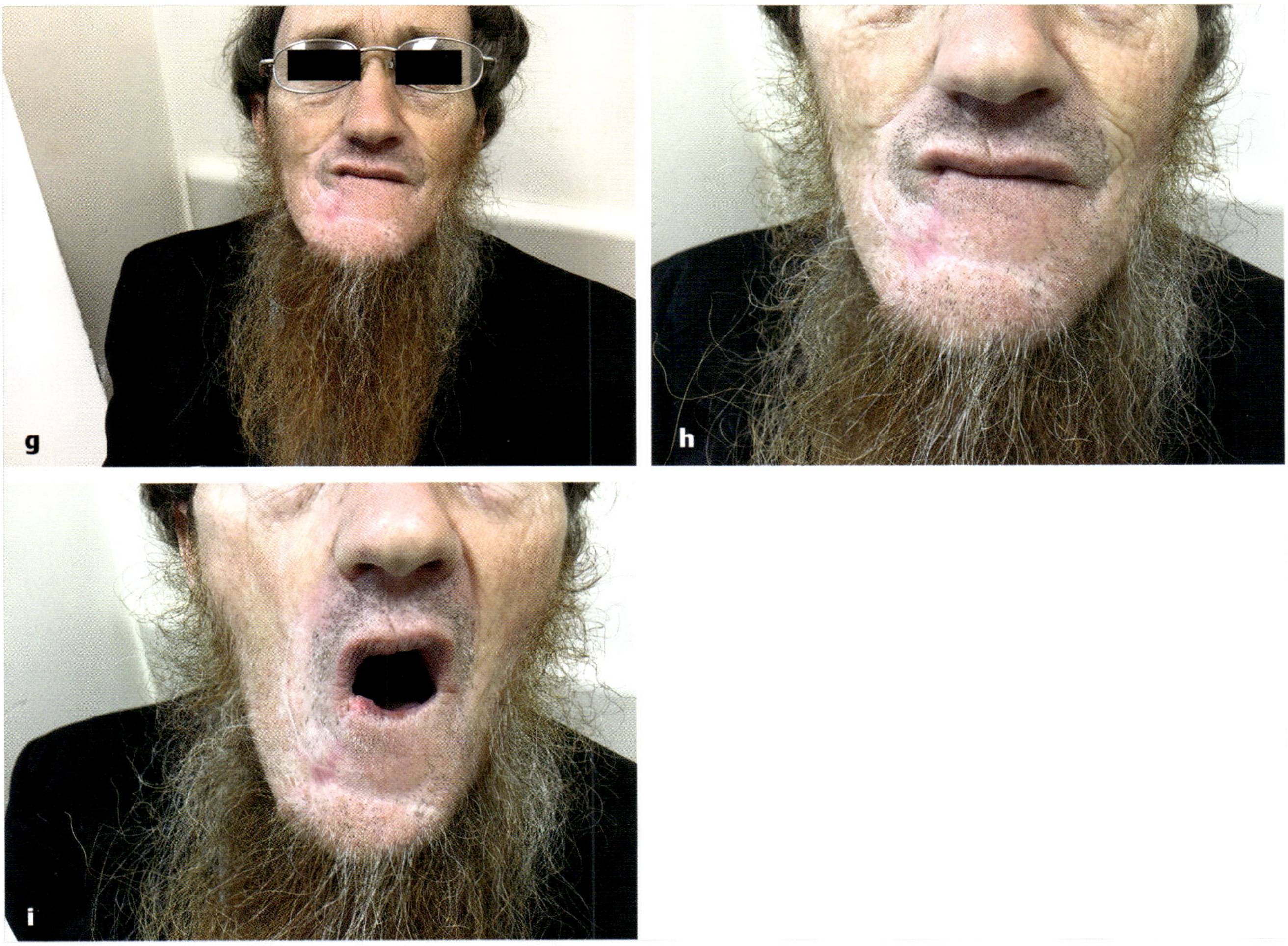

Fig. 9.10 (*continued*)

cartilage, are required to be removed during the extirpation. These defects are often not the situation when discussing nasal cutaneous malignancies. As such, we will not discuss, in-depth, wounds that involve cartilaginous and mucosa reconstruction because they are beyond the scope of this chapter.

While the workhorse of cutaneous nasal reconstruction stems from local flaps, full-thickness skin grafts (FTSGs) are of instrumental assistance to provide a reconstructive modality that is time efficient, which is a substantial benefit in patients who have a multitude of comorbidities. One of the key benefits of FTSGs is the ability to reconstruct nasal defect of almost any size. The most common locations for donor sites for color match include the pre- and postauricular skin as well as the supraclavicular skin. Additional sites, including the medial arm and groins, can also be used if there is substantial actinic damage or prior scarring to the aforementioned locations. Ideally, the nasal defect would be superficial as well as smaller than an aesthetic unit. Superficial wounds have improved vascularity, which increases the likelihood of graft take. Furthermore, the lateral aspects of the nose, which are thin by nature, tend to fill in well. This is an important characteristic given there is a wide variation in the nasal skin thickness among individuals. As a broad rule of thumb, skin grafting can be utilized to reconstruct the cranial nose. Typically, because the tip skin is thicker, grafting may not provide as ideal an outcome as a local flap. FTSGs are utilized instead of split-thickness skin grafts (STSGs) due to the improved color and texture match with nasal skin. The main drawbacks are the requirement of a donor-site repair and decreased graft take compared to STSGs. Furthermore, skin grafting on areas near the nostrils can lead to upturning due to contracture of the nostril; thus, flap reconstruction near this area is more often considered the norm.

While small defects of around 1.0 cm in size can be closed primarily—either in the transverse or vertical dimension—wounds of up to 1.5 cm often benefit from closure using a bilobed flap.[27] The bilobed flap is a random-pattern, single-stage flap that rotates two adjacent lobes about a pivot point.[28] The first lobe of the flap is rotated into the defect and the second lobe is rotated into the wound created by the movement of the first lobe. The defect left by the second lobe is closed primarily (▸ Fig. 9.11). The key concept is in the planning and design. The markings begin by drawing a perpendicular to the wound along the axis that is planned—typically in the vertical dimension. The first lobe is drawn adjacent to the wound and

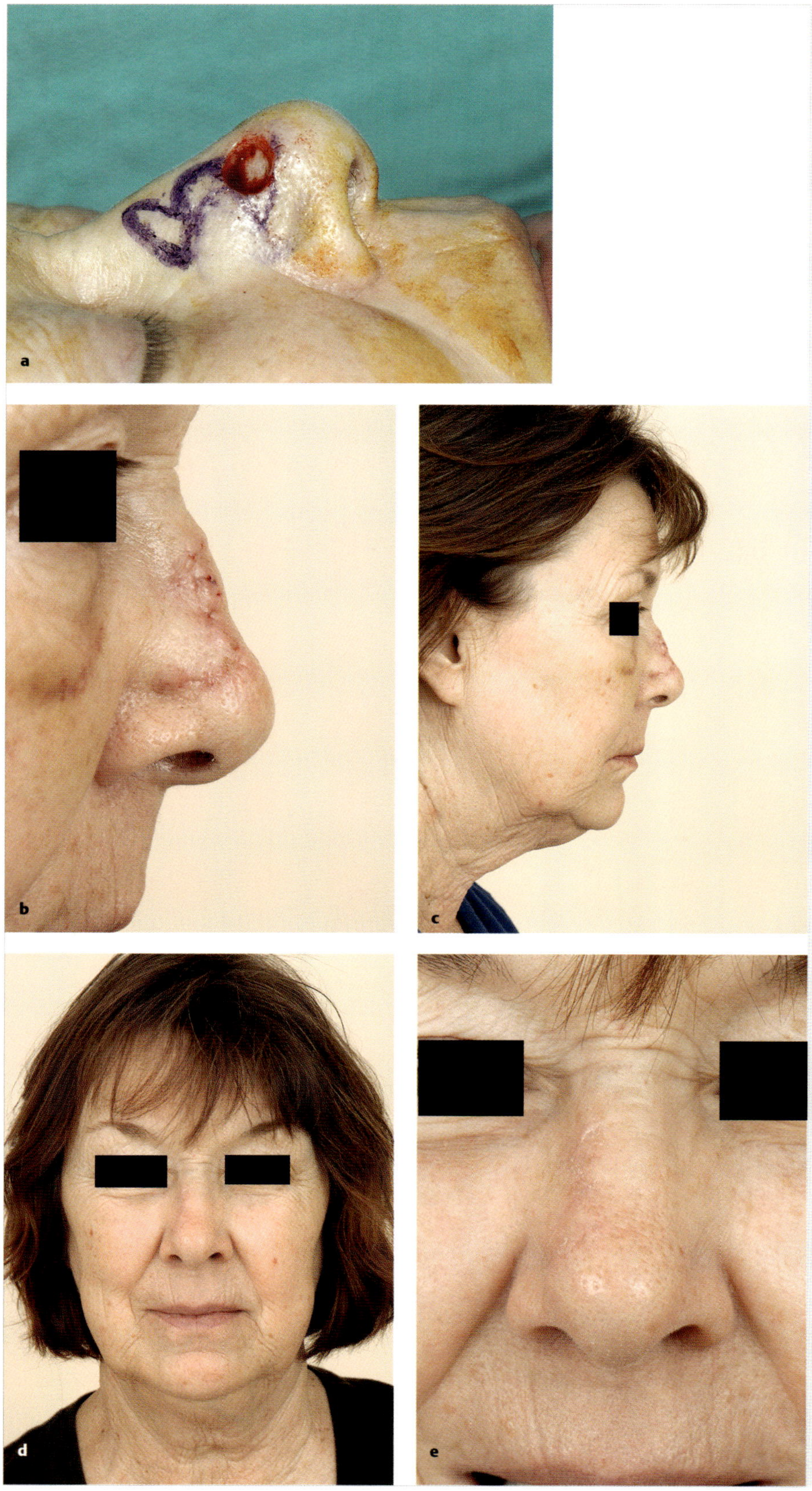

Fig. 9.11 A bilobed flap can be used for nasal reconstruction in wounds up to 1.5 cm.

designed to be slightly smaller than the defect. The second lobe is drawn approximately 45 degrees from the first lobe with the primary lobe axis positioned 45 degrees from the axis of the defect, ideally within the sidewall or upper dorsum. Zitelli stated that no more than 50 degrees of rotation should be designed for each lobe. Additionally, the burrow triangle between the defect and the pivot point should be excised prior to rotation.[27] The elevation of the flap is supraperichondrial plane. One needs to ensure that there is appropriate dissection —oftentimes more than one would think—to ensure adequate rotation of the flap without tension. The first lobe is rotated in place to close the defect followed by the second lobe rotation. The wound is closed in an interrupted manner using 6–0 monofilament sutures.

For defects that are between 1.5 and 2.5 cm in size, dorsal nasal flaps provide the ability to recruit the redundant skin of the glabella and can be used for defects of the tip, dorsum, and sidewall (▶ Fig. 9.12). It is based laterally and elevated on the angular arteries. This flap is ideal in older patients given it maximizes the laxity of their skin.[29] Like the bilobed flap, the plane of dissection is above the perichondrium. The superior triangle is removed, and after the flap is elevated, it is rotated in place with a broad base. The common disadvantages of this flap are tip elevation/rotation and elevation of the ala in lateral nasal defects.

The nasal ala is a critical structure in nasal reconstruction because notching can be seen readily. This can be avoided with the use of a nasolabial advancement flap. Additionally, the caudal one-third of the nose—which is the area of the highest concentration of cutaneous malignancies—can be reconstructed almost entirely by this flap, though additional cartilage grafting may be required for alar support.[30] The nasolabial flap is versatile in that it can be designed either superiorly or inferiorly based on the branches of the facial artery. When placed within the nasolabial fold, the donor site is provided excellent camouflage for an ideal cosmetic result (▶ Fig. 9.13 and ▶ Fig. 9.14).

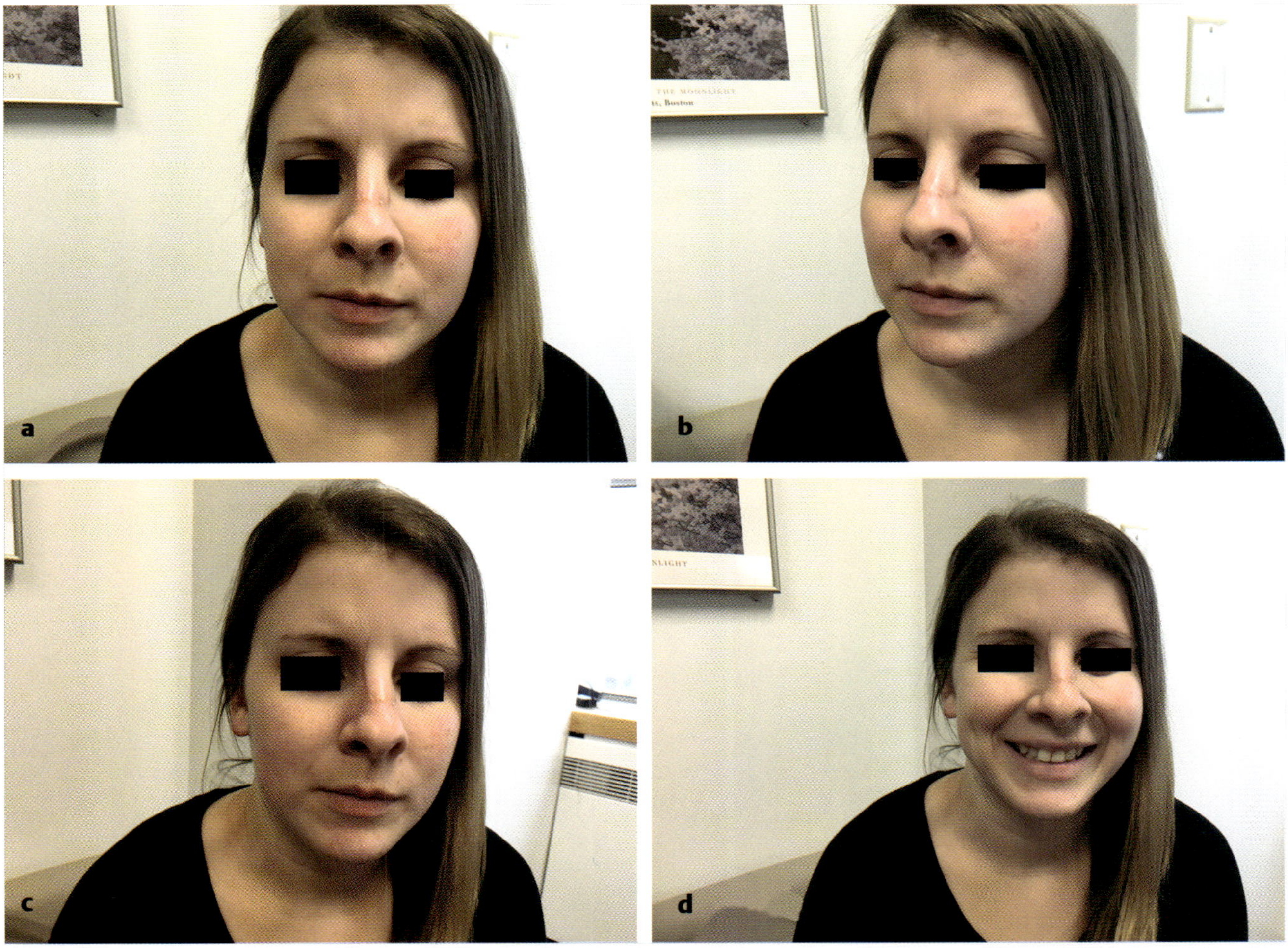

Fig. 9.12 A dorsal nasal flap can achieve excellent aesthetic results for appropriate defects. Here are multiple views of an early follow-up patient.

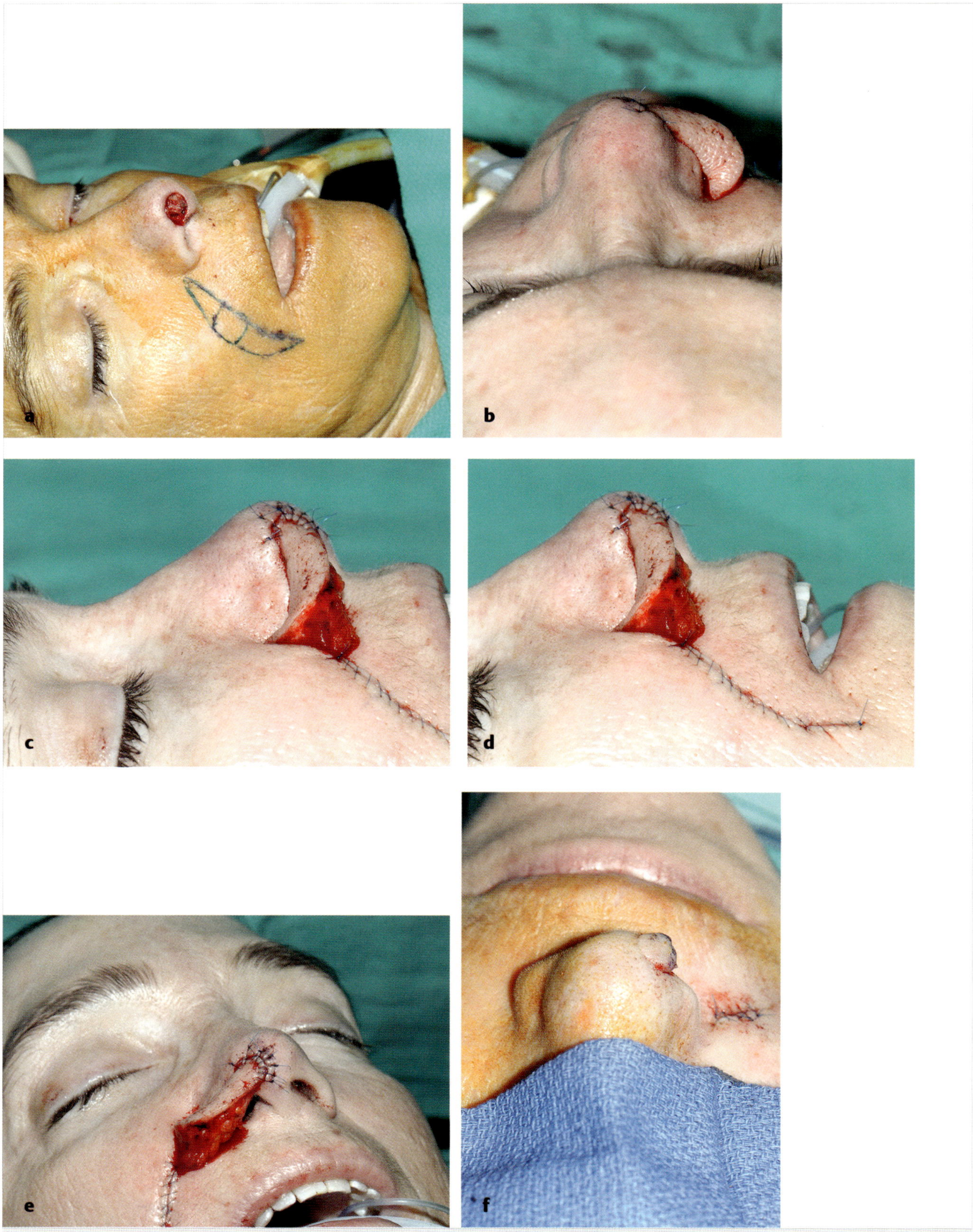

Fig. 9.13 Nasolabial fold flaps allow for excellent camouflage for nasal reconstruction.

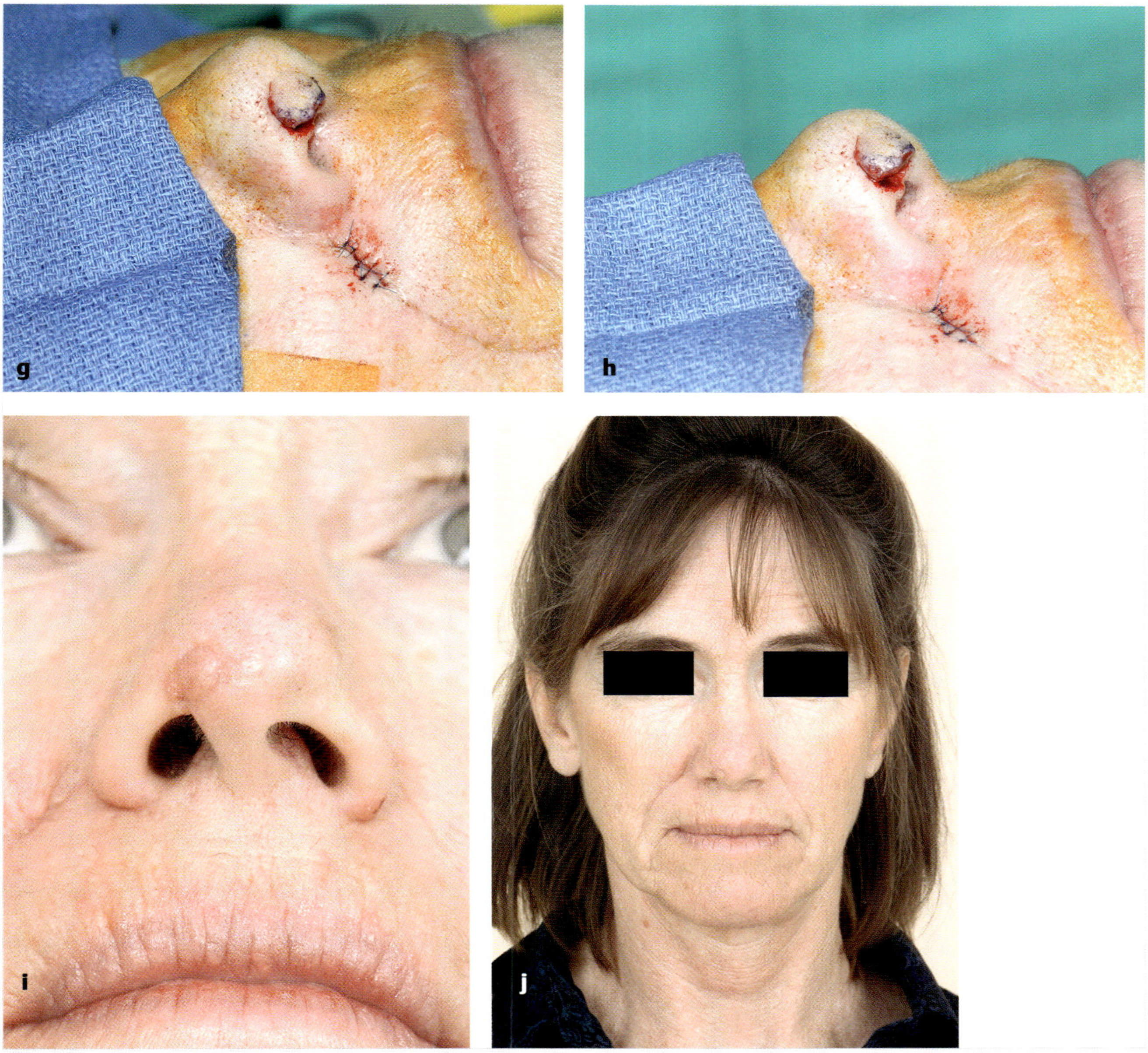

Fig. 9.13 (*continued*)

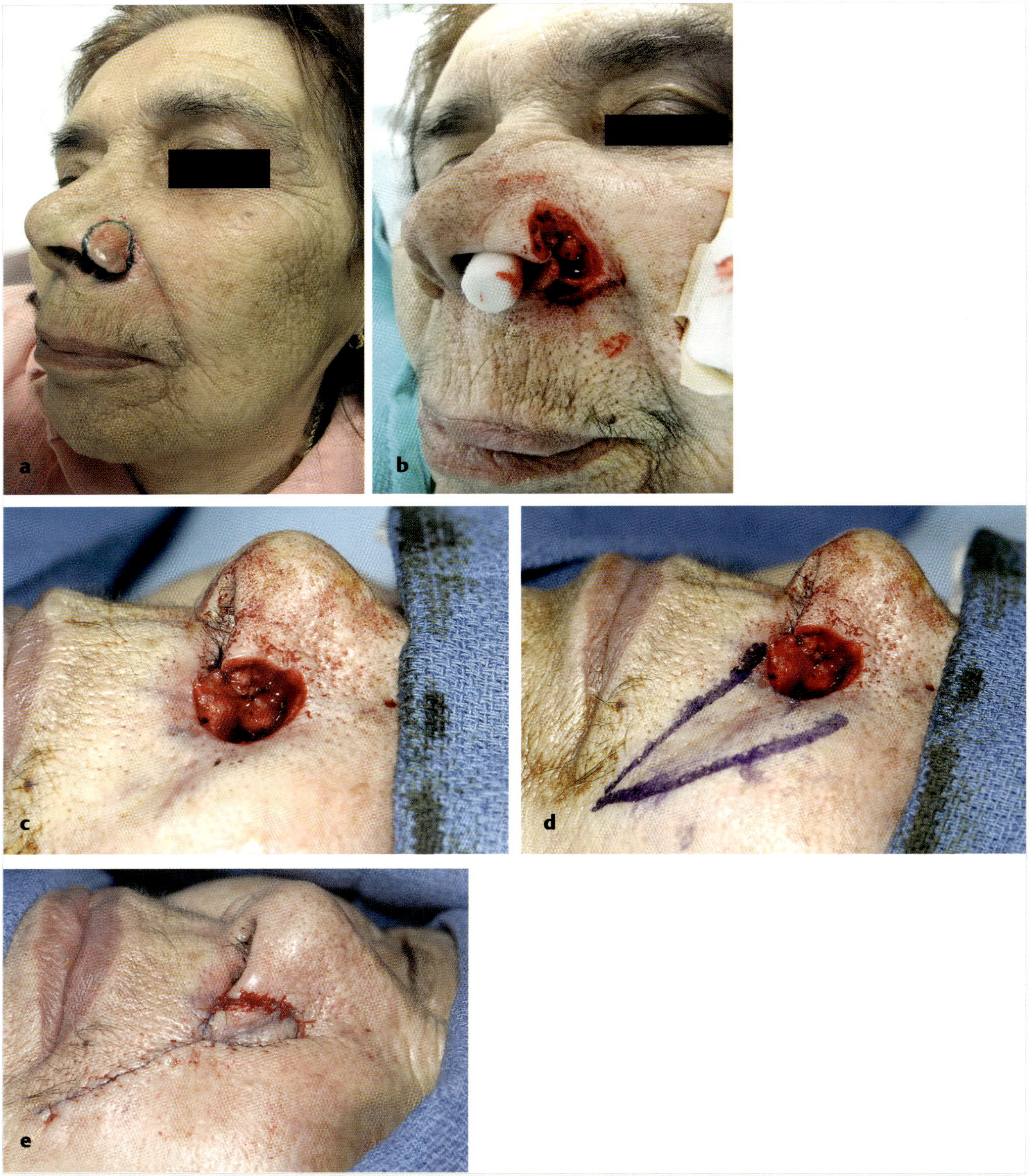

Fig. 9.14 Another patient with a nasolabial fold flap, which provides versatile soft tissue coverage for alar rim reconstruction.

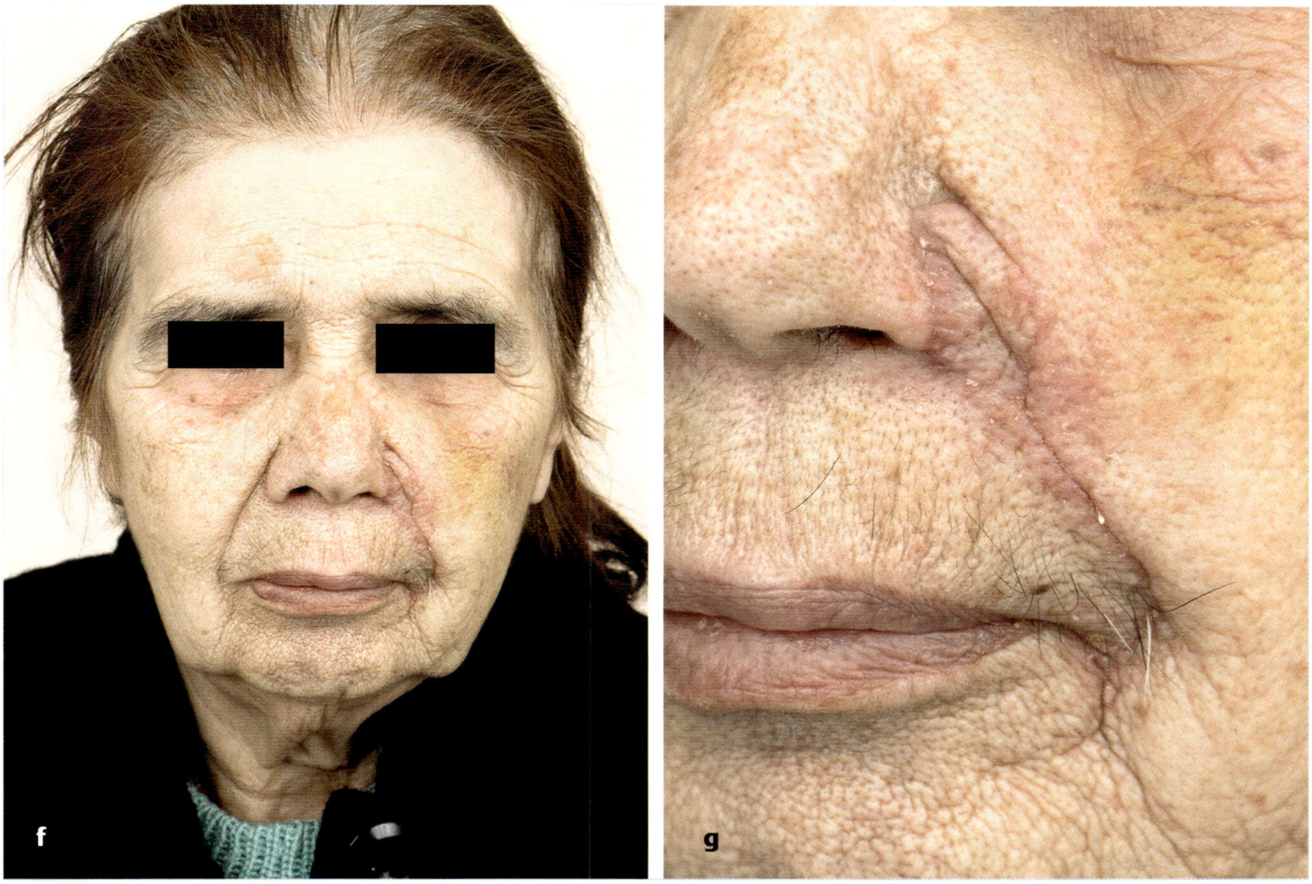

Fig. 9.14 *(continued)*

The key tenet of reconstruction using this flap is to ensure that the fold is positioned above the horizontal plane of the lateral oral commissure.

Large nasal defects—including near-total nasal reconstruction of the soft tissue—can be performed using a paramedian forehead flap. This well-known flap in plastic surgery can trace its roots to ancient India in the medial treatise, the *Sushruta Samita*, in 700 BC.[31] The flap is based on the supratrochlear vessels, which are branches of the ophthalmic artery from the internal carotid artery system (▸ Fig. 9.15). The defect has a template created which is placed onto the superior aspect of the forehead near the hairline in the plane of the supratrochlear

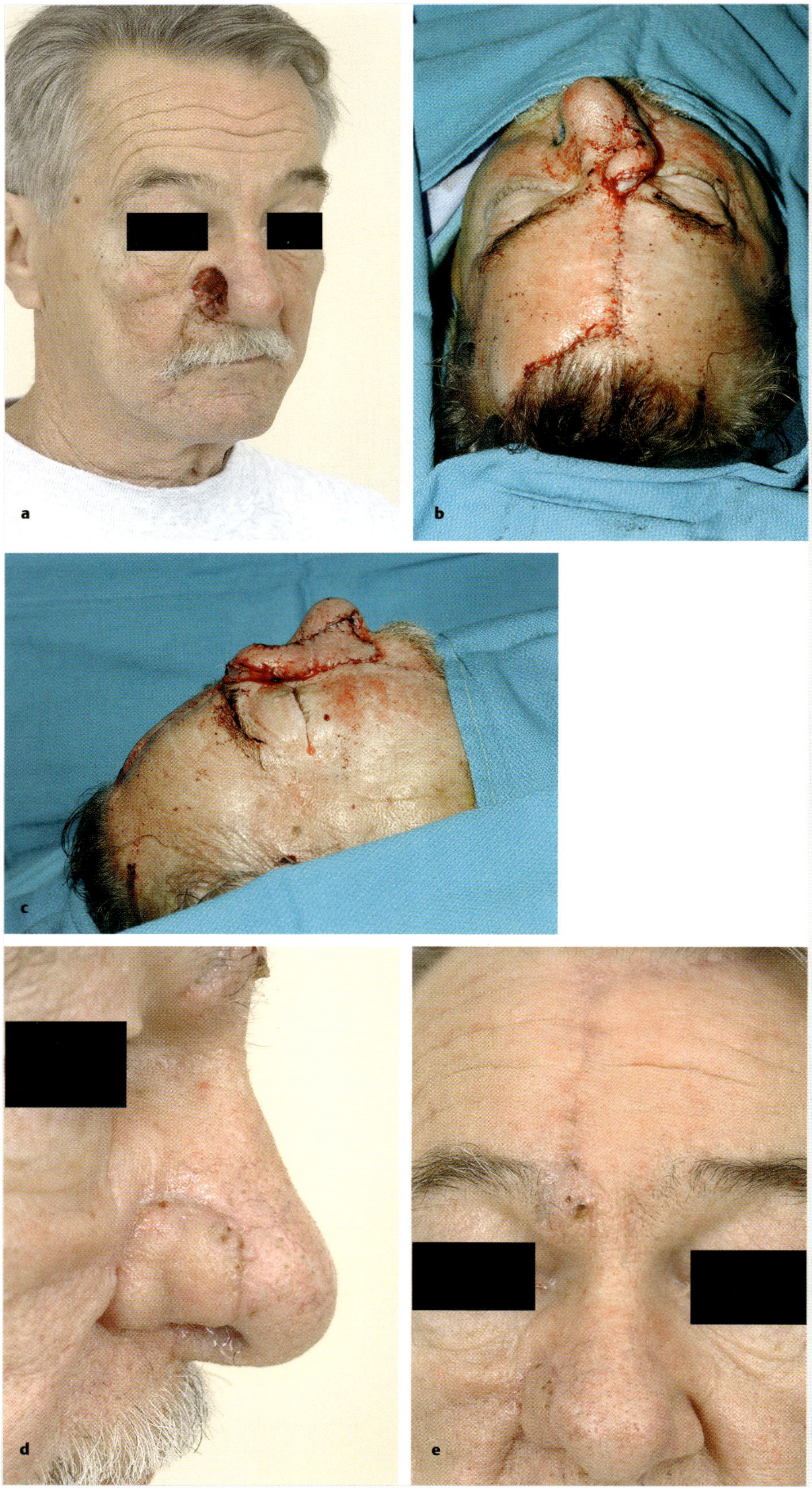

Fig. 9.15 Paramedian forehead flaps allow for reconstruction of large nasal defects.

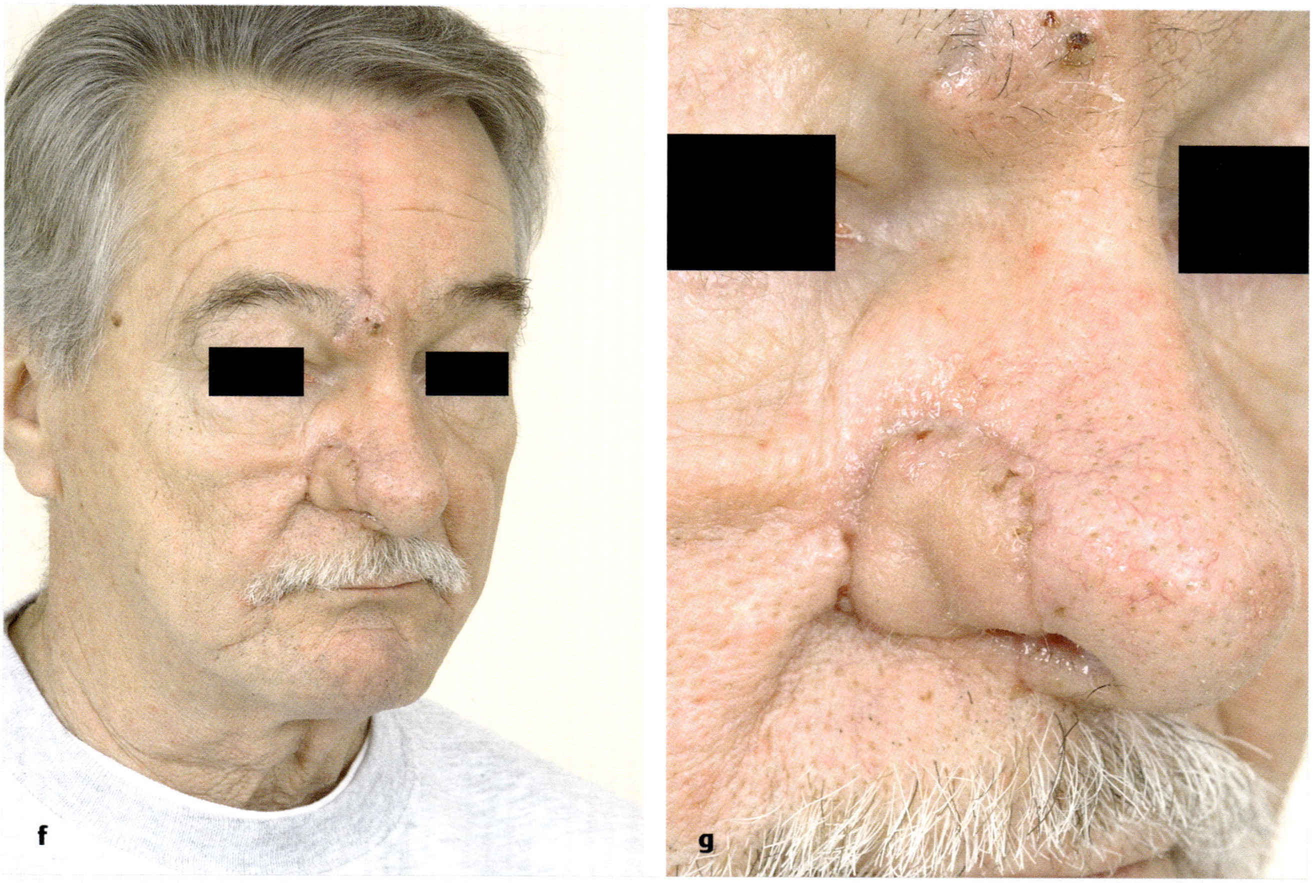

Fig. 9.15 (*continued*)

vessels. The supratrochlear vessels can be found between 1.7 and 2.2 cm lateral to the midline above the eyebrows.[32] The flap is designed such that the templated aspect is superior to the supratrochlear vessels. Dissection is performed down to the level of the frontalis muscle. The flap is then rotated on itself and sutured in place to cover the defect. Most of the donor site can be closed primarily; however, areas can be left to heal with secondary intention with outstanding cosmetic results (see Forehead section earlier). Flaps with a base of only 1.2 cm are capable of survival.

One of the largest downsides of the forehead flap for nasal reconstruction stems from the need to have multiple stages. Variations to provide the superior aesthetic outcomes of the forehead flap—due to the similar color and texture—without

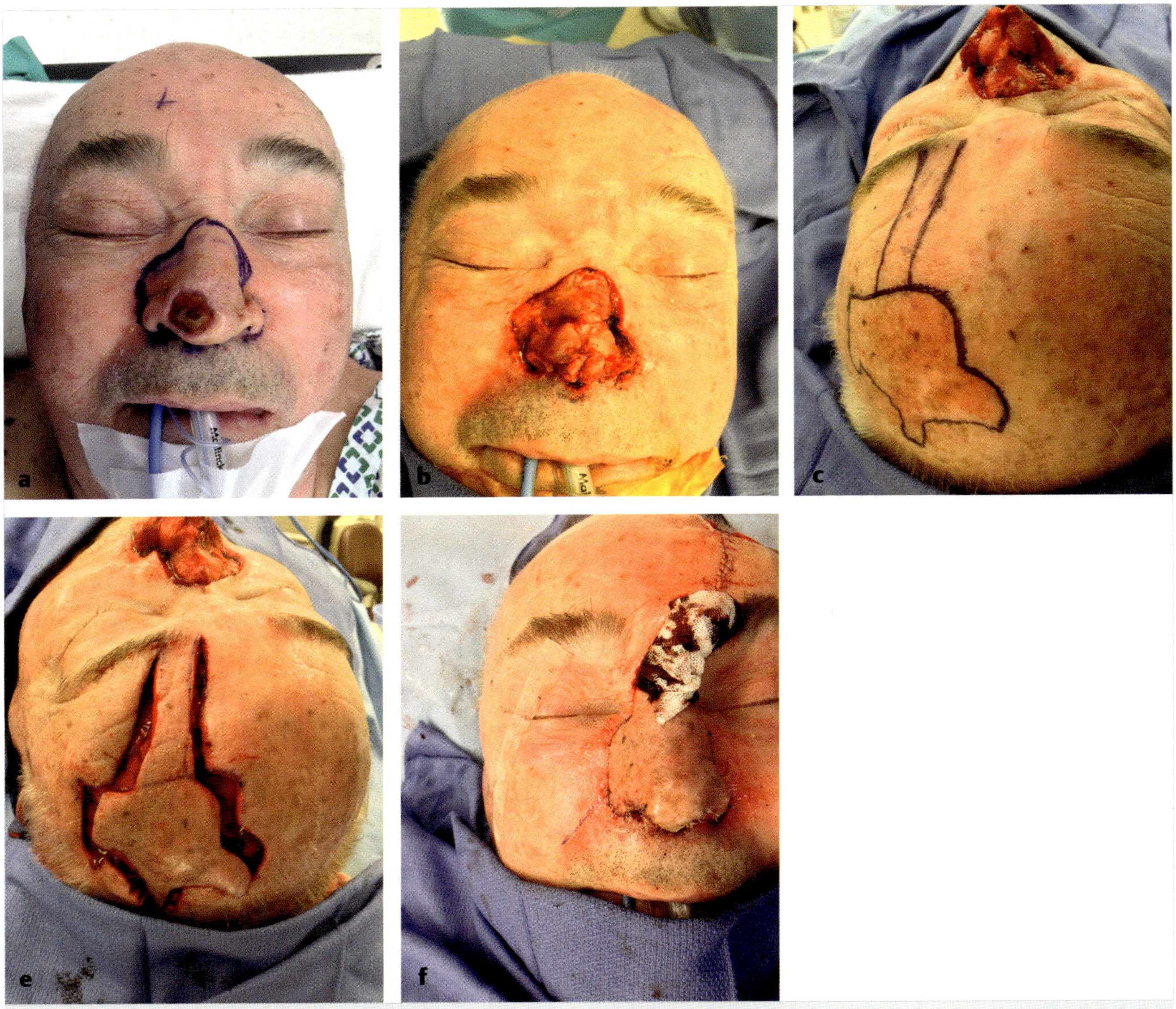

Fig. 9.16 Total nasal reconstruction can be performed using a paramedian forehead flap in a single-staged manner.

the multiple staged approach have been identified. Authors have described a single-stage paramedian forehead flap for nasal reconstruction that initially was utilized for small nasal defects.[33,34,35,36] However, total nasal reconstruction can be achieved in the single-staged manner (▶ Fig. 9.16). The flap is designed and elevated in a manner that is similar to the staged approach. However, the difference lies in creating a tunnel using the glabellar subunit. To decrease the potential for venous congestion by compression of the pedicle, corrugator muscles are resected and the flap tissue that is to be inset underneath the tunnel is de-epithelialized. As with the staged approach, the forehead donor site can be approximated until the tension is too great and the residual area can be left to heal with secondary intention. This method of reconstruction can be utilized in either the pediatric or elderly population as well as those with many comorbidities.

9.7 Conclusion

Facial reconstruction maintains several principles—maintenance of the aesthetic subunits as well as replacing "like with like" whenever possible. Following these basic tenets allows for the majority of wounds due to cutaneous malignancy extirpation to be reconstructed with cosmetically satisfactory results. While not an encyclopedic compilation of all flaps or specific areas of the face that can be performed, these common, workhorse flaps will allow the reconstructive surgeon to provide exceptional care for those afflicted with these wounds.

References

[1] Guy GP, Jr, Thomas CC, Thompson T, Watson M, Massetti GM, Richardson LC, Centers for Disease Control and Prevention (CDC). Vital signs: melanoma incidence and mortality trends and projections - United States, 1982–2030. MMWR Morb Mortal Wkly Rep. 2015; 64(21):591–596

[2] Guy GP, Jr, Machlin SR, Ekwueme DU, Yabroff KR. Prevalence and costs of skin cancer treatment in the U.S., 2002–2006 and 2007–2011. Am J Prev Med. 2015; 48(2):183–187

[3] Tagliacozzi G. De Curtorum Chirurgia per Insitionem, 1597.

[4] Nadol JB, Galla RJ, Fabian RL, Montgomery WW. Surgical Anatomy of the Head and Neck. Philadelphia, PA: Lippincott Williams & Wilkins; 2001

[5] Burget GC, Menick FJ. The subunit principle in nasal reconstruction. Plast Reconstr Surg. 1985; 76(2):239–247

[6] Seline PC, Siegle RJ. Forehead reconstruction. Dermatol Clin. 2005; 23(1):1–11, v

[7] Trussler AP, Stephan P, Hatef D, Schaverien M, Meade R, Barton FE. The frontal branch of the facial nerve across the zygomatic arch: anatomical relevance of the high-SMAS technique. Plast Reconstr Surg. 2010; 125(4):1221–1229

[8] Ebrahimi A, Nejadsarvari N. Upper forehead skin reconstruction with h-flap. J Cutan Aesthet Surg. 2013; 6(3):152–154

[9] La Trenta GS. Atlas of Aesthetic Face and Neck Surgery. Philadelphia, PA: Saunders; 2004

[10] Roth DA, Longaker MT, Zide BM. Cheek surface reconstruction: best choices according to zones. Oper Tech Plast Reconstr Surg.. 1998; 5(1):26–36

[11] Rapstine ED, Knaus WJ, II, Thornton JF. Simplifying cheek reconstruction: a review of over 400 cases. Plast Reconstr Surg. 2012; 129(6):1291–1299

[12] Mustarde JC. Repair and Reconstruction in the Orbital Region. 2nd ed. London: Churchill-Livingstone; 1980

[13] Austen WG, Jr, Parrett BM, Taghinia A, Wolfort SF, Upton J. The subcutaneous cervicofacial flap revisited. Ann Plast Surg. 2009; 62(2):149–153

[14] Boyette JR, Vural E. Cervicofacial advancement-rotation flap in midface reconstruction: forward or reverse? Otolaryngol Head Neck Surg. 2011; 144 (2):196–200

[15] Fralick FB. Anatomy and physiology of the eyelid. Trans Am Acad Ophthalmol Otolaryngol. 1962; 66:575–581

[16] Spinelli HM. Atlas of aesthetic eyelid and periocular surgery. Philadelphia, PA: Saunders; 2004

[17] Neligan PC. Strategies in lip reconstruction. Clin Plast Surg. 2009; 36(3):477–485

[18] Boutros S, Thorne CH, Beasley RW, et al. Grabb & Smith's Plastic Surgery. 6th ed. Philadelphia, PA: Lippincott Williams & Wilkins; 2007

[19] Ishii LE, Byrne PJ. Lip reconstruction. Facial Plast Surg Clin North Am. 2009; 17(3):445–453

[20] Behmand RA, Rees R. Reconstructive lip surgery. In: Achauer BM, Eriksson E, Guyuron B, et al., eds. Plastic Surgery: Indications, Operations, and Outcomes. Philadelphia, PA: Mosby-Year Book; 2000

[21] Sasidaran R, Zain MA, Basiron NH. Lip and oral commissure reconstruction with the radial forearm flap. Natl J Maxillofac Surg. 2012; 3(1):21–24

[22] Fernandes R, Clemow J. Outcomes of total or near-total lip reconstruction with microvascular tissue transfer. J Oral Maxillofac Surg. 2012; 70 (12):2899–2906

[23] Abbe RA. A new plastic operation for the relief of deformity due to double hairlip. Med Rec. 1898; 53:477

[24] Ebrahimi A, Maghsoudnia GR, Arshadi AA. Prospective comparative study of lower lip defects reconstruction with different local flaps. J Craniofac Surg. 2011; 22(6):2255–2259

[25] Degala S, Shetty SK, Monalisha. The karapandzic flap in lower lip reconstruction. J Maxillofac Oral Surg. 2015; 14 Suppl 1:421–425

[26] Menick FJ. Reconstruction of the nose. In: Baker SR, Swanson NA, eds. Local Flaps in Facial Reconstruction. St. Louis, MO: Mosby; 1995:305–307

[27] Zitelli JA. The bilobed flap for nasal reconstruction. Arch Dermatol. 1989; 125 (7):957–959

[28] Zoumalan RA, Hazan C, Levine VJ, Shah AR. Analysis of vector alignment with the Zitelli bilobed flap for nasal defect repair: a comparison of flap dynamics in human cadavers. Arch Facial Plast Surg. 2008; 10(3):181–185

[29] Rohrich RJ, Muzaffar AR, Adams WP, Jr, Hollier LH. The aesthetic unit dorsal nasal flap: rationale for avoiding a glabellar incision. Plast Reconstr Surg. 1999; 104(5):1289–1294

[30] Levy RM, Hanke CW. The nose: a high risk area for skin cancer. www.skincancer.org/skin-cancer-information/basal-cell-carcinoma/the-nose. Accessed May 1, 2015.

[31] Millard DR, Jr. Hemirhinoplasty. Plast Reconstr Surg. 1967; 40(5):440–445

[32] Shumrick KA, Smith TL. The anatomic basis for the design of forehead flaps in nasal reconstruction. Arch Otolaryngol Head Neck Surg. 1992; 118(4):373–379

[33] Har-El G. Single-stage paramedian forehead flap for nasal reconstruction. Oper Tech Otolaryngol-Head Neck Surg. 1999; 10:127–130

[34] Park SS. The single-stage forehead flap in nasal reconstruction: an alternative with advantages. Arch Facial Plast Surg. 2002; 4(1):32–36

[35] Fudem GM, Montilla RD, Vaughn CJ. Single-stage forehead flap in nasal reconstruction. Ann Plast Surg. 2010; 64(5):645–648

[36] Park SS. Revisiting the single-stage forehead flap in nasal reconstruction. JAMA Facial Plast Surg. 2013; 15(5):383–384

10 Operative Lymphadenectomy

Calvin J. Young, Amrita Pandit, and Deepak Narayan

10.1 Operative Lymphadenectomy

10.1.1 Introduction

Malignant melanoma is the cutaneous malignancy that most often mandates an operative lymphadenectomy. The presence or absence of a positive lymph node in the draining basin is one of the most important prognostic factors in this disease. The rationale for a sentinel lymph node biopsy (SLNB) is discussed elsewhere in this text. For melanoma patients with positive SLNBs, lymph node dissection of the entire nodal basin is currently the standard of care in the United States. Other cutaneous malignancies for which a sentinel node biopsy and lymphadenectomy may be performed include Merkel's cell carcinomas,[1,2] high-risk squamous cell carcinomas (SCCs),[3] cutaneous apocrine adenocarcinoma,[4] and digital papillary adenocarcinomas.[5]

10.2 Sentinel Node Biopsy: Technical Aspects

The concept of SLNB, as a minimally invasive technique to assess nodal involvement, was developed in 1977 by Cabanas, for the management of penile SCC.[6] In 1992, Morton et al applied the same concept to the management of cutaneous melanoma, with the objective to reduce the morbidity related to lymph node dissection in these patients. The SLNB protocol is currently applied to other cutaneous malignancies as well.[7] The assumption is that early detection of tumor cells in lymph nodes leads to a better prognosis by assisting in appropriate management by aiding the expeditious removal of other diseased lymph nodes in the affected basin. It also hones the indications for lymphadenectomy, by limiting the procedure only to those situations where an involved node has been definitively identified. This helps to limit the number of lymphadenectomies performed, consequently limiting the morbidity that they entail. In cutaneous melanomas, a completion lymphadenectomy performed for a positive SLN will reveal that only a small percentage of the dissection specimens examined will harbor more involved nodes—that is, nodes other than the sentinel node(s) containing malignant deposits. A representative figure of 15% was quoted by Elias et al from the Massachusetts General Hospital.[8] Thus, there is scope for further refinement of this particular intervention. One idea is to use the SLNB as a standalone therapeutic procedure. This concept is currently being tested out in clinical trials.

10.3 Lymphoscintigraphy

The concept of lymphoscintigraphy began with cadaveric studies in the 1800s when Cruickshank used intradermal mercury injections to demonstrate lymphatic drainage patterns.[9] It was later discovered that lymphatic drainage is not as dogmatic and predictable as once thought. Although it is possible, based on population studies, to predict which basin a particular cutaneous zone will drain into, a great deal of variability exists, especially in the head/neck and trunk.[10]

Lymphoscintigraphy allows noninvasive preoperative identification of the primary nodal basin for cutaneous neoplasms.[11] This imaging modality is especially valuable in lesions that have the potential to drain to several nodal basins. For example, lesions of the lower extremity can drain to the popliteal, femoral, inguinal, or iliac regions. In a similar fashion, lesions of the anterior scalp can drain to the intraparotid lymph nodes or levels I to V of the anterior cervical chain.

In current practice, lymphoscintigraphy is performed by injecting a radiolabeled substance into the intradermal space around the tumor site so that the tracer can be taken up into the lymphatic system. The ideal radiolabeled injectable substance should have the following characteristics[12]:

- It locates and demonstrates the sentinel lymph node without migrating further into the lymphatic chain.
- It rapidly clears from the injection site to optimize ease of imaging the draining nodal basin.
- The radiotracer should have a high detection rate but a short half-life and low particulate emission to minimize radiation dosage to health care personnel.

Radiopharmaceuticals used for lymphoscintigraphy are principally technetium (Tc)-based labels and include 99m-Tc antimony sulfide, 99m-Tc rhenium sulfur colloid, and 99m-Tc albumin nanocolloid.

In the United States, 99m-Tc sulfur colloid (50–2,000 nm particle size) is the most popular radiopharmaceutical. Typically, the filtered form of the compound is used. The use of a 0.2-µm filter eliminates particles larger than 200 nm, which allows for optimal uptake and transmission to the primary nodal basin for the lesion (▶ Fig. 10.1).

Identification of a sentinel node, however, does not mandate a lymphoscintigram. Vital dyes (isosulfan blue, methylene blue) have been used to duplicate the results of their radioactive counterparts. In this case, however, the identification of the sentinel lymph node cannot be performed in a noninvasive manner since the process of identification requires making an incision and visually identifying the appropriately stained node. A combination of 99m-Tc sulfur colloid and a blue dye has been reported to yield the best detection of sentinel nodes.[13]

A recent innovation has been the use of fluorescent imaging in the detection of sentinel lymph nodes.[14,15,16] Indocyanine green (ICG), a tricarbocyanine dye with a molecular weight of 751.4 Da, is the most commonly used compound for this purpose. ICG has been widely used for a variety of human studies, most commonly in ophthalmology, where it helps in delineating the retinal vasculature. In the context of sentinel node biopsies, the dye is injected in a peritumoral fashion analogous to its radioactive counterpart. The dye track and sentinel node are subsequently visualized using special imaging devices. The principle of fluorescence imaging is based on illuminating the target tissue with light at the excitation wavelength (□750–800 nm) while observing it at longer emission wavelengths,

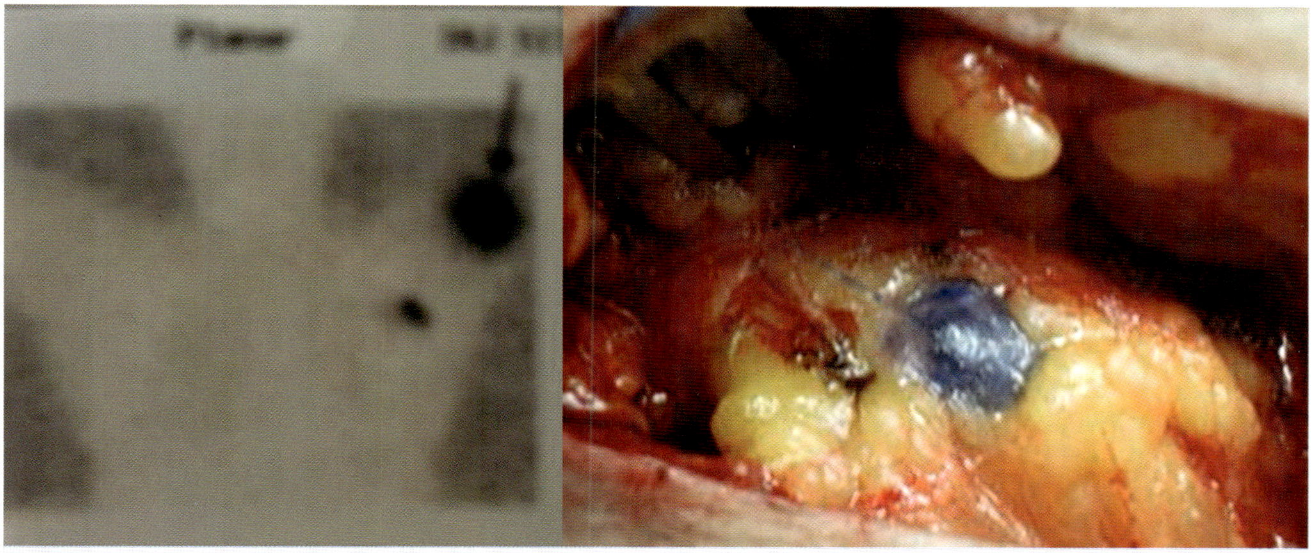

Fig. 10.1 The injection site (small arrow) and the uptake in the axilla. Concurrent use of isosulfan blue confirmed the presence of the sentinel node. Note blue lymphatic vessel leading into node.

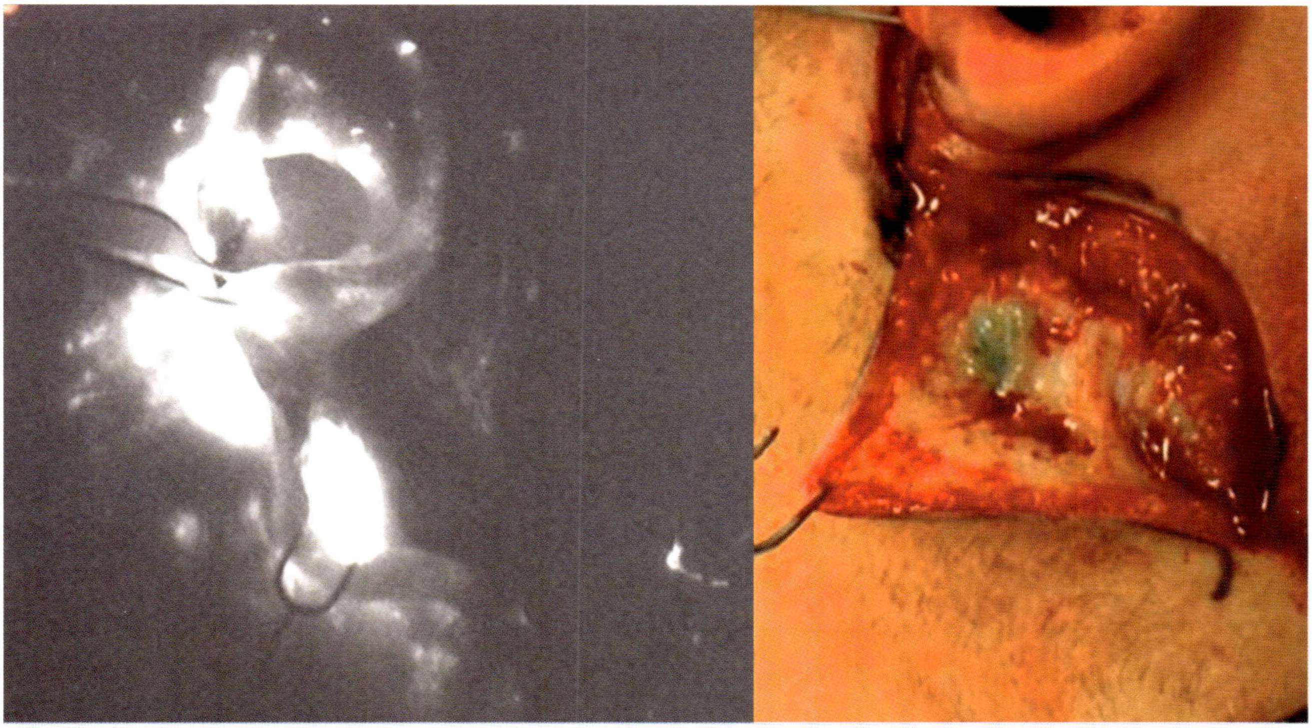

Fig. 10.2 The injection site of ICG in front of the ear (held by forceps) and the uptake in the node adjacent to the skin hook. The visualized node is also stained green.

that is, greater than 800 nm. An additional benefit is that the green color of the dye can provide visual confirmation of the node (► Fig. 10.2). Further research is warranted to reliably establish the efficacy and utility of ICG for SLNB.

A variety of other techniques such as quantum dots, receptor binding agents, and nanospheres have been used to visualize sentinel nodes on an experimental basis but have not yet been used routinely in the clinical arena.

10.4 Performance of Lymphoscintigram

As previously mentioned, the sulfur colloid is injected intradermally to mimic lymphatic drainage of the primary lesion. Using a 25-gauge needle, the tracer is injected to surround the lesion or on both sides of the center of the incisional scar (if the primary tumor has already been excised) in four to six sites. Dynamic and static images are then obtained, 1 to 2 hours after injection, such that all potential nodal basins within the field are visualized. Each static image collection time should last approximately 5 to 10 minutes so that faintly labeled lymph nodes can be detected. The static images are obtained in standard views to allow adequate anatomic localization. Markers can be used to identify stable anatomic landmarks such as the ear canal or clavicle.

The addition of SPECT/CT (single-photon emission computed tomography/computed tomography) allows tracer imaging to be superimposed on to the anatomic information obtained by CT and can be useful in head and neck primary melanomas.[17]

10.4.1 Timing of the Lymphoscintigram

It is worthwhile to consider the timing of preoperative lymphoscintigraphy given that it can be obtained either days in advance of the proposed sentinel node biopsy or on the day of the procedure. Given the logistical issues described earlier regarding timing delays of image acquisition, it can be difficult to schedule lymphoscintigraphy on the day of the procedure. Obtaining imaging in advance of the operative intervention allows for review and confirmation with the interpreting nuclear medicine specialist. The other side of this argument is that a vast majority of these studies are straightforward and do not require detailed analysis. The typical practice is to inject the patient with the radionucleotide on the day of surgery. This obviates loss of the signal and any false positives that might result from the migration of the label into secondary or tertiary lymph nodes.

10.4.2 Aberrant or Interval Drainage Patterns

Drainage patterns that do not conform to the norm are significantly more common in the head/neck and trunk.[18,19] Interval nodes refer to the presence of nontraditional nodes situated in line of the drainage path between the site of the tumor and the main (traditional) drainage basin.

In the head and neck, these patterns include drainage to the postauricular nodes from the anterior forehead or drainage to the occipital nodes from the scalp. Truncal melanomas may drain to the triangular intermuscular space, interpectoral nodes, interval nodes over the costal margin, or even retroperitoneal nodes. The epitrochlear and popliteal regions are a part of the normal lymphatic drainage patterns in the upper and lower limb, respectively, but their involvement is seen in less than 1% of cases (▶ Fig. 10.3).

10.5 Performance of the Sentinel Node Biopsy

As with the lymphoscintigram, the radiopharmaceutical is injected in four to six sites intradermally in a peritumoral location. This injection, depending on the institution, is done either by radiologists in the nuclear medicine suite or in the operating room by the surgeon. The uptake in the appropriate basin(s) is confirmed by a Geiger counter prior to the start of the procedure. Occasionally, this may take longer than 5 minutes, especially in the elderly with lower extremity melanomas. The vital dye, if used, can be injected in the operating room, after the induction of anesthesia to prevent unnecessary discomfort to the patient.

In the interests of patient comfort, our practice is to inject the dye and the radiopharmaceutical after the induction of anesthesia. The site of the biopsy is included in the operating field and is appropriately prepared. If access to the node

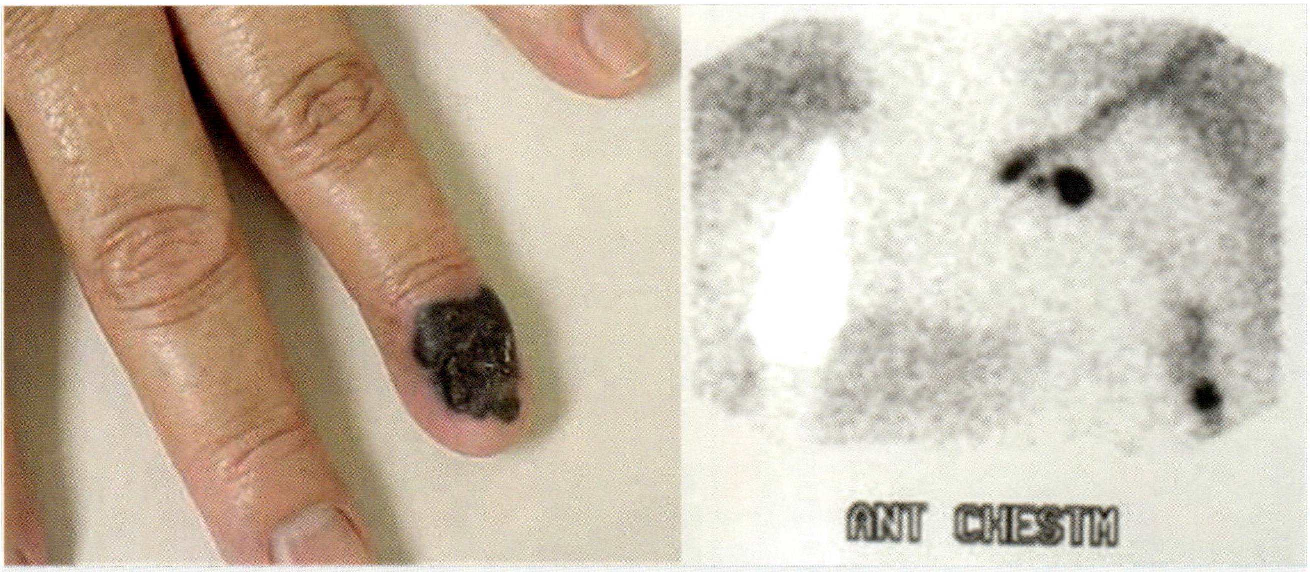

Fig. 10.3 A subungual melanoma draining to epitrochlear node (smaller inferior dark circle) and a high axillary node (large dark circle) seen below left clavicular marker. The epitrochlear node contained metastatic melanoma.

involves nerve stimulation, the anesthesiologist is informed, so that appropriate short-acting muscle relaxants are used, if indicated. We use prophylactic antibiotics that are administered immediately prior to the start of the procedure.

The resection of the primary tumor site is carried out first. This is done in order to minimize background radiation that might interfere with the location of the sentinel lymph node. The incision for the SLNB is centered over the node directly or in a site that gives the best access to other nodes that may be harvested as sentinel nodes. Care must be taken to site SLNB incisions appropriately. In general, the incisions are designed such that they can be extended into a larger access incision, should an operative lymphadenectomy prove necessary. For analogous reasons, the SLNB incisions must be placed in such a way so as not to compromise the flaps that will be raised if a subsequent lymphadenectomy is to be performed. Using the handheld gamma probe and a small incision, the bed is explored and the nodes are harvested. The use of a vital dye and its coloration of the sentinel node may aid in this process. Some surgeons tabulate the baseline counts in a nonaffected area as well as a non-node-bearing area and remove all nodes using the 10% rule (see later).The appropriate nodal counts are also documented. Care is taken to ligate the lymphatics to prevent a seroma postoperatively. The placement of a drain after this procedure is a matter of surgical judgment. While we have a low threshold for drain placement, we do not use antibiotics postoperatively, regardless of whether a drain is placed or not. The sentinel nodes are appropriately marked and the pathologist is informed about the use of radioactivity in the node harvest.

10.5.1 Identification of the True Sentinel Node

The experience of the last two decades has shown that the "hottest" node, that is, the node with the highest amount of radioactivity, does not translate into a guarantee that the malignant deposit will be found within it. In other words, a less radioactive lymph node may well be the abode of tumor cells.

In 2008, Chung et al established 10% rule for SLN for breast cancer.[20] These authors suggest that the removal of all the nodes with > 10% of radioactivity of the "hottest node" minimizes the false-negative rate of SLNB. The same criteria have been applied for SLNB in melanoma. Some other criteria used include radioactivity of 10 × background and even 3 × background.[11] The sensitivity after removal of three "hot nodes" is 93 to 99% and that after removal of four nodes is 100%.[21] The false-negative rate is 1 to 10% using the combined method (dye plus radionucleotide).[22]

10.5.2 Difficulties in Sentinel Node Identification

Nonvisualization of sentinel lymph nodes may occur in some cases. In our experience, this has usually been seen in elderly men in the head and neck region.

The proximity of the sentinel node site to the primary tumor may obscure the visualization of the sentinel node (▶ Fig. 10.4). In this scenario, it may be helpful to excise the primary lesion (and the principal source of the obscuring radioactivity) before looking for the sentinel node as mentioned earlier. Another solution to the problem is to combine the use of vital dye with the radioactive tracer such that the sentinel lymph node can be visually confirmed without the distraction of heightened background radioactivity.

The presence of previous flap surgery may alter the flow pattern of the draining lymph vessels and thus yield false-negative results. In an analogous problem, the presence of a large scar (from an ill-advised attempt at an excisional biopsy) can generate misleading results if the entire length of the scar is included in the injection of the radiopharmaceutical. Under these circumstances, injecting the central part of the scar, the presumed site of the primary lesion, can yield satisfactory results

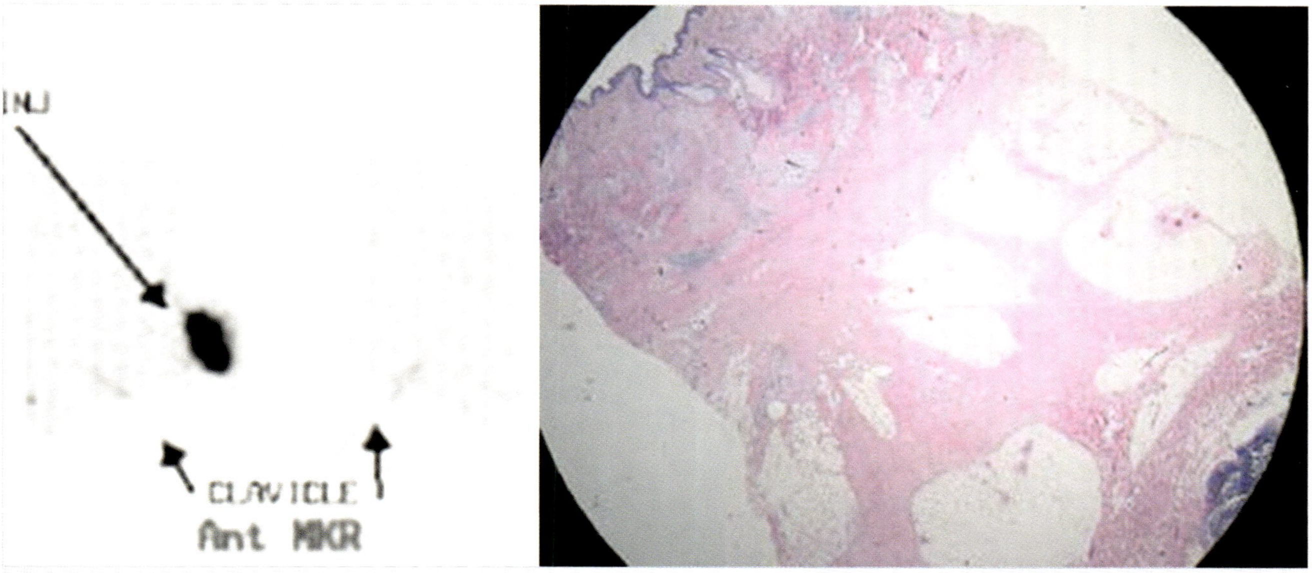

Fig. 10.4 Intense radioactivity at site of injection of right mandibular melanoma obscuring sentinel node (left). Low-power histological section depicting resected skin at the 11 o'clock position and the rim of the lymph node (blue) at the 4 o'clock position.

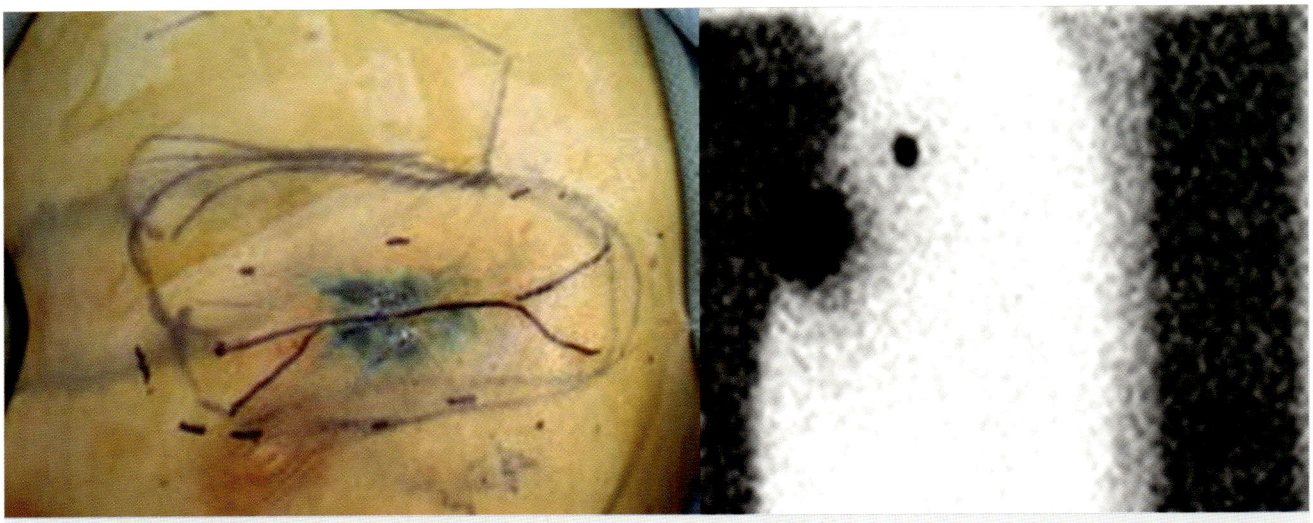

Fig. 10.5 Previous ill-advised excisional biopsy (8-mm depth melanoma) and scar indicated by the marked double Y on the left chest wall. This is encircled by the marking that shows presumed area of mobilization for closure. Injection of blue dye and 99m-Tc in the central part of the scar identified a single axillary sentinel node that was positive for melanoma.

(▸ Fig. 10.5). The presence of tattoos in the catchment area of the lymph node may lead to confusion with melanoma cells in the sentinel lymph nodes (▸ Fig. 10.6). The presence of concurrent melanomas of differing prognostic significance, in the same anatomic region, may mandate the sequential lymphoscintigraphic assessment to accurately delineate the lymph nodal basins involved (▸ Fig. 10.7).

Occasionally, anatomic or surgical constraints may dictate whether a sentinel node is accessible (▸ Fig. 10.8).

10.5.3 Special Considerations in the Head and Neck Region

The presence of a rich lymphatic network in and around the parotid gland complicates the harvest of sentinel nodes in the head and neck region.[23] The preauricular lymph nodes, situated in the sulcus between the external auditory meatus and the parotid gland, are usually small and are therefore difficult to detect. This difficulty increases when the sentinel node is detected within the substance of the parotid gland. Based on traditional teaching, the recommended method of harvesting these nodes is via a superficial parotidectomy with a formal identification of the facial nerve in order to minimize the chances of damaging it. Another option is to directly access the sentinel node in the parotid using a classic facelift incision and carefully dissecting through the substance of the gland, using a nerve stimulator if necessary, to harvest the node.[24] At our center, we have used both methods and currently prefer the technique of directly harvesting the sentinel node without a formal parotidectomy. In our series of 58 patients, we did not encounter a single case of facial nerve palsy. Interestingly, a survey of Head and Neck surgeons emphasized the wide variability in approaches to this problem, with as many as 48% of the surgeons surveyed opting for a superficial parotidectomy.[25]

It must be emphasized that the parotid sparing approach for sentinel node harvest should only be undertaken by experienced surgeons, failing which a parotidectomy is always the safer option.

10.5.4 Frozen Sections in the Identification of Sentinel Nodes

Frozen sections, in general, are not recommended for the analysis of sentinel nodes in melanomas.[26] These require a special expertise on the part of the examining pathologists which may not be universally available. The presence of benign nevus cells in the subcapsular region that may be mistaken for cells of metastatic melanoma further heightens the degree of uncertainty during such analyses.

A final consideration for lymphoscintigraphy in melanoma (and other malignancies) is how lymphatic drainage and therefore radiotracer localization may be affected by regional metastatic disease. There is evidence that micrometastases do not affect mapping techniques or SLNB identification. Additionally, there are some studies that demonstrate normal or near-normal lymphatic drainage patterns despite lymph node metastases.

10.5.5 Complications of Sentinel Node Biopsy

Sentinel node biopsies, generally speaking, are very safe procedures. Seromas and hematomas probably constitute the most common problems. To limit the occurrence of the former problem, we are liberal in the use of drains in our practice. Wound-healing problems such as infection and wound dehiscence are similarly rare. There have been reports of lymphedema occurring after the harvest of sentinel nodes alone but these situations, too, are extremely rare.

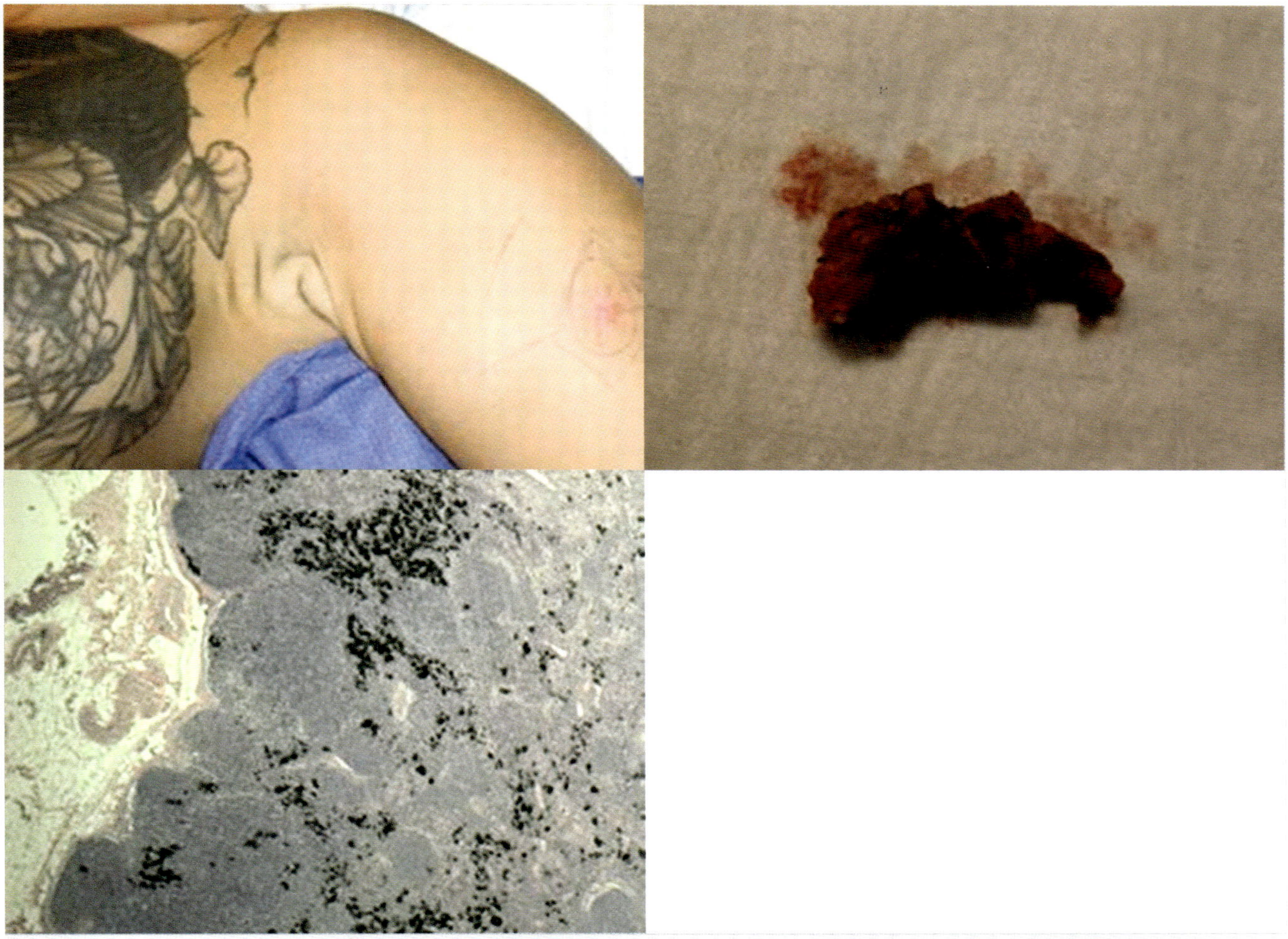

Fig. 10.6 Top left panel: extensive tattoo on chest wall and melanoma at the midarm. Top right panel: harvested lymph node with multiple dark areas suggestive of deposits of malignant melanoma. Bottom panel: histological evidence of iron pigment from tattoo stained with Prussian blue.

10.6 Operative Lymphadenectomy

Planning for operative lymphadenectomy begins with thorough history and physical exam at the initial encounter with the patient. Neck, groin, or axillary bulges, masses, or discomfort can be the first presentation of a clinically positive regional lymph node in a patient with melanoma and rarely in other cutaneous cancers. Physical exam should include examination of all possible drainage basins based on tumor location. Factors in this exam might be of considerable importance in the conduct of these procedures. Some examples include the presence of previous scars that might modify placement of incisions or impact the vascularity of poorly placed ones, problems affecting the cervical spine or the shoulder which might limit optimal positioning and exposure of the operative site of the patient, or the presence of inguinal of femoral hernias that might go unnoticed or unrecognized leading to possible damage in the dissections of this area.

10.6.1 General Considerations

Certain common features apply to the dissection of the major lymph nodal basins, that is, cervical, axillary, and inguinofemoral and pelvic basins.

- Positioning is of utmost importance. A poorly positioned patient can significantly add to operating time.
- Communication with the anesthesia team is critical if nerve testing is to be performed so that long-acting paralytic agents are not administered.
- The resection of large tumor masses that may result in significant bleeding should necessitate a preoperative type and cross-match of blood, if this is not routinely performed.
- Along the same lines, if an unusually long or bloody procedure is anticipated, the preoperative placement of a Foley catheter may be helpful. This is mandatory in patients with pelvic or groin dissection to prevent inadvertent damage to the bladder, especially in the elderly.

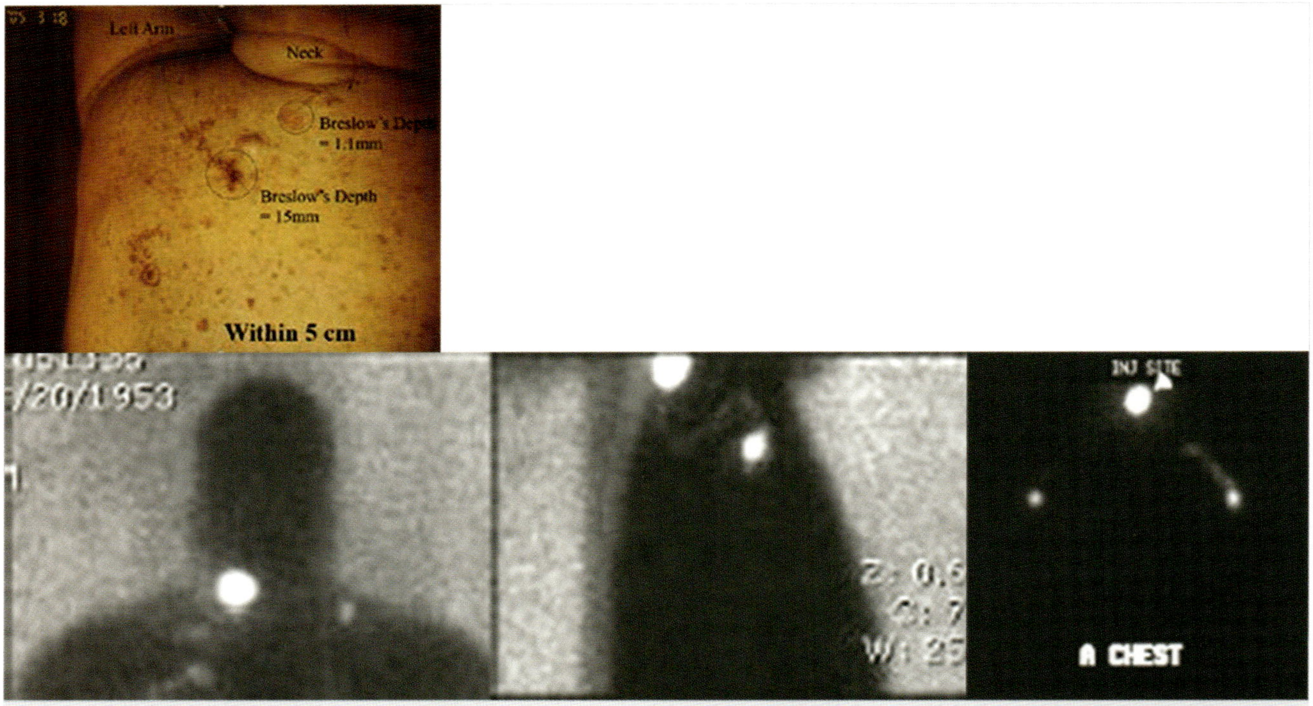

Fig. 10.7 Top panel: the location of two concurrent melanomas on the back—the superior melanoma of 1.1-mm depth and the inferior one of 15-mm depth. Lymphoscintigrams of the lesions on two separate days revealed that the superior lesion (situated on the right of the midline) drained to the left supraclavicular region (left and central panel), while the lower melanoma drained to both axillae (right inferior panel).

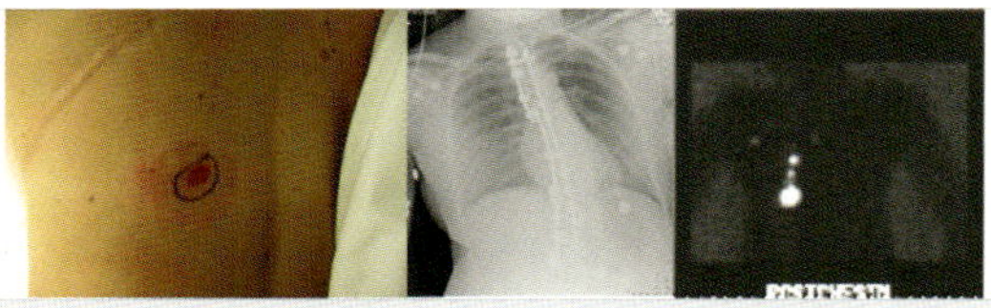

Fig. 10.8 Melanoma (circled) in a patient with history of spinal fusion with rib harvest from left chest wall and a midline incision over the spinous processes for Harrington's rod placement. Lymphoscintigram revealed drainage to paravertebral nodes. An attempt at biopsy was abandoned owing to difficulty of access under Harrington's rods.

- Sequential compression devices are routinely used on the lower extremities to prevent deep vein thrombosis.
- Postoperatively, one must be vigilant about lymphedema, especially with the lower limb, pelvic, and groin dissection and to a lesser degree in the upper limb. The importance of this preoperative discussion cannot be overemphasized. The prophylactic use of controlled pressure stockings may be of some benefit in high-risk patients, such as the obese ones.
- The adequacy of the lymphadenectomy can be judged using the number of nodes harvested during the procedure. Thus, Spillane and colleagues from the Sydney Melanoma Unit offer the following benchmarks.[27] Axillary dissections should aim for a minimum of 10 nodes, inguinal and ilioinguinal dissections for a minimum of 7 nodes, and cervical lymph node dissections involving 4 or more levels should aim for a minimum of 20 nodes.

10.7 Neck Dissection

The cervical lymph nodes are the most common initial site of regional metastases for melanomas of the head and neck. As mentioned previously, patterns of lymphatic spread can generally be predicted based on the location of the primary tumor. The anterior scalp, ear, and face typically drain first to the intraparotid node. These structures as well as the anterior neck can also drain to the cervical nodes including levels I to V (▶ Fig. 10.9). A complete (radical) neck dissection has become standard of care in patients with melanomas of the head and neck who have a positive SLNB or those patients with clinically positive lymph nodes.

The posterior scalp and posterior neck typically drain to level V cervical nodes as well as the retroauricular and suboccipital node. The discussion of head and neck lymphadenectomy is incomplete without a mention of SCCs of the lip and cheek. SCCs account for nearly 95% of lip cancers. The size of the primary tumor is one of the most significant predictors for prognosis.[28] For example, T2 lesions have a 5-year survival rate of approximately 90%, while T3 lesions have a 40 to 60% survival rate at 5 years.

Regional metastases to the lymphatic system seem to occur less frequently in SCCs of the lip as compared to other SCCs of the head and neck. Lower lip SCCs metastasize to the submandibular nodes in 70 to 90% of cases of regional spread.[28] Isolated nodal spread is present in 75% of regional metastases for SCCs of the lip, and 25 to 45% of these cases involved the submental,

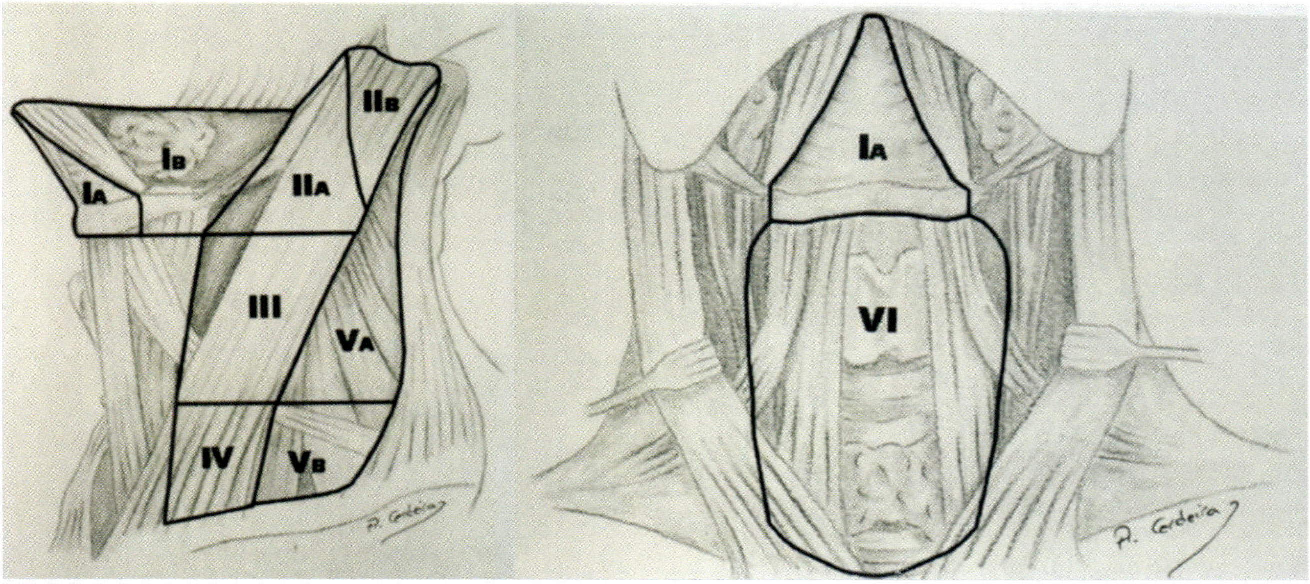

Fig. 10.9 Division of nodal groups by subzones in both lateral (left) and anterior view (right). Level I: Submental and submandibular nodes. This group includes the lymph nodes located within the submental triangle, bounded by the anterior belly of the digastric muscle and the hyoid bone. The submandibular group includes the lymph nodes located within the boundaries of the anterior and posterior bellies of the digastric muscle, the stylohyoid muscle, and the body of the mandible. The submandibular gland, which is located within this cervical space, should be removed when this nodal group is included in the resection. IA, submental nodes; IB, submandibular nodes. Level II: Upper jugular nodes. This group contains the lymph nodes located around the upper third of the internal jugular vein and the spinal accessory nerve. It goes from the level of the skull base superiorly to the level of the inferior border of the hyoid bone and carotid bifurcation inferiorly. The posterior boundary is the posterior border of the sternocleidomastoid muscle, and the anterior boundary is the lateral border of the sternohyoid and stylohyoid muscles. IIA, upper jugular nodes anterior to the XI nerve; IIB, upper jugular nodes posterior to the XI nerve. Level III: Middle jugular nodes. This group includes the lymph nodes located around the middle third of the internal jugular vein. The boundaries of this space are the inferior border of the hyoid bone and the carotid bifurcation superiorly, the inferior border of the cricoid cartilage, and the junction of the omohyoid muscle with the internal jugular vein inferiorly, the posterior border of the sternocleidomastoid muscle posteriorly, and the lateral border of the sternohyoid muscle anteriorly. Level IV: Lower jugular nodes. This nodal group contains the lymphatic structures located around the lower third of the internal jugular vein. Its boundaries are the inferior border of the cricoid cartilage and the omohyoid muscle superiorly, the clavicle inferiorly, the posterior border of the sternocleidomastoid muscle posteriorly, and the lateral border of the sternohyoid muscle anteriorly. Level V: Posterior triangle. This group includes the lymph nodes located along the transverse cervical artery and lower half of the spinal accessory nerve as well as the supraclavicular lymph nodes. The boundaries are the anterior border of the trapezius muscle posteriorly, the posterior border of the sternocleidomastoid muscle anteriorly, the clavicle inferiorly, and the convergence of the sternocleidomastoid and trapezius muscles superiorly. VA, lymph nodes in the posterior triangle located above the level of the inferior border of the cricoid cartilage; VB, lymph nodes in the posterior triangle located below the level of the inferior border of the cricoid cartilage. Level VI: Anterior compartment. This level contains the pre- and paratracheal nodes, precricoid (Delphian) node, perithyroidal nodes, and the lymph nodes along the recurrent laryngeal nerves. The boundaries are the hyoid bone superiorly, the suprasternal notch inferiorly, and the carotid arteries laterally.

level I nodes. SCCs of the upper lip typically spread to the submandibular or lower intraparotid nodes.

For SCCs of the lip and cheek, the presence of clinically evident, metastatic nodal disease mandates an ipsilateral complete neck dissection. It is possible to preserve structures within the lateral neck but preservation should not compromise lymphatic excision.

Some have advocated elective lymph node dissection in a clinically negative neck for SCCs of the lip and cheek.[28] However, 80% of clinically negative patients will not go on to develop cervical lymph node metastases during the course of their disease. This finding has led some to the supraomohyoid lymphatic dissection as a technique for assessing the lymph node status of the patient's neck given that the submandibular lymph nodes are the most frequently involved level. If the primary SCC is midline on the lower lip, bilateral levels I and II lymph nodes will need to be excised and examined.

10.7.1 Terminology

The term "neck dissection" has undergone many permutations over the last few decades. The classic radical neck dissection sacrificed the internal jugular vein, the sternocleidomastoid muscle, and the spinal accessory nerve. Based on the landmark studies of Bocca et al, the modified radical neck dissection or the functional neck dissection is now accepted as being oncologically equivalent to its more radical predecessor.[29] This dissection preserves the aforementioned structures and will be described in the following.

10.7.2 Modified Radical Neck Dissection (Anterior Cervical Chain Levels I–IV, Posterior Level V)

The following is standard technique for lymphadenectomy of the anterior and posterior cervical chain and includes levels I to V.

Access to the cervical group of lymph nodes can be obtained by means of a variety of incisions (▶ Fig. 10.10). Our preference is for the one popularized by Ariyan, which allows the incision to be hidden by regular clothing, as well as preventing the placement of a suture line over the major blood vessels.[25] The latter issue a matter of some concern in the face of postoperative radiation (for SCC or Merkel's cell tumors), which might result in exposure of the great vessels. A summary of our operative technique is presented in ▶ Fig. 10.11.

The patient is brought to the operating room and placed in the supine position on the operating room table. The head is rotated comfortably away from the lesion for exposure. A shoulder roll is placed to add to the ease of exposure.

The head end is elevated to approximately 20 degrees to collapse the veins and prevent venous oozing. The entire neck including the lower face to the angle of the mandible and chest is prepped and draped in a standard sterile fashion. The edge of the orbit and the modiolus are left visible by means of cover with a transparent dressing. This enables the visualization of the muscles innervated by the branches of the facial nerve, if nerve stimulation is employed. The incision begins by palpating the anterior border of the trapezius. The incision is made just behind the border of the trapezius so as not to inadvertently damage the spinal accessory nerve. This line is marked in a curvilinear fashion such that the inferior extent of the incision

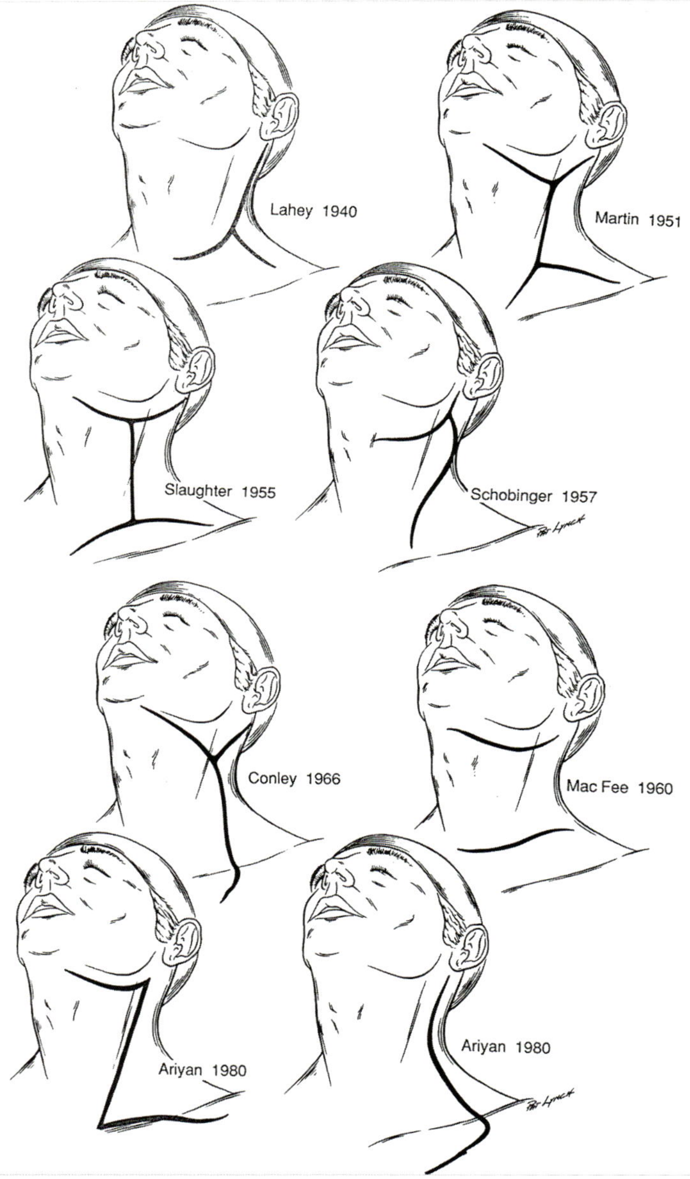

Fig. 10.10 Access incisions for neck dissection. (This image is provided courtesy of Stephan Ariyan, MD.)

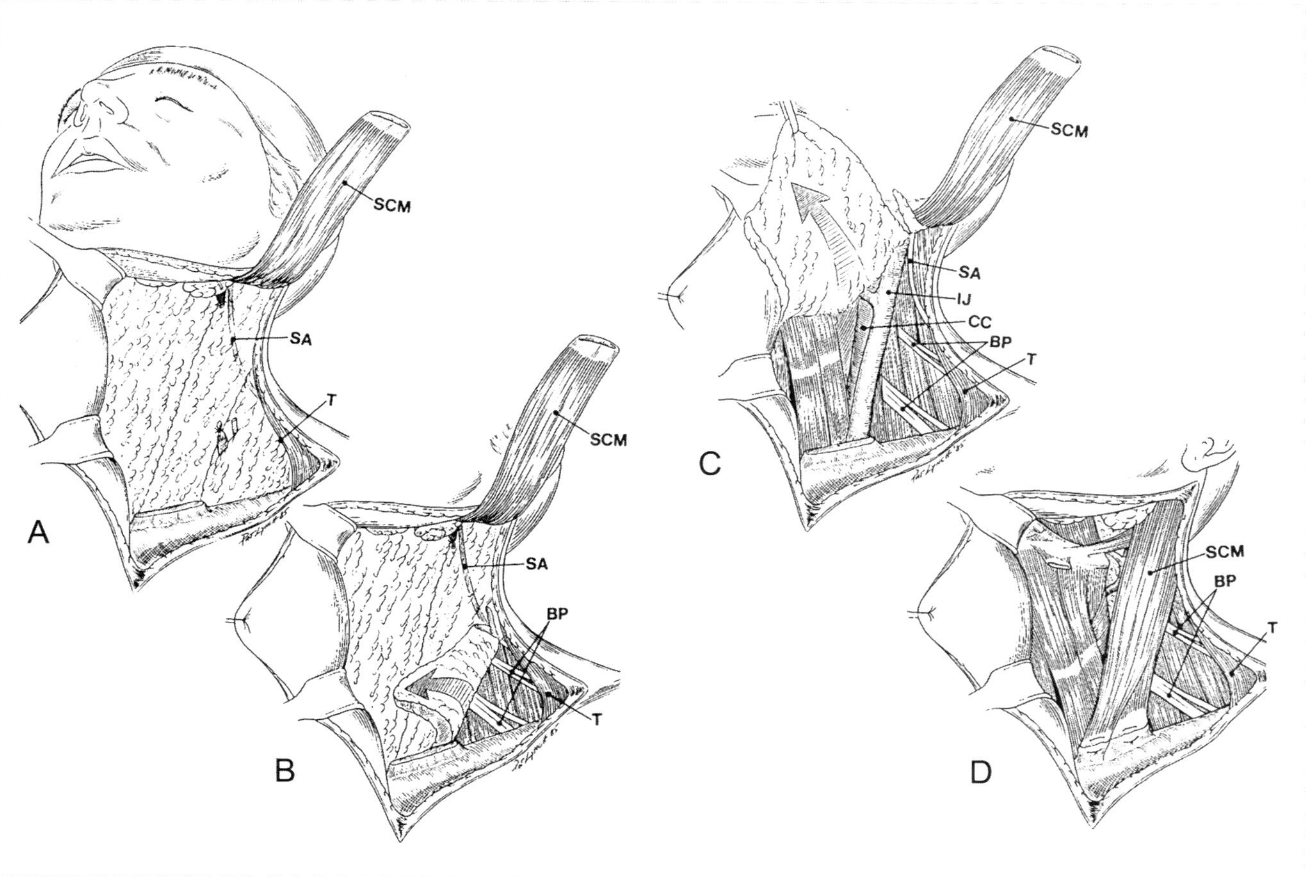

Fig. 10.11 Steps of neck dissection. See text for details. BP, brachial plexus; CC, common carotid; IJ, internal jugular; SA, spinal accessory; SCM, sternocleidomastoid; T, trapezius. (This image is provided courtesy of Stephan Ariyan, MD.)

moves gradually toward midline (▶ Fig. 10.12). The skin is incised sharply with a #15 blade. Electrocautery is used to carry the dissection through the platysma, the first muscular layer encountered. The platysma is raised with the medial skin flap both medially and superiorly. The two heads of the sternocleidomastoid muscles are identified, marked with heavy sutures, and transected, protecting the underlying structures with a wooden tongue blade. The investing layer of the deep cervical fascia is incised and the transected sternocleidomastoid is reflected upward. Thus, the entire lymph nodal packet is exposed. All lymphatic tissue is resected en bloc encompassing levels I to V, as shown in ▶ Fig. 10.12. This dissection can be modified according to the preference of the operator.

If alternate incisions, such as the ones shown are used, the above-mentioned principles are utilized. Classically trained Head and Neck surgeons may choose to leave the attachment of the sternocleidomastoid muscle intact and proceed with the dissection around the muscle.

We prefer to start the dissection inferiorly and move cranially and medially, since the plane here is easily found and there is a lesser density of vital structures. The identification of the spinal accessory nerve is easily accomplished first owing to its very superficial location. Erb's point on the middle of the posterior border of the sternocleidomastoid is a useful landmark for the spinal accessory and the great auricular nerves. We use the handheld nerve stimulator for ease of identification of motor nerves.

As this dissection moves medially, the omohyoid and the transverse cervical vessels are identified and transected. The carotid sheath is incised and the sheath attached to the lymph nodal packet is swept underneath the blood vessels. Superiorly, the dissection always includes the jugulodigastric nodes. If level I nodes are being dissected, the marginal mandibular nerve is identified deep to the fascia and the dissection proceeds anteriorly. If the nodal involvement of the submandibular gland is noted, removal of the submandibular salivary gland is recommended for oncologic clearance. The facial artery, which is intimately involved with the gland, is doubly ligated and care taken to preserve the lingual and hypoglossal nerves. Within the carotid sheath, the vagus nerve and the sympathetic trunk are encountered. Careful dissection preserves these vital structures and allows for adequate resection of all lymphatic tissue. The phrenic nerve lying on the scalene muscle is identified and preserved. Finally, the dissection continues to the inferior-most aspect of the neck where the thoracic duct is encountered as it joined the internal jugular vein (predominantly for dissections of the left neck). Once all the lymphatic tissue is excised and meticulous hemostasis is achieved, a closed suction drain is placed in the wound bed and brought out through the skin by a

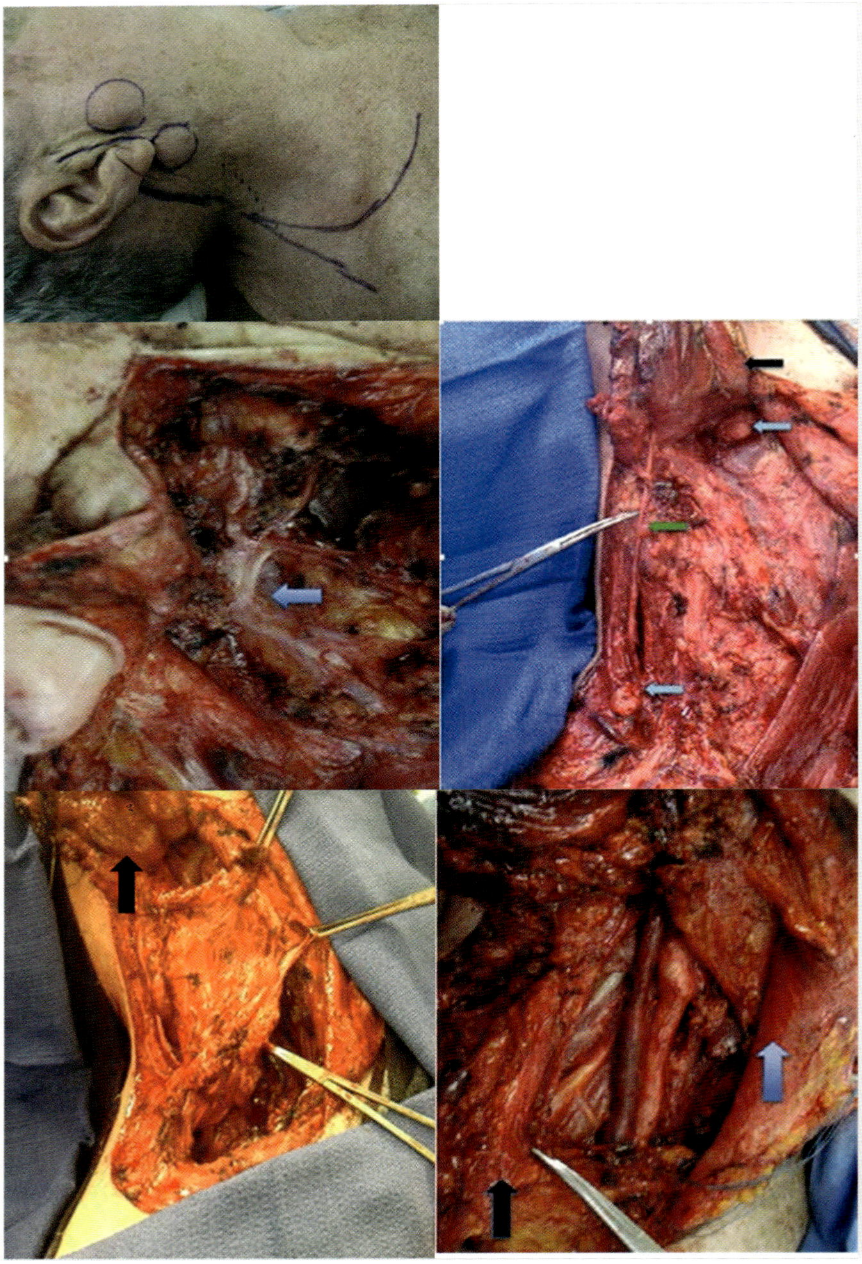

Fig. 10.12 Neck dissection. Top panel: Patient with metastatic melanoma lesions in parotid. Note preauricular incision carried out behind the neck and thence in a curvilinear fashion across the supraclavicular region. The dotted line represents the surface marking of the XI cranial nerve and the diagonal line the anterior border of the trapezius. Central panel (left): Completed superficial parotidectomy with blue arrow pointing to main trunk of the facial nerve. Central panel (right): Green arrow points to spinal accessory. Blue arrows point to lymph nodes that are often harvested as sentinel lymph nodes Black arrow points to reflected sternocleidomastoid muscle. Bottom panel (left): Lymphoid content of neck being removed en bloc. Note reflected sternocleidomastoid muscle in upper left corner. Bottom panel (right): Neck dissection just prior to completion. Note preserved internal jugular vein with common carotid adjacent to it. The green sutures (no. 1 Ethibond) at the inferior end of the incision will be used to resecure the sternocleidomastoid to its attachments. Blue arrow shows platysma incorporated in the reflected flap to improve vascularity. Black arrow points to lymphovascular packet. Note reflected sternocleidomastoid muscle in upper left corner (different case).

separate stab incision. The wound is then closed in layers with interrupted absorbable sutures.

Postoperatively, it is vital to initiate range of motion exercises for the neck. The drain can be removed either as an inpatient or upon follow-up, depending on the quantity and quality of the output.

10.7.3 Parotidectomy and Neck Dissection

The finding of a positive sentinel lymph node in the immediate vicinity of the parotid or in the substance of the gland mandates the removal of the parotid gland in continuity (en bloc) with a modified neck dissection. Failure to remove the parotid gland results in an unacceptably high recurrence rate. The same is true of palpable nodes or in-transit metastases in this region. The description that follows highlights our technique for a parotidectomy.

The positioning and general comments that apply to a neck dissection apply in their entirety to a parotidectomy. In most instances, the operative term refers to the removal of the gland anterior or superficial to the branches of the facial nerve. Rarely, an invasive tumor may mandate removal of the deeper part of the lobe, along with a possible resection of the facial nerve branch or branches.

In the case of a combined procedure, our preference is to start with the parotidectomy part since this is the more demanding half of the surgical exercise. Access to the parotid is obtained by a face-lift incision in the preauricular area. This incision can easily be extended into the neck as described earlier.

The skin flap is raised using skin hooks for traction. The dissection plane anterior to the parotid fascia (which is marked by a whitish hue) is easily found. The flap is raised to the anterior border of the parotid gland remembering that the facial nerve branches emerge immediately under the cover of this landmark. Dissection then proceeds in the interspace between the parotid gland and the external auditory meatus. Small nodes in this area are included in the final specimen. The use of a headlight and loupes is invaluable in dissecting this anatomically constrained area. Small crossing veins are sealed off with the bipolar cautery. Blunt self-retaining retractors are placed to maximize exposure. It is important to keep in mind that the anatomic landmark for intraoperative identification of the facial nerve (posterior belly of the digastric muscle, mastoid process, tympanic bone, and external auditory cartilage). The use of the "tragal pointer" is a very useful and reliable landmark in the identification of the trunk of the facial nerve. The nerve lies approximately 1-cm deep and slightly anterior and inferior to the tip of the external canal cartilage (also called "pointer"). Alternatively, the nerve can be identified as it lies approximately 1-cm deep to the medial attachment of the posterior belly of the digastric muscle to the digastric groove of the mastoid bone. In elderly men and those prone to alcohol abuse and diabetes, the diffuse enlargement of the parotid gland (sialosis) may make this tedious. The use of a nerve stimulator cannot be overemphasized while conducting this dissection. If an in-continuity dissection is to be performed, the dissection proceeds in a cranial to caudal direction. The gland is painstakingly dissected off the nerve using a combination of blunt and sharp dissection. We use the bipolar cautery at low settings, exclusively, to obtain hemostasis during this part of the procedure.

10.7.4 Posterior Cervical Chain Dissection

On occasion, only a posterior chain neck dissection is required if a pre- or intraoperative localizing study indicates that only the posterior triangle lymphatic tissue is involved. The following is an example of a standard technique for posterior cervical chain lymph node dissection.

The patient is brought to the operating room and placed in the supine position on the operating room table. The head is rotated comfortably away from the lesion for exposure of the posterior cervical chain. The entire neck including the lower face to the angle of the mandible and chest is prepped and draped in the standard sterile fashion. The anatomic borders of this lymphatic dissection are the most superior portion of the posterior border of the sternocleidomastoid muscle and the anterior aspect of the trapezius. The clavicle defines the inferior extent of the dissection. An incision is made 2 cm posterior to the anterior border of the trapezius. The incision is carried out inferiorly in a linear fashion such that each border of the dissection is accessible in the wound. Care is taken inferiorly as the brachial plexus is identified as it emerged between the anterior and middle scalene muscles. Once all the lymphatic tissue is excised and meticulous hemostasis was achieved, a closed suction drain is placed in the wound bed and brought out through the skin by a separate stab incision. The wound is then closed in layers with interrupted absorbable sutures. Postoperatively, the same considerations mentioned earlier apply.

10.7.5 Complications of Head and Neck Lymphadenectomy

Complications specific to the location are damage to the major motor nerves (marginal mandibular branch of the facial nerve, the phrenic nerve, and the spinal accessory nerves), chylous leak commonly seen on the left side due to damage of the thoracic duct, and potential exposure of the great vessels (with blowout) if working in a patient with compromised circulation and/or radiation.[30]

10.8 Selective Nodal Dissections

In general, the concept of selective nodal dissections has been advocated principally for low-risk SCCs involving the face or cheek. We have noted that a selective approach sparing level I nodes may be feasible in melanomas when lymphoscintigraphic studies do not indicate that the dye traverses a path through the level I tissue.[23] It must be emphasized that this is performed only in the absence of palpable nodal disease in melanoma, that is, a completion lymphadenectomy for an SLNB positive for melanoma. Similar studies have not been performed for Merkel's cell tumors and other rare cutaneous cancers.

10.8.1 Axillary Node Dissection

Therapeutic lymph node dissection of the axilla is most often performed in the surgical treatment melanoma metastatic to the lymph nodes and less frequently for Merkel's cell tumors or metastatic SCCs.[30] The following is a standard technique for approach to axillary lymphadenectomy.

The patient is brought to the operating room and positioned on the operative table in a supine position. The ipsilateral upper extremity is abducted on an arm board, while close attention is paid to positioning and padding of bony prominences, such that position-based neuropathies is minimized. A roll under the axilla thrusts the contents forward and makes dissection easier. The axilla is clipped and the chest wall, axilla, and circumferential arm and hand are prepped and draped in a standard sterile fashion. We administer preoperative antibiotics.

Several incisions are possible based on physician and patient preference. One option is to make a transverse incision in the axillary fold and opposing vertical incisions along the posterior arm and anterior chest wall near the border of the pectoralis major, thus opening the axilla in a Z fashion.

Alternatively, the incision is made starting at the superior and lateral edge of the pectoralis major muscle within the axillary hairline. This incision is continued posteriorly to the border of the latissimus dorsi in a curvilinear fashion. A final option is to place the incision in the same position within the axillary hairline and continue the incision inferiorly along the lateral border of the pectoralis major muscle.

We prefer to use the Z pattern for exposure of the axillary contents for the following reasons:

- It allows excellent access to the deeper reaches of the axilla with minimal retraction.
- Excision of cutaneous nodules or compromised scars can easily be incorporated without difficulty in subsequent closure (▶ Fig. 10.13).
- It minimizes the possibility of axillary contractures by redistributing tension across different planes.

This access incision creates medial and lateral flaps which are sutured to the skin by means of temporary silk sutures, which provide stable retraction. The flaps are raised in the subcutaneous plane, maintaining a thickness compatible with good vascularity. We have found that it is useful to keep the base of these flaps thick, in order to prevent ischemic compromise at the distal ends. The use of a lighted retractor (or headlights) and a handheld nerve stimulator is extremely valuable in this dissection.

Our practice is to commence the dissection by identifying the perimeter of the axillary contents to be removed. The superior border is defined by the length of the axillary vein. The posterior boundary corresponds to the anterior margin of the latissimus dorsi muscle, while the anterior counterpart is the lateral margin of the pectoralis major muscle. Inferiorly, the dissection is carried down to the junction of the latissimus dorsi and serratus anterior muscles, which usually correspond to the fifth intercostal space.

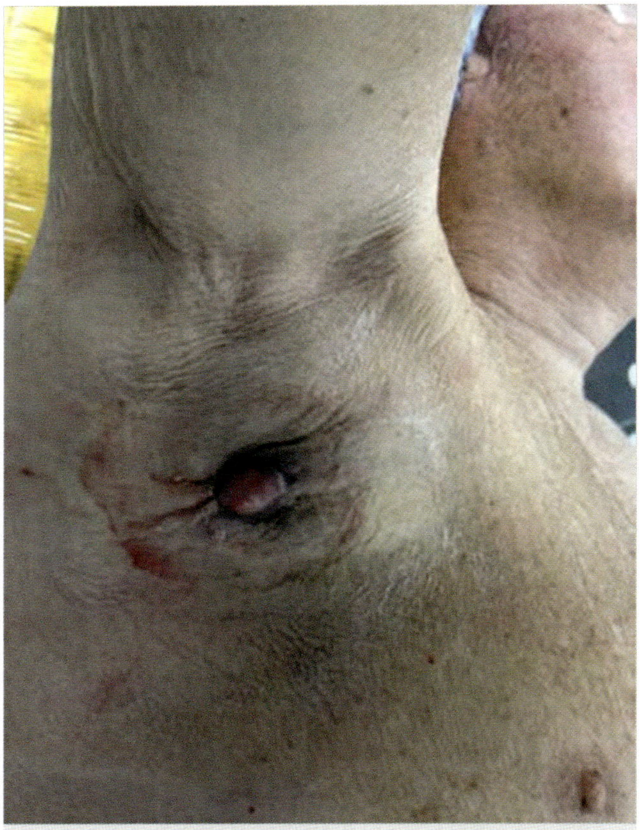

Fig. 10.13 Involvement of the skin of the axilla, as in the case of this squamous cell carcinoma metastatic to the lymph nodes, mandates resection of the overlying skin with tissue rearrangement to prevent axillary contracture.

In this context, it is useful to recollect the conventional nomenclature of axillary node levels[31]:

- Level 1 nodes: below (inferior to) the pectoralis minor.
- Level 2 nodes: behind (posterior to) the pectoralis minor.
- Level 3 nodes: above (superior to) the pectoralis minor.

In contrast to the breast lymphadenectomies, removal of involved nodes for melanomas encompasses all three levels.

The location of the axillary artery is first palpated to orient the operator to the axillary contents. The axillary vein lies immediately in front of this important landmark.

We begin the dissection superiorly by sharply incising the fascia over the axillary vein along its length. The dissection is kept anterior to the anterior surface of the axillary vein. Smaller vessels or tributaries are ligated or cauterized. As the dissection proceeds inferiorly, the subscapular vein (thoracodorsal vein) is identified on the inferior surface of the axillary vein.

Occasionally, multiple tributaries of the axillary vein are noted, which may prove confusing (▶ Fig. 10.14). It is important to dissect out all the tributaries to accurately identify the true subscapular vein, which helps in identifying the thoracodorsal artery and nerve.

Following the identification of these structures, the artery and nerve are dissected down to their point of entry into the substance of the latissimus dorsi muscle. Once this has been accomplished, the lateral component of the dissection begins on the anterior surface of the latissimus muscle. The dissection is first carried out medially until the previously dissected thoracodorsal neurovascular bundle is reached. The dissection is then carried out inferiorly, freeing up the base of the cone of the axillary contents until the chest wall is reached medially.

The medial aspect of the dissection starts at the lateral border of the pectoralis major muscle by incising the clavipectoral fascia. It is then carried out along laterally and superiorly until

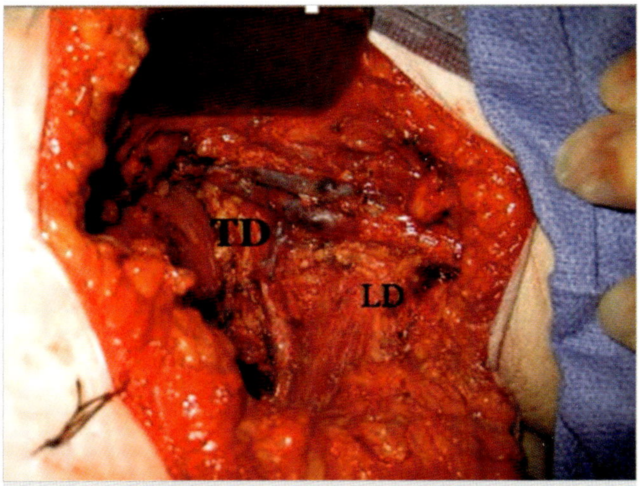

Fig. 10.14 Completed axillary dissection showing two tributaries of the axillary vein in the left axilla. These variants may pose difficulty in identification of the true thoracodorsal (TD) vasculature, which arises from the lower of the two tributaries descending into the latissimus dorsi (LD) muscle.

connected with the medial end of the superior dissection, that is, the medial part of the axillary vein. The dissection on the chest wall is now continued posteriorly. At this point, the intercostobrachial nerve is encountered and may be preserved or transected depending on the preference of the operator. On the undersurface of the pectoralis major muscle, the medial pectoral nerve is identified as it comes through or just medial to the pectoralis minor muscle. This is preserved to maintain the innervation of the pectoralis major muscle. The specimen is dissected off the lateral border of the pectoralis minor muscle incorporating the interpectoral nodes. The lateral pectoral nerve, which may have a variable course, is generally seen running along the lateral border of the pectoralis minor muscle. This muscle may be divided or resected if bulky nodal disease mandates better exposure or complete oncologic clearance.

At this point, it is mandatory to identify the long thoracic nerve. This can be done in two ways. In the first, the previously dissected thoracodorsal vascular bundle is identified. In most, if not all, cases, a venous branch can be seen extending medially to the chest wall. This vein is carefully followed to the chest wall. The long thoracic nerve is usually located posterior to this branch hugging the chest wall. The second method is to dissect posteriorly along the contour of the chest wall, putting gentle downward and lateral traction on the fibrofatty contents. The long thoracic nerve can be palpated as a taut cord at the upper end of the axilla or rolled along and/or visualized on the chest wall. The use of a handheld nerve stimulator can significantly speed up the process.

Once this structure is identified, the entire base of the cone representing the bulk of the axillary contents is rendered free. Dissection now proceeds superiorly toward the axillary apex. The insertion of the pectoralis minor may be detached to provide better access. Larger lymphatic trunks may be encountered which merit careful ligation. Level II lymph nodes are now dissected off the axillary vein and bluntly dissected downward. A centrally located vein in this fat pad must be identified and ligated before it causes troublesome bleeding. Removal of the level III nodes involves completion of the dissection from the thoracic inlet laterally to the pectorals minor medially.

This dissection technique allows excision of all lymphatic tissue in axillary levels I to III. The wound is then copiously irrigated and hemostasis is ensured. A closed suction drain is left in the wound bed and the wound is closed in layers with interrupted sutures.

Postoperatively, elevation of the extremity and avoidance of peripheral intravenous catheters on the ipsilateral arm will reduce edema. An arm sling can be maintained for comfort but range of motion exercises for the upper extremity should be started as soon as feasible for the patient.

10.8.2 Inguinofemoral Node Dissection (Groin Dissection)[32]

The term groin dissection generally refers to the removal of the superficial inguinal and femoral nodes. This can be combined with an iliac node dissection if needed or indicated.

The patient is placed in the supine position with the ipsilateral leg externally rotated and the knee slightly flexed. A Foley catheter is placed and body hair is clipped from the skin of the operative field including the groin, upper leg, and lower abdomen. The entire abdomen below the umbilicus to the knee, including bilateral groins, is prepped and draped in a sterile fashion. A modesty towel is placed. The options of incisions for inguinal–femoral node dissection are shown in ▸ Fig. 10.15. If the inguinal dissection has been combined with a femoral and iliac dissection, one can perform the dissection from both incisions (described elsewhere) with an elevated skin bridge by leaving 4 to 5 mm of subcutaneous tissue. If the inguinal dissection is to be performed as the sole procedure, a single incision is made from superior and lateral to the anterior superior iliac spine and continued inferiorly and medially until 1 to 2 cm below the inguinal crease (▸ Fig. 10.16). The borders of the dissection include all fatty and lymphatic tissue between Scarpa's fascia and the external oblique fascia from the inguinal ligament to 5 to 6 cm superiorly. A closed suction drain is left in place. The wound is then closed with interrupted sutures in Scarpa's fascia and a running subcuticular suture for the skin.

For the femoral part of the dissection, the lymphoid tissue and the fat contents of the femoral triangle are removed. The boundaries of the triangle are the sartorius laterally, the adductor longus medially, and the inguinal ligament as the base of the triangle. The femoral vessels within the femoral sheath and

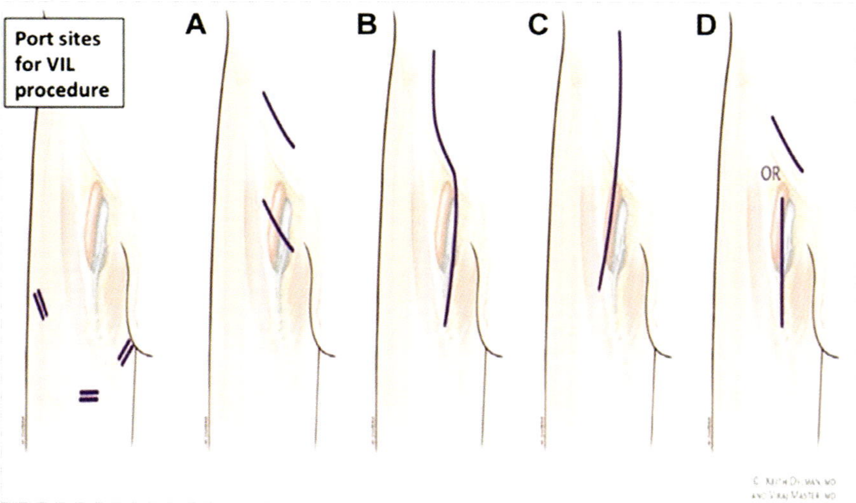

Fig. 10.15 Different access incisions for groin dissection. VIL, video inguinal lymphadenectomy. (This image is provided courtesy of Viraj Master, MD, PhD, FACS, and Keith Delman, MD, FACS.)

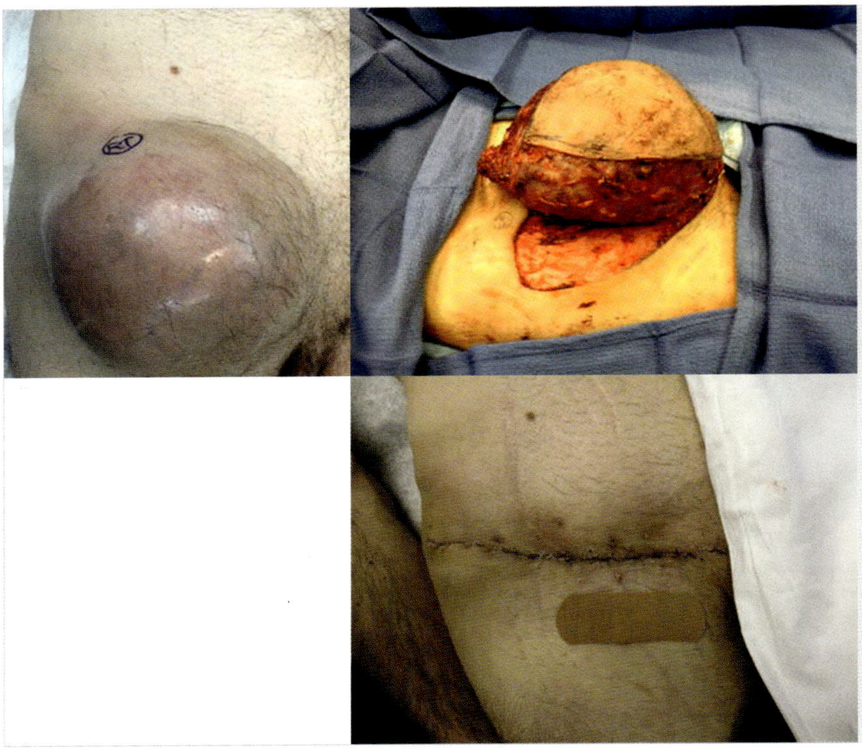

Fig. 10.16 Neglected metastatic melanoma (right groin). Groin dissection with resection of involved skin and reconstruction with advancement flap closure. Dressing is at drain site.

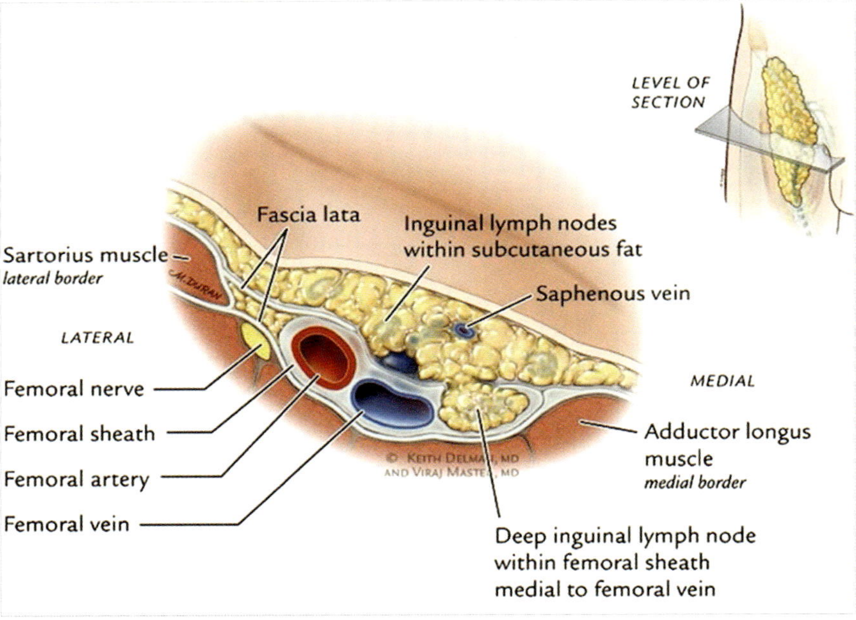

Fig. 10.17 Contents of the femoral triangle. (This image is provided courtesy of Viraj Master, MD, PhD, FACS, and Keith Delman, MD, FACS.)

the femoral nerve, lateral to the vascular structures, are important structures to be preserved in the dissection (▶ Fig. 10.17). The removal of these contents can be done en bloc with the inguinal part regardless of the incisions chosen and is important if there is extracapsular spread (▶ Fig. 10.18).

The course of the femoral artery is palpated and a vertical incision is marked from two fingerbreadths inferior to the inguinal ligament inferiorly to the femoral triangle apex. Alternatively, a single oblique incision along the inguinal crease can be used. The borders of this dissection are from level of the inguinal ligament to the apex of the femoral triangle formed by the junction of the adductor longus and the sartorius where they cross inferiorly.

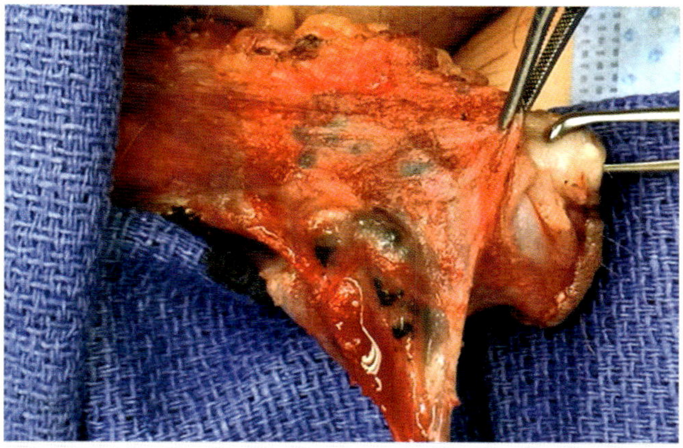

Fig. 10.18 The presence of extracapsular spread and in-transit metastases in this case of groin dissection emphasizes the need for en bloc resection.

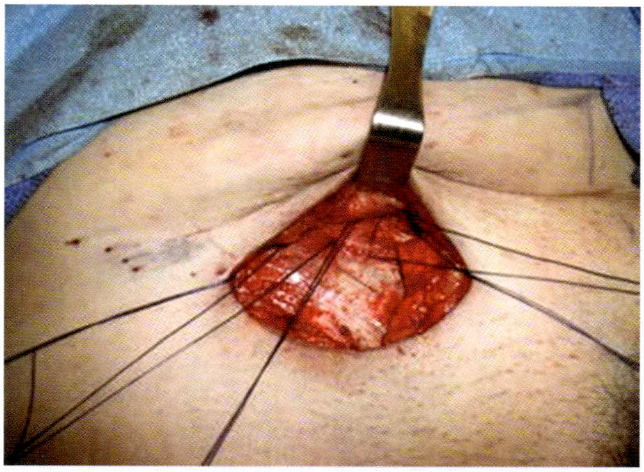

Fig. 10.19 Placement of heavy absorbable sutures to obliterate dead space in groin dissection field to prevent seroma formation.

The marked incision is carried out down sharply until Scarpa's fascia is encountered. The fascia is incised and included in the medial and lateral skin flaps. Dissection is carried out medially until the femoral vein is identified and preserved. The medial border—the border of the adductor longus—is then identified. Our practice then is to identify the lateral border of the dissection, that is, the sartorius muscle. The dissection is then carried out on the surface of the muscles, sparing the deep fascia on these muscles (to decrease the chances of lymphedema), until the apex is reached. Thus, the fat pad and the lymph nodes to be removed have been outlined. The saphenous vein is transected and securely ligated.

The saphenous vein and the adjacent tissue are carefully dissected heading cranially. Large lymphatics are seen alongside this vein and must be securely ligated or coagulated. The vein is followed superiorly sweeping all lymphatic tissue and the femoral sheath off the femoral vessels until the saphenofemoral junction is identified on the anterior surface of the femoral vein. The saphenous vein is ligated here. It is critically important to identify the femoral vein prior to ligating the saphenous for fear of confusing the femoral vein for the saphenous vein. The dissection is carried out medially from the adductor longus to the femoral vessels, and laterally from the sartorius to the same junction. The removal of the lymph node of Cloquet can be performed while moving from the medial border of the dissection to the femoral vessels. The dissection is completed while sweeping the lymphatic tissue off the femoral vessels. This dissection allows for the identification and preservation of the femoral vessels and femoral nerve. A closed suction drain is placed and the wound is closed in layers with interrupted sutures. Deep absorbable sutures are placed to obliterate the dead space (▶ Fig. 10.19). The skin is closed with a running subcuticular suture.

Postoperatively, it is important to stress elevation of the lower extremity and early ambulation. Lower extremity compression may be required for a short time postprocedure to alleviate edema.

10.8.3 Variations of Technique

Minimally Invasive Groin Dissections[33,34,35]

The previously described groin dissection techniques are effective for management of regional metastases of malignant skin neoplasms of the lower extremity, lower abdomen, and perineum. However, these traditional incisions have the potential to lead to undesired complications such as seroma formation, skin flap necrosis, wound infection, and wound dehiscence. In fact, groin lymph node dissection is associated with a 50 to 75% complication rate in some series. Recently, there has been interest in applying laparoscopic principles to groin dissections in an effort to decrease operative morbidity. Indeed, these techniques can reduce the degree of tissue injury and postoperative pain. Additionally, laparoscopic techniques can decrease the required dissection of important structures such as the abdominal wall musculature or the inguinal ligament.

Finally, there is an improved cosmetic result with minimally invasive techniques. Minimally invasive techniques generally use three smaller incisions with one camera port and two instrument ports (▶ Fig. 10.15). We have described a minimally invasive method using a small incision used for the sentinel node biopsy and a lighted retractor (▶ Fig. 10.20). Several groups, including ourselves, have described laparoscopic iliac lymphadenectomy either alone or in combination with superficial groin dissection.

Sartorius Flap

In order to prevent exposure of the femoral vessels, some surgeons transpose the sartorius muscle over the vessels (▶ Fig. 10.21). It is important to remember that the sartorius has a segmental blood supply (type IV in the Mathes–Nahai classification). For this reason, we recommend that not more than two segmental vessels be divided when mobilizing this muscle in an effort to maintain its viability.

Removal of the Lymph Node of Cloquet

There is significant variation in practice regarding the removal of Cloquet's node in the femoral canal. Some surgeons routinely remove and use it as an indicator of deeper involvement and a guide to iliac node dissection if positive for disease (melanoma). This practice, however, is not universal.

10.8.4 Iliac Node Dissection (Including Obturator Nodes)[36]

Based on pre- and intraoperative localization studies, iliac (pelvic) lymph node dissection may be required singly or in combination with other groin dissections for malignant melanoma of the lower extremity or torso. If combined with a femoral dissection, the lymph nodal packet can be removed en bloc by incising the inguinal ligament (followed by its repair) using a single incision or through a discontinuous incision. Our preference is for the latter as it avoids the morbidities commonly associated with these procedures, such as skin flap necrosis. Of note, it is useful to have muscle relaxants on board during the intra-abdominal part of the procedure to provide ease of access to deeper structures. A standard technique for iliac lymphadenectomy is described in the following.

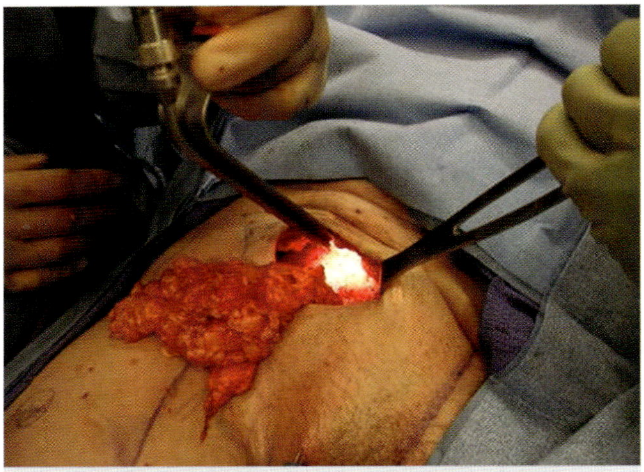

Fig. 10.20 The use of a lighted retractor as shown here can be used in the performance of a minimally invasive groin dissection.

The patient is placed in the supine position on the operative table with the leg ipsilateral to the dissection externally rotated and the knee slightly flexed. A Foley catheter is placed and the body hair clipped from the operative field including the groin, upper leg, and lower abdomen to the umbilicus. The entire abdomen below the umbilicus to the knee including bilateral groins is prepped and draped in a sterile fashion. A modesty towel is placed. The dissection described here ultimately allows for excision of all fatty tissue and lymphatics from the bifurcation of the common iliac artery to the fascia over the obturator foramen. A curvilinear incision is made approximately 5 cm above the inguinal ligament from the pubic tubercle to the anterior superior iliac spine. The external oblique aponeurosis is bluntly dissected off the subcutaneous tissue until the inguinal ligament is identified. This allows for easier reapproximation at the end of the operation as well as facile access to the femoral artery should it be required emergently. The fascia of the external oblique is incised along the length of the incision. The internal oblique muscle is split along its fibers, as is the transversalis muscle. In doing so, the deep circumflex iliac artery is ligated. Once through the transversalis fascia, the peritoneum is identified and bluntly swept cephalad until the common iliac vessels are identified. Care is taken to preserve the peritoneum to prevent the annoying intrusion of bowel loops into the field. The ureter is also identified and preserved as it crosses the common iliac just superior to the vessels' bifurcation. This allows for safe dissection of all lymphatic tissue from the level of the bifurcation inferiorly. It may be necessary to ligate the inferior epigastric artery as it comes off the external iliac artery for ease of dissection. This allows exposure of the vas and the testicular vessels (round ligament in females) and aids in placing them out of harm's way.

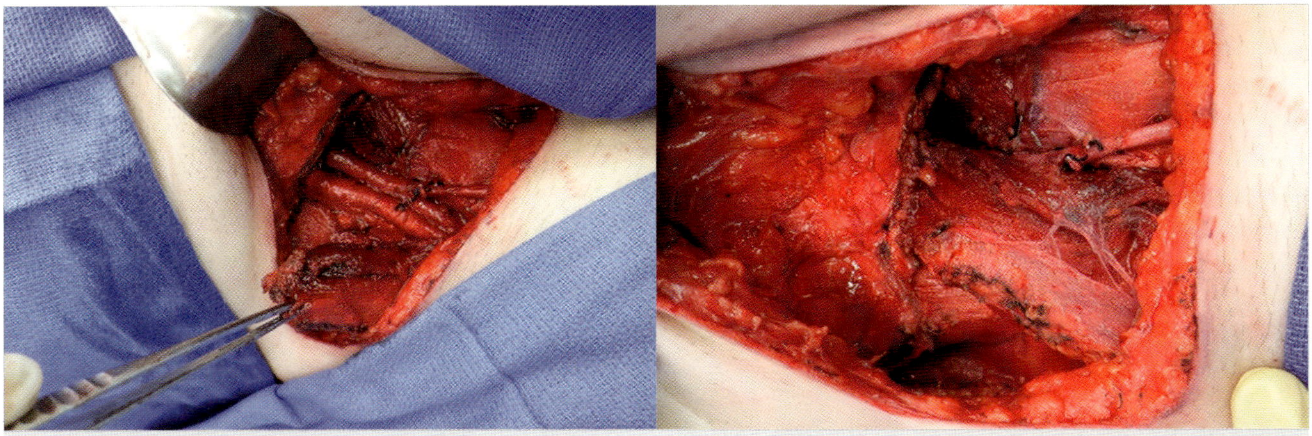

Fig. 10.21 Sartorius flap. The first panel shows the harvest of the sartorius muscle after a right groin dissection. Note the relatively short length mobilized (held by forceps) to preserve the vascularity of the muscle, which is segmental. The second panel shows the muscle transposed over the femoral vessels and secured to the inguinal ligament.

A self-retaining retractor (Bookwalter) is placed. We prefer to start the dissection superiorly using sharp dissection over the vessels. All lymphatic vessels are either clipped or ligated. The use of sealing devices (Ligasure, Medtronic) can significantly increase the speed of the procedure. The lymph nodes are swept off the artery and vein, peeling them off with a sheath over the vessels. This is continued inferiorly between the vessels to the level of the obturator fascia. The nodes overlying the obturator fascia are best dissected bluntly since palpation of the tissue in this area reveals the obturator nerve as a taut cordlike structure which is preserved. At this point, the iliac and obturator nodes are removed en bloc and the dissection is complete. The retroperitoneum is packed and reinspected for hemostasis No drain is left in the pelvis. Again, it is important to stress elevation of the lower extremity and early ambulation postoperatively. Lower extremity compression may be required for a short time postprocedure to alleviate edema.

10.8.5 Rare Locations[37]

There are other less frequently used lymph node dissections with which the melanoma surgeon should be familiar. These are the dissections of the epitrochlear basin and the popliteal fossa.

Epitrochlear lymph node dissection may be required for melanoma of the hand, subungual region, or skin of the forearm to the elbow (▶ Fig. 10.22). The incidence is infrequent. A rate of 3.7% for clinically apparent metastases to this region has been quoted. The following is a description of our technique for the epitrochlear dissection.

The patient is placed in the supine position on the operating table. An arm board is positioned appropriately. The entire arm and hand up to and including the axilla are prepped and draped in a sterile fashion. A curvilinear incision is made from 5 cm proximal to the medial epicondyle in an inferior and lateral fashion such that it traverses the antecubital fossa to the brachioradialis muscle. This pattern is critical to avoid a contracture in the region of the elbow. Skin flaps are raised such that the biceps and brachioradialis muscles are identified laterally and the medial head of the triceps and the flexor origin on the medial epicondyle are identified medially. Any superficial veins that are encountered are ligated. The borders of this dissection are the medial head of the triceps, the short head of the biceps, the musculature overlying the medial epicondyle (the common flexor origin), and the brachialis muscle. After the skin flaps are raised, dissection progressed from distal to proximal as outlined earlier, such that all adipose tissue is included. The superior cubital lymph node is encountered in its anatomic position deep to the biceps aponeurosis where the brachial artery bifurcates. This is included in the specimen. Additionally, the median nerve is identified in its anatomic position deep the biceps tendon and is preserved.

Proximally, the dissection is concluded once the intersection of the brachial artery and the medial intermuscular septum is reached. The inferior ulnar collateral artery and vein are ligated and divided and the specimen is delivered from the wound. A closed suction drain is placed in the wound bed. The wound is closed in layers and the skin is closed with a running subcuticular suture.

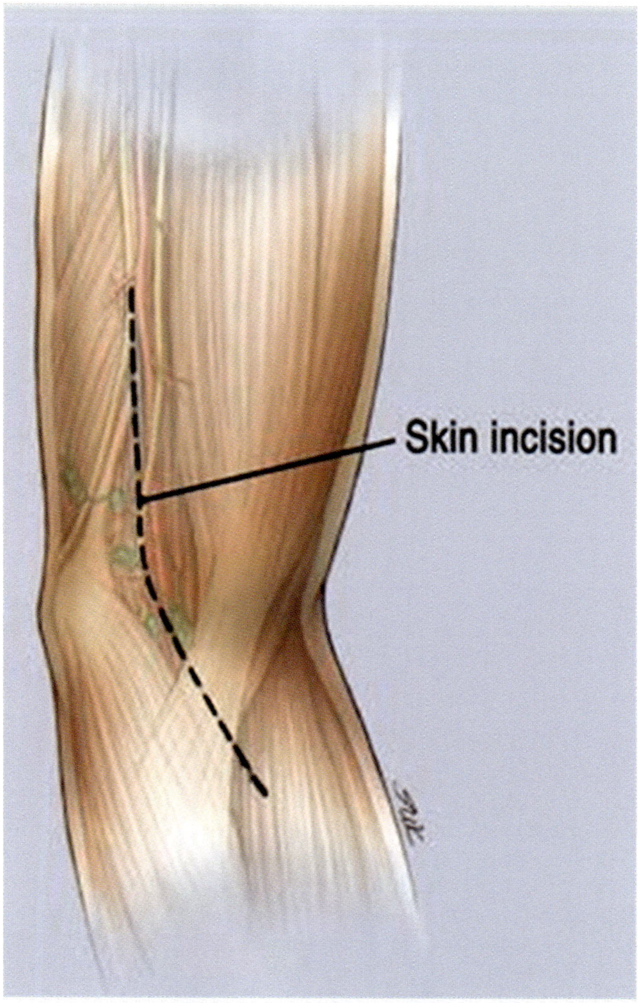

Fig. 10.22 Incision for access. Epitrochlear nodes shown in blue. (This image is provided courtesy of Viraj Master, MD, PhD, FACS, and Keith Delman, MD, FACS.)

Postoperatively, it is important to remember arm elevation and range of motion exercises.

10.8.6 Popliteal Lymphadenectomy[38]

Involvement of the popliteal lymph node is rare even in patients with primary lesions of the foot or posterior leg. One case series demonstrated clinically involved popliteal lymph nodes at a rate of 0.3%. As such, indications for popliteal lymphadenectomy are limited to SLNB-positive lymph nodes in this area or clinically apparent metastatic disease. A standard description of popliteal lymphadenectomy is as follows.

The patient is placed in the prone position on the operating table. The leg and foot are prepped and draped in a sterile fashion to the gluteal fold. To maximize exposure and minimize future scar contracture across the popliteal fossa, a Z-plasty-type incision is made within the flexor crease. The interior angle of the incision can be between 75 and 100 degrees. To prevent flap ischemia, we routinely raise skin flaps sharply using a knife, maintaining an even flap thickness. We also advocate the use of bipolar cautery for hemostasis for the same

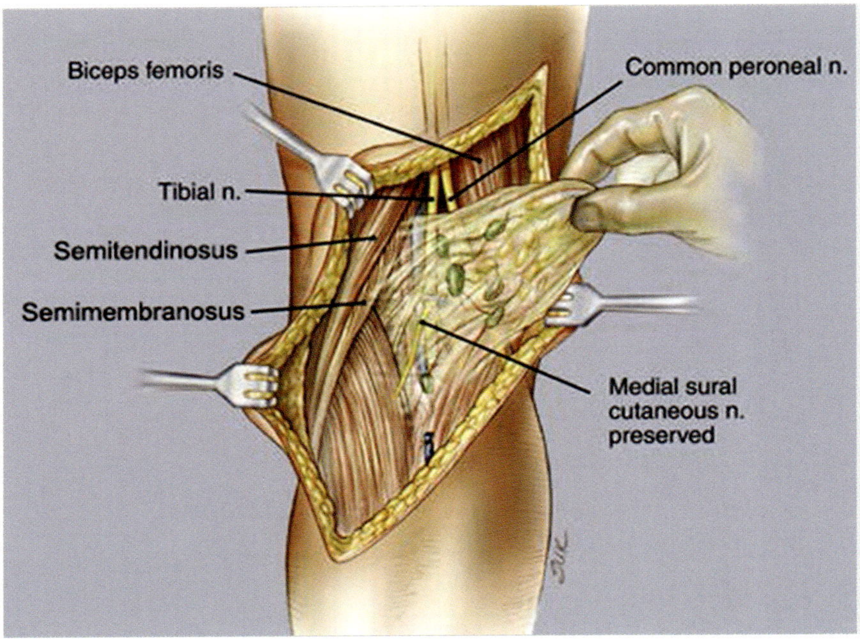

Fig. 10.23 Popliteal node dissection. (This image is provided courtesy of Viraj Master, MD, PhD, FACS, and Keith Delman, MD, FACS.)

reason. Once the flaps are raised, it is useful for the surgeon to orient himself/herself by palpating the popliteal artery.

The distal perimeter of the dissection is defined by the medial and lateral heads of the gastrocnemius muscle. Superiorly, the dissection is carried out up to the bifurcation of the common peroneal and tibial nerves from sciatic trunk.

We prefer to start the dissection distally. The lesser saphenous vein is identified, ligated, and divided to improve exposure. The small cutaneous nerve branches that are identified are preserved if possible. Next, the posterior fascia is incised in a vertical manner. Dissection of the lymphatic tissue within in the popliteal fossa is carried out using a combination of blunt and sharp dissection. The tibial nerve is identified as the most superficial midline structure and is gently retracted laterally. The peroneal nerve is identified as it courses along the biceps femoris and semimembranosus before it turns obliquely and laterally toward the fibula. It is gently retracted and protected. All lymphatic tissue from the bifurcation of the sciatic nerve to the heads of the gastrocnemius is excised en bloc (▶ Fig. 10.23). In doing so, the popliteal vessels are identified and exposed, with the artery being medial and deeper than the vein. A drain is left in the wound bed and placed to self-suction. The wound is closed with interrupted sutures in layers and a running subcuticular suture is used for the skin.

10.9 Conclusion

While the roles of sentinel node biopsy and completion lymphadenectomies in melanomas have been more clearly delineated and refined in recent years, the situation is far from being settled. The principal controversy has centered on the benefits of elective versus prophylactic node dissection as guided by the sentinel node status.

The final report of the MSLT I trial issued in 2014 indicated that biopsy-based staging of intermediate thickness (defined as 1.20–3.50 mm) or thick melanomas (3.50 mm) provides important prognostic information and prolongs disease-free survival.[39] However, in keeping with earlier studies (in the presentinel node era), the overall survival rates were not affected. The MSLT II trial that is currently ongoing should resolve some of the criticisms leveled against the previous study.[40] This is a phase III, multicenter, randomized trial of sentinel lymphadenectomy and complete lymph node dissection versus sentinel lymphadenectomy alone, in cutaneous melanoma with evidence of metastases in sentinel nodes. Unfortunately, the results of this study will not bear fruit until 2022. In the interim, the statistics of the low yield of additional positive lymph nodes, harvested at the time of completion lymphadenectomy, has led to carefully controlled ongoing studies in Europe using the sentinel node harvest alone as a *therapeutic* intervention. This minimalist approach resembles the evolution of treatment in breast cancer.[41] The results of these trials are eagerly awaited by surgeons and patients alike.

References

[1] Ortin-Perez J, van Rijk MC, Valdes-Olmos RA, et al. Lymphatic mapping and sentinel node biopsy in Merkel's cell carcinoma. Eur J Surg Oncol. 2007; 33 (1):119–122

[2] Shnayder Y, Weed DT, Arnold DJ, et al. Management of the neck in Merkel cell carcinoma of the head and neck: University of Miami experience. Head Neck. 2008; 30(12):1559–1565

[3] Zwald FO, Brown M. Skin cancer in solid organ transplant recipients: advances in therapy and management: part II. Management of skin cancer in solid organ transplant recipients. J Am Acad Dermatol. 2011; 65 (2):263–279, quiz 280

[4] Hollowell KL, Agle SC, Zervos EE, Fitzgerald TL. Cutaneous apocrine adenocarcinoma: defining epidemiology, outcomes, and optimal therapy for a rare neoplasm. J Surg Oncol. 2012; 105(4):415–419

[5] Hsu HC, Ho CY, Chen CH, Yang CH, Hong HS, Chuang YH. Aggressive digital papillary adenocarcinoma: a review. Clin Exp Dermatol. 2010; 35 (2):113–119

[6] Cabanas RM. An approach for the treatment of penile carcinoma. Cancer. 1977; 39(2):456–466

[7] Morton DL, Wen DR, Wong JH, et al. Technical details of intraoperative lymphatic mapping for early stage melanoma. Arch Surg. 1992; 127(4):392–399

[8] Elias N, Tanabe KK, Sober AJ, et al. Is completion lymphadenectomy after a positive sentinel lymph node biopsy for cutaneous melanoma always necessary? Arch Surg. 2004; 139(4):400–404, discussion 404–405

[9] Cruickshank W, ed. The Anatomy of the Absorbing Vessels of the Human Body. London: G. Nicol; 1790

[10] Bergqvist L, Strand SE, Hafström L, Jönsson PE. Lymphoscintigraphy in patients with malignant melanoma: a quantitative and qualitative evaluation of its usefulness. Eur J Nucl Med. 1984; 9(3):129–135

[11] Alex JC, Krag DN. Gamma-probe guided localization of lymph nodes. Surg Oncol. 1993; 2(3):137–143

[12] Vera DR, Hoh CK, Hall DJ, Tokin CA, Wallace AM. Technetium-99 m tilmanocept: a synthetic receptor targeted molecule for SLNM. In: Radiopharmaceuticals for Sentinel Lymph Node Detection: Status and Trends. Vienna: International Atomic Energy Agency; 2015:73–75

[13] Somasundaram SK, Chicken DW, Keshtgar MR. Detection of the sentinel lymph node in breast cancer. Br Med Bull. 2007; 84(1):117–131

[14] Cloyd JM, Wapnir IL, Read BM, Swetter S, Greco RS. Indocyanine green and fluorescence lymphangiography for sentinel lymph node identification in cutaneous melanoma. J Surg Oncol. 2014; 110(7):888–892

[15] Korn JM, Tellez-Diaz A, Bartz-Kurycki M, Gastman B. Indocyanine green SPY elite-assisted sentinel lymph node biopsy in cutaneous melanoma. Plast Reconstr Surg. 2014; 133(4):914–922

[16] Stoffels I, Dissemond J, Pöppel T, Schadendorf D, Klode J. Intraoperative fluorescence imaging for sentinel lymph node detection: prospective clinical trial to compare the usefulness of indocyanine green vs technetium Tc 99 m for identification of sentinel lymph nodes. JAMA Surg. 2015; 150(7):617–623

[17] Lerman H, Lievshitz G, Zak O, Metser U, Schneebaum S, Even-Sapir E. Improved sentinel node identification by SPECT/CT in overweight patients with breast cancer. J Nucl Med. 2007; 48(2):201–206

[18] Agnese DM, Maupin R, Tillman B, Pozderac RD, Magro C, Walker MJ. Head and neck melanoma in the sentinel lymph node era. Arch Otolaryngol Head Neck Surg. 2007; 133(11):1121–1124

[19] Lagier A, Pénicaud M, Le Corroller T, et al. Lymphatic drainage of skin areas of head and neck: in vivo approach by the location of the sentinel node [in French]. Morphologie. 2014; 98(320):32–39

[20] Chung A, Yu J, Stempel M, Patil S, Cody H, Montgomery L. Is the "10% rule" equally valid for all subsets of sentinel-node-positive breast cancer patients? Ann Surg Oncol. 2008; 15(10):2728–2733

[21] McCarter MD, Yeung H, Fey J, Borgen PI, Cody HS, III. The breast cancer patient with multiple sentinel nodes: when to stop? J Am Coll Surg. 2001; 192 (6):692–697

[22] Chao C, Wong SL, Edwards MJ, et al. Sunbelt Melanoma Trial Group. Sentinel lymph node biopsy for head and neck melanomas. Ann Surg Oncol. 2003; 10 (1):21–26

[23] Sawh-Martinez R, Salameh B, Colebunders B, et al. Level I sparing radical neck dissections for cutaneous melanoma in the lymphoscintigram era. Ann Plast Surg. 2012; 69(4):422–424

[24] Samra S, Sawh-Martinez R, Tom L, et al. A targeted approach to sentinel lymph node biopsies in the parotid region for head and neck melanomas. Ann Plast Surg. 2012; 69(4):415–417

[25] Sawh-Martinez R, Douglas S, Pavri S, Ariyan S, Narayan D. Management of head and neck melanoma: results of a national survey. Ann Plast Surg. 2014; 73 Suppl 2:S175–S177

[26] Tanis PJ, Boom RP, Koops HS, et al. Frozen section investigation of the sentinel node in malignant melanoma and breast cancer. Ann Surg Oncol. 2001; 8 (3):222–226

[27] Spillane AJ, Cheung BL, Stretch JR, et al. Proposed quality standards for regional lymph node dissections in patients with melanoma. Ann Surg. 2009; 249(3):473–480

[28] Renner GJ, Zitsch RP. Cancer of the lip. In: Myers EN, Suen JY, Myers JN, Hanna E, eds. Cancer of the Head and Neck. Philadelphia, PA: WB Saunders; 2003:294–320

[29] Bocca E, Pignataro O, Sasaki CT. Functional neck dissection. A description of operative technique. Arch Otolaryngol. 1980; 106(9):524–527

[30] Lawton GP, Ariyan S. Regional lymph node dissections in malignant melanoma. Clin Plast Surg. 2000; 27(3):431–440, ix

[31] Bland KI, Copeland EM. Breast. In: Schwartz SI, Shires GT, Spencer FC, eds. Principles of Surgery. 6th ed. New York, NY: McGraw-Hill; 1994:531–594

[32] Spratt J. Groin dissection. J Surg Oncol. 2000; 73(4):243–262

[33] Delman KA, Kooby DA, Ogan K, Hsiao W, Master V. Feasibility of a novel approach to inguinal lymphadenectomy: minimally invasive groin dissection for melanoma. Ann Surg Oncol. 2010; 17(3):731–737

[34] Spock CR, Smith DA, Narayan D. Minimally invasive groin dissection. Conn Med. 2012; 76(5):273–277

[35] Hoang D, Roberts KE, Teng E, Narayan D. Laparoscopic iliac and iliofemoral lymph node resection for melanoma. Surg Endosc. 2012; 26(12):3686–3687

[36] Ichimiya M, Goishi K, Muto M. Endoscopic groin lymph node dissection as a preferable technique for malignant skin neoplasms. J Plast Surg Hand Surg. 2013; 47(4):248–251

[37] McMasters KM, Wong SL, Tyler DS, Balch CM, Thompson JF. Axillary and epitrochlear lymph node dissection for melanoma. In: Balch CM, Houghton AN, Sober AJ, Soong S, Atkin MB, Thompson JF, eds. Cutaneous Melanoma. 5th ed. St. Louis, MO: CRC Press; 2009:397–404

[38] Hatta N, Morita R, Yamada M, Takehara K, Ichiyanagi K, Yokoyama K. Implications of popliteal lymph node detected by sentinel lymph node biopsy. Dermatol Surg. 2005; 31(3):327–330

[39] Morton DL, Thompson JF, Cochran AJ, et al. MSLT Group. Final trial report of sentinel-node biopsy versus nodal observation in melanoma. N Engl J Med. 2014; 370(7):599–609

[40] Morton DL. Overview and update of the phase III Multicenter Selective Lymphadenectomy Trials (MSLT-I and MSLT-II) in melanoma. Clin Exp Metastasis. 2012; 29(7):699–706

[41] Leiter U, Stadler R, Mauch C, et al. Survival of SLNB-positive melanoma patients with and without complete lymph node dissection: A multicenter, randomized DeCOG trial. 2015 ASCO Annual Meeting. Abstract LBA9002. Presented May 30, 2015

11 Role of Dermatopathology in the Surgical Management of Skin Cancer

Jennifer S. Ko, Eugen C. Minca, and Klaus J. Busam

11.1 Introduction

The role of dermatopathology in the surgical management of cutaneous malignancy mirrors the role of pathology in the management of most cancers. The goal is to establish an accurate diagnosis, provide prognostic information, and determine the surgical margin status. Dermatopathology is somewhat unique in that many tumors are caught at very early stages; thus, these patients are typically expected to do well compared to patients with tumors occurring at visceral sites. Also unique is the variety of benign and malignant cutaneous neoplasms with a broad spectrum of histopathologic features and clinical behaviors. For example, there is no other type of benign human tumor which displays as great a spectrum in features as melanocytic nevi. Additionally, there is no other benign tumor, which can be as difficult to distinguish from its malignant counterpart as an atypical nevus from melanoma. This chapter is intended to highlight the particularities found in the most common types of cutaneous malignancies as they relate to the vital diagnostic, prognostic, and predictive information contained within the pathology report.

The need for improved completeness in cancer pathology reporting to improve patient care has been recently recognized. In response to this need, pathology organizations have published recommended reporting protocols for various tumor types. Much of what is included in the pathology cancer reports generated in the United States is guided by the College of American Pathologists (CAP)-produced cancer Protocols, which reflect current updates to the American Joint Committee on Cancer (AJCC) Cancer Staging Manual and the most recent WHO tumor classification systems.[1] The CAP cancer protocols serve as a resource for pathologists to aid in effective reporting of surgical pathology findings necessary to provide quality patient care, and can additionally include optional cancer biomarker reporting templates. Biomarker reporting templates establish reporting guidance for commonly ordered biomarkers (e.g., estrogen receptor, progesterone receptor, and human epidermal growth factor receptor 2 in breast cancer) and improve consistency and completeness of results reporting. Currently, there are no such biomarker reporting templates for primary cutaneous neoplasms, yet this may change in the coming years. The American College of Surgeons Commission on Cancer (ACS CoC) has recognized the value of such protocols, and it has been mandated that pathologists at CoC-approved cancer programs include the scientifically validated or regularly used data elements of the protocols in their surgical pathology reports on cancer specimens, as of January 1, 2004.

11.2 Basal Cell Carcinoma

Basal cell carcinoma (BCC) derives its name from its resemblance to the basal layer keratinocytes of the epidermis. It is thought to originate from the lowest layers of the epidermis or the outer root sheath of the pilosebaceous unit. This carcinoma shares many features with follicular matrix epithelium, including their immunophenotypic-staining pattern. BCC is the most common cancer in humans,[2] and yet the CAP does not include specific cancer reporting protocols for BCC, due to its overall excellent prognosis. That said, appropriate management is necessary to avoid local tissue destruction and tissue disfigurement while preserving cosmesis and function. To this aim, pathologic parameters in the biopsy specimen can help determine the potential for subclinical extension beyond a clinically defined border, and thus are commented on.

The pathologic risk factors which define high-risk versus low-risk primary BCC relate to tumor size, depth of invasion, histologic tumor subtype, perineural invasion, and vascular invasion (very rarely seen, but unfavorable if present). Studies have shown that the gross size of tumor impacts the risk for depth of invasion, subclinical extension, and recurrence-free survival, with ≥ 2 cm appearing to confer increased risk to trunk and extremity lesions; ≥ 6 mm for face, genitalia, hands/feet; and ≥ 10 mm for all other anatomic locations.[3] The histologic tumor subtype of BCC is a predictor of risk of recurrence and metastasis. Indeed, studies list the strongest predictors for recurrence to be aggressive histologic tumor type, along with positive excision margins.[4] While there are many types of BCC recognized, most can be grouped as nonaggressive, aggressive, or indifferent (▶ Table 11.1), and often there are mixed types within one tumor. Nodular (▶ Fig. 11.1a) and superficial (▶ Fig. 11.1b) BCCs are common forms falling into the nonaggressive category. Nodular BCC grows in large dermal tumor nodules, often with connection to the overlying epidermis.

Table 11.1 Histologic subtypes of basal cell carcinoma according to aggressiveness and risk of recurrence

Aggressiveness/ Risk of recurrence	Low/Low	Low/High	High/High
Basal cell carcinoma histologic subtype (most common in bold)	**Nodular** Adenoid Keratotic Pleomorphic (giant cell) Clear cell Signet ring With adnexal differentiation Infundibulocystic	**Superficial** (multicentric)	**Micronodular** **Infiltrative** **Morpheaform** **Metatypical** (basosquamous)

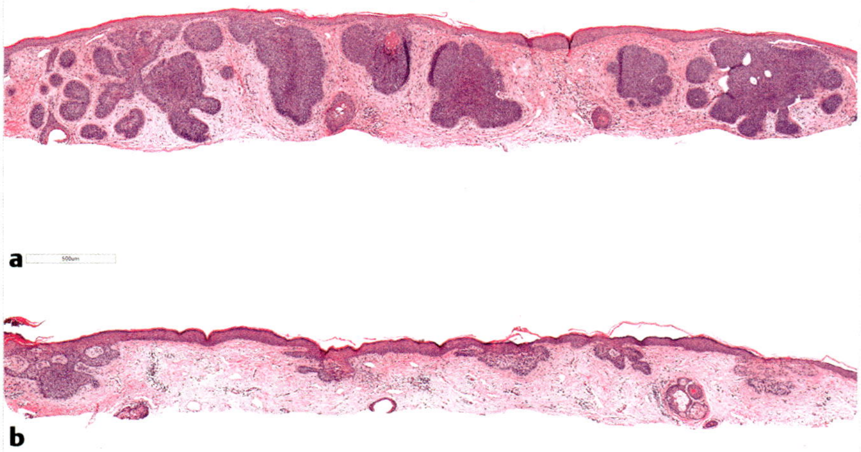

Fig. 11.1 **(a)** BCC, nodular. **(b)** BCC, superficial, multifocal.

Within these nodules, cells can form into trabeculae or pseudoglandular spaces. The perimeter of tumor nodules shows nuclear palisading and often retraction artifact from the surrounding myxoid stroma by a cleft-like space. Superficial BCCs are multifocal in nature and hang off the epidermis. For this reason, they show a higher rate of local recurrence compared to nodular subtype alone. Infundibulocystic BCC is the most indolent variant of BCC, and some argue it may not be a real carcinoma, thus referring to it as "basaloid follicular hamartoma." Micronodular (▶ Fig. 11.2a), infiltrative (▶ Fig. 11.2b, c), and morpheaform (▶ Fig. 11.2d) subtypes of BCC are associated with a higher incidence of positive margins and thus tumor recurrence.[5,6] For this reason, BCC subtyping is important information to be included in the pathology report. The micronodular pattern shows small tumor nodules (< 0.15 mm) and lacks circumscription. Micronodular BCC (▶ Fig. 11.2e) usually shows at least focal retraction artifact, stromal mucin, increased mitosis, and a lack of papillary mesenchymal bodies, as distinguishing factors from trichoepitheliomas (▶ Fig. 11.3a–c). Infiltrative BCCs show thin, linear basaloid tumor strands growing in an infiltrative pattern. When the same type of growth becomes even more spiked and associated with a densely sclerotic stroma, tumors are called morpheaform BCC. Perineural invasion is another important pathologic prognostic feature in BCC, and BCC tumors with this feature (▶ Fig. 11.3d) have higher rates of recurrence and morbidity. While studies on treatment protocols in this setting are relatively limited, Mohs surgery appears to confer better outcome, and adjuvant radiotherapy may be considered.[7]

The vast majority of BCCs do not require immunohistochemical (IHC) staining for diagnosis. In rare BCCs, such as the so-called trichoepitheliomatous types (▶ Fig. 11.2e), or clear cell types, IHC staining may be required. BCC stains in a pattern similar to the follicular infundibulum and will be positive for both high- and low-molecular-weight cytokeratins, BerEP4, Bcl-2 (diffuse), and Ki-67 (20–40% proliferative index), and will show exclusion of CK20 + Merkel's cells.[8] A recent study by Nedved et al revealed that while there is only fair concordance between dermatopathologists with regard to specific BCC typing, there is substantial agreement when tumors were reclassified into a two-tiered system of high- and low-risk phenotypes.[9] As such, BCCs often do not require a second pathologic opinion.

BCC is typically thought to be a continuously growing tumor; yet, reports of "skip" lesions still exist, especially with regard to superficial BCC. For the purposes of surgical and pathologic margins, however, BCCs can be considered a continuously growing tumor. Current practice guidelines from the National Comprehensive Cancer Network suggest a 4-mm lateral clinical margin for BCCs ≤ 2 cm diameter treated with elliptical excision, based on studies which showed a 98% histologic cure rate in this setting.[10] This may not always be desirable given the cosmetically and functionally sensitive location. As such, Mohs' micrographic surgery or surgical excision with complete, circumferential, peripheral, and deep margin assessment (CCPDMA) or "slow Mohs" is often undertaken.[11] Some studies suggest that traditional paraffin-fixed serial cross-sectioning (bread loafing) techniques can miss positive surgical margins in up to 56% of cases.[12] In addition, although the pathology report will include the positivity or negativity of the surgical margins, the distance of the margin to tumor may or may not be reported. Margins can only be partially examined in shave "saucerization" and punch biopsy specimens, and thus are typically not discussed. In rare circumstances in which surgical treatment is not feasible for BCC, systemic therapy has become available. Options include vismodegib (BMS-833923), saridegib (IPI-926), and sonidegib/erismodegib (LDE225), which target the activating mutations in the hedgehog signaling pathway that are known to drive BCCs.[13]

11.3 Squamous Cell Carcinoma

Cutaneous squamous cell carcinoma (cSCC) is the second most common skin cancer, and is formed from the keratinizing cells of the epidermis. SCC is typically classified as high risk or low risk depending on the risk for local recurrence and metastasis. The tumor size and anatomic location criteria for risk

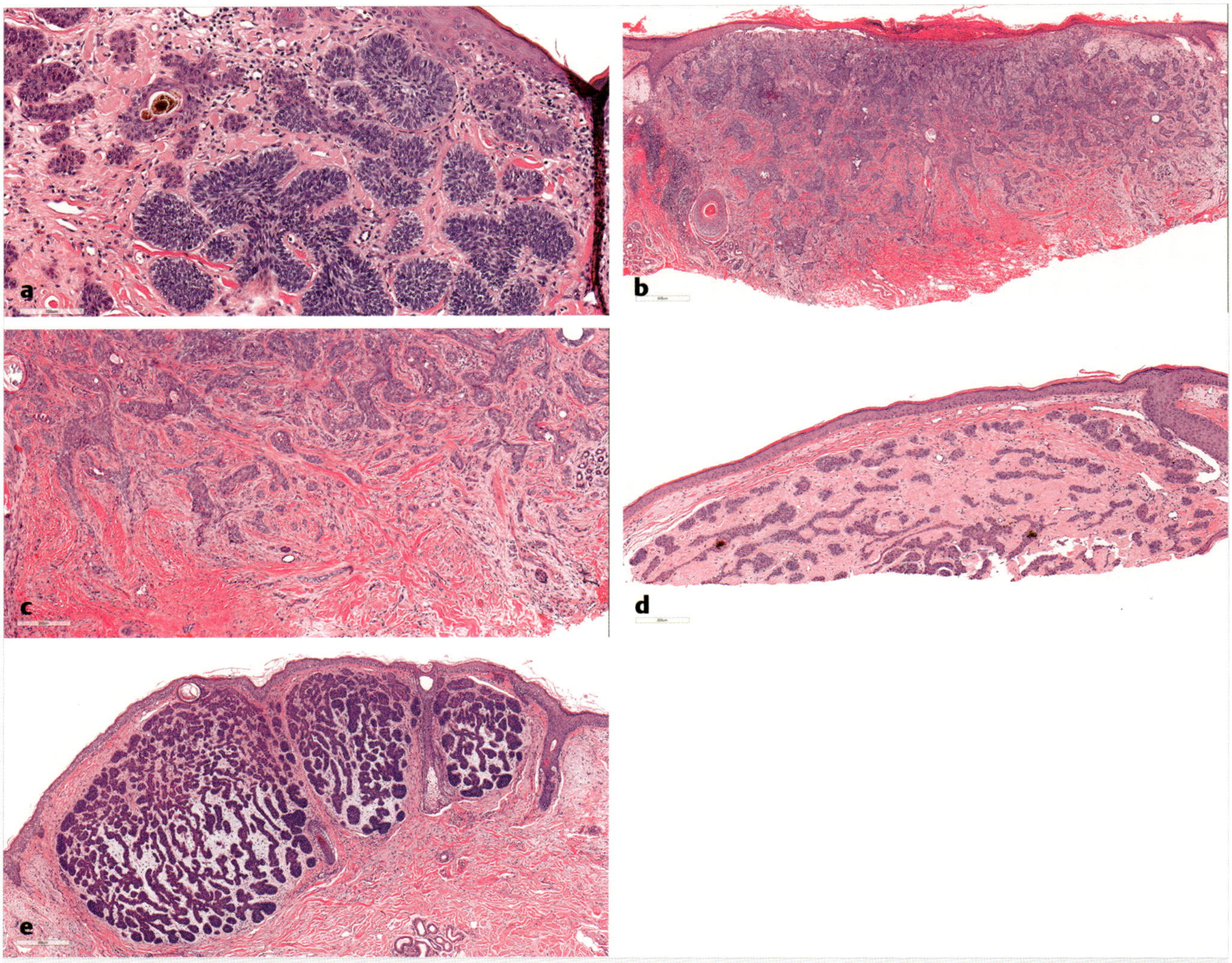

Fig. 11.2 **(a)** BCC, micronodular. **(b)** BCC, infiltrative (low power). **(c)** BCC, infiltrative (high power). **(d)** BCC, morpheaform. **(e)** BCC, trichoepitheliomatous (alternative).

stratification are identical to those used for BCC. CAP requires reporting of invasive squamous cell carcinomas greater than 2 cm in greatest dimension (which are automatically a minimum of pT2 pathologic tumor stage) to be performed in a templated manner,[1] due to the doubled risk for local recurrence and tripled risk for metastasis in this setting.[14] The templated pathologic report should contain all histopathologic parameters associated with a worse prognosis, defined as high-risk features by the AJCC-7 staging criteria. These include tumor size and site (greatest dimension: > 2 cm; ear or non–hair-bearing lip), histologic grade (poor or undifferentiated), maximum tumor thickness (> 2 mm), anatomic level (Clark IV or V), and perineural or vascular involvement (present).[14,15] The caliber and location of the involved nerve is prognostically relevant. Local recurrence is more likely if the involved nerve is located in the subcutis or muscle and when the caliber exceeds 0.2 mm.

While various subtypes of squamous cell carcinoma are recognized, including acantholytic (▶ Fig. 11.4a), Bowenoid (▶ Fig. 11.4b), and verrucous (▶ Fig. 11.4c), such typing is not necessary to include (though often incorporated) in the reporting template. The histologic grade, rather, is the required information because decreasing levels of differentiation are associated with increasing risk of recurrence. Well-differentiated cSCC will closely resemble normal epithelium, but often shows an irregular border of invasive islands with a desmoplastic host response, paradoxical maturation with descent into the dermis, and subtle nuclear atypia (▶ Fig. 11.5a). Keratoacanthomas (▶ Fig. 11.5b) appear to represent a unique form of invasive, well-differentiated squamous cell carcinoma that will often involute on its own, possibly due to the relatively increased expression of apoptotic genes.[16] As such, well-differentiated SCC and keratoacanthomas perform the best clinically. Moderately differentiated cases show less obvious squamous features (▶ Fig. 11.5c). Poorly differentiated (▶ Fig. 11.5d, e) squamous cell carcinoma, which may require IHC staining for confirmation (▶ Fig. 11.5f), and undifferentiated, sarcomatoid (▶ Fig. 11.6a-BSCC) squamous cell carcinoma, which requires clinical correlation, a precursor lesion, or focal IHC staining

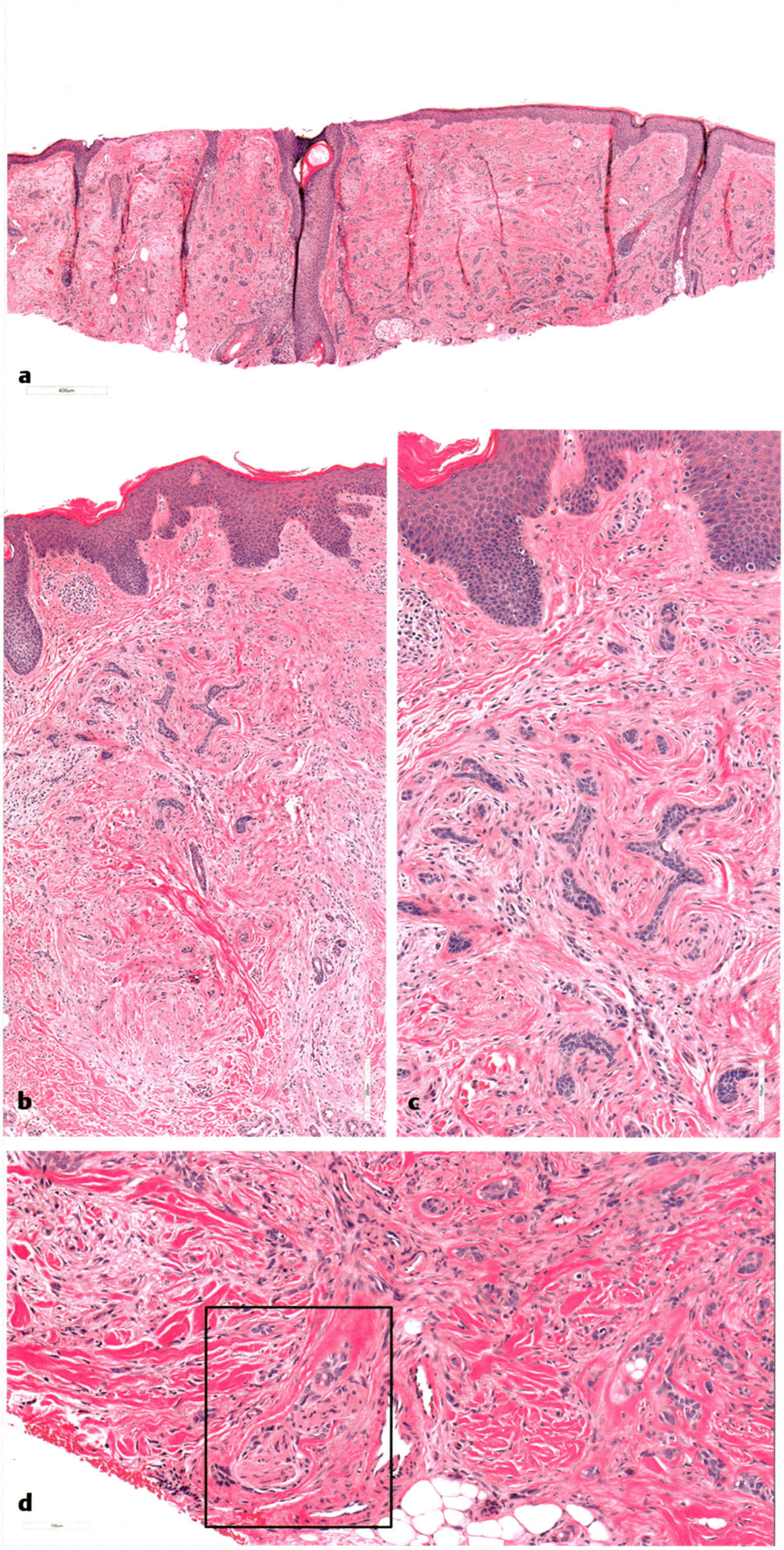

Fig. 11.3 (a) Desmoplastic trichoepithelioma. (b, c) Desmoplastic trichoepithelioma (low and high power, alternative). (d) BCC, infiltrative with perineural invasion.

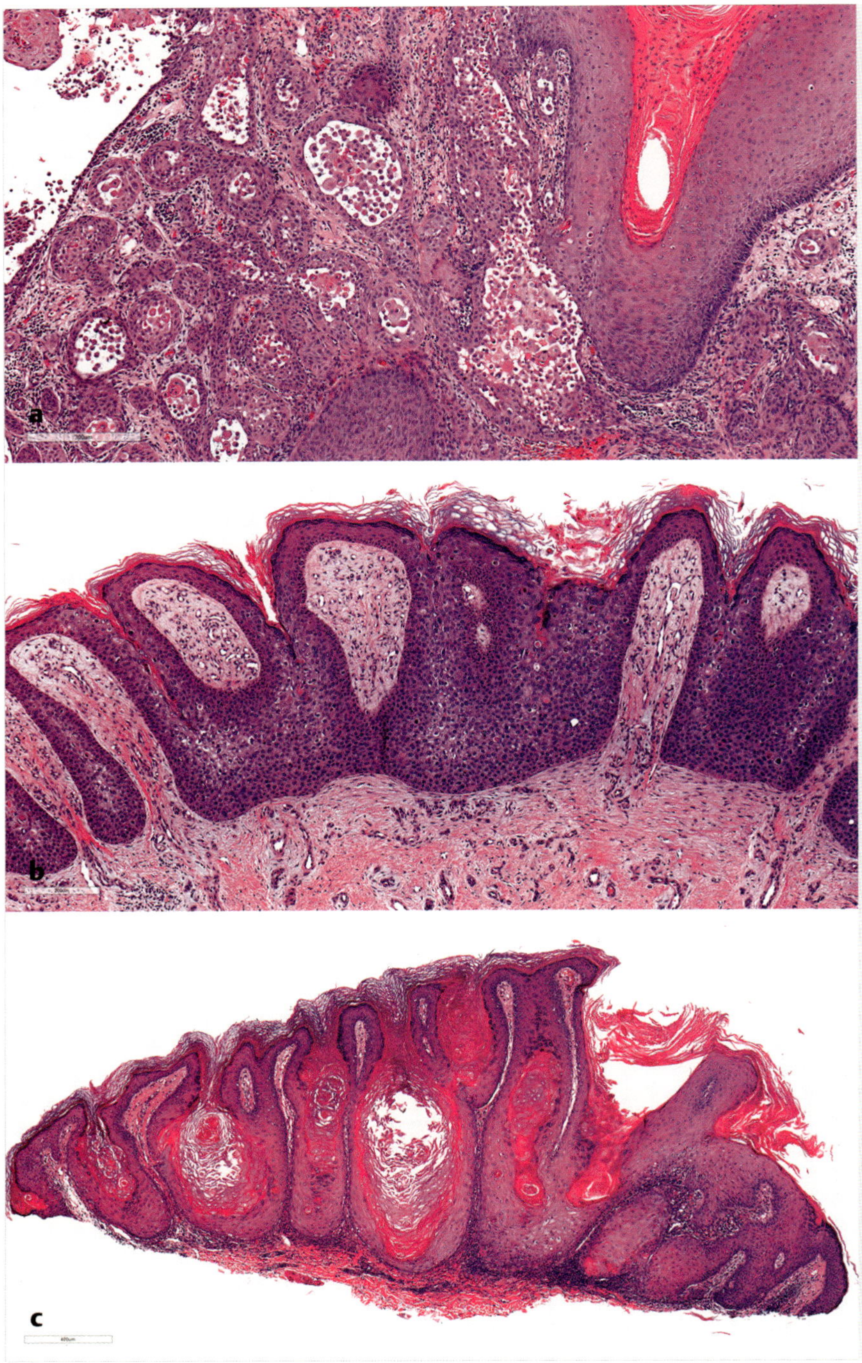

Fig. 11.4 **(a)** Cutaneous squamous cell carcinoma (cSCC), acantholytic. **(b)** cSCC, Bowenoid. **(c)** cSCC, verrucous.

positivity by definition, have increased risk for recurrence. As such, both poor and de-differentiation are histologic features which upstage a patient from a pT1 to a pT2 tumor.[14]

Maximum tumor thickness (Breslow's thickness) is measured with a calibrated ocular micrometer, which is a glass disk that fits in the microscope eyepiece. It has a ruled scale used to measure the size of magnified objects. The physical length of the marks on the scale varies depending on the degree of magnification. Breslow's tumor thickness is measured from the granular layer of the epidermis, or the base of the ulcer in ulcerated lesions, to the deepest extent of tumor. Increasing Breslow's thickness is associated with increased risk, as is increasing Clark's level of invasion (▶ Table 11.2). Perineural invasion is more common in larger tumors (▶ Fig. 11.7a), as is lymphovascular invasion.

Often, tumors with high-risk features are treated with Mohs micrographic surgery or resection with CCPDMA. Tumors with perineural invasion especially benefit from intraoperative margin control and possibly adjuvant radiation therapy. The size of the involved nerve should be included in the pathology report, as diameter 0.1-mm or greater increases risk of recurrence and metastasis.[16]

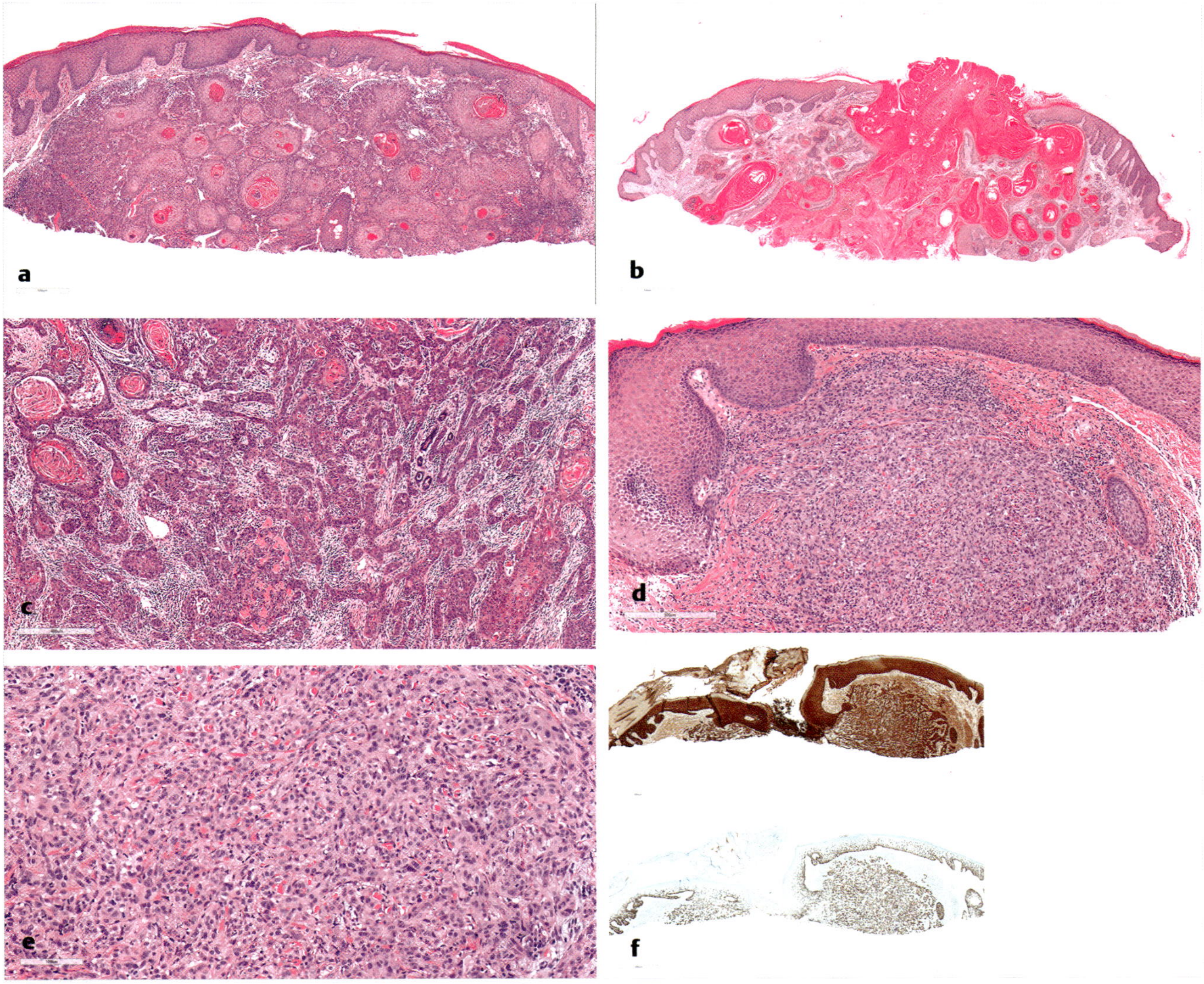

Fig. 11.5 **(a)** Cutaneous squamous cell carcinoma (cSCC), well-differentiated. **(b)** cSCC, keratoacanthoma. **(c)** cSCC, moderately differentiated. **(d)** cSCC, poorly differentiated (low power). **(e)** cSCC, poorly differentiated (high power). **(f)** cSCC, poorly differentiated (CK5/6 and p63).

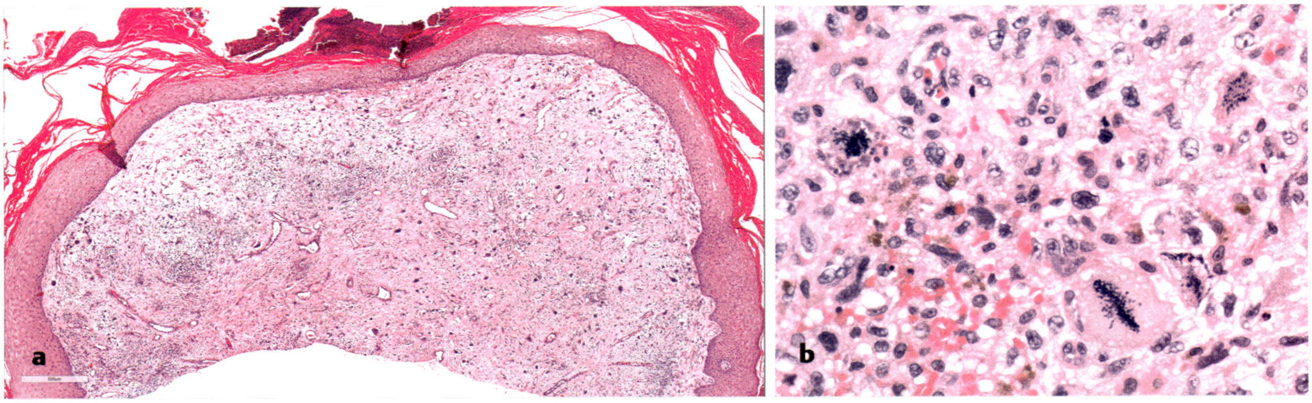

Fig. 11.6 **(a)** Cutaneous squamous cell carcinoma (cSCC), sarcomatoid, spindle cell (H&E low power). **(b)** cSCC, sarcomatoid, epithelioid (high power).

Incomplete removal of primary cSCC makes subsequent therapies much less likely to succeed.[17] If a lesion is removed by elliptical excision, the surgical specimen should be oriented and bread-loafed sections submitted at 2- to 3-mm intervals with marginal involvement reported. The best clear indicator of a positive margin is tumor with either ink or cautery artifact on it (► Fig. 11.7b). If positive margins are found after initial excision, then Mohs micrographic surgery or resection with CCPDMA is typically indicated, especially if graft placement is necessary. Measurement of distance to the margin is not required information, but is often reported.

Sentinel lymph node biopsy (SLNBx) is considered in patients with high-risk cSCC and clinically negative lymph nodes because approximately 12% of these nodes will be positive.[18,19] Sentinel and regional lymph node detection of cSCC is usually possible using hematoxylin and eosin (H&E) stains alone, due to the significantly different morphology of this carcinoma compared to normal lymph node constituents (► Fig. 11.7c). The size, number, and site (ipsilateral or bilateral) of lymph node involvement is associated with clinical outcome, with metastatic deposit size the most important factor.[20,21] As such, these are required components of the templated pathology report.

Table 11.2 Risk of recurrence and metastases in cutaneous squamous cell carcinomas based on Clark's level of invasion

Clark's level		cSCC risk of recurrence and metastases
I	Tumor confined to the epidermis (in situ)	Low
II	Tumor invasion into the papillary dermis	
III	Tumor at the junction of the papillary and reticular dermis	
IV	Tumor invasion into the reticular dermis	High
V	Tumor invasion into the subcutaneous fat	

Abbreviation: cSCC, cutaneous squamous cell carcinoma.

11.4 Malignant Melanoma

Although malignant melanoma (MM) is much less common than BCC and cSCC, no other diagnosis lends itself to as much difficulty, subjectivity, and lack of agreement among dermatopathologists.[22,23,24,25,26] This may be due to the large degree of histologic overlap of melanoma with various benign mimickers, and due to the limited spectrum of cytologic atypia in melanomas compared to other malignancies. For instance, superficial spreading (► Fig. 11.8a), nevoid (► Fig. 11.8b, c), and Spitzoid (► Fig. 11.8d, e) melanomas can show histopathologic overlap with dysplastic nevi (► Fig. 11.9a) or recurrent nevi (► Fig. 11.9b-d) and Spitz nevi (► Fig. 11.9e), respectively.[21] Meanwhile, the so-called atypical Spitz tumor/nevus is a diagnosis that often requires ancillary testing for confirmation due to the lack of consistent distinguishing histologic features from melanoma. Farmer et al illustrated that within a panel of eight expert pathologists, diagnostic discordance between two or more panel members was observed in 38% of melanocytic lesions.[25] The experimental design and premise of this study has been questioned by some who insist that the majority of cases can be accurately classified; and that descriptive reporting

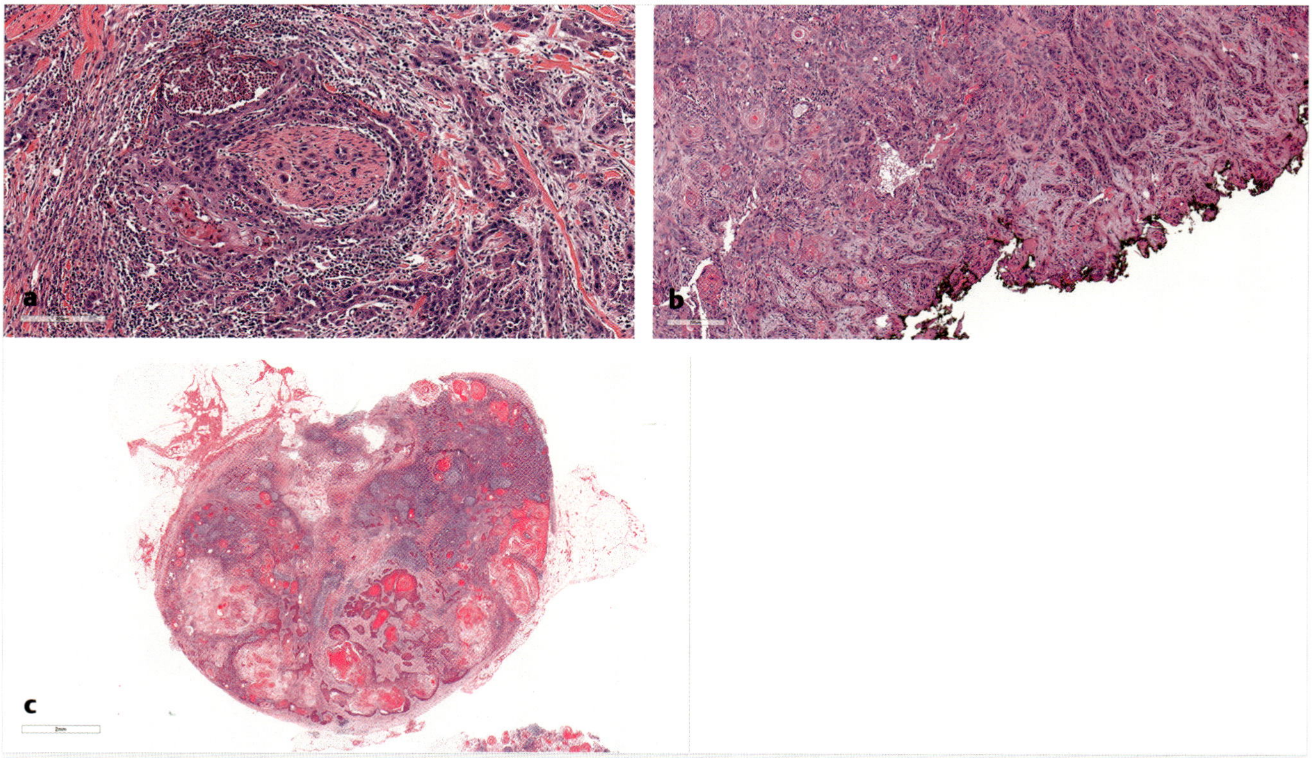

Fig. 11.7 **(a)** Cutaneous squamous cell carcinoma (cSCC), perineural invasion. **(b)** cSCC, positive inked margin. **(c)** cSCC, lymph node metastasis.

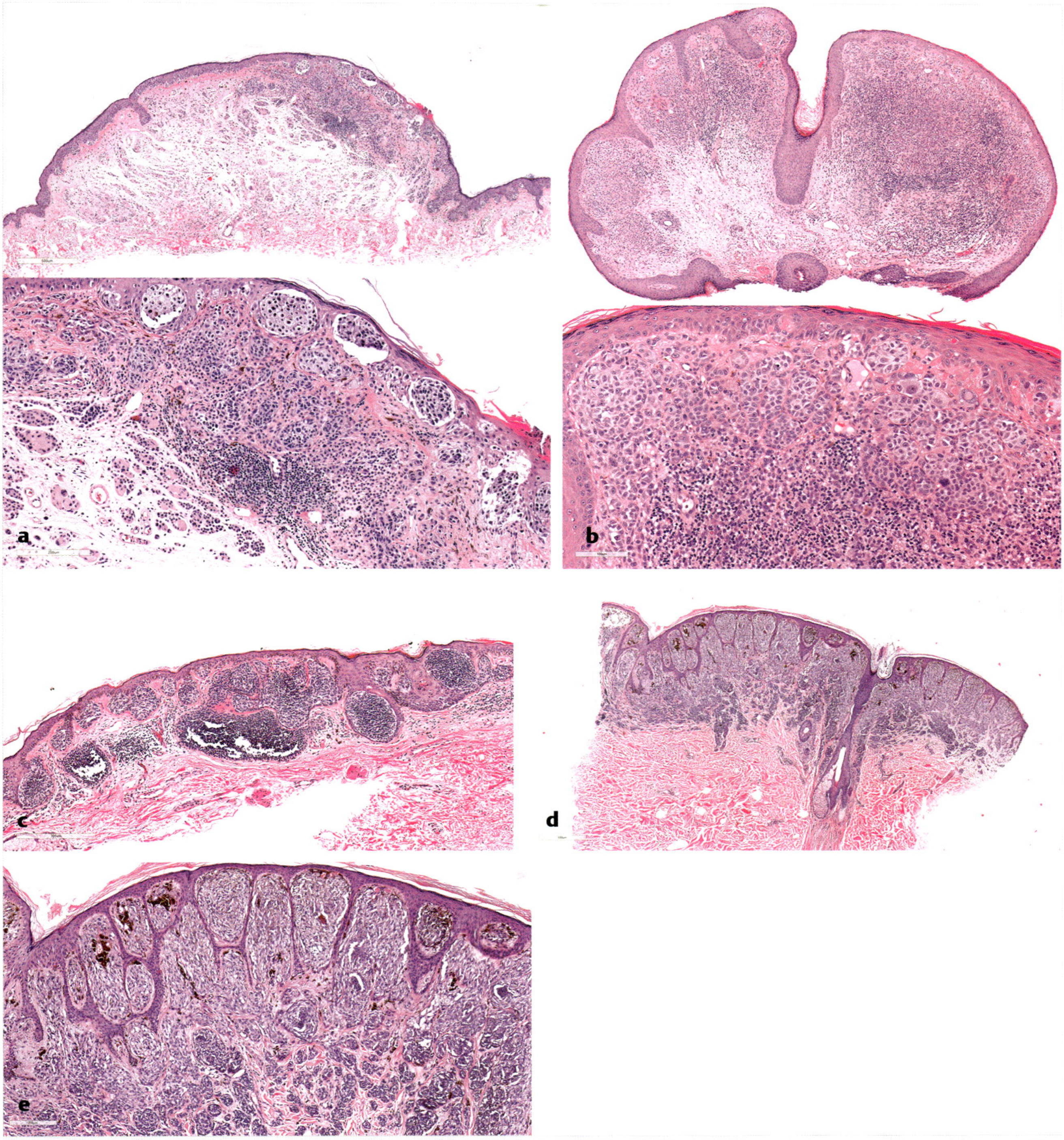

Fig. 11.8 **(a)** Melanoma, superficial spreading, arising in a nevus. **(b)** Melanoma, Spitzoid and nevoid (low power). **(c)** Melanoma, nevoid (low power). **(d)** Melanoma, spitzoid, with epidermal consumption (low power). **(e)** Melanoma, spitzoid, with epidermal consumption (high power).

on the uncertain malignant potential of particular lesions is in fact permissible.[27] Contemporary studies done by Niebling et al at the Melanoma Institute Australia (MIA) on 5,011 MIA and non–MIA-matched reports on the same primary melanomas found significant changes in the diagnosis, AJCC-T classification, and treatment recommendations after pathology review by melanoma pathologists, with moderate concordance demonstrated for various tumor staging parameters. Because of this, the recommendation that pathology review be considered for all patients attending specialist melanoma treatment centers has been made.[28,29] Needless to say, it is important to trust the dermatopathologist diagnosing melanocytic lesions. Likewise, it is important that pathology reports of at least borderline melanocytic lesions document key diagnostic criteria

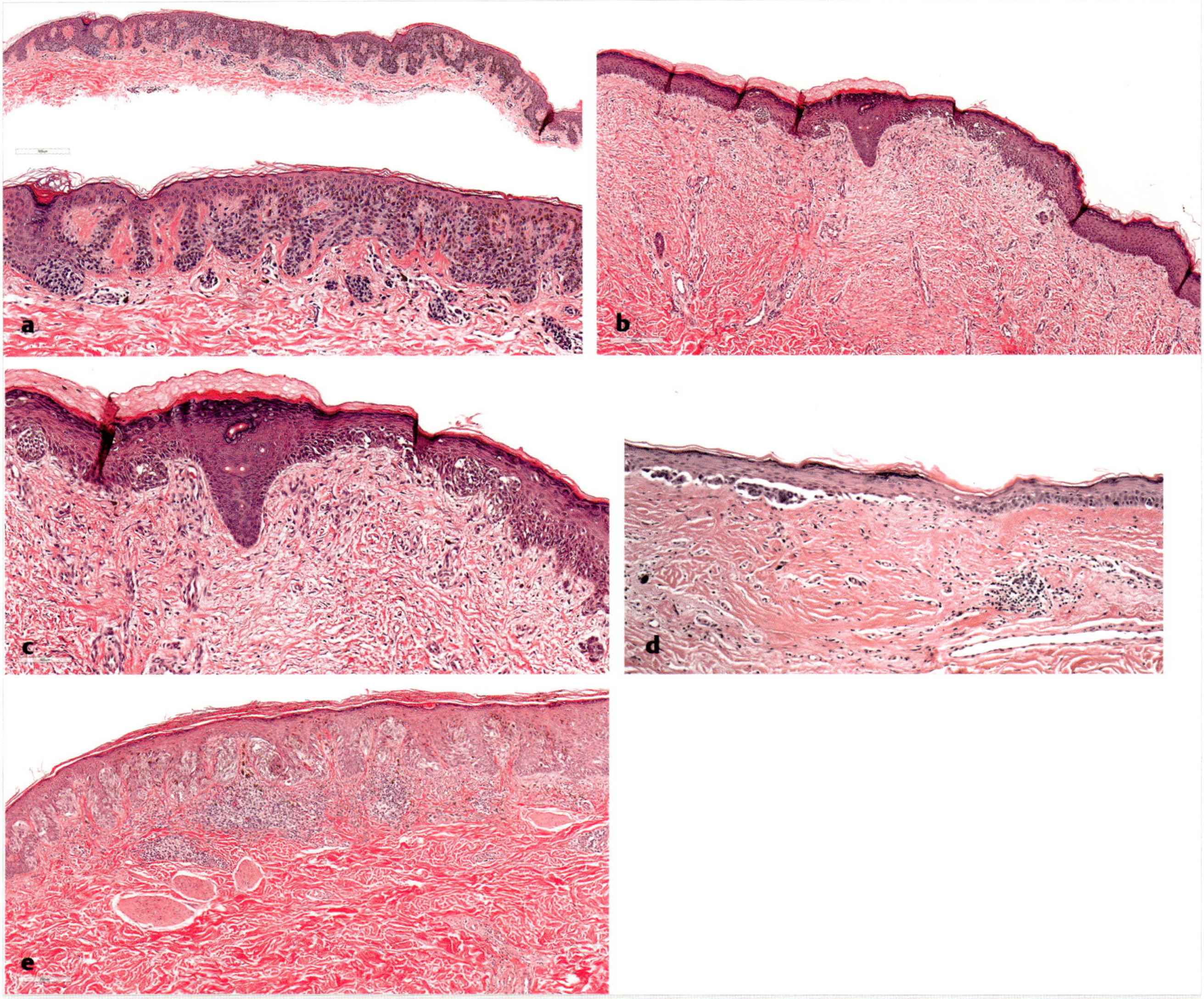

Fig. 11.9 **(a)** Dysplastic nevus (mild melanocytic atypia). **(b)** Recurrent nevus versus melanoma (nevus), low power. **(c)** Recurrent nevus versus melanoma (nevus), high power. **(d)** Recurrent nevus versus melanoma (melanoma). **(e)** Spitz nevus.

(microscopic features) on which the diagnosis was based, and describe any areas of uncertainty.

Clinical information can be crucially important in the diagnosis of melanoma. Older patient age, increased signs of solar damage, and large lesional diameter (> 6 mm) will immediately alter the perspective through which a biopsy is reviewed. Numerous criteria are considered, both in number and severity, in the assessment for malignancy. In general, melanomas tend to show many forms of asymmetry. These include asymmetry of low power silhouette, lateral border cell distribution, cytologic features, pigmentation, inflammatory host response, and nesting architecture. Consumption of the epidermis (▶ Fig. 11.8e) and pagetoid spread of melanocytes (▶ Fig. 11.10) are emblematic clues to melanoma.[30]

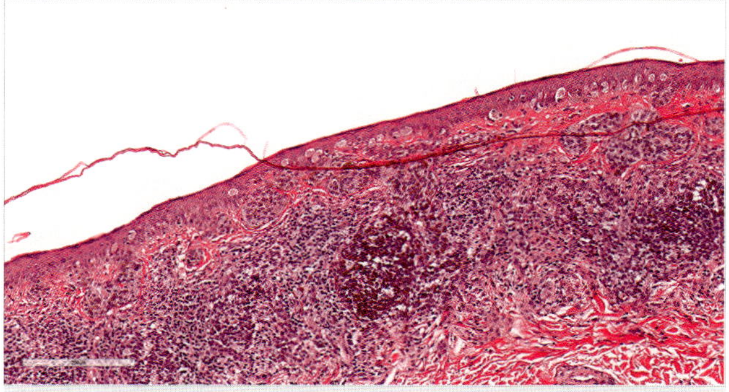

Fig. 11.10 Melanoma, superficial spreading with pagetoid spread.

Owing to the diagnostic difficulty sometimes associated with melanoma and its capacity to spread relatively early in evolution, it is our practice that all melanomas diagnosed by outside pathologists be reviewed by pathologists within our institution prior to definitive treatment at our institution. For those surgeons treating patients in the community, it is likely not practical to have every melanoma reviewed by an outside

Table 11.3 Common scenarios for requesting a second opinion in the diagnosis of melanocytic lesions

Lesions with overlapping or ambiguous histopathologic features	Dysplastic nevi Spitzoid lesions
Obscuring histopathologic features	Inflammation Regression Melanocytic lesions arising in association with a previous biopsy
Unusual clinical features	Young age, unusual location

pathologist. However, there are certain red flags that surgeons can be aware of which should reflexively lead to a second pathologist's opinion (▶ Table 11.3). When a second opinion is sought, it should often be from a dermatopathology group at a tertiary-care center who more regularly diagnose melanomas, and who has access to ancillary diagnostic tests which can aid in the differential diagnosis.

11.4.1 Diagnostic Aids in Melanoma

Comparative Genomic Hybridization

Ancillary tests that assist in distinguishing potentially lethal melanomas from benign melanocytic nevi with atypical histopathologic features are available. The arguably most robust ancillary method that has emerged over the past decade is cytogenetic analysis. Based on the pioneering work by Bastian and colleagues, melanomas were found to commonly carry chromosomal copy number changes, while these are absent or rare in nevi. The preferred cytogenetic method is comparative genomic hybridization (CGH), because it tests all chromosomes. CGH determines DNA copy number by the competitive hybridization of two differentially labeled DNA populations (tumor DNA and normal control DNA) hybridized to a substrate (representing the genome). The ratio of the two differentially labeled signals is used to determine increases and decreases in copy number of tumoral DNA at a given genomic coordinate. Multiple studies have shown semi-characteristic chromosomal gains and losses in melanomas that were not seen in nevi.[31,32] Isolated 11p gains were seen in Spitz nevi and not melanomas.[32] Higher resolution array-based CGH studies have allowed for the identification of recurrent genetic abnormalities more common in unique types of melanomas arising in various contexts (▶ Table 11.4).[33]

Table 11.4 Recurrent genomic/genetic abnormalities in unique melanoma types

Melanoma subtype	Cutaneous non-chronic sun damage	Cutaneous chronic sun damage	Acral	Mucosal	Uveal
Chromosome gains/amplification	1q, 6p, 7, 8q, 17q, 20q	1q, 6p, 7, 8q, 11q, 17q, 20q	4q, 6p, 7, 8q, 17q, 20q 5p15, 11q13, 12q14	1q, 6p, 7, 8q, 11q13, 17q, 20q 1q31, 4q12, 12q14	6p, 8q
Chromosome losses	6q, 9p, 10	6q, 9p, 13	6q, 9p, 10, 11q, 15q, 16q, 21q	3q, 4q, 6q, 8p, 9p, 10, 11p, 11q, 21q	1p, 3, 6q, 8p
Gene alteration	$BRAF^{mut}$ $NRAS^{mut}$ $PTEN^{del}$	$NRAS^{mut}$ KIT^{mut} $CCND1^{mut}$	KIT^{mut} $p16^{del}$ $CDK4^{amp}$	KIT^{mut} $p16^{del}$ $CDK4^{amp}$	$GNAQ^{mut}$ $GNA11^{mut}$ $BAP1^{del}$

Abbreviations: mut, mutation; del, deletion; amp, amplification.

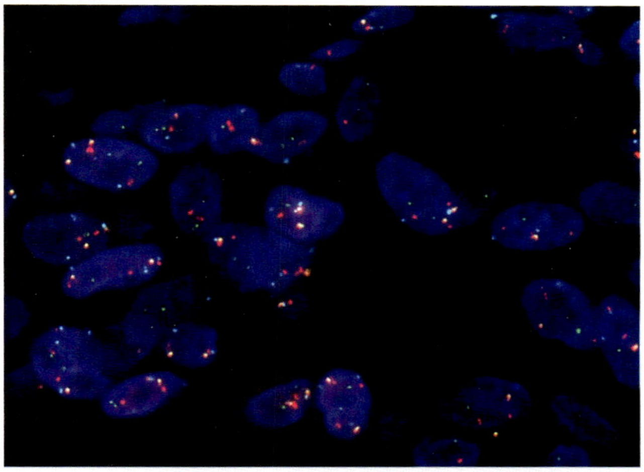

Fig. 11.11 Melanoma fluorescence in situ hybridization: Most cells show three red signals (6p), two green (11q), two cyan (CEP6), and one to two gold (6q).

Fluorescence In Situ Hybridization

Multiprobe fluorescence in situ hybridization (FISH) assays, which were based on existing CGH data, have been tested in their ability to discriminate melanomas and nevi. Of the various combinations tested, those probes to loci 6p25 (RREB1), 6p23 (MYB), CEP6 (Centromere 6, for discrimination of aneuploidy and polyploidy), and 11q13 (CCND1) proved to have the highest sensitivity and specificity (▶ Fig. 11.11 and ▶ Table 11.5).[34] This probe set shows a range of reported sensitivities and specificities depending on the diagnostic problem and particular study (▶ Table 11.6[35]). Multiple studies using the same four-probe FISH set have reported

Table 11.5 Cutoffs of four-probe FISH criteria for genomic abnormalities consistent with melanoma

FISH criterion	6p25 (RREB1) absolute gain (>2 signals/cell)	6p25 (RREB1) relative gain (6p25/CEP6 > 1)	6q23 (MYB) relative loss (6q23/CEP6 < 1)	11q13 (CCND1) absolute gain (>2 signals/cell)
Cutoff	> 29% tumor cells	> 55% tumor cells	> 40% tumor cells	> 38% tumor cells

Abbreviation: FISH, fluorescence in situ hybridization.

Table 11.6 Utility of FISH in the diagnosis of melanocytic lesions

Diagnostic problem	FISH sensitivity/specificity
Nevus vs. Melanoma	80–95%; 90–98%
Histopathologically ambiguous melanocytic tumors	43–100%; 50–80%
Subcapsular nodal nevus vs. metastatic melanoma	
Microstaging primary melanomas arising in precursor nevi	
Primary nevus vs. nevus-like metastatic melanoma	
Prognosis of melanoma	

Abbreviation: FISH, fluorescence in situ hybridization.

diagnostic utility for distinguishing melanoma from nevi,[36,37,38] and particular utility in various diagnostically difficult circumstances (▶ Table 11.6). Of note, pigmented spindle cell nevi-like[39] and desmoplastic melanoma[40] have reduced FISH sensitivity (73 and 47%, respectively). Homozygous loss of 9p21 (CDKN2A) and gains in 8q24 (MYC) are additional FISH parameters for the diagnosis of cutaneous melanoma. When such probes are used in combination with the previously mentioned four probes, the sensitivity and specificity of the test is improved to 94 and 98%, respectively, in unambiguous lesions.[41,42,43,44,45] Additional studies will be needed to determine the sensitivity and specificity in ambiguous lesions. Due to the possibility of false-negative or false-positive cytogenetic test results, CGH and, in particular, FISH data need to be carefully correlated with clinical and histopathologic findings. A diagnosis should not solely be based on cytogenetic results.

Myriad MyPath

In addition to FISH, gene expression microarray studies have attempted to distinguish primary cutaneous melanomas from various types of nevi. Myriad Genetics, Inc. has developed a 23-gene expression signature clinically validated to differentiate benign nevi from MM with a sensitivity of 89% and a specificity of 93%.[46] The genes in this expression signature include those involved in immune function and those involved in cell differentiation and cell cycle. However, this test is currently of unproved value for ambiguous lesions, since the test has so far only been compared to consensus diagnoses of the diagnostically straightforward nevi and melanoma.

Immunohistochemical Stains in Melanoma

Although various investigators have at various times claimed that immunohistochemistry can aid in the distinction of nevus from melanoma, there are no robust data available, and we caution against using staining patterns, such as for HMB-45 and p16 for diagnosis.[47] It is also questionable whether immunohistochemistry, such as for p16, has independent prognostic significance.[48] The main value of immunohistochemistry is to verify the line of differentiation of amelanotic tumors, such as for the distinction of melanoma from sarcoma, and better visualization of melanocytes in the context of inflammation (e.g., lentigo maligna with lichenoid inflammatory reaction) or improved detection of small melanocyte deposits in the sentinel lymph node. More recently, immunohistochemistry has also become relevant for a quick assessment of mutation status, such as by using the antibody VE1 to detect the most common form of *BRAF* gene mutation—BRAFV600E.[49]

11.4.2 Histologic Subtypes of Melanoma

The common melanoma histologic subtypes, superficial spreading melanoma, nodular melanoma, and desmoplastic and lentigo maligna melanoma, show fairly good clinicopathologic and molecular concordance, but have no prognostic significance beyond that afforded by Breslow's thickness. Their categorically discrepant clinical presentations and skewed molecular signatures are of interest, however, in so much as they may lead to variant algorithms for treatment when additional targeted therapies become available. This histologic subclassification also brings to light various clinical and histologic mimickers, and they are included below for interest.

Superficial Spreading Melanoma

MM is typically characterized by a proliferation of malignant melanocytes, which begins to grow horizontally along the dermal–epidermal junction and within the epidermis, as part of the radial growth phase, prior to entering the vertical growth phase characterized by progressively thicker dermal involvement. This relationship shows a broader intraepidermal component than dermal component. The most common of melanoma subtypes, these lesions are often characterized by pagetoid spread of melanocytes above the dermal–epidermal junction; irregularly shaped, sized, and placed melanocytic nests; and consumption of and clefting from the epidermis. Superficial spreading melanoma is typically found on intermittently sun-exposed areas as well as arising from pre-existing nevi. The main differential diagnosis is with dysplastic nevi; nevi of special sites such as scalp, breast, or genitals; traumatized nevi; or persistent/recurrent nevi. The most common genetic driver in superficial spreading melanomas is *BRAF* mutation, which appears to correlate with more epithelioid cytology in tumor cells and more pagetoid scatter of tumor cells.[50,51,52]

Superficial spreading melanoma will typically show mostly epithelioid cytomorphology. In banal nevi, melanocytes are often more epithelioid the younger the patient's age is. Indeed, Spitz nevi, which occur mostly in children and young adults, are the most epithelioid of all nevi. Congenital nevi are typically very epithelioid superficially, often with patchy single cells in the epidermis. However, their overall architecture is very orderly with marked maturation upon descent into the dermis. Epithelioid cytomorphology in older individuals with background sun damage should cause pause and closer examination to exclude a nevoid melanoma.

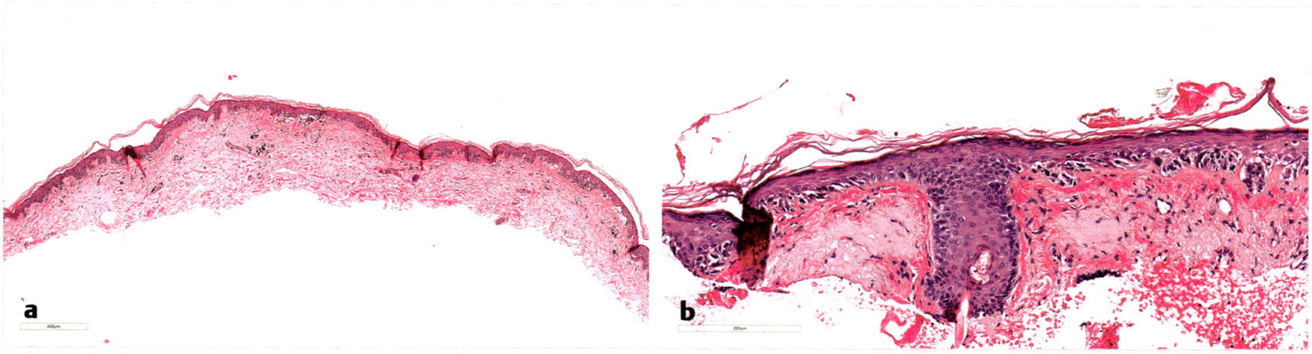

Fig. 11.12 (a) Lentigo maligna melanoma (low power). (b) Lentigo maligna melanoma (high power).

Nodular Melanoma

The nodular subtype of melanoma contains, by definition, a larger, broader, dermal component of malignant melanocytes than that in the epidermis. It suggests loss of senescence, and proliferative advantage early on in the neoplastic process. The main differential diagnosis in these types of melanoma includes intradermal or primarily intradermal Spitz nevi and metastatic melanoma. The diagnosis of intradermal Spitz nevus should only comfortably be made when the histologic criteria are perfect for Spitz nevi, the patient is young (< 40 years old), and histologic evidence of significant sun damage is lacking. The distinction between metastatic melanoma is often a clinical one, based on patient history. It should be noted, however, that cutaneous metastases can show significant epidermotropism, mimicking a primary melanoma.

According to some reports, nodular melanomas are more common on intermittently sun-exposed areas in patients with pale skin and few nevi.[53] Some reports also suggest a worse outcome in nodular subtype that is independent of tumor thickness, ulceration, Clark's level, and mitotic count.[54] The main genetic drivers of these lesions are NRAS or BRAF mutations, which are mutually exclusive in melanoma in general.[55]

Lentigo Maligna Melanoma

Lentigo maligna melanomas typically develop on the face or other sun-exposed areas in elderly patients and are related to a history of chronic sun exposure. As such, biopsy specimens show abundant solar elastosis and actinic changes in keratinocytes. Melanocytes are arranged in a lentiginous or "lining up" pattern along the dermal–epidermal junction (► Fig. 11.12), with frequent involvement of hair follicles and frequent upward migration in the epidermis. Cytologically, the cells typically show high nuclear to cytoplasmic ratios, with increased retraction artifact from surrounding keratinocytes and nuclear hyperchromasia with irregular nuclear contours. Epithelioid morphology with vesicular chromatin and enlarged nucleoli can also be seen. The main differential diagnosis is with actinic melanocytic hyperplasia, pigmented actinic keratosis, dysplastic nevi, and even lichenoid keratosis. Genetic drivers in LMM most commonly include NRAS mutations, and rarely c-kit mutations.[53,55]

Because most melanocytic nevi are known to regress as we age, the diagnosis of an atypical or "dysplastic" junctional lentiginous nevus on sun-damaged skin in elderly patients (especially when the lesion is clinically at least 6 mm in diameter) is rarely to be made. Clinicopathologic experience has trained dermatopathologists to have a low threshold for calling lentigo maligna in this setting, especially considering the low degree of cytologic atypical often seen in these lesions, and their propensity to show field effect, skipping around the dermal–epidermal junction quite broadly.

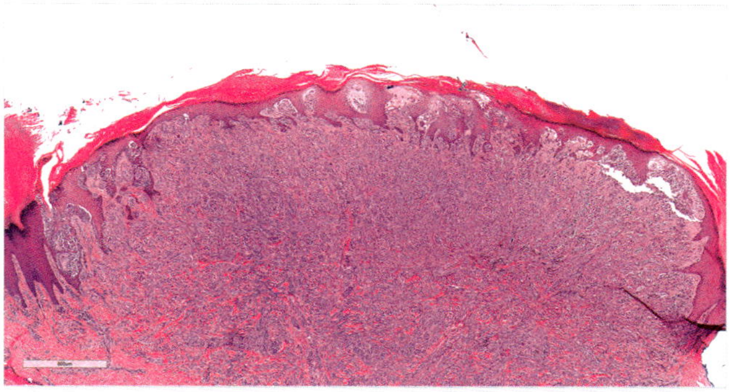

Fig. 11.13 Acral melanoma.

Acral Lentiginous Melanoma

Acral lentiginous melanoma (ALM) occurs on the palms, soles, and nail beds, and is named based on both its location and its histologic pattern of growth. This melanoma subtype is the most common type to occur in dark-skinned patients, and is not thought to be related to sun exposure. As such, biopsy specimens show a somewhat similar arrangement to that seen in lentigo maligna, that is, lentiginous growth of atypical melanocytes along the dermal–epidermal junction, with disorganized nest size and placement, and frequent upward migration of nests and single cells within the acral epidermis. Cytologically, the cells typically can resemble those seen in lentigo maligna with high nuclear to cytoplasmic ratios, increased retraction artifact, and nuclear hyperchromasia with irregular nuclear contours. Epithelioid morphology with vesicular chromatin and enlarged nucleoli can also be seen (► Fig. 11.13). The main differential diagnosis is with acral nevi, which notoriously show overlapping architectural features of melanoma, possibly related to trauma. Genetic drivers in ALM can include BRAF, NRAS, and KIT. BRAF mutations were identified in 17% of the primary ALMs; and both NRAS and KIT mutations were found at a similar frequency of 15% in a study of 88 ALMs by Zebary

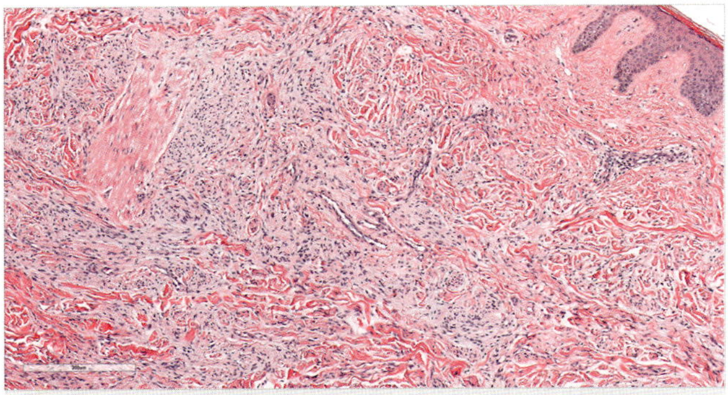

Fig. 11.14 Desmoplastic melanoma.

et al.[56] Similar rates of BRAF mutations were found in a Japanese cohort in a study by Hong et al, where BRAF-positive tumors showed improved outcome as well.[57]

Because of the overlapping, particularly architectural, features of acral melanoma and acral nevi, the increased fear of overdiagnosis due to functional location, and the often incomplete biopsy sampling of lesions, acral melanomas have increased potential for misdiagnosis. As such, a low threshold for a second pathologist's opinion is prudent, especially in new lesions in adults.

Desmoplastic Melanoma

Desmoplastic melanomas are the rarest subtype. They are characterized by narrow, spindled melanocytes with subtle nuclear atypia, associated with a fibrotic stroma (▶ Fig. 11.14). Tumor cells often extend deeply into the subcutis along fibrous septae, but can be difficult to delineate without the help of IHC stains, due to histologic overlap with scar and other neurofibromatous proliferations. Some reports suggest that these lesions do better clinically, compared to their similarly staged counterparts, with increased tendency for local recurrence and decreased tendency for metastatic spread.[58]

Desmoplastic melanomas need not have an epidermal component, but when they do, it is often lentigo maligna, which is known to frequently invade in a desmoplastic fashion. The main differential diagnosis for DM includes atypical neurofibromas, malignant peripheral nerve sheath tumors, and nonspecific increases in dermal fibroblasts. Desmoplastic melanomas usually lack BRAF mutations.[59] Rare cases may carry NRAS mutations. Mutations of TP53 and NF1 are common in desmoplastic melanoma.[60]

11.4.3 Pathologic Parameters for Melanoma Management

Beyond general clinical data elements including tumor site, laterality, and specimen type, the pathologic data elements required or recommended for inclusion in the structured reporting protocol for cutaneous melanoma are listed in ▶ Table 11.7 and highlighted below. In addition, some have argued for the presence and amount of desmoplastic melanoma to be included as core requirements in the reporting of melanoma due to the evidence showing this type to have improved survival and reduced rate of lymph node metastasis.[58]

Table 11.7 Pathologic data elements included in the structured reporting protocol for cutaneous melanomas

Required pathologic data	Recommended pathologic data
• Procedure (e.g., biopsy, excision) • Specimen laterality • Tumor site • Tumor size (required only if tumor is grossly present) • Presence of macroscopic satellite nodule(s) (required for excision specimens only) • Histologic type (e.g., superficial-spreading, nodular, lentigo maligna) • Maximum tumor thickness (Breslow) • Presence of ulceration • Margins (including distance of margin uninvolved by invasive or in situ tumor) • Mitotic rate (per mm^2) • Presence of microsatellitosis • Presence of lymph-vascular invasion • Lymph nodes (required only if lymph nodes are present in the specimen) • Pathologic staging (pTNM)	• Macroscopic pigmentation (e.g., none, diffuse, patchy) • Anatomic level (Clark's level) • Presence of perineural invasion • Presence of tumor-infiltrating lymphocytes • Presence of tumor regression • Growth phase (e.g., radial, vertical) • Additional pathologic findings (e.g., nevus remnant)

Abbreviation: pTNM, pathologic, tumor, lymph nodes, metastasis.

Source: Adapted from www.cap.org

11.4.4 Breslow's Thickness

Of all the parameters reported for cutaneous melanoma, Breslow's thickness holds the most prognostic significance for localized melanoma. It is the primary determinant of tumor stage within the TNM staging system. Breslow's thickness is determined by measuring the distance of the deepest invasive tumor cell across the broad tumor base from the top of the overlying granular layer of the epidermis. Breslow's thickness is only accurate in sections cut perpendicular to the epidermis. However, in some tangentially sectioned specimens, Breslow's thickness can be measured tangentially, given that it can typically be inferred that the true Breslow's thickness is not greater than the tangential measurement. A statement to this effect can be included in the report. In the case that the epidermis is ulcerated in the region overlying the deepest tumor extent, the measurement is taken from the ulcer base. Deep vertical tumor extensions perpendicular to the tumor base are assumed to be periadnexal and are not included in Breslow's thickness, except if they are the only invasive focus. In that particular case, the Breslow's thickness may be measured from the inner layer of the outer root sheath of the follicular epithelium or the inner luminal surface of sweat glands. Microsatellites and areas of tumor regression without visible tumor are not to be included in Breslow's thickness.[61,62] Although controversy exists, tumor regression in melanoma has not consistently proven to have an independently positive or negative impact on melanoma-specific disease-free survival or overall survival.[62]

The Breslow's thickness is measured with an ocular micrometer in millimeters. Tumors less than 1 mm thickness have traditionally been considered "thin melanomas," and are Stage 1 by definition (either 1A or 1B depending on additional factors). Depending on the look of the sampled tumor, the dermatopathologist may decide to cut deeper levels into the paraffin tissue block to ensure the deepest extent of tumor is available for measuring, permitting accurate staging.

Because of the importance of Breslow's thickness, punch biopsy for suspected melanomas has been advocated. From the dermatopathologists' perspective, this approach should only be employed if the diameter of the lesion is smaller than the diameter of the punch biopsy piercing tool. It is important for the entire breadth of the lesion to be available for examination in order to evaluate symmetry, nest placement, and many of the other features that discriminate melanomas from dysplastic nevi or Spitz nevi. If the lesion is clinically too large, two alternative biopsy approaches include a "scoop shave" or saucerization biopsy technique, or an excisional biopsy. Scoop shave biopsies typically allow for complete visualization of the lesion across the horizontal plane, and allow many different cuts into the tumor, facilitating the evaluation of depth, ulceration, mitoses, etc. That said, scoop shave biopsies risk transecting the tumor at the biopsy base, thus precluding accurate measurement of Breslow's thickness, and hence tumor staging. When strong clinical suspicion for melanoma exists, a small excisional biopsy may be the best method. In this way, the tumor can be visualized across its entire breadth, and depth, with little chance of transection at the base. Large primary excisions should be avoided due to the theoretical risk of lymphatic drainage disruption with healing and hence impaired accuracy of SLNBx that may follow. In addition, when larger tissue samples are submitted, less cuts through the center of the lesion may be histologically visualized following biopsy bread loafing.

A majority of studies show that melanoma biopsies are submitted fairly evenly as punch biopsies shave biopsies and excisional biopsies. Published reports appear to show no difference in patient outcome based on the biopsy type.[63] Often times, regardless of the biopsy type, and regardless of whether tumor was present at the peripheral or deep aspects of the biopsy margins, residual tumor is not found in the wide excision specimen. Whether this is a function of residual tumor destruction by tissue macrophages during wound healing, or of the propensity for bread loafing of large excisional specimens to miss microscopic residual disease that may remain within the paraffin block, is unclear and has not been studied.

11.4.5 Ulceration

Primary melanoma tumor ulceration, as defined by intraepidermal tumor growth which leads to denudation/erosion of the epidermis with consequent exposure of lesional cells to the external environment, ranks second to Breslow's thickness in primary tumor prognostic factors. Within a given pathologic T stage, ulceration will upstage a lesion from an A to B, which can consequently lead to clinical upstaging, and hence worse prognosis. The mechanism behind the conferred worse prognosis is proposed to relate to an implied increase in tumor proliferative index.[64] Additionally, there is potential for artificial reductions in Breslow's thickness, due to erosion of the granular epidermal layer and the practice of tumor measurement from the ulcer base in these instances. Finally, ulceration induces a host response characterized by the formation of granulation tissue and wound healing processes also reported to facilitate metastasis.[65] Indeed, ulcerated lesions show a relative increase in hematogenous spread compared to nonulcerated lesions.[66]

While there appears to be agreement among dermatopathologists for Breslow's thickness, more subjectivity appears to exist in the assessment of ulceration. Within the differential diagnosis for tumor ulceration is tumor traumatization. True tumor ulceration with its prognostic implications should show thinning of the epidermis to the side of the epidermal defect, otherwise known as "consumption of the epidermis" which leads to "attenuative ulceration." Such findings would not be expected in ulceration resulting from trauma alone.

11.4.6 Mitotic Count

The newest prognostic tumor feature to be included in the AJCC staging system is tumor dermal mitoses per square millimeter. The tumor mitotic count should be initiated in the most mitotically active area or "hot spot" and continued in adjacent fields until an area corresponding to 1 mm^2 is assessed. Depending on the type of microscope, 1 mm^2 corresponds to approximately 4 to 6 adjacent high power fields at 400 × –40 × objective with 10 × ocular. If no hot spot can be found, then several randomly chosen areas can be counted and summed. When the intradermal component is less than 1 mm^2, a single mitotic figure is classified as "at least 1/mm^2."[67]

The mitotic rate, according to some studies, has been independently associated with outcome in melanoma, with the difference being most marked with increasing mitotic counts.[68] The most important implication to this approach, however, is that previously staged T1a melanoma tumors with any dermal mitotic activity (>0 Mit/mm^2) are now classified as stage T1b tumors according to the 2009 revision of the AJCC staging system.[65] As such, patients who would not have been previously considered for SLNBx are now often undergoing this procedure in many centers.[69,70] Some have argued that the evaluation of mitoses is too subjective and confounded by variability in tissue processing, number of histologic levels obtained, and time spent searching, for example, to be bestowed with such impact on management.[71] As such, attempts at standardization of this procedure have been made which include recommendation for mitotic figures to be sought in the original two levels obtained with multiple cuts on each level. Additional sections for the purpose of mitotic count should not be obtained.[67] The impact that this change ultimately has on primary tumor staging, management, and outcome in thin melanomas will be an interesting area of future investigation.

11.4.7 Lymph Node Biopsy

It is required that the number of sentinel and nonsentinel lymph nodes received and the number with tumor be reported. The lymph node status is the strongest pathologic predictor of outcome for cutaneous melanoma patients. Unfortunately, the method in which sentinel and nonsentinel lymph nodes are processed varies between medical centers, with SLNBx processing being one of the most nonstandardized processes.[72] Dekker and Duncan found that uniform processing practices included[1] processing (for paraffin) all of the lymph node tissue rather than submitting representative sections and[2] use of IHC stains if no tumor was identified on the H&E-stained sections. They found significant variability regarding the method of sectioning lymph nodes at grossing and in the histology laboratory (e.g., thickness in mm of lymph node sections at grossing and number of cuts into the paraffin block examined histologically). Most laboratories bisect nodes longitudinally (94%) and place at least some deeper levels into the block (67%), but these were not uniform practices. S-100 was the most commonly used IHC stain (78%), followed by Melan-A (56%), MART-1 (50%), HMB-45 (44%), tyrosinase (33%), MiTF (11%), and pan-melanoma (6%).[73]

Interestingly, at least two large studies have shown that the amount of tumor burden seen in SLNBx following routine processing (typically two H&E levels, and two to four levels for IHC staining per LN) tends to underestimate the tumor burden present in the SL, when the paraffin block is more thoroughly sectioned into.[74,75,76] This may help explain why rare isolated melanoma tumor cells found in SLNs retain prognostic significance regardless of the minute size of tumor involvement. More intriguing, perhaps, is the fact that patients with SLNBx positivity detected with enhance pathologic analysis (EPA) which included at least 20 sections (250 µM apart), as well as those with negative SLNs by EPA demonstrated improved recurrence-free and disease-specific survival compared with patients with SLN disease detected by routine pathologic analysis (RPA).[74] This may be due to the fact that most outcome and management studies have been conducted using RPA. Furthermore, when Li et al re-reviewed the histopathology of negative SLNs from patients who developed regional node field recurrence after a negative SLN biopsy (2.7% of cases total in a median follow-up of 35.7 months) via multiple further sections cut from each block and stained with H&E, S-100, HMB45, and Melan A, they revealed occult tumor in approximately 25% of the cases available for examination.[76] While this study depicts the inherent inaccuracy in SLNBx evaluation due to the impracticality of histologically evaluating the entire LN, it also points to the relative rarity of clinical consequence of this inaccuracy, as well as additional mechanisms which may lead to nodal recurrence in this setting.

11.4.8 Additional Prognostic Features

While the type of biopsy technique—scoop shave, punch, or excisional—used in primary melanoma diagnosis does appear to impact the rate of residual tumor found in the wide excision specimen, it does not appear to have any impact on SLNBx accuracy, rate of positivity, tumor recurrence, or disease-specific survival.[76] Likewise, the length of time between primary biopsy and definitive treatment has been shown not to impact overall survival, disease-free survival, and recurrence-free survival within a 56-day window for definitive surgery.[77,78] The presence of residual tumor in the wide excision specimen does not appear to impact survival independently from other poor pathologic factors. The detection of perineural invasion is associated with tumor ulceration, desmoplastic and acral lentiginous histologic subtype, and head/neck/hands/feet tumor location. Although detection of perineural invasion is enhanced by the use immunohistochemistry, it does not appear to impact disease-free or overall survival. Routinely detected (H&E stains) perineural invasion, but not immunohistochemically detected perineural invasion, was associated with increased risk of local tumor recurrence.[79] In contrast to perineural invasion, immunohistochemistry-aided detection of lymphovascular space invasion (LVSI;D2–40 and CD34 antibodies) was found by Rose et al to be a significant marker of both reduced disease-free survival and overall survival.[80] However, Storr et al did not find significant and independent association with clinical outcome using the same IHC markers, although LVSI was positively associated with known markers of aggressive disease, including Breslow's thickness, ulceration, and mitotic count.[81]

Distance to the surgical margin is included in pathology reports to ensure that definitive treatment is achieved. Involvement of the surgical margin is known to result in tumor regrowth and to poorly affect patient outcome. Wide excision margin recommendations are based on the tumor thickness of the primary cutaneous melanoma, and are derived from the results of numerous randomized controlled trials done in several countries.[82,83,84,85]

Melanoma is known to be one of the most immunogenic tumors, and is frequently associated with histologic evidence of a host immune response. Tumor-infiltrating lymphocytes (TIL) can be characterized based on their level of tumor infiltration and disruption. Historically, an infiltrate has been considered "brisk" if it surrounds and infiltrates the tumor base leaving less than a 0.3-mm defect in the bandlike infiltrate. An infiltrate that is "present, non-brisk" has a defect that is greater than 0.3 mm. Around 50% of tumors will show "absent" TIL. The factors which dictate such host recognition warrant investigation for two basic reasons. First, numerous studies have shown that patients whose tumors are briskly infiltrated by TIL have superior clinical outcome and reduced sentinel lymph node tumor spread, and that this relationship is independent of other primary tumor factors.[86,87,88,89] Second, the magnitude of immune infiltration of tumors is positively associated with programmed death 1 receptor and its ligand (PD-1 and PD-1L) expression in the tumor microenvironment, and responsiveness to the newly approved PD-1 inhibitor therapies, pembrolizumab and nivolumab.[90,91] The assessment and grading of TIL currently remains somewhat subjective. That said, the superior efficacy of immunotherapy in melanoma will likely demand the development of methods for pathologic quantification and characterization of the tumor-infiltrating immune signature in the future.

Although lymphatic spread at the time of melanoma diagnosis can be fairly successfully detected with SLNBx, there is currently no way to detect whether or not hematogenous spread has occurred at the time of diagnosis. With improved molecular techniques to detect circulating, cell-free DNA, it is expected that hematogenously disseminated tumor cells may one day be detected and intervention be initiated prior to clinical manifestation. This is an area of ongoing investigation.[92,93]

Castle Biosciences Inc. (Friendswood, TX) has developed a prognostic test for melanoma, also known as DecisionDx-Melanoma, which is a gene expression–profiling (GEP) test that looks at the messenger RNA expression profile of 28 genes to identify patients at risk for tumor spread. The data are reported as either a class I (low risk) or class II (high risk) signature. This assay has been shown to be an independent prognostic marker for cutaneous melanoma in multivariate analysis[94] and may one day be adopted as a frontline test to identify Stage I–II patients who may benefit from adjuvant systemic therapy following wide excision.

11.5 Merkel's Cell Carcinoma

Merkel's cell carcinoma is a primary neuroendocrine tumor of the skin, derived from Merkel's cells, which are inconspicuously distributed among basal keratinocytes in the epidermis and are involved in discrimination of light touch. Although still relatively rare, MCC appears to be increasing in incidence. The rise in incidence is thought to be due to the larger population of patients who are elderly and who are immunosuppressed, and relates to the mechanistic initiation of carcinogenesis by the Merkel's polyomavirus in approximately 80% of cases in the United States.[95] This virus is one of the thirteen known polyomaviruses that naturally infect humans,[96] and one of six viruses thus far implicated in human malignancy. While approximately 60% of patients have the MPV in their skin flora, most of these do not develop MCC.[97]

Histologically, MCC is typically a dermal-based proliferation of small to medium-sized cells with scant cytoplasm, high nuclear to cytoplasmic ratio, finely clumped, salt and pepper chromatin, and no nucleoli (▶ Fig. 11.15a, b). The main morphologic differential diagnosis is with metastatic small cell carcinoma of the lung, BCC, and lymphoma. As such, confirmation with IHC staining is almost always required. MCC will stain positively with pan-cytokeratin markers such as CAM5.2 and AE1/3, typically in a perinuclear dot-like pattern, and negatively for the follicular epithelial marker characteristic of BCC (BerEP4), and the lymphoid marker CD45. To rule out cutaneous involvement by metastatic small cell lung carcinoma, it is prudent to always stain MCC with TTF-1 and CK20. MCC will be negative for TTF-1 and CK7, and positive for CK20 in more than 95% of cases, although rare CK20-negative cases exist. Meanwhile, small cell lung carcinoma will be positive for TTF-1 and CK7 in

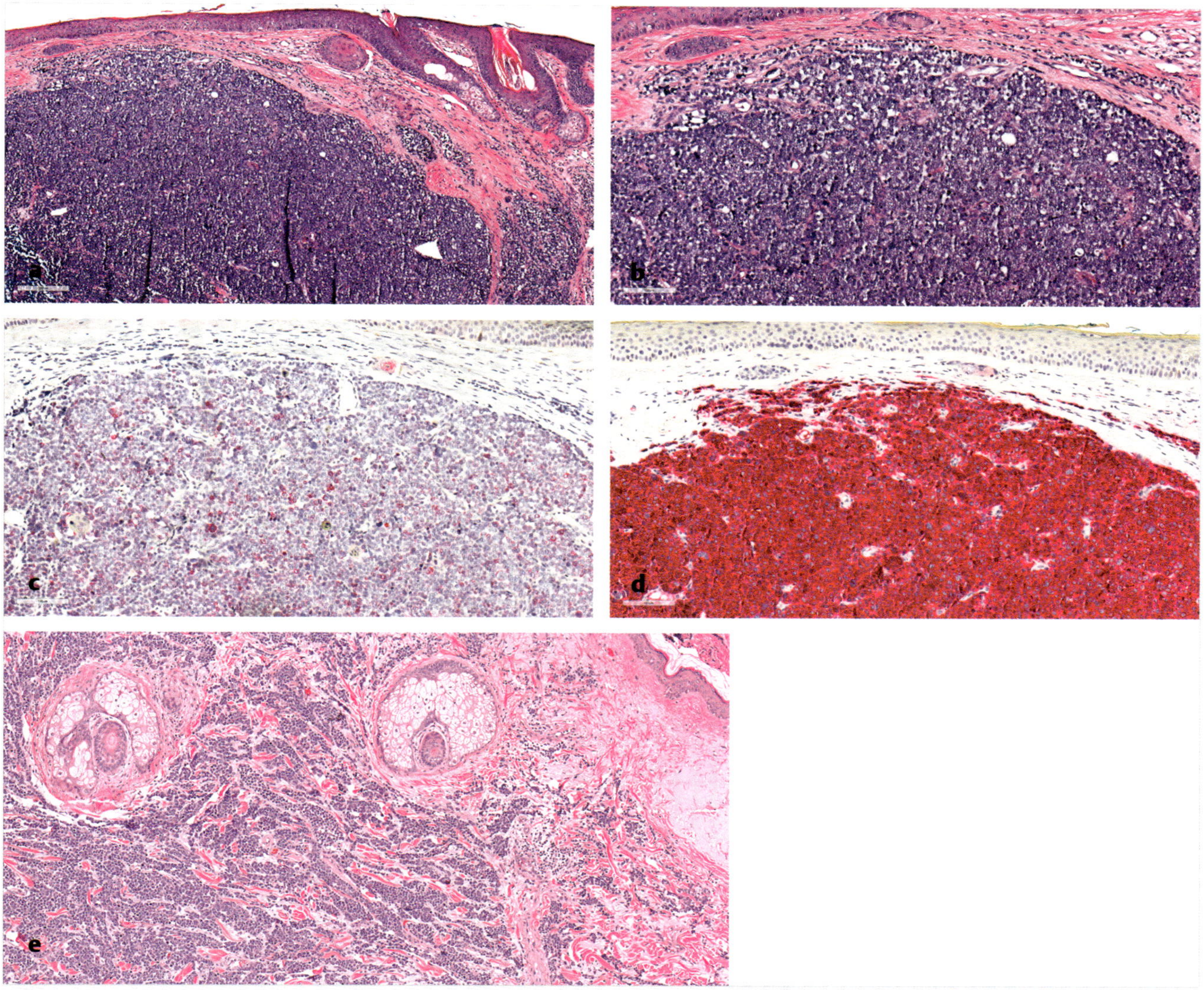

Fig. 11.15 (a) Merkel's cell carcinoma, nodular (H&E, low power). **(b)** Merkel's cell carcinoma, nodular (high power). **(c, d)** Merkel's cell carcinoma, nodular (CK20, synaptophysin). **(e)** Merkel's cell carcinoma, infiltrative (low power).

more than 80% of cases, and negative for CK20. Perinuclear staining with CK20 is particularly specific for MCC in this setting, and neuroendocrine markers, such as synaptophysin, will also be positive (▶ Fig. 11.15c, d). Indeed, NCCN guidelines call for confirmatory immunostains to establish the diagnosis of MCC, preferable with CK20 and TTF-1.[98]

11.6 Prognostic Features Reported

The only relevant features to be reported for Merkel's cell carcinoma beyond the diagnosis include tumor size, the presence or absence of lymphatic invasion, and margin status.[99,100,101,102,103] It is possible that in the future, knowledge of the viral status and CD8-positive TILs may be clinically relevant and therefore beneficial to report. Virus-positive tumors tend to be mutation-poor. Virus-negative tumors often occur in older individuals, are more common in areas of high UV exposure, such as Australia, and are rich in mutations typical of a UV signature. Virus-negative tumors may be pure or associated with squamous cell or other carcinomas. Studies mostly suggest that MCPyV DNA-positive tumors are associated with relatively improved clinical outcome compared to virus-negative tumors, although not all studies confirm this.[103,104,105] Superior outcome in virus-positive tumors would seem to parallel data in head and neck squamous cell carcinomas, for instance, where human papilloma virus–associated tumors have improved outcome. It is postulated that the improved survival in this setting is related to increased tumor recognition by host immune cells, and therefore increased tumor control, and increased synergy with chemotherapy and radiation.[106] As such, further reports have shown that increasing density of tumor-infiltrating CD8+T-lymphocytes (TIL) is associated with improved survival in MCC.[107,108,109] For this reason, viral status testing and TIL quantification may one day become a part of the tumor report. The tumor growth pattern (nodular or infiltrative) and the presence of secondary malignancy (typically squamous cell carcinoma) are other pertinent pieces of information typically reported, with some reports showing survival advantage with nodular (▶ Fig. 11.15a) compared to infiltrative (▶ Fig. 11.15e) growth pattern.[99]

11.6.1 SLNBx Evaluation

As with most other tumors, SLNBx has been increasingly utilized in the management of MCC. There have been conflicting reports as to the utility of this procedure, and the information gained from it, to direct management decisions or aid in prognostication.[110,111,112,113,114,115] There is conflicting evidence on the prognostic value of the SLNBx in patients with MCC.[114,115] A therapeutic benefit by the procedure has not been proven. For histopathologic analysis of the SLN status, pathologists often use CK20[116] for best identification of tumor cells in the lymph node. Recent studies by our group suggest that patients with microscopic stage III disease may be prognostically stratified based on a solid versus non-solid pattern of sentinel lymph node involvement by MCC, among other factors.[117] Confirmatory studies in a larger cohort are needed.

11.7 Cutaneous Sarcomas

Cutaneous sarcomas vary widely in both their histomorphology and clinical outcome, and are relatively rare. For this reason, they are often and should often result in diagnostic consultation within pathology. Due to the histologic overlap with various benign and malignant processes, as well as the varied morphologic subtypes within each tumor type, IHC staining may be a requisite for almost all cutaneous sarcomas for correct identification (▶ Table 11.8). Compared to sarcomas located in the deep soft tissues, dermal sarcomas can show significant nuclear pleomorphism and still behave in a relatively indolent fashion.[118]

11.7.1 Angiosarcoma

Angiosarcoma is a malignant sarcoma derived from vascular endothelial cells. Cutaneous angiosarcoma comprises approximately half of all angiosarcomas, and occurs in two basic settings. Primary angiosarcoma occurs on sun-exposed areas, primarily head and neck, of older individuals. While primary angiosarcoma is thought to be related to sun exposure, due to the strong predilection to affect sun-exposed skin of older Caucasians, this has not been directly proven. Secondary angiosarcoma occurs following surgery, in the setting of Stewart-Treves syndrome due to chronic lymphedema, and following radiation, as postradiation angiosarcoma.[119] Up to 100% of secondary angiosarcomas may show amplification in the MYC oncogene.[120,121] Angiosarcoma, although always considered biologically high grade, can show variable degrees of vascular differentiation, and the amount of differentiation in a given tumor will dictate which other conditions come into the differential diagnosis. Highly differentiated tumors can be difficult to distinguish from unusual benign hemangiomas, because they

Table 11.8 Immunohistochemical stains useful in the diagnosis of cutaneous spindle cell lesions and sarcomas

	Immunohistochemical stain					
Tumor	**Cytokeratin**	**S-100**	**Melanocytic markers (Melan-A, HMB-45)**	**SMA**	**Desmin**	**Endothelial markers (CD31, CD34)**
Sarcomatoid SCC	+	-	-	-	-	-
Spindle cell melanoma	-	+	-/+	-	-	-
AFX	-	-	-	-/+	-	-
Leiomyosarcoma	-/+	-	-	+	+	-
Angiosarcoma	-/+	-	-	-	-	+

Abbreviations: AFX, atypical fibroxanthoma; SCC, squamous cell carcinoma; SMA, smooth muscle actin.

form distinct vascular channels lined by mildly atypical endothelial cells which, nevertheless, show an infiltrative pattern of growth (▶ Fig. 11.16a). Most angiosarcomas show moderate differentiation and consist of irregularly shaped and sized vascular channels which travel in unique planes and wrap around and splay collagen bundles. These channels often anastomose in an irregular, sieve-like fashion and can be filled with erythrocytes or clear fluid (▶ Fig. 11.16b). Poorly differentiated tumors may not be distinguishable from poorly differentiated carcinomas, melanoma, or other sarcomas, and may consist of sheets of highly atypical, epithelioid cells with significant nuclear pleomorphism (▶ Fig. 11.16c). In this setting, more well-differentiated areas may provide diagnostic clues, and IHC staining specific for vascular endothelial cells, CD31, CD34, and ERG, provide confirmation (▶ Fig. 11.16d-g). Extravasated erythrocytes can be an additional diagnostic clue.

Outcome in angiosarcoma is linked to a number of factors, including patient age, tumor size, and surgical margin status. In general, outcome in angiosarcoma may be more closely linked to clinical factors compared to histologic factors, because the systems commonly used in tumor grading do not lend themselves well to angiosarcoma. The various subtypes of angiosarcoma, including soft-tissue angiosarcomas, are often grouped together for study purposes, due to the rarity of the disease, and this may confound precise prognostic categorization. That said, older patients have a worse prognosis than their younger counterparts; tumor size is strongly linked to outcome, clinical extent of disease, and tumor resectability; and margin status is

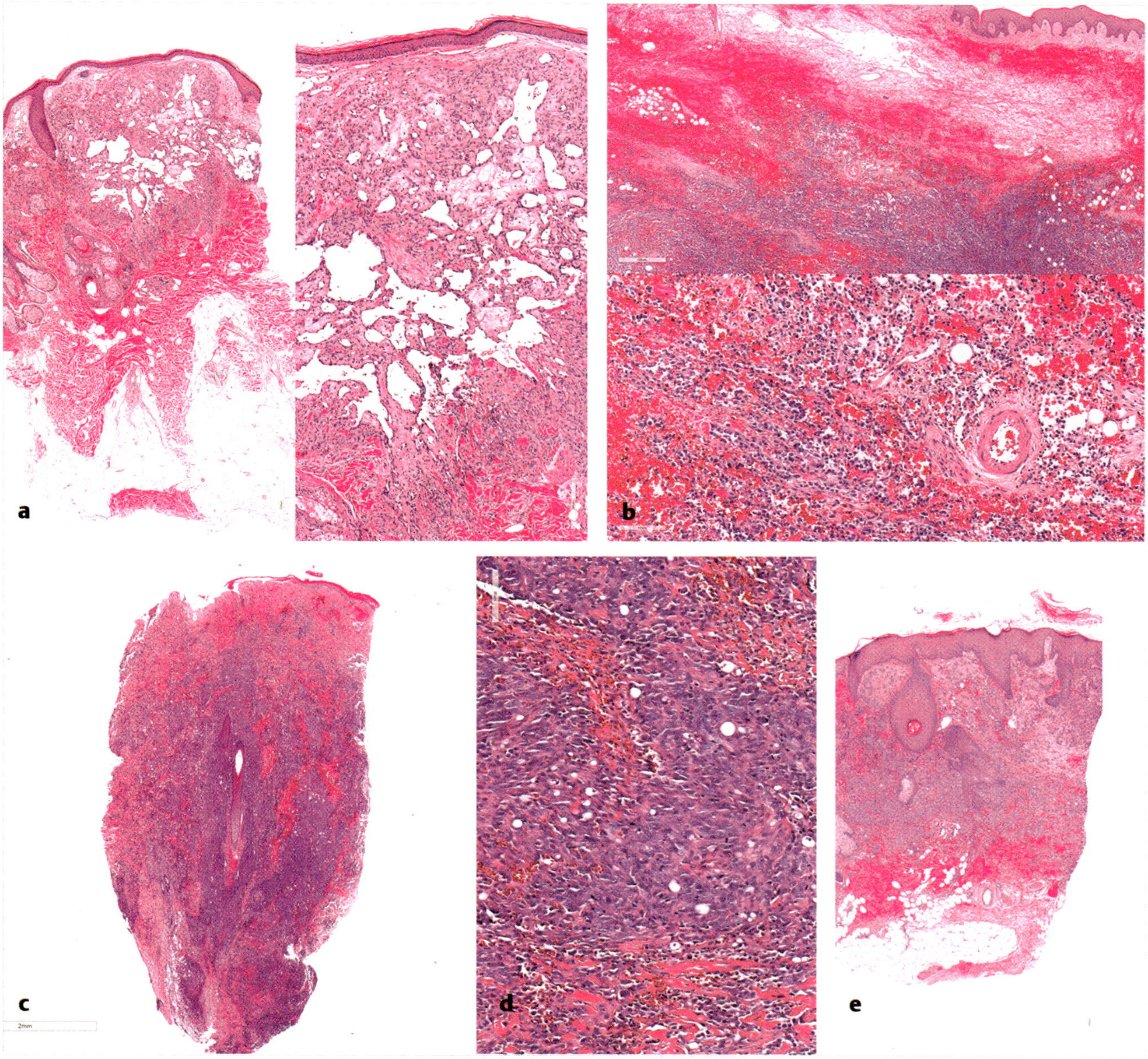

Fig. 11.16 **(a)** Angiosarcoma, well-differentiated (low and high power). **(b)** Angiosarcoma, moderately-differentiated. **(c, d)** Angiosarcoma, epithelioid. **(e, f, g)** Angiosarcoma, epithelioid, with ERG nuclear staining positivity.

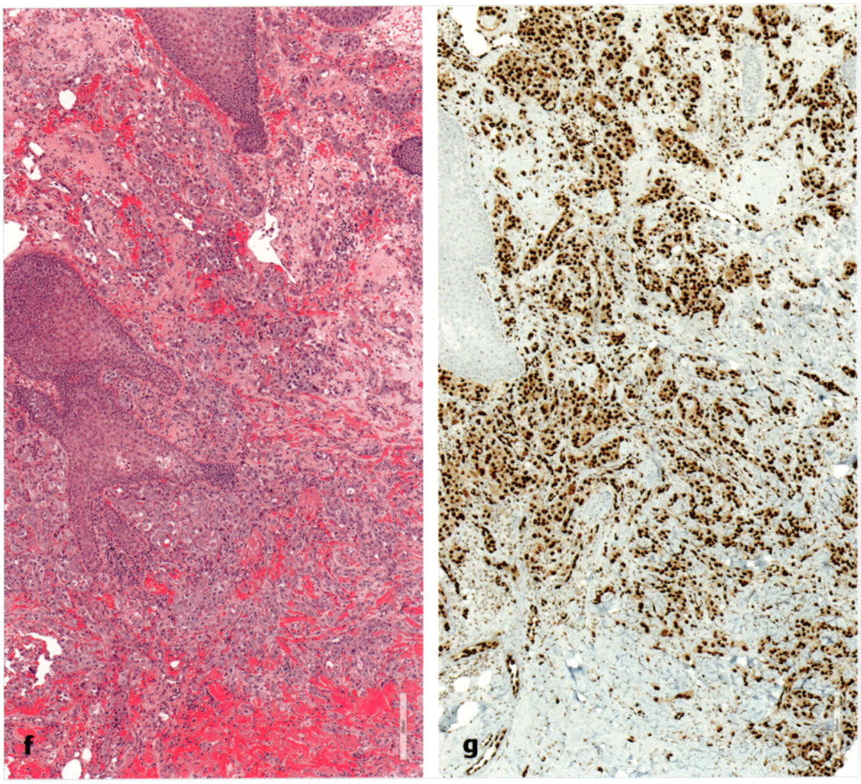

Fig. 11.16 *(continued)*

an important determinant of outcome, based on several studies.[122,123,124,125] Patients whose tumors are less than 5 cm and completely excised with negative margins have improved prognosis. As such, the most important part of the pathology report for angiosarcoma will be histologic margin status (in addition to tumor size which may be clinically apparent). Margin status will become more difficult to evaluate with increasing differentiation of the tumor, especially considering the subtle and far-reaching manner in which angiosarcomas can travel. For this reason, Mohs surgery may be technically unsatisfactory, while CCPDMA is a practical alternative. Due to the known hematogenous, rather than lymphangitic manner in which angiosarcoma disseminates, lymph node biopsy has not been employed in this disease.

Atypical Fibroxanthoma

Atypical fibroxanthoma (AFX) is an undifferentiated tumor, typically occurring in sun-damaged skin, often with some fibrohistiocytic/myofibroblastic features. By definition, the tumor does not involve the subcutis or deeper structures. Because of the presence of mesenchymal cell malignant atypia and associated genomic aberrations, AFX is in essence a sarcoma. That said, the term "AFX" is preferable to avoid overtreatment, since strictly defined tumors (no extension beyond the dermis on multiple levels) tend to be indolent following complete excision. A tumor with the appearance of an AFX that involves the subcutis or deeper structures is best reported as pleomorphic dermal-based sarcoma and is clinically/surgically managed more aggressively. Histologically, the cells of an AFX are arranged in fascicles or sheets. Rarely, a storiform pattern is evident. The cells are spindled to round, with multinucleation, pleomorphism, and numerous typical and atypical mitotic figures (► Fig. 11.17a, b). Immunohistochemically, AFX is typically negative for both S-100 protein and cytokeratins, allowing distinction from melanoma and spindled squamous cell carcinoma, respectively. In addition, pleomorphic leiomyosarcoma and angiosarcoma can be ruled out with desmin and ERG negativity as needed. Most cases of AFX also show strong expression of CD10, but this is not specific. Some cases express smooth muscle actin, although desmin is typically negative, consistent with myofibroblastic differentiation. Aside from these aforementioned entities, which can be ruled out using immunohistochemistry, it is important that AFX be distinguished from a superficial or dermal undifferentiated pleomorphic sarcoma, due to the risk of recurrence and metastasis in the latter compared with the nearly uniform excellent prognosis in the former.[126] Aside from correct diagnosis and categorization of AFX, margin status is the most important prognostic variable to be included in the pathology report.

Dermatofibrosarcoma Protuberans

Dermatofibrosarcoma protuberans (DFSP) is a cutaneous fibrohistiocytic tumor of intermediate malignant potential which can recur locally and rarely metastasizes. It typically presents in early or middle adult life, although it does affect pediatric patients. Histologically, the tumor consists of a uniform dermal proliferation of spindled cells arranged in a storiform pattern (► Fig. 11.18a, b). The tumor typically extends into the subcutaneous fat in an infiltrative pattern, imparting a lace or sieve-like appearance. The most common entity which enters into the

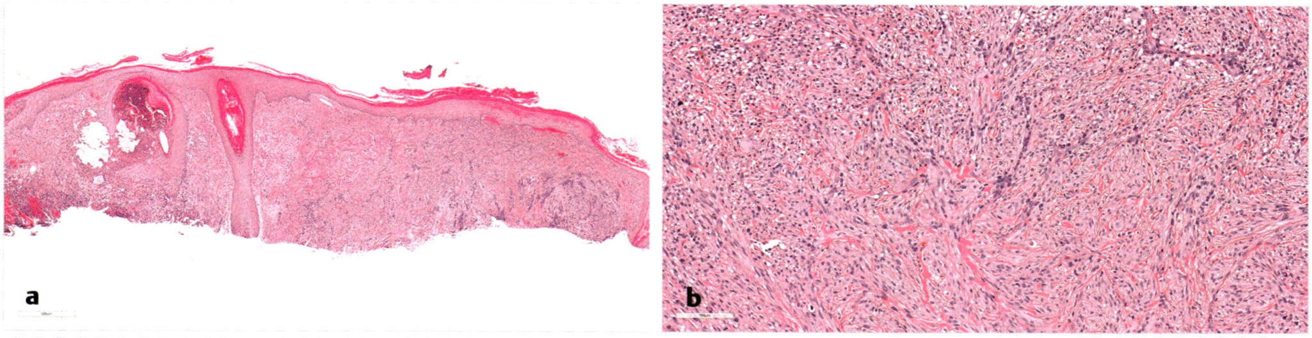

Fig. 11.17 **(a)** Atypical fibroxanthoma (low power). **(b)** Atypical fibroxanthoma (high power).

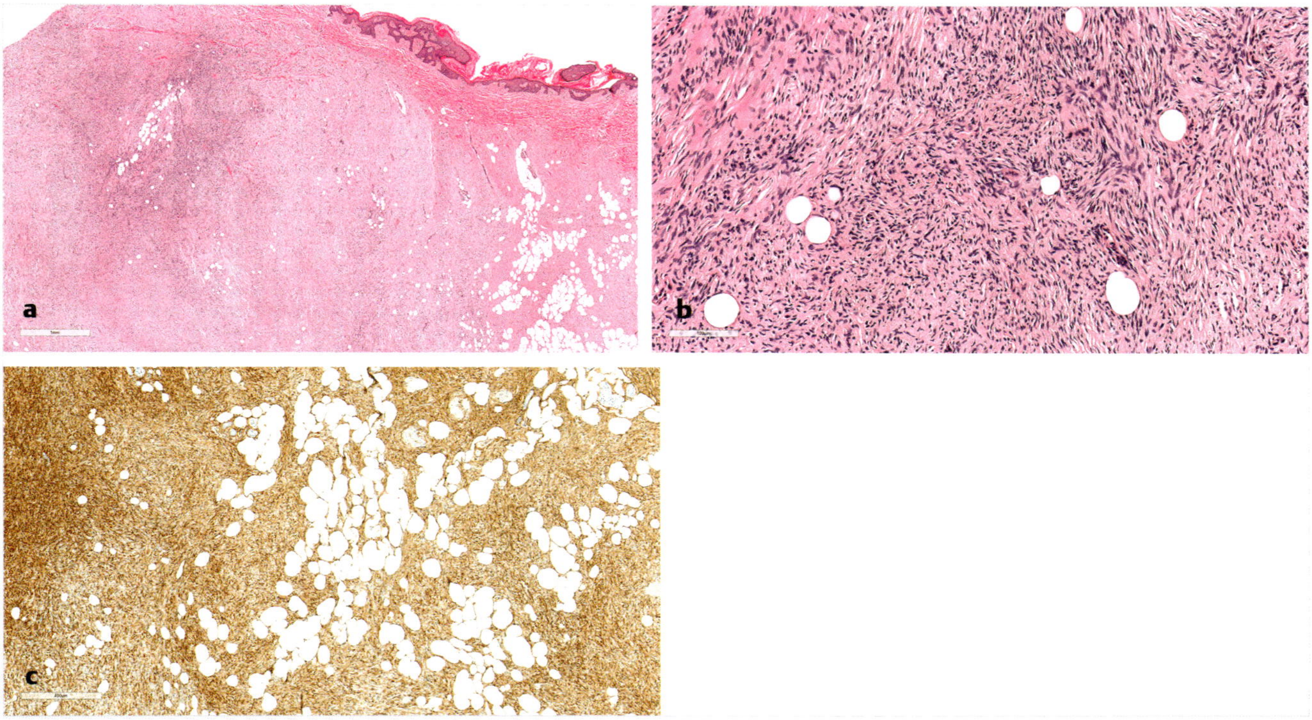

Fig. 11.18 **(a)** Dermatofibrosarcoma (low power). **(b)** Dermatofibrosarcoma (high power). **(c)** Dermatofibrosarcoma (CD34).

differential diagnosis includes benign fibrous histiocytoma (i.e., dermatofibroma), especially the cellular variant. Importantly, DFSPs will stain diffusely positive for CD34 (▶ Fig. 11.18c), and contain a translocation which results in fusion between the collagen gene *COL1A1* on chromosome 17 and the platelet-derived growth factor-beta gene *PDGFβ* on chromosome 22 [t(17;22)]. This translocation can be detected by FISH studies, and can be targeted with the drug imatinib.[118,127,128,129]

Surgical margin status is the most important predictor of outcome in DFSP, as well as the presence or absence of fibrosarcomatous transformation.[127] Negative margins can be technically difficult to achieve due to the tendency of this tumor to infiltrate with multiple irregular extensions. CD34 staining may be used to aid in the assessment of margin status, especially in cases where wide margins are less possible due to cosmetic locations, etc. In addition, Mohs and CCPDMA approaches have been used for complex cases, especially in cosmetic areas.[129,130,131]

References

[1] CAP Cancer Protocol Templates. http://www.cap.org/apps/docs/committees/cancer/cancer_protocols. Accessed December 29, 2014

[2] Randle HW. Basal cell carcinoma. Identification and treatment of the high-risk patient. Dermatol Surg. 1996; 22(3):255–261

[3] Weinstein MC, Brodell RT, Bordeaux J, Honda K. The art and science of surgical margins for the dermatopathologist. Am J Dermatopathol. 2012; 34 (7):737–745

[4] Kyrgidis A, Vahtsevanos K, Tzellos TG, et al. Clinical, histological and demographic predictors for recurrence and second primary tumours of head and neck basal cell carcinoma. A 1062 patient-cohort study from a tertiary cancer referral hospital. Eur J Dermatol. 2010; 20(3):276–282

[5] Preston DS, Stern RS. Nonmelanoma cancers of the skin. N Engl J Med. 1992; 327(23):1649–1662
[6] Sexton M, Jones DB, Maloney ME. Histologic pattern analysis of basal cell carcinoma. Study of a series of 1039 consecutive neoplasms. J Am Acad Dermatol. 1990; 23(6, Pt 1):1118–1126
[7] Geist DE, Garcia-Moliner M, Fitzek MM, Cho H, Rogers GS. Perineural invasion of cutaneous squamous cell carcinoma and basal cell carcinoma: raising awareness and optimizing management. Dermatol Surg. 2008; 34 (12):1642–1651
[8] Alsaad KO, Obaidat NA, Ghazarian D. Skin adnexal neoplasms–part 1: an approach to tumours of the pilosebaceous unit. J Clin Pathol. 2007; 60 (2):129–144
[9] Nedved D, Tonkovic-Capin V, Hunt E, et al. Diagnostic concordance rates in the subtyping of basal cell carcinoma by different dermatopathologists. J Cutan Pathol. 2014; 41(1):9–13
[10] Wolf DJ, Zitelli JA. Surgical margins for basal cell carcinoma. Arch Dermatol. 1987; 123(3):340–344
[11] Flohil SC, van Dorst AM, Nijsten T, Martino Neumann HA, Munte K. Mohs micrographic surgery for basal cell carcinomas: appropriateness of 'Rotterdam' criteria and predictive factors for three or more stages. J Eur Acad Dermatol Venereol. 2013; 27(10):1228–1235
[12] Kimyai-Asadi A, Goldberg LH, Jih MH. Accuracy of serial transverse cross-sections in detecting residual basal cell carcinoma at the surgical margins of an elliptical excision specimen. J Am Acad Dermatol. 2005; 53(3):469–474
[13] Justilien V, Fields AP. Molecular pathways: novel approaches for improved therapeutic targeting of Hedgehog signaling in cancer stem cells. Clin Cancer Res. 2015; 21(3):505–513
[14] National Comprehensive Cancer Network (NCCN). Clinical practice guidelines in oncology, basal and squamous cell skin cancers. V. 1. 2015. Available at: www.nccn.org. Accessed December 29, 2014
[15] NCCN Clinical Practice Guidelines in Oncology (NCCN Guidelines) Squamous Cell Skin Cancer Version 1.2017-October 3, 2016. http://www.nccn.org/professionals/physician_gls/pdf/squamous.pdf. Accessed December 29, 2014
[16] Jacobs MS, Persons DL, Fraga GR. EGFR and MYC gene copy number aberrations are more common in squamous cell carcinoma than keratoacanthoma: a FISH study. J Cutan Pathol. 2013; 40(5):447–454
[17] Jambusaria-Pahlajani A, Miller CJ, Quon H, Smith N, Klein RQ, Schmults CD. Surgical monotherapy versus surgery plus adjuvant radiotherapy in high-risk cutaneous squamous cell carcinoma: a systematic review of outcomes. Dermatol Surg. 2009; 35(4):574–585
[18] Brodland DG, Zitelli JA. Surgical margins for excision of primary cutaneous squamous cell carcinoma. J Am Acad Dermatol. 1992; 27(2, Pt 1):241–248
[19] Schmitt AR, Brewer JD, Bordeaux JS, Baum CL. Staging for cutaneous squamous cell carcinoma as a predictor of sentinel lymph node biopsy results: meta-analysis of American Joint Committee on Cancer criteria and a proposed alternative system. JAMA Dermatol. 2014; 150(1):19–24
[20] Andruchow JL, Veness MJ, Morgan GJ, et al. Implications for clinical staging of metastatic cutaneous squamous carcinoma of the head and neck based on a multicenter study of treatment outcomes. Cancer. 2006; 106 (5):1078–1083
[21] Buethe D, Warner C, Miedler J, Cockerell CJ. Focus issue on squamous cell carcinoma: practical concerns regarding the 7th edition AJCC staging guidelines. J Skin Cancer 2011:1–9
[22] van Dijk MC, Aben KK, van Hees F, et al. Expert review remains important in the histopathological diagnosis of cutaneous melanocytic lesions. Histopathology. 2008; 52(2):139–146
[23] Shoo BA, Sagebiel RW, Kashani-Sabet M. Discordance in the histopathologic diagnosis of melanoma at a melanoma referral center. J Am Acad Dermatol. 2010; 62(5):751–756
[24] Hawryluk EB, Sober AJ, Piris A, et al. Histologically challenging melanocytic tumors referred to a tertiary care pigmented lesion clinic. J Am Acad Dermatol. 2012; 67(4):727–735
[25] Farmer ER, Gonin R, Hanna MP. Discordance in the histopathologic diagnosis of melanoma and melanocytic nevi between expert pathologists. Hum Pathol. 1996; 27(6):528–531
[26] Ackerman AB. Discordance among expert pathologists in diagnosis of melanocytic neoplasms. Hum Pathol. 1996; 27(11):1115–1116
[27] Okun MR. There are standards for the proper evaluation and reporting of moles and melanoma. Hum Pathol. 1998; 29(1):100–102
[28] Niebling MG, Haydu LE, Karim RZ, Thompson JF, Scolyer RA. Pathology review significantly affects diagnosis and treatment of melanoma patients: an analysis of 5011 patients treated at a melanoma treatment center. Ann Surg Oncol. 2014; 21(7):2245–2251
[29] Niebling MG, Haydu LE, Karim RZ, Thompson JF, Scolyer RA. Reproducibility of AJCC staging parameters in primary cutaneous melanoma: an analysis of 4,924 cases. Ann Surg Oncol. 2013; 20(12):3969–3975
[30] Massi G, LeBoit PE. Histological Diagnosis of Nevi and Melanoma, 2nd ed. New York, NY: Springer; 2014
[31] Bastian BC, LeBoit PE, Hamm H, Bröcker E-B, Pinkel D. Chromosomal gains and losses in primary cutaneous melanomas detected by comparative genomic hybridization. Cancer Res. 1998; 58(10):2170–2175
[32] Bastian BC, Olshen AB, LeBoit PE, Pinkel D. Classifying melanocytic tumors based on DNA copy number changes. Am J Pathol. 2003; 163(5):1765–1770
[33] North JP, Vemula SS, Bastian BC. Chromosomal Copy Number Analysis in Melanoma Diagnostics. In: Thurin M, Marincola FM, eds. Molecular Diagnostics for Melanoma: Methods and Protocols, Methods in Molecular Biology, Vol. 1102. New York, NY: Springer; 2014
[34] Gerami P, Jewell SS, Morrison LE, et al. Fluorescence in situ hybridization (FISH) as an ancillary diagnostic tool in the diagnosis of melanoma. Am J Surg Pathol. 2009; 33(8):1146–1156
[35] Gerami P, Busam K, et al. Utility of FISH in the diagnosis of melanocytic lesions. Dermatol Clin. 2012; 30:555–566
[36] Clemente C, Bettio D, Venci A, et al. A fluorescence in situ hybridization (FISH) procedure to assist in differentiating benign from malignant melanocytic lesions. Pathologica. 2009; 101(5):169–174
[37] Morey AL, Murali R, McCarthy SW, Mann GJ, Scolyer RA. Diagnosis of cutaneous melanocytic tumours by four-colour fluorescence in situ hybridisation. Pathology. 2009; 41(4):383–387
[38] Newman MD, Lertsburapa T, Mirzabeigi M, Mafee M, Guitart J, Gerami P. Fluorescence in situ hybridization as a tool for microstaging in malignant melanoma. Mod Pathol. 2009; 22(8):989–995
[39] Diaz A, Valera A, Carrera C, et al. Pigmented spindle cell nevus: clues for differentiating it from spindle cell malignant melanoma. A comprehensive survey including clinicopathologic, immunohistochemical, and FISH studies. Am J Surg Pathol. 2010; 34:816–821
[40] Gerami P, Beilfuss B, Haghighat Z, Fang Y, Jhanwar S, Busam KJ. Fluorescence in situ hybridization as an ancillary method for the distinction of desmoplastic melanomas from sclerosing melanocytic nevi. J Cutan Pathol. 2011; 38(4):329–334
[41] Gammon B, Beilfuss B, Guitart J, Gerami P. Enhanced detection of spitzoid melanomas using fluorescence in situ hybridization with 9p21 as an adjunctive probe. Am J Surg Pathol. 2012; 36(1):81–88
[42] Gerami P, Li G, Pouryazdanparast P, et al. A highly specific and discriminatory FISH assay for distinguishing between benign and malignant melanocytic neoplasms. Am J Surg Pathol. 2012; 36(6):808–817
[43] Vergier B, Prochazkova-Carlotti M, de la Fouchardière A, et al. Fluorescence in situ hybridization, a diagnostic aid in ambiguous melanocytic tumors: European study of 113 cases. Mod Pathol. 2011; 24(5):613–623
[44] Moore MW, Gasparini R. FISH as an effective diagnostic tool for the management of challenging melanocytic lesions. Diagn Pathol. 2011; 6:76
[45] Gaiser T, Kutzner H, Palmedo G, et al. Classifying ambiguous melanocytic lesions with FISH and correlation with clinical long-term follow up. Mod Pathol. 2010; 23(3):413–419
[46] Cassarino DS, Lewine N, Cole D, Wade B, Gustavsen G. Budget impact analysis of a novel gene expression assay for the diagnosis of malignant melanoma. J Med Econ. 2014; 17(11):782–791
[47] Tuthill RJ, Reed RJ. Failure of senescence in the dysplasia-melanoma sequence: demonstration using a tissue microarray and a revised paradigm for melanoma. Semin Oncol. 2007; 34(6):467–475
[48] Lade-Keller J, Riber-Hansen R, Guldberg P, Schmidt H, Hamilton-Dutoit SJ, Steiniche T. Immunohistochemical analysis of molecular drivers in melanoma identifies p16 as an independent prognostic biomarker. J Clin Pathol. 2014; 67(6):520–528
[49] Ponti G, Tomasi A, Maiorana A, et al. BRAFp.V600E, p.V600K, and p.V600R mutations in malignant melanoma: do they also differ in immunohistochemical assessment and clinical features? Appl Immunohistochem Mol Morphol. 2016; 24(1):30–34
[50] Lee JH, Choi JW, Kim YS. Frequencies of BRAF and NRAS mutations are different in histological types and sites of origin of cutaneous melanoma: a meta-analysis. Br J Dermatol. 2011; 164(4):776–784
[51] Broekaert SM, Roy R, Okamoto I, et al. Genetic and morphologic features for melanoma classification. Pigment Cell Melanoma Res. 2010; 23(6):763–770
[52] Viros A, Fridlyand J, Bauer J, et al. Improving melanoma classification by integrating genetic and morphologic features. PLoS Med. 2008; 5(6):e120

[53] Scolyer RA, Long GV, Thompson JF. Evolving concepts in melanoma classification and their relevance to multidisciplinary melanoma patient care. Mol Oncol. 2011; 5(2):124–136
[54] Mar V, Roberts H, Wolfe R, English DR, Kelly JW. Nodular melanoma: a distinct clinical entity and the largest contributor to melanoma deaths in Victoria, Australia. J Am Acad Dermatol. 2013; 68(4):568–575
[55] Bastian BC. The molecular pathology of melanoma: an integrated taxonomy of melanocytic neoplasia. Annu Rev Pathol. 2014; 9:239–271
[56] Zebary A, Omholt K, Vassilaki I, et al. KIT, NRAS, BRAF and PTEN mutations in a sample of Swedish patients with acral lentiginous melanoma. J Dermatol Sci. 2013; 72(3):284–289
[57] Hong JW, Lee S, Kim DC, Kim KH, Song KH. Prognostic and clinicopathologic associations of BRAF mutation in primary acral lentiginous melanoma in Korean patients: a preliminary study. Ann Dermatol. 2014; 26(2):195–202
[58] Miller DD, Emley A, Yang S, et al. Mixed versus pure variants of desmoplastic melanoma: a genetic and immunohistochemical appraisal. Mod Pathol. 2012; 25(4):505–515
[59] Coupelon S, Franck F, Jarrousse AS, Déchelotte P, Souteyrand P, D'Incan M. Desmoplastic malignant melanoma: a study of ten cases and status of BRAF mutation. Dermatology. 2012; 225(2):168–171
[60] Wiesner T, Kiuru M, Scott SN, et al. NF1 mutations are common in desmoplastic melanoma. Am J Surg Pathol. 2015; 39(10):1357–1362
[61] Scolyer RA, Judge MJ, Evans A, et al. International Collaboration on Cancer Reporting. Data set for pathology reporting of cutaneous invasive melanoma: recommendations from the international collaboration on cancer reporting (ICCR). Am J Surg Pathol. 2013; 37(12):1797–1814
[62] Burton AL, Gilbert J, Farmer RW, et al. Regression does not predict nodal metastasis or survival in patients with cutaneous melanoma. Am Surg. 2011; 77(8):1009–1013
[63] Mills JK, White I, Diggs B, Fortino J, Vetto JT. Effect of biopsy type on outcomes in the treatment of primary cutaneous melanoma. Am J Surg. 2013; 205(5):585–590, discussion 590
[64] Azzola MF, Shaw HM, Thompson JF, et al. Tumor mitotic rate is a more powerful prognostic indicator than ulceration in patients with primary cutaneous melanoma: an analysis of 3661 patients from a single center. Cancer. 2003; 97(6):1488–1498
[65] Meng X, Zhong J, Liu S, Murray M, Gonzalez-Angulo AM. A new hypothesis for the cancer mechanism. Cancer Metastasis Rev. 2012; 31(1–2):247–268
[66] Ria R, Reale A, Castrovilli A, et al. Angiogenesis and progression in human melanoma. Dermatol Res Pract. 2010; 2010:185687
[67] Balch CM, Gershenwald JE, Soong SJ, et al. Final version of 2009 AJCC melanoma staging and classification. J Clin Oncol. 2009; 27(36):6199–6206
[68] Thompson JF, Soong S-J, Balch CM, et al. Prognostic significance of mitotic rate in localized primary cutaneous melanoma: an analysis of patients in the multi-institutional American Joint Committee on Cancer melanoma staging database. J Clin Oncol. 2011; 29(16):2199–2205
[69] de Waal AC, van Harten-Gerritsen AS, Aben KK, Kiemeney LA, van Rossum MM, Blokx WA. Impact of mitotic activity on the pathological substaging of pT1 cutaneous melanoma. Br J Dermatol. 2014; 170(4):874–877
[70] Chu VH, Tetzlaff MT, Torres-Cabala CA, et al. Impact of the 2009 (7th edition) AJCC melanoma staging system in the classification of thin cutaneous melanomas. BioMed Res Int. 2013; 2013:898719
[71] Weyers W. The magic of numbers: malignant melanoma between science and pseudoscience. Am J Dermatopathol. 2011; 33(4):371–378
[72] Cole CM, Ferringer T. Histopathologic evaluation of the sentinel lymph node for malignant melanoma: the unstandardized process. Am J Dermatopathol. 2014; 36(1):80–87
[73] Dekker J, Duncan LM. Lack of standards for the detection of melanoma in sentinel lymph nodes: a survey and recommendations. Arch Pathol Lab Med. 2013; 137(11):1603–1609
[74] Spanknebel K, Coit DG, Bieligk SC, Gonen M, Rosai J, Klimstra DS. Characterization of micrometastatic disease in melanoma sentinel lymph nodes by enhanced pathology: recommendations for standardizing pathologic analysis. Am J Surg Pathol. 2005; 29(3):305–317
[75] Murali R, DeSilva C, McCarthy SW, Thompson JF, Scolyer RA. Sentinel lymph nodes containing very small (< 0.1 mm) deposits of metastatic melanoma cannot be safely regarded as tumor-negative. Ann Surg Oncol. 2012; 19 (4):1089–1099
[76] Li LX, Scolyer RA, Ka VS, et al. Pathologic review of negative sentinel lymph nodes in melanoma patients with regional recurrence: a clinicopathologic study of 1152 patients undergoing sentinel lymph node biopsy. Am J Surg Pathol. 2003; 27(9):1197–1202
[77] McKenna DB, Lee RJ, Prescott RJ, Doherty VR. The time from diagnostic excision biopsy to wide local excision for primary cutaneous malignant melanoma may not affect patient survival. Br J Dermatol. 2002; 147(1):48–54
[78] Carpenter S, Pockaj B, Dueck A, et al. Factors influencing time between biopsy and definitive surgery for malignant melanoma: do they impact clinical outcome? Am J Surg. 2008; 196(6):834–842, discussion 842–843
[79] Scanlon P, Tian J, Zhong J, et al. Enhanced immunohistochemical detection of neural infiltration in primary melanoma: is there a clinical value? Hum Pathol. 2014; 45(8):1656–1663
[80] Rose AE, Christos PJ, Lackaye D, et al. Clinical relevance of detection of lymphovascular invasion in primary melanoma using endothelial markers D2-40 and CD34. Am J Surg Pathol. 2011; 35(10):1441–1449
[81] Storr SJ, Safuan S, Mitra A, et al. Objective assessment of blood and lymphatic vessel invasion and association with macrophage infiltration in cutaneous melanoma. Mod Pathol. 2012; 25(4):493–504
[82] Pasquali S, Haydu LE, Scolyer RA, et al. The importance of adequate primary tumor excision margins and sentinel node biopsy in achieving optimal locoregional control for patients with thick primary melanomas. Ann Surg. 2013; 258(1):152–157
[83] McKinnon JG, Starritt EC, Scolyer RA, McCarthy WH, Thompson JF. Histopathologic excision margin affects local recurrence rate: analysis of 2681 patients with melanomas < or = 2 mm thick. Ann Surg. 2005; 241 (2):326–333
[84] Thompson JF, Ollila DW. Optimum excision margins for melanoma. Lancet. 2011; 378(9803):1608–1610
[85] Sladden MJ, Balch C, Barzilai DA, et al. Surgical excision margins for primary cutaneous melanoma. Cochrane Database Syst Rev. 2009(4):CD004835
[86] Tuthill RJ, Unger JM, Liu PY, Flaherty LE, Sondak VK, Southwest Oncology Group. Risk assessment in localized primary cutaneous melanoma: a Southwest Oncology Group study evaluating nine factors and a test of the Clark logistic regression prediction model. Am J Clin Pathol. 2002; 118(4):504–511
[87] Taylor RC, Patel A, Panageas KS, Busam KJ, Brady MS. Tumor-infiltrating lymphocytes predict sentinel lymph node positivity in patients with cutaneous melanoma. J Clin Oncol. 2007; 25(7):869–875
[88] Azimi F, Scolyer RA, Rumcheva P, et al. Tumor-infiltrating lymphocyte grade is an independent predictor of sentinel lymph node status and survival in patients with cutaneous melanoma. J Clin Oncol. 2012; 30(21):2678–2683
[89] Thomas NE, Busam KJ, From L, et al. Tumor-infiltrating lymphocyte grade in primary melanomas is independently associated with melanoma-specific survival in the population-based genes, environment and melanoma study. J Clin Oncol. 2013; 31(33):4252–4259
[90] Taube JM, Klein A, Brahmer JR, et al. Association of PD-1, PD-1 ligands, and other features of the tumor immune microenvironment with response to anti-PD-1 therapy. Clin Cancer Res. 2014; 20(19):5064–5074
[91] Topalian SL, Hodi FS, Brahmer JR, et al. Safety, activity, and immune correlates of anti-PD-1 antibody in cancer. N Engl J Med. 2012; 366 (26):2443–2454
[92] Lipson EJ, Velculescu VE, Pritchard TS, et al. Circulating tumor DNA analysis as a real-time method for monitoring tumor burden in melanoma patients undergoing treatment with immune checkpoint blockade. J Immunother Cancer. 2014; 2(1):42
[93] Sanmamed MF, Fernández-Landázuri S, Rodríguez C, et al. Quantitative cell-free circulating BRAFV600E mutation analysis by use of droplet digital PCR in the follow-up of patients with melanoma being treated with BRAF inhibitors. Clin Chem. 2015; 61(1):297–304
[94] Gerami P, Cook RW, Wilkinson J, et al. Development of a prognostic genetic signature to predict the metastatic risk associated with cutaneous melanoma. Clin Cancer Res. 2015; 21(1):175–183
[95] Feng H, Shuda M, Chang Y, Moore PS. Clonal integration of a polyomavirus in human Merkel cell carcinoma. Science. 2008; 319(5866):1096–1100
[96] Erstad DJ, Jr JC. Mutational analysis of Merkel cell carcinoma. Cancers (Basel). 2014; 6(4):2116–2136
[97] Foulongne V, Sauvage V, Hebert C, et al. Human skin microbiota: high diversity of DNA viruses identified on the human skin by high throughput sequencing. PLoS One. 2012; 7(6):e38499
[98] Bichakjian CK, Olencki T, Alam M et al. NCCN Clinical Practice Guidelines in Oncology: Merkel Cell Carcinoma. Version 2. 2015. Available at: NCCN.org. Accessed January 2, 2015
[99] Andea AA, Coit DG, Amin B, Busam KJ. Merkel cell carcinoma: histologic features and prognosis. Cancer. 2008; 113(9):2549–2558
[100] Skelton HG, Smith KJ, Hitchcock CL, McCarthy WF, Lupton GP, Graham JH. Merkel cell carcinoma: analysis of clinical, histologic, and immunohistologic

features of 132 cases with relation to survival. J Am Acad Dermatol. 1997; 37 (5, Pt 1):734–739
[101] Llombart B, Monteagudo C, López-Guerrero JA, et al. Clinicopathological and immunohistochemical analysis of 20 cases of Merkel cell carcinoma in search of prognostic markers. Histopathology. 2005; 46(6):622–634
[102] Schwartz JL, Griffith KA, Lowe L, et al. Features predicting sentinel lymph node positivity in Merkel cell carcinoma. J Clin Oncol. 2011; 29 (8):1036–1041
[103] Fields RC, Busam KJ, Chou JF, et al. Five hundred patients with Merkel cell carcinoma evaluated at a single institution. Ann Surg. 2011; 254(3):465–473, discussion 473–475
[104] Sihto H, Kukko H, Koljonen V, Sankila R, Böhling T, Joensuu H. Merkel cell polyomavirus infection, large T antigen, retinoblastoma protein and outcome in Merkel cell carcinoma. Clin Cancer Res. 2011; 17(14):4806–4813
[105] Marcoval J, Ferreres JR, Penín RM, Pérez D, Viñals JM. Merkel cell carcinoma: differences between sun-exposed and non-sun-exposed variants–a clinical analysis of 36 cases. Dermatology. 2014; 229(3):205–209
[106] Higaki-Mori H, Kuwamoto S, Iwasaki T, et al. Association of Merkel cell polyomavirus infection with clinicopathological differences in Merkel cell carcinoma. Hum Pathol. 2012; 43(12):2282–2291
[107] Paulson KG, Iyer JG, Tegeder AR, et al. Transcriptome-wide studies of Merkel cell carcinoma and validation of intratumoral CD8+lymphocyte invasion as an independent predictor of survival. J Clin Oncol. 2011; 29(12):1539–1546
[108] Sihto H, Böhling T, Kavola H, et al. Tumor infiltrating immune cells and outcome of Merkel cell carcinoma: a population-based study. Clin Cancer Res. 2012; 18(10):2872–2881
[109] Sihto H, Joensuu H. Tumor-infiltrating lymphocytes and outcome in Merkel cell carcinoma, a virus-associated cancer. OncoImmunology. 2012; 1 (8):1420–1421
[110] Mott RT, Smoller BR, Morgan MB. Merkel cell carcinoma: a clinicopathologic study with prognostic implications. J Cutan Pathol. 2004; 31(3):217–223
[111] Fritsch VA, Camp ER, Lentsch EJ. Sentinel lymph node status in Merkel cell carcinoma of the head and neck: not a predictor of survival. Head Neck. 2014; 36(4):571–579
[112] Fields RC, Busam KJ, Chou JF, et al. Recurrence and survival in patients undergoing sentinel lymph node biopsy for Merkel cell carcinoma: analysis of 153 patients from a single institution. Ann Surg Oncol. 2011; 18 (9):2529–2537
[113] Sattler E, Geimer T, Sick I, et al. Sentinel lymph node in Merkel cell carcinoma: to biopsy or not to biopsy? J Dermatol. 2013; 40(5):374–379
[114] Sadeghi R, Adinehpoor Z, Maleki M, Fallahi B, Giovanella L, Treglia G. Prognostic significance of sentinel lymph node mapping in Merkel cell carcinoma: systematic review and meta-analysis of prognostic studies. BioMed Res Int. 2014; 2014:489536
[115] Tseng J, Dhungel B, Mills JK, et al. Merkel cell carcinoma: what makes a difference? Am J Surg. 2015; 209(2):342–346
[116] NCCN Clinical Practice Guidelines in Oncology (NCCN Guidelines) Merkel Cell Carcinoma Version 1.2017-October 3, 2016. http://www.nccn.org/professionals/physician_gls/pdf/mcc.pdf Accessed January 21, 2015
[117] Ko JS, Prieto VG, Elson PJ, et al. Histological pattern of Merkel cell carcinoma sentinel lymph node metastasis improves stratification of Stage III patients. Mod Pathol. 2016; 29(2):122–130
[118] Brenn T. Pleomorphic dermal neoplasms: a review. Adv Anat Pathol. 2014; 21(2):108–130
[119] Weiss SW, Goldblum JR. Malignant vascular tumors. In: Enzinger and Weiss's Soft Tissue Tumors. 5th ed. Philadelphia, PA: Mosby; 2008: 703–32
[120] Ko JS, Billings SD, Lanigan CP, Buehler D, Fernandez AP, Tubbs RR. Fully automated dual-color dual-hapten silver in situ hybridization staining for MYC amplification: a diagnostic tool for discriminating secondary angiosarcoma. J Cutan Pathol. 2014; 41(3):286–292
[121] Antonescu C. Malignant vascular tumors–an update. Mod Pathol. 2014; 27 Suppl 1:S30–S38
[122] Deyrup AT, McKenney JK, Tighiouart M, Folpe AL, Weiss SW. Sporadic cutaneous angiosarcomas: a proposal for risk stratification based on 69 cases. Am J Surg Pathol. 2008; 32(1):72–77
[123] Perez MC, Padhya TA, Messina JL, et al. Cutaneous angiosarcoma: a single-institution experience. Ann Surg Oncol. 2013; 20(11):3391–3397
[124] Seinen JM, Styring E, Verstappen V, et al. Radiation-associated angiosarcoma after breast cancer: high recurrence rate and poor survival despite surgical treatment with R0 resection. Ann Surg Oncol. 2012; 19(8):2700–2706
[125] Albores-Saavedra J, Schwartz AM, Henson DE, et al. Cutaneous angiosarcoma. Analysis of 434 cases from the Surveillance, Epidemiology, and End Results Program, 1973–2007. Ann Diagn Pathol. 2011; 15(2):93–97
[126] Miller K, Goodlad JR, Brenn T. Pleomorphic dermal sarcoma: adverse histologic features predict aggressive behavior and allow distinction from atypical fibroxanthoma. Am J Surg Pathol. 2012; 36(9):1317–1326
[127] Liang CA, Jambusaria-Pahlajani A, Karia PS, Elenitsas R, Zhang PD, Schmults CD. A systematic review of outcome data for dermatofibrosarcoma protuberans with and without fibrosarcomatous change. J Am Acad Dermatol. 2014; 71(4):781–786
[128] Ugurel S, Mentzel T, Utikal J, et al. Neoadjuvant imatinib in advanced primary or locally recurrent dermatofibrosarcoma protuberans: a multicenter phase II DeCOG trial with long-term follow-up. Clin Cancer Res. 2014; 20 (2):499–510
[129] Fields RC, Hameed M, Qin LX, et al. Dermatofibrosarcoma protuberans (DFSP): predictors of recurrence and the use of systemic therapy. Ann Surg Oncol. 2011; 18(2):328–336
[130] Farma JM, Ammori JB, Zager JS, et al. Dermatofibrosarcoma protuberans: how wide should we resect? Ann Surg Oncol. 2010; 17(8):2112–2118
[131] DuBay D, Cimmino V, Lowe L, Johnson TM, Sondak VK. Low recurrence rate after surgery for dermatofibrosarcoma protuberans: a multidisciplinary approach from a single institution. Cancer. 2004; 100(5):1008–1016

12 High-Risk Cutaneous Malignancies

Sashank K. Reddy and Anthony P. Tufaro

12.1 Introduction

While the incidence of cutaneous malignancies has been rising in the general population, it has been particularly notable in certain groups, whom we term high-risk patients. Broadly, these patients can be divided into two categories: (1) those with genetic syndromes conferring a predisposition to skin cancer and (2) immunosuppressed patients. The types and numbers of malignancies acquired, the aggressiveness of tumors, the age of onset, their management, and their ultimate outcome differ in important ways in high-risk patients and in the general population. Here, we review contemporary understanding of the etiologies of and approaches to cutaneous malignancies in high-risk patients.

12.2 Genetic Syndromes

Several genetic syndromes increase the risk of developing cutaneous malignancies. These include xeroderma pigmentosum (XP), Gorlin's syndrome, Fanconi anemia, Bazex's syndrome, and Bloom's syndrome, among others.[1] Below we focus on two of these rare conditions—XP and Gorlin's syndrome—that confer a predilection for nonmelanoma skin cancers, and we also consider genetic predisposition to melanoma.

12.2.1 Xeroderma Pigmentosum

XP comprises a group of disorders with autosomal recessive inheritance and a prevalence in the United States of 1:250,000 individuals. It is characterized by defects in genes involved in the nucleotide excision repair (NER) pathway of deoxyribonucleic acid (DNA) repair. This pathway is critical for resolving mutagenic adducts in DNA that result from ultraviolet (UV) exposure. Since the pathway is defective in XP patients, their keratinocytes accumulate numerous mutations, leading to accelerated tumorigenesis.

Clinically, XP patients have normal skin at birth, but most show extreme photosensitivity with sunburn occurring even in infancy.[2] Affected children develop innumerable freckles and other areas of hypopigmentation and hyperpigmentation. Such patients have a 10,000-fold increase in incidence of developing nonmelanoma skin cancer and a 2,000-fold increase in incidence of melanoma.[2] Nonmelanoma skin cancers mainly occur on sun-exposed regions, with 80% occurring on the face, head, and neck.[3] By contrast, approximately 45% of melanomas in these patients occur in the extremities. Not only do cutaneous malignancies occur more frequently in XP patients, but they also occur at an earlier age. The median age of onset for nonmelanoma skin cancer and melanoma are 9 and 22 years, respectively.[2] Both are several decades earlier than in the general population.

The most important step in management of XP patients is vigorous sun protection including avoiding peak sun exposure, use of UV-protective clothing and sunglasses, and window tinting. This should be complemented by vitamin D supplementation. If patients develop cutaneous malignancies, they are managed through disease- and stage-appropriate surgical and medical therapies. With these measures, some patients with XP live well into adulthood.[4]

12.2.2 Gorlin's Syndrome

Gorlin's syndrome, or nevoid basal cell carcinoma (BCC) syndrome, is a rare autosomal dominant disorder in which patients develop BCCs, odontogenic keratocysts, and palmar or plantar pits. Affected patients can also show various bony developmental defects. Patients with Gorlin's syndrome develop numerous BCCs in their lifetime—up to thousands in some cases.[5] Gorlin's syndrome patients with fairer skin are at particularly high risk.[5,6,7]

Alterations in the Hedgehog (Hh) pathway—a developmental cascade involved in cell growth and differentiation—underlie Gorlin's syndrome in many patients. Specifically, germline mutations in the pathway inhibitor Patched (*PTCH1*) are the most commonly identified molecular lesions in patients with Gorlin's syndrome.[8] In the absence of *PTCH1* activity, the protein smoothened (SMO) becomes constitutively active, leading to transcription of Hh pathway effectors. This is turn leads to dysregulation of cell growth and tumorigenesis. The recent clinical development of inhibitors of the Hh pathway, including several small molecule SMO inhibitors, provides hope for more efficacious treatment of patients with Gorlin's syndrome. Indeed, these agents not only reduce BCC tumor burden, but also remedy the odontogenic keratocysts and palmoplantar pits characteristic of the disorder.[8] Based on early clinical efficacy, vismodegib became the first SMO inhibitor to gain the approval of Food and Drug Administration (FDA) for patients with Gorlin's syndrome in 2012. Better handling of treatment-related adverse events and methods to combat resistance will be required, however, before these novel agents achieve their full promise.

12.2.3 Melanoma

Patients with familial atypical multiple mole melanoma (FAMMM) syndrome are at a greatly increased risk of developing melanoma and pancreatic cancer. The disease is defined by (1) melanoma in one or more first- or second-degree relatives, (2) high total body nevus count, including atypical nevi, and (3) specific histologic features of the nevi. FAMMM is inherited in autosomally dominant fashion with variable penetrance. In up to 40% of affected patients, mutations can be found in the *CDKN2A* gene which encodes the tumor suppressors p16INK4A and p14ARF.[9] These genes are important for establishing cell cycle arrest or senescence in damaged cells. In the absence of *CDKN2A* gene product activity, incipient tumor cells may be allowed to progress in the evolution to melanoma.

The large number of nevi that FAMMM patients develop increases the risk of malignant degeneration. Such patients should be screened at least every 6 months to document evolution of nevi. Total body photography and self-examination can be valuable adjuncts to identifying nevi requiring further investigation. Nevi whose appearance changes according to the asymmetry, border irregularity, color variegation, diameter, elevation or evolution (ABCDE) criteria should prompt early biopsy. Patients and their immediate family members should also be referred for genetic counseling. As the number of targeted therapies for melanoma increases, genetic sequencing may become part of the standard of care for such patients as well. As with spontaneously occurring melanomas, surgical excision is the mainstay of management when these lesions occur in FAMMM patients. Novel immunomodulatory agents for the treatment of aggressive melanomas will be discussed later.

12.3 Immunosuppression

The number of patients who are chronically immunosuppressed has increased markedly in recent decades. This reflects both natural and iatrogenic causes. The emergence and rapid spread of human immunodeficiency virus (HIV) since the 1980s has produced millions of people with severe immunosuppression worldwide. Autoimmune diseases have also increased in prevalence over the past few decades, particularly in the developed world.[10] This fact, coupled with the use of immunosuppressive medications, has left many people relatively immunosuppressed during the chronic courses of these diseases. The development of effective immunosuppressive agents has also heralded a large increase in organ transplantation since the pioneering operations of the 1960s. While allogeneic transplants have saved or improved thousands of lives, the requirement for lifelong immunosuppression has deleterious consequences. Most notably, patients with long-term natural or therapeutical immunosuppression show an increased incidence of cutaneous malignancies and other cancers. Indeed, the spectrum of malignancies encountered in patients with HIV/acquired immune deficiency syndrome (AIDS) parallels that of patients on chronic immunosuppression. One recent meta-analysis found an increased incidence of 20 of 28 cancer types in transplant and HIV/AIDS patients when compared with the general populace.[11] This suggests that immunosuppression itself can contribute to the development of cancer. Below, we first consider the mechanisms by which immunosuppression may promote cutaneous malignancy. Then we review specific cases of natural and iatrogenic immunosuppression and consider implications for the emergence and management of cutaneous malignancies.

12.4 Basic Science

12.4.1 Immune Surveillance

The concept that the immune system may control or eliminate malignancies was formally proposed by Thomas and Burnet more than five decades ago.[12,13] Burnet argued that since cells of long-lived animals naturally accumulate mutations, some of which are tumorigenic, it is evolutionarily advantageous for the immune system to eliminate these cells.[13] In its strictest form, this tumor surveillance concept remains controversial, in part because of the difficulty of proving a negative—incipient tumors eliminated by the immune system are not detected in the clinic. However, a number of lines of evidence at least indirectly support the notion that the immune system suppresses cancer development.

If the immune system naturally suppresses cancer growth or spread, one would predict that patients with impaired immunity would be at higher risk of developing malignancy. This is indeed the case, both in patients with inherited and acquired immunodeficiency. Patients with common variable immunodeficiency (CVID) who have deficits in antibody-mediated immunity display an increased risk for lymphoma and various carcinomas.[14,15] Patients with X-linked immunodeficiency with hyper-IgM (immunoglobulin M) and those with selective IgA (immunoglobulin A) deficiency are at higher risk for a variety of gastrointestinal malignancies.[15,16] These examples demonstrate that severe, inherited immunodeficiency predisposes patients to cancer development, but the rarity of these genetic syndromes limits the generalizability of this finding. Just because some patients with inherited immunodeficiency develop cancer more frequently, it does not follow that the immune system in the much larger group of healthy individuals naturally prevents tumor development.

More persuasive evidence in this regard comes from patients who are therapeutically immunosuppressed for autoimmune disease or for transplantation. It is estimated that over half a million patients have received organ transplants in the United States and the increased incidence of various malignancies in these patients has been amply documented. A recent study of 175,000 solid organ transplant recipients in the United States revealed an increased risk for 32 types of cancer in patients who had undergone lung, liver, heart, and kidney transplantation.[17] Notably, the risk was increased both for tumors known to be caused by oncogenic viruses (implying that a decrease in antiviral immunity may contribute) and for those in which no viral cause is known (suggesting that impaired immune surveillance may play a role).[17] Strikingly, in a prospective trial of kidney transplant patients on cyclosporine, the incidence of malignancies increased in a dose-dependent fashion and the majority of these were cutaneous malignancies.[18]

The increased risk of carcinogenesis in this group is not solely explained by decreased tumor surveillance, however. Several of the agents used in immunosuppressive regimens are themselves carcinogenic. In experimental studies, cyclosporine was shown to increase adenocarcinoma invasiveness and tumor growth even in mice that are already immunocompromised.[19] Similarly, in squamous cell carcinoma (SCC) samples from patients treated with cyclosporine, there was a significant increase in the level of activating transcription factor 3 (ATF3), a transcription factor that can impair p53-dependent cellular senescence and thereby promote tumorigenesis.[20] As with cyclosporine, use of the immunosuppressive drug azathioprine is associated with an increased risk of malignancy, in this case SCC.[21] It is thought that azathioprine enhances photosensitivity, leading to a direct increase in mutagenic adducts in the deoxyribonucleic acid (DNA) of keratinocytes.[22] In summary, the greater propensity for tumorigenesis in transplant recipients likely reflects an interplay between impaired immune surveillance, long-term exposure to carcinogenic drugs, and heightened sensitivity to environmental carcinogens such as UV light and oncogenic viruses.

Further evidence for the tumor surveillance hypothesis can be gleaned from studies on patients infected with HIV. If untreated, these patients have decreased numbers of circulating $CD4^+$ (cluster of differentiation 4+) T cells and consequent deficits in adaptive immunity. Patients with HIV show an increased propensity to develop malignancies that are both related and unrelated to oncogenic viruses. Risks of Kaposi's sarcoma (KS), lymphoma, and cervical, anal, and hepatocellular carcinoma are all elevated in patients with HIV.[23,24,25] Lung cancer and multiple myeloma risks are also elevated.[23,24,25] KS, non-Hodgkin's lymphoma, and cervical cancer become much more prevalent as $CD4^+$ counts drop and are therefore among the AIDS-defining illnesses.[26] Interestingly, even lung cancer incidence is inversely correlated to $CD4^+$ counts, despite the lack of a known viral etiology.[25,27] This last fact in particular supports the notion that the immune system naturally suppresses cancer development.

Perhaps, the most striking evidence of tumor surveillance is provided by the presence of immune cell infiltrates in many tumors and the ability of these cells to clear even advanced disease when sufficiently activated. Increasing numbers of infiltrating T cells have been shown to correlate with improved prognosis in a number of cancers, including those of lung, breast, and colon.[26,28,29,30] Similarly, it had long been clinically observed that some melanomas spontaneously regress. Upon pathologic sampling of these tumors, dense infiltrates of T cells were found to be attacking melanoma cells.[31]

These observations coupled with the knowledge of cell surface proteins that downregulate T cell function led to the development of a novel class of cancer therapeutics aimed at activating the immune system. These immunostimulatory medications are monoclonal antibodies that target one of two cell surface proteins—cytotoxic T-lymphocyte associated protein 4 (CTLA4) or programmed death 1 protein (PD1). Ipilimumab, the first anti-CTLA4 monoclonal antibody to reach the market, was FDA approved on the strength of phase III clinical trials in patients with metastatic melanoma. In patients with stage III or IV melanoma who had failed previous therapies, treatment with ipilimumab improved overall survival, with a median overall survival of 10 months.[32] A second phase III trial in previously untreated patients showed improved overall survival with ipilimumab plus dacarbazine versus dacarbazine alone.[33] Recent long-term analysis of patients in this trial showed a 5-year survival of 18.2% in patients treated with ipilimumab plus dacarbazine versus only 8.8% for patients treated with dacarbazine alone.[34] Two anti-PD1 monoclonal antibodies have been recently approved in patients with advanced melanoma. Pembrolizumab was approved in an accelerated fashion in 2014 for patients with unresectable or metastatic melanoma. Preliminary results from a phase III trial presented at the 2014 Society of Melanoma Research Congress revealed that patients treated with pembrolizumab had improved progression-free survival and an overall response rate of at least 21 to 24%. Nivolumab, another humanized monoclonal antibody to PD-1, was approved for patients with melanoma that has progressed during treatment with ipilimumab. It showed strong efficacy in the Checkmate 066 Phase III trial in which 1-year survival was 73% compared to 42% for patients treated with dacarbazine.[35] Progression-free survival was also increased.

UV radiation has long been known to contribute to cutaneous malignancy. This is particularly true of UVB radiation, which has been shown to promote BCC or melanoma following intense exposure and SCC following more chronic exposure.[36,37] Irradiation by UVB has direct carcinogenic effects through the formation of mutagenic photoadducts in DNA as well as through generation of reactive oxygen species that attack DNA. Not surprisingly, a number of UV-associated mutations in oncogenes and tumor suppressors are found in the tumors of patients with cutaneous malignancies as well as in surrounding premalignant skin. A less appreciated role of UV radiation in promoting tumorigenesis is its contribution to immunosuppression. Seminal animal studies in the 1970s demonstrated that cutaneous malignancies in mice could be rejected when grafted onto immunocompetent recipients, but not by syngeneic animals first exposed to UV irradiation.[38,39] Subsequent studies revealed that irradiation induced regulatory T cells (Tregs) that can impair the immune system's ability to destroy tumor cells. The extension of these findings to the development of cutaneous malignancies in humans is plausible, but remains to be formally demonstrated. UV irradiation has been shown to decrease propensity for allergic responses such as delayed-type hypersensitivity or contact dermatitis, and indeed UV light exposure has been used as a therapy in atopic dermatitis. While this demonstrates that UV irradiation in humans can weaken allergic immune responses, these responses are not thought to be involved in controlling malignancies. Nonetheless, there is an indirect link between UV-mediated suppression of allergic responses and the development of cutaneous malignancies. Patients with a history of skin cancer were much more likely to have decreased contact hypersensitivity to a chemical irritant following UV irradiation compared to patients without skin cancer.[40] Thus, impaired allergic responses correlate with a history of cutaneous malignancy, but any causal link remains to be demonstrated. Mechanisms proposed to contribute to UV-induced immunosuppression include induction of the anti-inflammatory cytokine interleukin-10 as well as the depletion of antigen presenting cells in the skin.[41,42]

Taken together, the above findings demonstrate that patients with impaired immunity are at higher risk of developing a variety of malignancies, likely through impaired tumor surveillance coupled with the direct oncogenic effect of some immunosuppressive medications, UV light, and oncogenic viruses. They also demonstrate the potential of the immune system to clear cutaneous malignancies when appropriately activated.

12.4.2 Oncogenic Viruses

A number of cancers are known to be caused, at least in part, by oncogenic viruses. In the setting of immunosuppression, latent viral infections can be reactivated and the ability to respond to ongoing infections is compromised. Therefore, some virally mediated cancers occur more frequently in immunosuppressed patients.[43] Cancers associated with viral infection include KS (human herpes virus 8), lymphoma (Epstein Barr virus), cervical and anal carcinoma (human papilloma virus [HPV]), and hepatocellular carcinoma (hepatitis B and C viruses). HPV DNA has been detected in patients with nonmelanoma skin cancer, in particular up to 80% of SCC samples in some studies.[44] Interestingly, HPV DNA is found more commonly in sun-exposed skin compared to protected skin, suggesting a potential synergy between UV irradiation and infection. However, the particularly high-risk serotypes of HPV are not always found in SCC lesions. These HPV serotypes express proteins that inactivate the tumor suppressors p53 and Rb, but SCCs often have direct mutations in p53 and Rb pathway components, obviating a need for the virally expressed proteins.[45] The exact contributions of decreased tumor surveillance, unchecked viral oncogenesis, or both to the increased incidence of nonmelanoma skin cancer in immunocompromised patients remain to be determined.

Further evidence of a viral contribution to skin cancer in immunosuppressed patients can be found from Merkel cell carcinoma (MCC). This rare, very aggressive neuroendocrine tumor of the skin is associated with Merkel cell polyomavirus (MCV). Immunocompromised patients are 15 times more likely to develop MCC than their immunocompetent counterparts and they are diagnosed with the malignancy an average of 10 years earlier.[46] As with nonmelanoma skin cancer, MCC is more aggressive in immunocompromised patients with 56% of patients succumbing to their disease in one study with a mean time from diagnosis to death of only 13 months.[47]

12.5 Mechanisms of Immunosuppression and Association with Cutaneous Malignancies

12.5.1 Human Immunodeficiency Virus

HIV is the leading cause of acquired immunodeficiency in the world with an estimated 35 million people infected as of 2013 (World Health Organization). HIV attacks $CD4^+$ T cells, the helper T cells that orchestrate immune responses to pathogens and also coordinate tumor surveillance. Untreated, HIV depletes the body of this vital cell population. When $CD4^+$ T cell counts fall sufficiently, a host of attendant illnesses and opportunistic infections occur. These define the AIDS.

The link between HIV infection and cutaneous malignancy is longstanding. The emergence of KS in immunosuppressed homosexual men in the early 1980s led to KS being among the original AIDS-defining illnesses. KS is associated with human herpes virus 8 (HHV8), with nearly all patients exhibiting viral DNA in tumor samples.[48,49,50,51] The inverse relationship between KS and $CD4^+$ cell counts provides powerful evidence that the immune system can suppress this malignancy. Consistent with this, the incidence of KS has declined dramatically since the advent of combination antiretroviral therapy (cART), which preserves functional $CD4^+$ levels.[52] Further, initiation of cART has been shown to decrease KS lesion size and number and represents a critical component of treatment.[53,54]

Nonmelanoma skin cancers are the most frequent non-AIDS-defining cancers in HIV^+ patients.[55] In a large, retrospective study of over 4,000 HIV-infected patients followed between 1988 and 2003, 32% of all malignancies were BCC and 16% were SCC. Patients who have progressed to AIDS have a threefold to fivefold higher risk of developing nonmelanoma skin cancers.[56,57] The high incidence of nonmelanoma skin cancers in HIV^+ patients may not be surprising since these are also the most common cancers in the general population. However, other characteristics of these tumors may differ in HIV^+ patients. One study from the University of California, San Francisco, found earlier age of onset, higher risk of local recurrence and metastasis, and a higher lethality of SCCs in patients with HIV. Interestingly, BCC is found more frequently than SCC in the HIV^+ patient population, mirroring the distribution of these tumors in the general populace. As discussed below, this is in contrast to transplant patients who show a relative propensity of SCC. Whether this reflects differences in virally versus chemically mediated immunosuppression or other factors remains to be seen.

The aggressive nature of SCC in HIV^+ patients necessitates vigilance and aggressive management. Wilkins and colleagues recommend early biopsy of suspicious cutaneous lesions along with frequent monitoring for possible recurrence or metastasis.[58] These patients should be considered for sentinel node mapping for tumors presenting with an aggressive clinical presentation. These include recurrent lesions, tumors with depth of invasion more than 2 mm, tumors that exhibit perineural or lymphatic/vascular invasion, and poorly differentiated tumors. Tumors more than 2 cm in diameter on the trunk and 0.6 cm on the "mask" areas of the face, genitalia, hands, and feet are more likely to behave aggressively as well. Adjunctive therapies such as chemotherapy or radiation may also be considered.[58] Patients with BCC should be treated in the standard fashion with wide local excision.[58]

Melanoma—already the most aggressive of common cutaneous malignancies—is even more lethal in patients with HIV. In a case control study of HIV^+ and HIV^- patients with melanomas of the same subtype and thickness, outcomes were significantly worse in patients with HIV.[59] Both disease-free survival and overall survival were reduced among HIV^+ patients. Further, the time to melanoma recurrence in treated patients was inversely related to $CD4^+$ counts. This fact coupled with the recent success of immunostimulatory medications in treating advanced melanoma suggests that the immune system may play an important role in controlling this malignancy even in immunocompetent people. Management of melanoma in patients with HIV should follow standard treatment protocols with an emphasis on restoring or preserving immune function through cART. Use of new immunostimulatory medications for melanoma treatment in HIV^+ patients is a promising area for the future.

12.6 Organ Transplantation

The development of effective immunosuppressive medications in the 1980s enabled an enormous increase in lifesaving organ transplantation. The need for replacement organs greatly outstrips supply with over 123,000 patients on waiting lists in the United States (Organ Procurement and Transplantation Network) and the gap continues to widen. Nearly 30,000 organ transplants were performed in the United States in 2013 (organdonor.gov). Further advances in immunosuppressive regimens, surgical technique, and posttransplant care have increased life expectancies for transplant recipients. Five-year survival approaches 85% for kidney transplant recipients, 48% for lung transplant, and 70% for liver and heart transplant.[60] These advances have led to a large number of patients living long term with organ transplants. An estimated 140,000 transplant recipients live in the United States currently.[60]

The requirement for lifelong immunosuppression to prevent transplant rejection leaves these patients in a state of chronic immune deficiency. The deleterious consequences of transplant-associated immunosuppression include cardiovascular disease, heightened susceptibility to infections, and increased incidence of malignancies. Studies across transplant registry cohorts have revealed a twofold to fourfold increased risk of developing cancer in transplant patients relative to matched controls.[17] A recent study examined more than 175,000 transplant recipients in the United States over an 11-year period, considering data from transplant and cancer registries.[17] These patients had twice the risk of developing malignancies compared to the general population. The risk of developing cutaneous malignancies is particularly elevated among transplant patients with an estimated cumulative risk as high as 70%.[61,62,63] This makes cutaneous malignancy the most frequently encountered cancer type in transplant recipients. These cancers include SCC, BCC, KS, MCC, and cutaneous lymphoma.[64]

12.6.1 Biology

Cutaneous malignancies are not only more frequent in organ transplant recipients, but also exhibit a more aggressive course (▶ Fig. 12.1). Data from the Cincinnati Transplant Registry demonstrate that 5% of transplant patients with cutaneous malignancies ultimately succumb to these tumors compared with 1 to 2% of patients who had not been transplanted.[65] In kidney transplant patients, 13% of patients exhibit SCC recurrence in the 6 months following excision.[61] Patients with metastatic cutaneous malignancies have overall and disease-free survivals at 3 years of only 48% and 56%, respectively.[66]

The increased aggressiveness of cutaneous malignancies in transplant patients may be explained by alterations in tumor biology, impaired antitumor responses, or both. Evidence for the former comes from the observation that matrix metalloproteinase expression is elevated in SCCs from transplant recipients.[67,68] These proteins degrade the extracellular matrix and may thereby provide a path for local invasion and ultimate metastasis. Interestingly, alterations in the matrix metalloproteinase (MMP) profile are also found in surrounding nonmalignant skin of transplant recipients. This finding may play a role in the "field cancerization" that contributes to the high ultimate lesional burden in these patients. It is also likely that impaired tumor surveillance and antitumor immune response allow incipient cutaneous malignancies to grow relatively unchecked. When combined with the direct carcinogenic role of some immunosuppressive medications, this decrease in antitumor response and increase in MMP activity create a vicious cycle that promotes carcinogenesis.

12.6.2 Epidemiology

Nonmelanoma skin cancers including SCC and BCC are the most frequent cutaneous malignancies in transplant patients, accounting for 95% of observed tumors.[60,69] Unlike the general population, transplant recipients have a preponderance of SCC over BCC in a 4:1 ratio. Interestingly, this represents an inversion of the usual findings.[70,71,72,73] The risk of developing SCC is elevated 65-fold and the risk of BCC is elevated 10-fold relative to the general population.[74] As in the general population, these cancers tend to occur in sun-exposed regions such as the head and neck and upper extremities.[74] Other markers of UV-associated skin damage such as actinic keratoses are associated with an increased risk of nonmelanoma skin cancer in transplant recipients.[75] Interestingly, heart and lung transplant recipients have a higher overall risk of SCC development than do kidney transplant recipients, likely reflecting the more potent immunosuppressive regimens required for organ preservation in the former group.[60]

Melanoma risk is also elevated in organ transplant recipients. A threefold to fivefold increased risk of melanoma is present compared to the general population. These lesions occur with a mean duration of 5 years posttransplant.[60] In a study of nearly 90,000 transplant recipients over a 10-year period, Hollenbeak and colleagues found an incidence of melanoma of 55.9 cases per 100,000 individuals on an age-adjusted basis, which corresponds to a 3.6-fold greater risk compared to the general population.[76] Strikingly, among

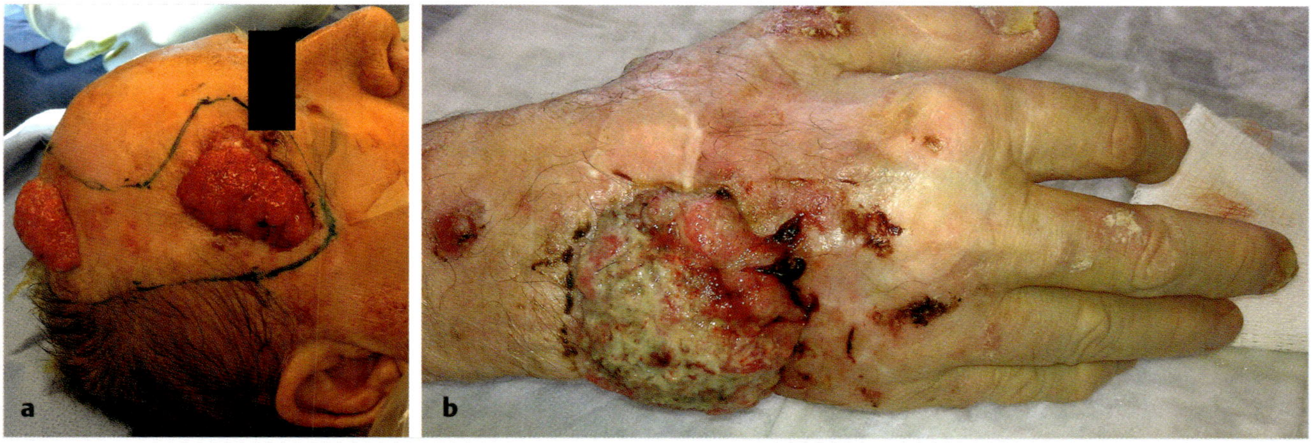

Fig. 12.1 Multifocal cutaneous malignancies in a transplant patient. This patient developed multiple aggressive squamous cell carcinoma (SCCs) of the face and hand after prolonged immunosuppression. **(a)** SCCs on the face. **(b)** SCC on the hand.

African-American kidney transplant recipients, the risk was 17.2-fold higher than in race-matched healthy counterparts. The remarkable success of immunostimulatory drugs in combating metastatic melanoma—a success all the more notable for the dismal natural history previously—points to an important interplay between the immune system and malignant melanocytes. Interestingly, oncogenic BRAF mutations appear less commonly in melanomas of transplant recipients.[77] This suggests that immunosuppressive medications may activate alternative pathways to promote melanomagenesis or that impaired immune surveillance abrogates the need for this oncogenic pathway.[77]

Other cutaneous malignancies are also found more commonly in transplant recipients. KS incidence in these patients occurs 84-fold to 500-fold more commonly, reflecting the extreme rarity of the tumor in immunocompetent people.[61,62,78] This lesion is more common among men and is found in regions of high HHV-8 seroprevalence including the Middle East and Central and Southern Africa.[79] MCC is found fivefold to 10-fold more frequently in organ transplant recipients, though the rarity of this malignancy overall makes reliable data difficult to obtain.[80,81] As is the case in immunocompetent people, MCC in transplant recipients is extremely aggressive. In a study of 41 solid organ transplant recipients who acquired MCC, the mean duration from transplantation to development of MCC was 7 to 8 years.[47] These tumors ultimately caused death in 56% of patients despite a mean follow-up period of only 18 months in the study.

The spectrum of cutaneous malignancies in transplant patients closely parallels that of patients infected with HIV.[11] A notable exception is the higher ratio of SCC to BCC, which is not found among HIV patients or among the general populace. Whether this reflects alterations in the etiology of these non-melanoma skin cancers by immunosuppressive drugs is an important area for future investigation.

12.6.3 Demographics

Incidence of cutaneous malignancies is positively correlated with the time since transplantation. In a study of transplant patients in the Netherlands, cumulative incidence of cutaneous malignancies increased from 10% at 10 years posttransplant to 40% after 20 years.[73] In the United States and Europe, SCC risk climbs from 10 to 27% at 10 years to 40 to 60% at 20 years.[60] Patients in Australia have a striking 80% incidence at 20 years.[60] The increased risk of skin cancer with time likely reflects the duration of immunosuppression as well as greater exposure to environmental carcinogens such as UV light.

Other characteristics that correlate with increased risk of cutaneous malignancy in transplant patients include male gender and older age.[82,83] Compared to the general population, however, skin cancers occur at a younger age in transplant recipients. Cutaneous malignancies are the second most frequently encountered cancers in pediatric transplant patients, following posttransplantation lymphoproliferative disorder (PTLD). These tumors typically manifest in young adulthood, with an average age of onset of 27 years.[84] Melanoma accounts for a proportionally higher percentage of skin cancers in pediatric transplant patients compared to adults.[85]

12.6.4 Risk Factors

Risk factors for developing cutaneous malignancies in transplant recipients parallel those in the general populace. History of a previous cutaneous malignancy places an individual at higher risk of acquiring another following organ transplantation.[75,82] Similarly, a history of actinic keratoses or leukemias and lymphomas also increase risk of cutaneous malignancy incidence following transplantation. UV radiation—particularly intense, intermittent exposure—has long been correlated with cutaneous malignancy risk and this risk is further elevated in transplant patients. Patients with light-colored eyes, hair, or skin such as those with Fitzpatrick types I to III are at higher risk because they are less shielded from the mutagenic effects of UV light.[59] As discussed above, infection with tumorigenic viruses increases the risk of cutaneous malignancy formation in transplant patients who are immunosuppressed.[43] These virus associated cancers include KS (HIV) and SCC (HPV). Finally, inherited cancer syndromes such as Gorlin's syndrome and XP increase incidence of cutaneous malignancies on their own and among transplant recipients.

12.6.5 Immunosuppressive Medications

To prevent rejection following solid organ transplantation, patients typically receive intense induction immunosuppression followed by a prolonged course of maintenance medications. Induction agents aim to deplete or impair T cell responses, which are critical to coordinating rejection. Biologic agents such as antithymocyte globulin (ATG), antilymphocyte globulin (ADG), muromonab (OKT3), or alemtuzumab (Campath) are used to deplete T cells. Other biologics include the anti-CD25 monoclonal antibodies basiliximab and daclizumab, which prevent interleukin-2 (IL-2) mediated T cell activation. Specific induction regimens vary between transplant centers, but they share the goal of preventing acute rejection and preparing the immune system for maintenance therapy. Some of these agents including ATG, OKT3, and anti-CD25 antibodies have been shown to increase the risk of cutaneous malignancy in heart transplant recipient.[86]

Traditional maintenance immunosuppression for most solid organ transplants requires three drugs: a calcineurin inhibitor (cyclosporine or tacrolimus), an antiproliferative agent (azathioprine, mycophenolate, sirolimus, or everolimus), and corticosteroids. These medications are typically taken for life. Acute rejection episodes require increases in immunosuppressive doses or the use of additional agents. If by contrast the graft is well tolerated, then maintenance dosing may be reduced or individual drugs may be eliminated. Many transplant centers are attempting minimal immunosuppressive strategies aimed at avoiding the deleterious consequences of long-term, high-dose immunosuppression. With respect to cutaneous malignancies, patients on traditional three drug regimens had an increased risk of cancer compared to patients treated with two drugs only.[71] Kidney transplant patients on triple therapy were 2.8 times more likely to acquire SCC than age-adjusted counterparts on azathioprine and prednisolone only.[71] This risk is further reduced when patients are treated on monotherapy with calcineurin inhibitors. In a retrospective study of kidney transplant patients over 40 years of age maintained on calcineurin inhibitors alone compared to those on dual or triple therapies, the former patients had a significantly decreased risk of developing SCC.[87] A trend toward decreased SCC risk was noted among patients of all ages, but this was not statistically significant. Patients on monotherapy had improved graft survival as well. Strikingly, the ratio of SCC to BCC was 1:2 in the monotherapy arm at the end of the 12-year observation period, approaching the 1:4 ratio observed in the general population. This is in contrast to patients on dual or triple therapy who showed the preponderance of SCC characteristic of transplant patients. Taken together, these data suggest that monotherapy with a calcineurin inhibitor ought to be preferred over dual and triple drug maintenance regimens in patients with a high risk of cutaneous malignancy. Nonetheless, even calcineurin inhibition alone carries a significant risk of cutaneous malignancy, particularly when accomplished by the drug cyclosporine. Cyclosporine has direct tumor-promoting properties in addition to inhibiting tumor surveillance. Thus, effective but safer maintenance strategies are still required.

One such approach is the use of immunosuppressive strategies incorporating inhibitors of the mammalian target of rapamycin (mTOR). These drugs—sirolimus and everolimus—accomplish immunosuppression by preventing the proliferation of T cells following antigenic challenge. Unlike cyclosporine, they are non-nephrotoxic, making them particularly valuable alternatives in the setting of kidney transplantation. Use of sirolimus is associated with a decreased risk of developing cutaneous malignancies when compared with cyclosporine. In kidney transplant recipients, the relative risk of developing both SCC and BCC was reduced in patients on sirolimus immunosuppression and the mean time to skin cancer appearance was increased.[88] Furthermore, conversion from calcineurin inhibitors to sirolimus in patients with known skin cancer may improve outcomes.[89,90] In one study of 53 kidney transplant patients with nonmelanoma skin cancer, 37 exhibited tumor regression.[90] Intriguingly, mTOR inhibitors have been shown to have direct antineoplastic effects in other cancer types. Numerous ongoing clinical trials aim to examine the efficacy of sirolimus and related inhibitors as cancer therapeutics. Early data from these trials have been encouraging for patients with metastatic renal cell carcinoma, neuroendocrine tumors of the pancreas, and certain kinds of breast cancers.[91] Prospective clinical trials to address the efficacy of sirolimus in treating cutaneous malignancies in transplant patients are ongoing.

Other minimal immunosuppressive or immunomodulatory strategies, such as the use of the CTLA4-Ig molecule belatacept as a single maintenance agent, have been attempted. These approaches are particularly valuable in life-enhancing transplants such as vascularized composite allotransplantation of hands or faces.[92] However, the benefit of these regimens in reducing cutaneous malignancy incidence remains to be demonstrated.

12.6.6 Patient Education and Prevention

The approach to cutaneous malignancies in transplant patients begins with prevention. Given the high propensity of these patients to develop skin cancer, every attempt must be made to address modifiable risk factors and to identify lesions early. Unfortunately, many transplant recipients do not remember being counseled on their increased risk for skin cancer.[93,94] These patients benefit from evaluation at dedicated transplant dermatology clinics before and after transplantation. Patients who are followed at such clinics have higher compliance with preventative measures and are more aware of the risks of cutaneous malignancy.[95,96] Pretransplantation visits should emphasize avoidance of intense sun exposure or tanning bed use, as well as use of sun-protective clothing and sunscreen. Existing skin lesions should be catalogued for future follow-up and suspicious lesions should be biopsied as warranted. This is particularly true in patients who show evidence of extensive cumulative exposure to UV light. These patients will have large areas of keratotic skin lesions including actinic keratoses, papillomas, and porokeratoses. Much of the skin in these areas will show evidence of epidermal dysplasia, which can be a precursor of epithelial malignancy. Thus, a large area of the skin in these patients is susceptible to malignant transformation—a concept termed "field cancerization." Keratotic skin lesions in these patients should be aggressively treated using cryosurgery, electrodessication and curettage, or topical 5-fluorouracil (5-FU).[97] Suspicious lesions should be biopsied early given that it can be difficult to distinguish premalignant lesions from SCC in areas of extensive damage.[98,99]

Transplant patients should be evaluated regularly in transplant dermatology clinics—at least yearly if there is no evidence of preexisting disease and as frequently as every 3 months in patients with aggressive SCC or melanoma.[93] There is evidence that exposure to preventative measures decreases the incidence of cutaneous malignancy. A prospective, case-control study of heart, kidney, or lung transplant patients compared patients who were given sun-protection education alone versus those given education and unlimited free sunscreen with instructions on application. Over the 2-year follow-up period, the latter group demonstrated statistically significantly fewer invasive SCCs and a nonsignificant trend toward decreased BCCs.[100]

12.6.7 Management of Cutaneous Malignancies in Transplant Patients

Once cutaneous malignancies appear, management is guided by their type and aggressiveness. Below we consider the role of destructive and extirpative modalities, sentinel lymph node biopsy (SLNB), radiation therapy, photodynamic therapy, and preventative and curative chemotherapy for various types of cutaneous malignancies.

12.6.8 Squamous Cell Carcinoma

A major meta-analysis by the Guidelines Committee of the International Transplant-Skin Cancer Collaborative divided SCC in transplant patients into less aggressive and more aggressive lesions, and established corresponding management strategies. Less aggressive lesions are defined as in ▶ Table 12.1.[97] Lesions with less aggressive characteristics on biopsy should be treated by destructive or excisional modalities. Destructive techniques include electrodessication and curettage or cryosurgery. These methods can be used alone or in combination and are particularly valuable in patients with multiple lesions. Excisional techniques include Mohs micrographic surgery and conventional resection with pathologic assessment of margins. Mohs surgery is the first choice for areas of high cosmetic sensitivity such as the face. It allows for high cure rates while minimizing resection of adjacent normal tissue.[97] Conventional surgical excision can be used in less critical anatomic regions or if the patient is not a candidate for Mohs surgery. In organ transplant patients, minimal margins are 4 to 6 mm.[101]

Aggressive SCCs are defined in ▶ Table 12.2. These are more common in transplant patients than in the general population. These lesions are best managed by a multidisciplinary team including surgical oncologists and plastic and reconstructive surgeons. At the time of presentation, a metastatic workup should first be performed for patients with aggressive SCCs. Ultimately, surgical excision by Mohs surgery or conventional methods is the mainstay of management. Numerous studies have documented the high cure rates achieved by Mohs surgery.[102,103,104] When Mohs surgery is not available or feasible, excision with intraoperative frozen section margin control is recommended. Excision with postoperative margin assessment only is not ideal, but when it is required, margins of 4 to 6 mm beyond surrounding erythema or subcutaneous invasion are required. The lymph node status of patients with aggressive SCCs should also be evaluated. Imaging with computed tomography (CT) or magnetic resonance imaging (MRI) can be useful in patients with high-thickness SCCs (> 6 mm) in high-risk areas.[93,105] Comprehensive regional lymph node dissection is recommended for patients with clinically palpable nodes. The role of sentinel node biopsy in patients with aggressive SCCs remains to be defined. One case series demonstrated a benefit to sentinel node biopsy in detecting early nodal metastases with a sensitivity of 88% and negative predictive value of 0.94.[106] These procedures can be performed with minimal morbidity by experienced practitioners and are therefore recommended in most cases. Further prospective studies are required, however, to determine which patients with aggressive SCCs would most benefit from sentinel node evaluation.

Numerous adjunctive modalities exist for patients with SCC. For patients with multiple lesions in areas of field cancerization, preventative therapies can be added following surgical excision. These include topical 5-FU, imiquimod, and photodynamic therapy.[93] Topical 5-FU can cause regression or elimination of premalignant lesions in some cases. Imiquimod is an immune modulator that has been approved for the treatment of SCCs

Table 12.1 Characteristics of less aggressive squamous cell carcinoma in transplant patients

Characteristic	
Size	< 0.6 cm on mask areas of face, genitalia, hands, feet < 1 cm cheeks, forehead, neck, scalp < 2 cm trunk and extremities
Growth rate	Static or slowly growing
Ulceration	No
Border	Distinct and well defined
Satellite lesions	No
Histology	In situ, keratoacanthoma type, well differentiated, invasion limited to papillary dermis, no neurotropism, no perivascular/intravascular invasion

Source: Adapted from Stasko T, Brown MD, Carucci JA, et al. Guidelines for the management of squamous cell carcinoma in organ transplant recipients. Dermatol Surg 2004;30(4, Pt 2):642–650.

Table 12.2 Characteristics of more aggressive squamous cell carcinoma (SCC) in transplant patients # M

Characteristic	
Number of lesions	Multiple SCCs
Size	> 0.6 cm on mask areas of face, genitalia, hands, feet > 1 cm cheeks, forehead, neck, scalp > 2 cm trunk and extremities
Growth	Rapid
Ulceration	Yes
Border	Indistinct clinical borders
Satellite lesions	Yes
Location	Central face, eyelids, eyebrows, periorbital, nose, lips, chin, mandible, preauricular or postauricular area, temple, ear, genitalia, digits
Occurrence in damaged skin	Occurrence in scar, area of chronic inflammation, or previous radiation
Recurrence	Tumor returns after previous treatment
Histology	Extension into subcutaneous fat, perineural invasion/inflammation, perivascular/intravascular infiltration, poorly differentiated

Source: Adapted from Stasko T, Brown MD, Carucci JA, et al. Guidelines for the management of squamous cell carcinoma in organ transplant recipients. Dermatol Surg 2004;30(4, Pt 2):642–650.

and BCCs. Several studies have documented its safety and efficacy in transplant patients. In treatment of actinic keratoses, for example, one multisite study found clearance rates of 62% for patients treated on imiquimod compared to 0% for controls.[107] Another study found a decrease in the incidence of SCCs in kidney transplant patients treated with imiquimod.[108]

Photodynamic therapy (PDT) is another adjunctive modality in the management of SCC. It entails topical application of a photosensitive chemical in affected areas of skin followed by light administration. Activation of the photosensitizer by light leads to formation of reactive oxygen species that destroy tumor cells. Perrett and colleagues compared PDT using the topical photosensitizer methyl aminolevulinate (MAL) to treatment with 5-FU in a small group of organ transplant recipients with epidermal dysplasia.[109] Nearly 90% of the lesions treated with PDT were cleared compared to only 11% treated with 5-FU. In addition, PDT was subjectively preferred by patients, and both patients and clinicians noted improved cosmetic outcome with PDT. This modality has also proven effective in the management of actinic keratoses in transplant recipients.[110] While PDT is effective in the management of premalignant lesions, whether it ultimately prevents the formation of SCC is less clear. One randomized controlled trial failed to demonstrate a benefit of PDT in SCC prevention at 2-year follow-up, while another smaller trial appeared to show a significant reduction in SCC incidence with PDT.[111,112] Firm conclusions on the role of PDT in preventing SCC in transplant patients will require larger studies. Nonetheless, the modality has a role in treating premalignant skin in these patients who are at high risk of developing cutaneous malignancy. In summary, for patients with less aggressive SCCs, 5-FU, imiquimod, and PDT can supplement surgical resection and treat premalignant epidermal dysplasia in areas of field cancerization.

Transplant patients with aggressive SCCs may benefit from other adjunctive modalities. Systemic retinoid administration can be used as a preventative measure for SCC in these patients. Due to the significant toxicities associated with this therapy, it should be reserved for patients with an extremely high propensity for SCC formation—5 to 10 lesions per year—or in those with particularly aggressive SCCs.[93] Retinoids such as acretin or isotretinoin are extremely teratogenic and are therefore absolutely contraindicated in women who are pregnant or may become pregnant. Acretin can lead to hyperlipidemia and liver dysfunction. These side effects must be carefully monitored and doses adjusted accordingly. Multiple studies have borne out the effectiveness of retinoids in preventing SCC in transplant recipients.[113,114,115,116,117] However, these medications must be continued indefinitely because treatment interruption can lead to more rapid and aggressive SCC formation.

Capecitabine—a prodrug of 5-FU—has also been used to good effect in patients with aggressive SCCs. In one small study of four patients with aggressive disease, complete regression was achieved in two patients.[118] Another case series of just three patients showed a decreased incidence of new SCCs over a 6-month period.[119] As with systemic retinoids, toxicities limit the use of capecitabine to patients with the most aggressive SCCs. Nephrotoxicity, neutropenia, and gastrointestinal toxicities require dose modification or elimination.

Radiotherapy can also be indicated in patients with aggressive SCCs or in patients in whom complete surgical resection cannot be achieved. Aggressive SCCs such as recurrent lesions, tumors with depth of invasion more than 2 mm, tumors more than 2 cm in diameter, tumors that exhibit perineural or lymphatic/vascular invasion, or poorly differentiated tumors all carry poorer prognosis and may benefit from radiotherapy. A review of 167 patients treated over 20 years with surgery and radiation or surgery alone demonstrated a clear benefit to multimodal therapy with such patients having lower recurrence and improved long-term survival.[120] As this study was carried out in immunocompetent patients, it remains to be seen whether similar improvements in outcome can be achieved in patients with SCCs following organ transplantation.

In transplant patients with SCC, alterations in immunosuppressive regimens may be warranted. Immunosuppression should always be reduced to the lowest level compatible with graft survival. Several studies have demonstrated the superiority of single or dual medication regimens over traditional triple immunosuppressive therapy in reducing risk of cutaneous malignancies.[71,87] In addition to reducing the number of agents, replacement of calcineurin inhibitors with mTOR inhibitors may further improve outcomes. Several studies have demonstrated decreased malignancy risk and improved outcomes in patients treated with the mTOR inhibitor sirolimus.[89,91] In one randomized, multicenter trial, patients with SCC who switched from calcineurin to sirolimus had longer cancer-free survival and an overall decreased incidence of new SCC development.[121] In addition, an ongoing clinical trial is testing whether sirolimus is effective in directly treating SCC among kidney transplant recipients.[122] For both decreasing the risk of new SCCs and potential treatment of existing SCCs, use of mTOR inhibitors in place of calcineurin inhibitors is recommended whenever feasible.

Transplant recipients who develop metastatic SCC fare more poorly than their immunocompetent counterparts.[66] Three-year disease-free survival is approximately 50%. Patients who are immunocompromised from transplantation or other malignancies have a higher rate of locoregional relapse following SCC treatment.[123] Adjunctive radiation therapy is of limited effectiveness in patients with metastatic SCC. Unlike patients with BCC, those with advanced SCC have a median time to recurrence of only 5 months in one study, and the majority of these patients succumb to their disease.[124] Traditional chemotherapeutic agents such as platinum-based compounds are also of limited efficacy.

Novel targeted therapeutics do show some promise in advanced SCC, however. One set of agents target epidermal growth factor receptor (EGFR) family members. These include the monoclonal antibodies cetuximab and panitumumab, and small molecules gefitinib and erlotinib. Cetuximab has been approved for the treatment of advanced SCC of the head and neck as a single agent and in combination with radiation and chemotherapy. Its role in the management of cutaneous SCC is being explored. A prospective phase II study of cetuximab in patients with unresecatable cutaneous SCC demonstrated an encouraging disease control rate at 6 weeks of nearly 70%.[125] It will be interesting to see if these results are confirmed in longer and larger phase III investigations. A phase II study of gefitinib revealed a complete response rate of 18% with acceptable tolerability, suggesting that this may be a useful agent alone or in combination with resection and/or radiotherapy.[126] Further studies to identify biomarkers predictive of response to gefitinib are also warranted.[122] Other molecular targets for advanced SCC such as the NOTCH and PI3K-AKT pathways are also being explored and may provide more therapeutic options in the future.[122]

12.6.9 Basal Cell Carcinoma

While BCC occurs much more frequently in transplant recipients compared to immunocompetent counterparts, it does not behave in a much more aggressive fashion. This is in contrast to SCC, which is more aggressive in transplant patients. Transplant patients with BCC are not more likely to succumb to their disease, nor do they suffer a higher incidence of metastasis.[127] Therefore, the management of BCC in these patients parallels the management in patients who are not immunosuppressed. A primary focus is on prevention, with counseling on sun avoidance and frequent surveillance being paramount. When locally contained BCCs do arise, destructive modalities such as electrodessication and curettage or cryoablation may suffice. Topical 5-FU can also be used for smaller lesions. Mohs micrographic surgery and conventional surgical resection offer an excellent chance of cure as well.

In patients who develop advanced disease, surgery with or without radiation is the traditional treatment of choice. Recently, targeted therapeutics that inhibit the Hh pathway have offered a medical alternative in patients with advanced BCC. These agents were developed following the discovery that mutations in the Hh pathway underlie familial BCC and many spontaneous cases.[128,129,130,131,132] Transplant recipients were excluded from the original trials establishing the efficacy of these agents, however. Recently, a case report documented the use of the Hh pathway inhibitor vismodegib in a heart transplant recipient with a history of multiply recurrent BCC.[133] After 24 weeks of therapy, he demonstrated stabilization of his disease and histologic evidence of tumor response to the agent. Further studies on the use of targeted therapies for BCC in transplant recipients are warranted.

12.6.10 Melanoma

Melanoma is among the most aggressive of cutaneous malignancies, and the clear role of the immune system in controlling melanoma makes the prospects of immunosuppression particularly fraught. The Melanoma Working Group of the International Transplant Skin Cancer Collaborative identifies three scenarios of particular concern: (1) patients with a history of melanoma who are contemplating organ transplantation, (2) potential donors with a history of melanoma, and (3) transplant recipients who develop melanoma de novo.[134] For patients with a history of melanoma, the decision to proceed with transplantation is in part based on Breslow thickness. Based on risk of recurrence, the Working Group suggest proceeding without delay in patients with melanoma in situ, waiting at least 2 years in patients with melanoma less than 2 mm and negative sentinel node biopsy, and waiting 5 years in patients with more than 2 mm lesions. Patients with nodal involvement or metastatic disease should not be transplanted. Of course, these recommendations must be tempered by the severity of the disease processes necessitating transplantation. Each situation should ideally be evaluated by a multidisciplinary team of transplant surgeons, immunologists, and dermatologists.

While rare, case reports of melanoma transmission from transplant donor to recipient have been published.[93] In one study, melanoma figured in 12 of 167 malignancies that were transferred from donor to recipient.[135] Clearly prevention should be paramount, with a whole-body skin examination performed prior to organ donation. When melanoma is passed from donor to recipient, consensus opinion favors removal of the transplanted organ and any resectable metastases coupled with discontinuation of immunosuppression.[134]

Once diagnosed, the mainstay of melanoma management in transplant recipients is surgical excision with margin control just as it is in immunocompetent individuals. Resection margins should follow guidelines based on Breslow thickness. Given the importance of lymph node status on prognosis and management in melanoma, patients with intermediate and thick melanomas should undergo SLNB at the time of tumor resection. Sentinel node sampling may even be considered in thinner melanomas given the more aggressive course of melanoma in transplant patients and the relatively low morbidity of SLNB. Lymph node dissection should be performed when feasible in patients with Stage III disease.[134]

Medical management of melanoma in transplant recipients begins with minimization of immunosuppression. Novel immunostimulatory molecules based on immune-checkpoint blockade should also be considered. As discussed earlier, these agents have shown encouraging results in patients with advanced disease. The first reports of immunostimulatory agents in treating melanoma among transplant recipients have been encouraging. Partial responses were achieved in two kidney transplant patients with metastatic melanoma who were treated with ipilimumab.[136] Interestingly, these patients did not develop episodes of acute rejection, which may reflect the longstanding nature of their transplants and possible tolerance to the grafts. These agents are beginning to be used in combination with molecularly targeted therapeutics such as BRAF inhibitors which aim to inhibit proteins critical to tumor progression.[137] If the toxicities associated with such combinations can be overcome, patients with advanced melanoma may achieve more durable responses to treatment.

12.7 Conclusion

Cutaneous malignancies are becoming more prevalent in developed countries. High-risk cutaneous malignancies resulting from inherited predisposition or immunosuppression are particularly devastating given their aggressive courses and propensity for recurrence. Prevention should be the foremost concern for providers who treat these patients. Sun avoidance and skin surveillance at dedicated dermatology clinics are critical. When cutaneous malignancies occur, prompt surgical and medical management, with alterations in immunosuppression when possible, is advised. The development of molecularly targeted therapies and immunomodulatory agents offers new hope to patients with these challenging conditions.

References

[1] Nikolaou V, Stratigos AJ, Tsao H. Hereditary nonmelanoma skin cancer. Semin Cutan Med Surg. 2012; 31(4):204–210

[2] DiGiovanna JJ, Kraemer KH. Shining a light on xeroderma pigmentosum. J Invest Dermatol. 2012; 132(3, Pt 2):785–796

[3] Kraemer KH, Lee MM, Andrews AD, Lambert WC. The role of sunlight and DNA repair in melanoma and nonmelanoma skin cancer. The xeroderma pigmentosum paradigm. Arch Dermatol. 1994; 130(8):1018–1021

[4] Oh KS, Emmert S, Tamura D, DiGiovanna JJ, Kraemer KH. Multiple skin cancers in adults with mutations in the XP-E (DDB2) DNA repair gene. J Invest Dermatol. 2011; 131(3):785–788

[5] Athar M, Li C, Kim AL, Spiegelman VS, Bickers DR. Sonic hedgehog signaling in Basal cell nevus syndrome. Cancer Res. 2014; 74(18):4967–4975

[6] Epstein EH. Basal cell carcinomas: attack of the hedgehog. Nat Rev Cancer. 2008; 8(10):743–754

[7] Kimonis VE, Mehta SG, Digiovanna JJ, Bale SJ, Pastakia B. Radiological features in 82 patients with nevoid basal cell carcinoma (NBCC or Gorlin) syndrome. Genet Med. 2004; 6(6):495–502

[8] Basset-Seguin N, Sharpe HJ, de Sauvage FJ. Efficacy of Hedgehog pathway inhibitors in Basal cell carcinoma. Mol Cancer Ther. 2015; 14(3):633–641

[9] Czajkowski R, Placek W, Drewa G, Czajkowska A, Uchańska G. FAMMM syndrome: pathogenesis and management. Dermatol Surg. 2004; 30(2, Pt 2):291–296

[10] Jacobson DL, Gange SJ, Rose NR, Graham NM. Epidemiology and estimated population burden of selected autoimmune diseases in the United States. Clin Immunol Immunopathol. 1997; 84(3):223–243

[11] Grulich AE, van Leeuwen MT, Falster MO, Vajdic CM. Incidence of cancers in people with HIV/AIDS compared with immunosuppressed transplant recipients: a meta-analysis. Lancet. 2007; 370(9581):59–67

[12] Burnet M. Cancer: a biological approach. III. Viruses associated with neoplastic conditions. IV. Practical applications. BMJ. 1957; 1(5023):841–847

[13] Burnet FM. The concept of immunological surveillance. Prog Exp Tumor Res. 1970; 13:1–27

[14] Kinlen LJ, Webster AD, Bird AG, et al. Prospective study of cancer in patients with hypogammaglobulinaemia. Lancet. 1985; 1(8423):263–266

[15] Mueller BU, Pizzo PA. Cancer in children with primary or secondary immunodeficiencies. J Pediatr. 1995; 126(1):1–10

[16] Hayward AR, Levy J, Facchetti F, et al. Cholangiopathy and tumors of the pancreas, liver, and biliary tree in boys with X-linked immunodeficiency with hyper-IgM. J Immunol. 1997; 158(2):977–983

[17] Engels EA, Pfeiffer RM, Fraumeni JF, Jr, et al. Spectrum of cancer risk among US solid organ transplant recipients. JAMA. 2011; 306(17):1891–1901

[18] Dantal J, Hourmant M, Cantarovich D, et al. Effect of long-term immunosuppression in kidney-graft recipients on cancer incidence: randomised comparison of two cyclosporin regimens. Lancet. 1998; 351 (9103):623–628

[19] Hojo M, Morimoto T, Maluccio M, et al. Cyclosporine induces cancer progression by a cell-autonomous mechanism. Nature. 1999; 397(6719):530–534

[20] Wu X, Nguyen BC, Dziunycz P, et al. Opposing roles for calcineurin and ATF3 in squamous skin cancer. Nature. 2010; 465(7296):368–372

[21] Bottomley WW, Ford G, Cunliffe WJ, Cotterill JA. Aggressive squamous cell carcinomas developing in patients receiving long-term azathioprine. Br J Dermatol. 1995; 133(3):460–462

[22] O'Donovan P, Perrett CM, Zhang X, et al. Azathioprine and UVA light generate mutagenic oxidative DNA damage. Science. 2005; 309(5742):1871–1874

[23] Clifford GM, Polesel J, Rickenbach M, et al. Swiss HIV Cohort. Cancer risk in the Swiss HIV Cohort Study: associations with immunodeficiency, smoking, and highly active antiretroviral therapy. J Natl Cancer Inst. 2005; 97(6):425–432

[24] Shiels MS, Cole SR, Kirk GD, Poole C. A meta-analysis of the incidence of non-AIDS cancers in HIV-infected individuals. J Acquir Immune Defic Syndr. 2009; 52(5):611–622

[25] Sigel K, Wisnivesky J, Gordon K, et al. HIV as an independent risk factor for incident lung cancer. AIDS. 2012; 26(8):1017–1025

[26] Corthay A. Does the immune system naturally protect against cancer? Front Immunol. 2014; 5:197

[27] Guiguet M, Boué F, Cadranel J, Lang JM, Rosenthal E, Costagliola D, Clinical Epidemiology Group of the FHDH-ANRS CO4 cohort. Effect of immunodeficiency, HIV viral load, and antiretroviral therapy on the risk of individual malignancies (FHDH-ANRS CO4): a prospective cohort study. Lancet Oncol. 2009; 10(12):1152–1159

[28] Al-Shibli KI, Donnem T, Al-Saad S, Persson M, Bremnes RM, Busund LT. Prognostic effect of epithelial and stromal lymphocyte infiltration in non-small cell lung cancer. Clin Cancer Res. 2008; 14(16):5220–5227

[29] Kawai O, Ishii G, Kubota K, et al. Predominant infiltration of macrophages and CD8(+) T Cells in cancer nests is a significant predictor of survival in stage IV nonsmall cell lung cancer. Cancer. 2008; 113(6):1387–1395

[30] Mahmoud SM, Paish EC, Powe DG, et al. Tumor-infiltrating CD8 + lymphocytes predict clinical outcome in breast cancer. J Clin Oncol. 2011; 29 (15):1949–1955

[31] Kluger HM, Zito CR, Barr ML, et al. Characterization of PD-L1 Expression and Associated T-cell Infiltrates in Metastatic Melanoma Samples from Variable Anatomic Sites. Clin Cancer Res. 2015; 21(13):3052–3060

[32] Hodi FS, O'Day SJ, McDermott DF, et al. Improved survival with ipilimumab in patients with metastatic melanoma. N Engl J Med. 2010; 363(8):711–723

[33] Robert C, Thomas L, Bondarenko I, et al. Ipilimumab plus dacarbazine for previously untreated metastatic melanoma. N Engl J Med. 2011; 364 (26):2517–2526

[34] Maio M, Grob JJ, Aamdal S, et al. Five-year survival rates for treatment-naive patients with advanced melanoma who received ipilimumab plus dacarbazine in a phase III trial. J Clin Oncol. 2015; 33(10):1191–1196

[35] Robert C, Long GV, Brady B, et al. Nivolumab in previously untreated melanoma without BRAF mutation. N Engl J Med. 2015; 372(4):320–330

[36] Rangwala S, Tsai KY. Roles of the immune system in skin cancer. Br J Dermatol. 2011; 165(5):953–965

[37] Kütting B, Drexler H. UV-induced skin cancer at workplace and evidence-based prevention. Int Arch Occup Environ Health. 2010; 83(8):843–854

[38] Kripke ML. Antigenicity of murine skin tumors induced by ultraviolet light. J Natl Cancer Inst. 1974; 53(5):1333–1336

[39] Kripke ML. Latency, histology, and antigenicity of tumors induced by ultraviolet light in three inbred mouse strains. Cancer Res. 1977; 37 (5):1395–1400

[40] Yoshikawa T, Rae V, Bruins-Slot W, Van den Berg JW, Taylor JR, Streilein JW. Susceptibility to effects of UVB radiation on induction of contact hypersensitivity as a risk factor for skin cancer in humans. J Invest Dermatol. 1990; 95 (5):530–536

[41] Cooper KD, Oberhelman L, Hamilton TA, et al. UV exposure reduces immunization rates and promotes tolerance to epicutaneous antigens in humans: relationship to dose, CD1a-DR + epidermal macrophage induction, and Langerhans cell depletion. Proc Natl Acad Sci U S A. 1992; 89(18):8497–8501

[42] Damian DL, Halliday GM, Barnetson RS. Broad-spectrum sunscreens provide greater protection against ultraviolet-radiation-induced suppression of contact hypersensitivity to a recall antigen in humans. J Invest Dermatol. 1997; 109(2):146–151

[43] Nindl I, Rösl F. Molecular concepts of virus infections causing skin cancer in organ transplant recipients. Am J Transplant. 2008; 8(11):2199–2204

[44] Dubina M, Goldenberg G. Viral-associated nonmelanoma skin cancers: a review. Am J Dermatopathol. 2009; 31(6):561–573

[45] Boukamp P. Non-melanoma skin cancer: what drives tumor development and progression? Carcinogenesis. 2005; 26(10):1657–1667

[46] Kassem A, Schöpflin A, Diaz C, et al. Frequent detection of Merkel cell polyomavirus in human Merkel cell carcinomas and identification of a unique deletion in the VP1 gene. Cancer Res. 2008; 68(13):5009–5013

[47] Penn I, First MR. Merkel's cell carcinoma in organ recipients: report of 41 cases. Transplantation. 1999; 68(11):1717–1721

[48] Antman K, Chang Y. Kaposi's sarcoma. N Engl J Med. 2000; 342 (14):1027–1038

[49] Moore PS, Chang Y. Detection of herpesvirus-like DNA sequences in Kaposi's sarcoma in patients with and without HIV infection. N Engl J Med. 1995; 332(18):1181–1185

[50] Dictor M, Rambech E, Way D, Witte M, Bendsöe N. Human herpesvirus 8 (Kaposi's sarcoma-associated herpesvirus) DNA in Kaposi's sarcoma lesions, AIDS Kaposi's sarcoma cell lines, endothelial Kaposi's sarcoma simulators, and the skin of immunosuppressed patients. Am J Pathol. 1996; 148 (6):2009–2016

[51] Ensoli B, Sgadari C, Barillari G, Sirianni MC, Stürzl M, Monini P. Biology of Kaposi's sarcoma. Eur J Cancer. 2001; 37(10):1251–1269

[52] Grabar S, Abraham B, Mahamat A, Del Giudice P, Rosenthal E, Costagliola D. Differential impact of combination antiretroviral therapy in preventing Kaposi's sarcoma with and without visceral involvement. J Clin Oncol. 2006; 24(21):3408–3414

[53] Cheung MC, Pantanowitz L, Dezube BJ. AIDS-related malignancies: emerging challenges in the era of highly active antiretroviral therapy. Oncologist. 2005; 10(6):412–426

[54] Di Lorenzo G, Konstantinopoulos PA, Pantanowitz L, Di Trolio R, De Placido S, Dezube BJ. Management of AIDS-related Kaposi's sarcoma. Lancet Oncol. 2007; 8(2):167–176

[55] Burgi A, Brodine S, Wegner S, et al. Incidence and risk factors for the occurrence of non-AIDS-defining cancers among human immunodeficiency virus-infected individuals. Cancer. 2005; 104(7):1505–1511

[56] Franceschi S, Dal Maso L, Arniani S, et al. Risk of cancer other than Kaposi's sarcoma and non-Hodgkin's lymphoma in persons with AIDS in Italy. Cancer and AIDS Registry Linkage Study. Br J Cancer. 1998; 78(7):966–970

[57] Goedert JJ, Coté TR, Virgo P, et al. Spectrum of AIDS-associated malignant disorders. Lancet. 1998; 351(9119):1833–1839

[58] Wilkins K, Turner R, Dolev JC, LeBoit PE, Berger TG, Maurer TA. Cutaneous malignancy and human immunodeficiency virus disease. J Am Acad Dermatol. 2006; 54(2):189–206, quiz 207–210

[59] Rodrigues LK, Klencke BJ, Vin-Christian K, et al. Altered clinical course of malignant melanoma in HIV-positive patients. Arch Dermatol. 2002; 138 (6):765–770

[60] Zwald FO, Brown M. Skin cancer in solid organ transplant recipients: advances in therapy and management: part I. Epidemiology of skin cancer in solid organ transplant recipients. J Am Acad Dermatol. 2011; 65 (2):253–261, quiz 262

[61] Euvrard S, Kanitakis J, Claudy A. Skin cancers after organ transplantation. N Engl J Med. 2003; 348(17):1681–1691

[62] Berg D, Otley CC. Skin cancer in organ transplant recipients: epidemiology, pathogenesis, and management. J Am Acad Dermatol. 2002; 47(1):1–17, quiz 18–20

[63] Parada MT, Sepúlveda C, Alba A, Salas A. Malignancy development in lung transplant patients. Transplant Proc. 2011; 43(6):2316–2317

[64] Otley CC, Pittelkow MR. Skin cancer in liver transplant recipients. Liver Transpl. 2000; 6(3):253–262

[65] Penn I. Neoplastic complications of transplantation. Semin Respir Infect. 1993; 8(3):233–239

[66] Martinez JC, Otley CC, Stasko T, et al. Transplant-Skin Cancer Collaborative. Defining the clinical course of metastatic skin cancer in organ transplant recipients: a multicenter collaborative study. Arch Dermatol. 2003; 139 (3):301–306

[67] Tufaro AP, Chuang JC, Prasad N, Chuang A, Chuang TC, Fischer AC. Molecular markers in cutaneous squamous cell carcinoma. Int J Surg Oncol. 2011; 2011:231475

[68] Prasad NB, Fischer AC, Chuang AY, et al. Differential expression of degradome components in cutaneous squamous cell carcinomas. Mod Pathol. 2014; 27(7):945–957

[69] Kasiske BL, Vazquez MA, Harmon WE, et al. American Society of Transplantation. Recommendations for the outpatient surveillance of renal transplant recipients. J Am Soc Nephrol. 2000; 11 Suppl 15:S1–S86

[70] Zavos G, Karidis NP, Tsourouflis G, et al. Nonmelanoma skin cancer after renal transplantation: a single-center experience in 1736 transplantations. Int J Dermatol. 2011; 50(12):1496–1500

[71] Jensen P, Hansen S, Møller B, et al. Skin cancer in kidney and heart transplant recipients and different long-term immunosuppressive therapy regimens. J Am Acad Dermatol. 1999; 40(2, Pt 1):177–186

[72] Lindelöf B, Sigurgeirsson B, Gäbel H, Stern RS. Incidence of skin cancer in 5356 patients following organ transplantation. Br J Dermatol. 2000; 143 (3):513–519

[73] Hartevelt MM, Bavinck JN, Kootte AM, Vermeer BJ, Vandenbroucke JP. Incidence of skin cancer after renal transplantation in The Netherlands. Transplantation. 1990; 49(3):506–509

[74] Yu SH, Bordeaux JS, Baron ED. The immune system and skin cancer. Adv Exp Med Biol. 2014; 810:182–191

[75] Bouwes Bavinck JN, Euvrard S, Naldi L, et al. EPI-HPV-UV-CA group. Keratotic skin lesions and other risk factors are associated with skin cancer in organ-transplant recipients: a case-control study in The Netherlands, United Kingdom, Germany, France, and Italy. J Invest Dermatol. 2007; 127(7):1647–1656

[76] Hollenbeak CS, Todd MM, Billingsley EM, Harper G, Dyer AM, Lengerich EJ. Increased incidence of melanoma in renal transplantation recipients. Cancer. 2005; 104(9):1962–1967

[77] Kanitakis J, Baldassini S, Lora V, Euvrard S. BRAF mutations in melanocytic tumors (nevi and melanomas) from organ transplant recipients. Eur J Dermatol. 2010; 20(2):167–171

[78] Woodle ES, Hanaway M, Buell J, et al. Israel Penn International Transplant Tumor Registry. Kaposi sarcoma: an analysis of the US and international experiences from the Israel Penn International Transplant Tumor Registry. Transplant Proc. 2001; 33(7–8):3660–3661

[79] Allen UD. Human herpesvirus type 8 infections among solid organ transplant recipients. Pediatr Transplant. 2002; 6(3):187–192

[80] Rockville Merkel Cell Carcinoma G, Rockville Merkel Cell Carcinoma Group. Merkel cell carcinoma: recent progress and current priorities on etiology, pathogenesis, and clinical management. J Clin Oncol. 2009; 27 (24):4021–4026

[81] Feng H, Shuda M, Chang Y, Moore PS. Clonal integration of a polyomavirus in human Merkel cell carcinoma. Science. 2008; 319(5866):1096–1100

[82] Ramsay HM, Fryer AA, Reece S, Smith AG, Harden PN. Clinical risk factors associated with nonmelanoma skin cancer in renal transplant recipients. Am J Kidney Dis. 2000; 36(1):167–176

[83] Dyall-Smith D, Ross JB. Cutaneous malignancies in renal transplant recipients from Nova Scotia, Canada. Australas J Dermatol. 1995; 36(2):79–82

[84] Euvrard S, Kanitakis J, Cochat P, Claudy A. Skin cancers following pediatric organ transplantation. Dermatol Surg. 2004; 30(4, Pt 2):616–621

[85] Penn I. De novo malignances in pediatric organ transplant recipients. Pediatr Transplant. 1998; 2(1):56–63

[86] Geusau A, Dunkler D, Messeritsch E, et al. Non-melanoma skin cancer and its risk factors in an Austrian population of heart transplant recipients receiving induction therapy. Int J Dermatol. 2008; 47(9):918–925

[87] Abou Ayache R, Thierry A, Bridoux F, et al. Long-term maintenance of calcineurin inhibitor monotherapy reduces the risk for squamous cell carcinomas after kidney transplantation compared with bi- or tritherapy. Transplant Proc. 2007; 39(8):2592–2594

[88] Campistol JM, Eris J, Oberbauer R, et al. Sirolimus therapy after early cyclosporine withdrawal reduces the risk for cancer in adult renal transplantation. J Am Soc Nephrol. 2006; 17(2):581–589

[89] Fernández A, Marcén R, Pascual J, et al. Conversion from calcineurin inhibitors to everolimus in kidney transplant recipients with malignant neoplasia. Transplant Proc. 2006; 38(8):2453–2455

[90] de Fijter JW. Use of proliferation signal inhibitors in non-melanoma skin cancer following renal transplantation. Nephrol Dial Transplant. 2007; 22 Suppl 1:i23–i26

[91] Sun SY. mTOR kinase inhibitors as potential cancer therapeutic drugs. Cancer Lett. 2013; 340(1):1–8

[92] Schneeberger S, Khalifian S, Brandacher G. Immunosuppression and monitoring of rejection in hand transplantation. Tech Hand Up Extrem Surg. 2013; 17(4):208–214

[93] Zwald FO, Brown M. Skin cancer in solid organ transplant recipients: advances in therapy and management: part II. Management of skin cancer in solid organ transplant recipients. J Am Acad Dermatol. 2011; 65 (2):263–279, quiz 280

[94] Seukeran DC, Newstead CG, Cunliffe WJ. The compliance of renal transplant recipients with advice about sun protection measures. Br J Dermatol. 1998; 138(2):301–303

[95] Ismail F, Mitchell L, Casabonne D, et al. Specialist dermatology clinics for organ transplant recipients significantly improve compliance with photoprotection and levels of skin cancer awareness. Br J Dermatol. 2006; 155 (5):916–925

[96] Clowers-Webb HE, Christenson LJ, Phillips PK, et al. Educational outcomes regarding skin cancer in organ transplant recipients: randomized intervention of intensive vs standard education. Arch Dermatol. 2006; 142(6):712–718

[97] Stasko T, Brown MD, Carucci JA, et al. International Transplant-Skin Cancer Collaborative, European Skin Care in Organ Transplant Patients Network. Guidelines for the management of squamous cell carcinoma in organ transplant recipients. Dermatol Surg. 2004; 30(4, Pt 2):642–650

[98] Blessing K, McLaren KM, Benton EC, et al. Histopathology of skin lesions in renal allograft recipients–an assessment of viral features and dysplasia. Histopathology. 1989; 14(2):129–139

[99] King GN, Healy CM, Glover MT, et al. Increased prevalence of dysplastic and malignant lip lesions in renal-transplant recipients. N Engl J Med. 1995; 332 (16):1052–1057

[100] Ulrich C, Jürgensen JS, Degen A, et al. Prevention of non-melanoma skin cancer in organ transplant patients by regular use of a sunscreen: a 24 months, prospective, case-control study. Br J Dermatol. 2009; 161 Suppl 3:78–84

[101] Brodland DG, Zitelli JA. Surgical margins for excision of primary cutaneous squamous cell carcinoma. J Am Acad Dermatol. 1992; 27(2, Pt 1):241–248

[102] Nguyen TH, Ho DQ. Nonmelanoma skin cancer. Curr Treat Options Oncol. 2002; 3(3):193–203

[103] Rowe DE, Carroll RJ, Day CL, Jr. Prognostic factors for local recurrence, metastasis, and survival rates in squamous cell carcinoma of the skin, ear, and lip. Implications for treatment modality selection. J Am Acad Dermatol. 1992; 26(6):976–990

[104] Sinclair RD, Dawber RP. Cryosurgery of malignant and premalignant diseases of the skin: a simple approach. Australas J Dermatol. 1995; 36(3):133–142

[105] Brantsch KD, Meisner C, Schönfisch B, et al. Analysis of risk factors determining prognosis of cutaneous squamous-cell carcinoma: a prospective study. Lancet Oncol. 2008; 9(8):713–720

[106] Wagner JD, Evdokimow DZ, Weisberger E, et al. Sentinel node biopsy for high-risk nonmelanoma cutaneous malignancy. Arch Dermatol. 2004; 140 (1):75–79

[107] Ulrich C, Busch JO, Meyer T, et al. Successful treatment of multiple actinic keratoses in organ transplant patients with topical 5% imiquimod: a report of six cases. Br J Dermatol. 2006; 155(2):451–454

[108] Brown VL, Atkins CL, Ghali L, Cerio R, Harwood CA, Proby CM. Safety and efficacy of 5% imiquimod cream for the treatment of skin dysplasia in high-risk renal transplant recipients: randomized, double-blind, placebo-controlled trial. Arch Dermatol. 2005; 141(8):985–993

[109] Perrett CM, McGregor JM, Warwick J, et al. Treatment of post-transplant premalignant skin disease: a randomized intrapatient comparative study of 5-fluorouracil cream and topical photodynamic therapy. Br J Dermatol. 2007; 156(2):320–328

[110] Piaserico S, Belloni Fortina A, Rigotti P, et al. Topical photodynamic therapy of actinic keratosis in renal transplant recipients. Transplant Proc. 2007; 39 (6):1847–1850

[111] de Graaf YG, Kennedy C, Wolterbeek R, Collen AF, Willemze R, Bouwes Bavinck JN. Photodynamic therapy does not prevent cutaneous squamous-cell carcinoma in organ-transplant recipients: results of a randomized-controlled trial. J Invest Dermatol. 2006; 126(3):569–574

[112] Willey A, Mehta S, Lee PK. Reduction in the incidence of squamous cell carcinoma in solid organ transplant recipients treated with cyclic photodynamic therapy. Dermatol Surg. 2010; 36(5):652–658

[113] Bavinck JN, Tieben LM, Van der Woude FJ, et al. Prevention of skin cancer and reduction of keratotic skin lesions during acitretin therapy in renal transplant recipients: a double-blind, placebo-controlled study. J Clin Oncol. 1995; 13(8):1933–1938

[114] Harwood CA, Leedham-Green M, Leigh IM, Proby CM. Low-dose retinoids in the prevention of cutaneous squamous cell carcinomas in organ transplant recipients: a 16-year retrospective study. Arch Dermatol. 2005; 141(4):456–464

[115] DiGiovanna JJ. Retinoid chemoprevention in the high-risk patient. J Am Acad Dermatol. 1998; 39(2, Pt 3):S82–S85

[116] McKenna DB, Murphy GM. Skin cancer chemoprophylaxis in renal transplant recipients: 5 years of experience using low-dose acitretin. Br J Dermatol. 1999; 140(4):656–660

[117] George R, Weightman W, Russ GR, Bannister KM, Mathew TH. Acitretin for chemoprevention of non-melanoma skin cancers in renal transplant recipients. Australas J Dermatol. 2002; 43(4):269–273

[118] Dooley M, Goa KL. Capecitabine. Drugs. 1999; 58(1):69–76, discussion 77–78

[119] Endrizzi BT, Lee PK. Management of carcinoma of the skin in solid organ transplant recipients with oral capecitabine. Dermatol Surg. 2009; 35 (10):1567–1572

[120] Veness MJ, Morgan GJ, Palme CE, Gebski V. Surgery and adjuvant radiotherapy in patients with cutaneous head and neck squamous cell carcinoma metastatic to lymph nodes: combined treatment should be considered best practice. Laryngoscope. 2005; 115(5):870–875

[121] Euvrard S, Morelon E, Rostaing L, et al. TUMORAPA Study Group. Sirolimus and secondary skin-cancer prevention in kidney transplantation. N Engl J Med. 2012; 367(4):329–339

[122] Bejar C, Maubec E. Therapy of advanced squamous cell carcinoma of the skin. Curr Treat Options Oncol. 2014; 15(2):302–320

[123] Southwell KE, Chaplin JM, Eisenberg RL, McIvor NP, Morton RP. Effect of immunocompromise on metastatic cutaneous squamous cell carcinoma in the parotid and neck. Head Neck. 2006; 28(3):244–248

[124] Kwan W, Wilson D, Moravan V. Radiotherapy for locally advanced basal cell and squamous cell carcinomas of the skin. Int J Radiat Oncol Biol Phys. 2004; 60(2):406–411

[125] Maubec E, Petrow P, Scheer-Senyarich I, et al. Phase II study of cetuximab as first-line single-drug therapy in patients with unresectable squamous cell carcinoma of the skin. J Clin Oncol. 2011; 29(25):3419–3426

[126] Lewis CM, Glisson BS, Feng L, et al. A phase II study of gefitinib for aggressive cutaneous squamous cell carcinoma of the head and neck. Clin Cancer Res. 2012; 18(5):1435–1446

[127] Brin L, Zubair AS, Brewer JD. Optimal management of skin cancer in immunosuppressed patients. Am J Clin Dermatol. 2014; 15(4):339–356

[128] Hahn H, Wicking C, Zaphiropoulous PG, et al. Mutations of the human homolog of Drosophila patched in the nevoid basal cell carcinoma syndrome. Cell. 1996; 85(6):841–851

[129] Xie J, Murone M, Luoh SM, et al. Activating Smoothened mutations in sporadic basal-cell carcinoma. Nature. 1998; 391(6662):90–92

[130] Johnson RL, Rothman AL, Xie J, et al. Human homolog of patched, a candidate gene for the basal cell nevus syndrome. Science. 1996; 272 (5268):1668–1671

[131] Gailani MR, Ståhle-Bäckdahl M, Leffell DJ, et al. The role of the human homologue of Drosophila patched in sporadic basal cell carcinomas. Nat Genet. 1996; 14(1):78–81

[132] Aszterbaum M, Rothman A, Johnson RL, et al. Identification of mutations in the human PATCHED gene in sporadic basal cell carcinomas and in patients with the basal cell nevus syndrome. J Invest Dermatol. 1998; 110(6):885–888

[133] Cusack CA, Nijhawan R, Miller B, et al. Vismodegib for locally advanced basal cell carcinoma in a heart transplant patient. JAMA Dermatol. 2015; 151 (1):70–72

[134] Zwald FO, Christenson LJ, Billingsley EM, et al. Melanoma Working Group of The International Transplant Skin Cancer Collaborative and Skin Care in Organ Transplant Patients, Europe. Melanoma in solid organ transplant recipients. Am J Transplant. 2010; 10(5):1297–1304

[135] Penn I. Transmission of cancer from organ donors. Ann Transplant. 1997; 2 (4):7–12

[136] Lipson EJ, Bodell MA, Kraus ES, Sharfman WH. Successful administration of ipilimumab to two kidney transplantation patients with metastatic melanoma. J Clin Oncol. 2014; 32(19):e69–e71

[137] Azijli K, Stelloo E, Peters GJ, VAN DEN Eertwegh AJ. New developments in the treatment of metastatic melanoma: immune checkpoint inhibitors and targeted therapies. Anticancer Res. 2014; 34(4):1493–1505

Index

Note: Page numbers set **bold** or *italic* indicate headings or figures, respectively.